Endoscopic Spine Surgery

Second Edition

Daniel H. Kim, MD, FAANS, FACS
The Nancy, Clive, and Pierce Runnells Distinguished Chair in Neuroscience
Professor, Director of Spinal Neurosurgery
Reconstructive Peripheral Nerve Surgery
Director of Microsurgical Robotic Lab
Department of Neurosurgery
University of Texas Health Science Center at Houston
Houston, Texas, USA

Gun Choi, MD, PhD
President
Pohang Wooridul Hospital
Pohang, South Korea

Sang-Ho Lee, MD, PhD
President and Chairman
Wooridul Spine Hospital
Seoul, South Korea

Richard G. Fessler, MD, PhD
Professor
Department of Neurosurgery
Rush University Medical Center
Chicago, Illinois, USA

1,094 illustrations

Thieme
New York • Stuttgart • Delhi • Rio de Janeiro

Executive Editor: Timothy Hiscock
Managing Editor: J. Owen Zurhellen IV
Director, Editorial Services: Mary Jo Casey
Production Editor: Kenny Chumbley
International Production Director: Andreas Schabert
Editorial Director: Sue Hodgson
International Marketing Director: Fiona Henderson
International Sales Director: Louisa Turrell
Director of Institutional Sales: Adam Bernacki
Senior Vice President and Chief Operating Officer: Sarah Vanderbilt
President: Brian D. Scanlan

Library of Congress Cataloging-in-Publication Data

Names: Kim, Daniel H., editor. | Choi, Gun, editor. |
   Lee, Sang-Ho, editor. | Fessler, Richard G., editor.
Title: Endoscopic spine surgery / [edited by] Daniel H. Kim, Gun Choi,
   Sang-Ho Lee, Richard G. Fessler.
Other titles: Endoscopic spine surgery and instrumentation.
Description: Second edition. | New York : Thieme, [2018] |
   Preceded by: Endoscopic spine surgery and instrumentation /
   [edited by] Daniel H. Kim, Richard G. Fessler, John J. Regan.
Identifiers: LCCN 2017039372| ISBN 9781626232648 (hardcover) |
   ISBN 9781626232655 (eBook)
Subjects: | MESH: Spine--surgery | Endoscopy--methods
Classification: LCC RD533 | NLM WE 725 | DDC 617.5/60597--dc23
LC record available at https://lccn.loc.gov/2017039372

Important note: Medicine is an ever-changing science undergoing continual development. Research and clinical experience are continually expanding our knowledge, in particular our knowledge of proper treatment and drug therapy. Insofar as this book mentions any dosage or application, readers may rest assured that the authors, editors, and publishers have made every effort to ensure that such references are in accordance with **the state of knowledge at the time of production of the book**.

Nevertheless, this does not involve, imply, or express any guarantee or responsibility on the part of the publishers in respect to any dosage instructions and forms of applications stated in the book. **Every user is requested to examine carefully** the manufacturers' leaflets accompanying each drug and to check, if necessary in consultation with a physician or specialist, whether the dosage schedules mentioned therein or the contraindications stated by the manufacturers differ from the statements made in the present book. Such examination is particularly important with drugs that are either rarely used or have been newly released on the market. Every dosage schedule or every form of application used is entirely at the user's own risk and responsibility. The authors and publishers request every user to report to the publishers any discrepancies or inaccuracies noticed. If errors in this work are found after publication, errata will be posted at www.thieme.com on the product description page.

Some of the product names, patents, and registered designs referred to in this book are in fact registered trademarks or proprietary names even though specific reference to this fact is not always made in the text. Therefore, the appearance of a name without designation as proprietary is not to be construed as a representation by the publisher that it is in the public domain.

© 2018 Thieme Medical Publishers, Inc.
Thieme Publishers New York
333 Seventh Avenue, New York, NY 10001 USA
+1 800 782 3488, customerservice@thieme.com

Thieme Publishers Stuttgart
Rüdigerstrasse 14, 70469 Stuttgart, Germany
+49 [0]711 8931 421, customerservice@thieme.de

Thieme Publishers Delhi
A-12, Second Floor, Sector-2, Noida-201301
Uttar Pradesh, India
+91 120 45 566 00, customerservice@thieme.in

Thieme Publishers Rio de Janeiro, Thieme Publicações Ltda.
Edifício Rodolpho de Paoli, 25º andar
Av. Nilo Peçanha, 50 – Sala 2508
Rio de Janeiro 20020-906, Brasil
+55 21 3172 2297

Cover design: Thieme Publishing Group
Typesetting by Prairie Papers

Printed in U.S.A. by King Printing Co., Inc.

ISBN 978-1-62623-264-8

Also available as an e-book:
eISBN 978-1-62623-265-5

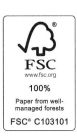

FSC
www.fsc.org
100%
Paper from well-managed forests
FSC® C103101

To my wife Anslie and to my children Elise, Rebecca, Sarah, and Isaiah.

—Daniel H. Kim, MD, FAANS, FACS

I would like to acknowledge my colleagues Alfonso Garcia, Akarawit Asawasaksakul, Ketan Dilip Deshpande, Chetan Pophale, and Leo Acedillo, who helped me to write this book, along with my always supportive family, my spouse and two sons, GangHyuk and Gangwoo.

I would also like to express my sincere gratitude to Daniel Kim for bestowing upon me the opportunity to be part of this book.

—Gun Choi, MD, PhD

I dedicate this book to my patients to whom I have given myself to lovingly learn and do all I can to treat their spinal disorder.

—Sang-Ho Lee, MD, PhD

This book is dedicated to all the pioneers who continue to look for ways to improve the care and outcome of their patients.

—Richard G. Fessler, MD, PhD

Contents

Contents

Video Menu

Preface

For decades, endoscopy has been widely embraced in many medical and surgical disciplines, but its use has lagged in the management of spine disorders. Now, with the refinement of endoscopic tools, it is possible to achieve the long-sought goals of minimally invasive procedures for spine patients: short hospital stays and early functional recovery. Endoscopic technology has advanced to the point where practitioners can now access, visualize, and treat spine pathologies that were previously accessible only by open surgical means. With the detailed step-by-step guides in this book, neurosurgeons can successfully use endoscopic skills in the treatment of their patients.

The intended audience for this text includes all surgeons interested in furthering their knowledge of diagnostic and treatment options available for spinal disorders, including practicing physicians, fellows, and residents. This book may also be of interest to nurses, physical therapists, chiropractors, and medical device professionals. With the detailed step-by-step guides in this book, surgeons can successfully learn and use endoscopic techniques in managing the spine disorders of their patients.

This second edition of *Endoscopic Spine Surgery* contains over 1,000 images, including photos of procedures and medical illustrations. In addition, the accompanying videos contain actual cases illustrating spinal pathologies and procedures. The videos range from case demonstrations to step-by-step technique demonstrations. The images, videos, and accompanying explanations supplement understanding and provide substantial insight for the nascent and seasoned surgeon alike.

This book is organized anatomically, starting with procedures for the lumbar spine and ending with procedures for the cervical spine. It offers an in-depth look into different approaches to endoscopic spine surgery as well as instruments used to treat various spinal diseases presented as step-by-step procedures. The text is organized in bullet points with numerous illustrations, making it easy to find specific information.

The cervical, thoracic, and lumbar regions have subtle microanatomical differences, and even a skilled surgeon can become disoriented because of the narrow endoscopic view. With this in mind, the book contains descriptions and images of what the surgical team will see when viewing various structures endoscopically. Other helpful information includes how to best surgically approach the thoracic spine and how to effectively remove pathologies, calcified disks, and osteophytes that can cause symptomatic foraminal stenosis. Not only are these procedures and techniques addressed, but each section offers suggestions on how to avoid surgical complications—knowledge as important as how to conduct the surgery itself.

Endoscopic Spine Surgery, Second Edition takes current and future surgeons caring for spine patients through the most up-to-date endoscopic spinal equipment, techniques, and skills one step at a time, allowing them to glean from the years of experience of the editors and authors.

Daniel H. Kim, MD, FAANS, FACS
Gun Choi, MD, PhD
Sang-Ho Lee, MD, PhD
Richard G. Fessler, MD, PhD

Contributors

Saleh Almenawer, MD
Staff Neurosurgeon
Hamilton Health Sciences
Hamilton, Ontario, Canada

Mohammed Aref, MD
Division of Neurosurgery
McMaster University Medical Centre
Hamilton, Ontario, Canada

Akarawit Asawasaksakul, MD
Spine Surgeon, MIS Spine Surgeon
Department of Orthopaedic
Paolo Memorial Hospital Paholyothin
Bangkok, Thailand

Jetan Badhiwala, MD
University of Toronto
Toronto, Ontario, Canada

Sarfaraz Mubarak Banglawala, MD, FRCSC
Assistant Professor (Clinical)
Department of Surgery–Otolaryngology/Head and Neck
    Surgery Division
McMaster University Medical Centre
Hamilton, Ontario, Canada
Lecturer, University of Toronto
Rhinology and Skull Base Surgery,
Otolaryngology–Head and Neck Surgery
William Osler Health System
Toronto, Ontario, Canada

Juan Barges Coll, MD, MSc
Co-Director, Education
Assistant Professor Neurosurgery
National Institute of Neurology and Neurosurgery "Manuel
    Velasco Suárez"
Mexico City, Mexico

Rudolf Beisse, MD
Medical Director
Chief Surgeon
Department of Spine Surgery
Benedictus Hospital Tutzing
Tutzing, Germany

Ashley E. Brown, BS
Department of Neurosurgery
University of Texas Health Science Center at Houston
Houston, Texas, USA

Benedikt W. Burkhardt, MD
Department of Neurosurgery
Saarland University Medical Center and Saarland University
    Faculty of Medicine
Homburg-Saar, Germany

Sebastián Casanueva Eliceiry, MD
Universidad Complutense de Madrid
Madrid, Spain
Clínica Kennedy of Endoscopic Spine Surgery
Santiago, Chile

Gabriel Armando Castillo Velázquez, MD
Neurosurgery Department
Centro Medico Puerta de Hierro
Guadalajara Jalisco, Mexico

Dragos Catana, MD
Division of Neurosurgery
McMaster University Medical Centre
Hamilton, Ontario, Canada

Gabriela C. Chica Heredia, MD
Universidad de Cuenca
Cuenca, Ecuador
Clinica Kennedy of Endoscopic Spine Surgery
Santiago, Chile

John C. Chiu, MD, FRCS, DSc
Diplomate American Board of Neurological Surgery
President
California Spine Institute
Thousand Oaks, California

Gun Choi, MD, PhD
President
Pohang Wooridul Hospital
Pohang, South Korea

Won-Suh Choi, MD
Department of Neurosurgery
Seoul St Mary's Hospital
The Catholic University of Korea
Seoul, South Korea

Chun Kee Chung, MD, PhD
Department of Neurosurgery
Seoul National University College of Medicine and Hospital
Seoul, South Korea

Nader S. Dahdaleh, MD
Department of Neurological Surgery
Northwestern University Feinberg School of Medicine
Chicago, Illinois, USA

Ketan Deshpande, MD
Endoscopic and Minimally Invasive Spine Surgeon
Saishree Hospital
Pune, India

Alvaro Dowling, MD
Orthopaedic and Traumatology Surgeon
Cape Town University
Cape Town, South Africa
Universidad de Chile
Clínica Kennedy of Endoscopic Spine Surgery
Santiago, Chile

Doniel Drazin, MD, MA
Department of Neurosurgery
Spine Center
Cedars-Sinai Medical Center
Los Angeles, California, USA

Jin Hwa Eum, MD
Neurosurgeon
Department of Neurosurgery
Kimhae Jungang Hospital
Kimhae, South Korea

Richard G. Fessler, MD, PhD
Professor
Department of Neurosurgery
Rush University Medical Center
Chicago, Illinois, USA

Ricardo B. V. Fontes, MD, PhD
Assistant Professor
Department of Neurosurgery
Rush University Medical Center
Chicago, Illinois, USA

Alfonso García, MD
Spine Surgeon
MK Spine Health
Tijuana, Mexico

Christopher C. Gillis, MD
Assistant Professor
Division of Neurosurgery
University of Nebraska Medical Center
Omaha, Nebraska, USA

Youssef J. Hamade, MD, MSCI
Department of Neurological Surgery
Mayo Clinic
Phoenix, Arizona, USA

Dong Hwa Heo, MD, PhD
Department of Neurosurgery
Spine Center
The Leon Wiltse Memorial Hospital
Suwon, South Korea

Jung-Woo Hur, MD
Assistant Professor
Department of Neurosurgery
Seoul St. Mary's Hospital
The Catholic University of Korea
Seoul, South Korea

Il Tae Jang, MD, PhD
Department of Neurosurgery
Nanoori Gangnam Hospital
Seoul, South Korea

Ji Soo Jang, MD, PhD
Department of Neurosurgery
Nanoori Suwon Hospital
Suwon, South Korea

R. Tushar Jha, MD
Department of Neurosurgery
Medstar Georgetown University Hospital
Washington, DC, USA

J. Patrick Johnson, MD
Director, Cedars-Sinai Institute for Spinal Disorders
University of California at Los Angeles
Los Angeles, California, USA

Chang Il Ju, MD, PhD
Department of Neurosurgery
College of Medicine, Chosun University
Gwangju, South Korea

Ricky Raj S. Kalra, MD
Department of Neurosurgery
University of Utah
Salt Lake City, Utah, USA

Manish Kasliwal, MD
Department of Neurosurgery
Rush University Medical Center
Chicago, Illinois, USA

Renée Kennedy, MD
Division of Neurosurgery
McMaster University Medical Centre
Hamilton, Ontario, Canada

Keith A. Kerr, MD
Department of Neurosurgery
University of Texas Health Science Center at Houston
Houston, Texas, USA

Ryan Khanna, BS
Department of Neurosurgery
Northwestern University Feinberg School of Medicine
Chicago, Illinois, USA

Chi Heon Kim, MD, PhD
Department of Neurosurgery
Seoul National University College of Medicine and Hospital
Seoul, South Korea

Daniel H. Kim, MD, FAANS, FACS
The Nancy, Clive, and Pierce Runnells Distinguished Chair in
   Neuroscience
Professor, Director of Spinal Neurosurgery
Reconstructive Peripheral Nerve Surgery
Director of Microsurgical Robotic Lab
Department of Neurosurgery
University of Texas Health Science Center at Houston
Houston, Texas, USA

Hyeun Sung Kim, MD, PhD
Department of Neurosurgery
Nanoori Suwon Hospital
Suwon, South Korea

Jin-Sung Luke Kim, MD, PhD
Associate Professor
Department of Neurosurgery
Seoul St. Mary's Hospital
The Catholic University of Korea
Seoul, South Korea

Leok-Lim Lau, MD
University Spine Centre
University Orthopaedics
Hand and Reconstructive Microsurgery Cluster
National University Hospital
Singapore

John Y. K. Lee, MD, MSCE
Associate Professor
Department of Neurosurgery
University of Pennsylvania
Philadelphia, Pennsylvania, USA

Jongsun Lee, MD, PhD
Department of Neurosurgery
Sewoori Spine and Joint Hospital
Daejeon, South Korea

Sang-Ho Lee, MD, PhD
President and Chairman
Wooridul Spine Hospital
Seoul, South Korea

Victor Lo, MD, MPH
Clinical Assistant Professor
Department of Neurosurgery
Mischer Neuroscience Associates
University of Texas Health Science Center at Houston
Houston, Texas, USA

Alejandro J. Lopez, BS
Department of Neurological Surgery
Northwestern University Feinberg School of Medicine
Chicago, Illinois, USA

Adam N. Mamelak, MD, FACS, FAANS
Professor
Director of Functional Neurosurgery
Co-Director of Pituitary Center
Cedars-Sinai Medical Center
Los Angeles, California, USA

Joachim M. Oertel, MD, PhD
Chief, Department of Neurosurgery
Saarland University Medical Center
Saarland University Faculty of Medicine
Homburg-Saar, Germany

Sung Hoon Oh, MD, PhD
Department of Neurosurgery
Nanoori Incheon Hospital
Incheon, South Korea

Luis Alberto Ortega-Porcayo, MD
Department of Neurological Surgery
National Institute of Neurology and Neurosurgery "Manuel
   Velasco Suárez"
Mexico City, Mexico

John O'Toole, MD, MS
Associate Professor
Department of Neurosurgery
Rush University Medical Center
Chicago, Illinois, USA

Choon Keun Park, MD, PhD
Department of Neurosurgery
The Wilste Memorial Hospital
Suwon, South Korea

Mick Perez-Cruet, MD, MS
Vice-Chairman and Professor
Department of Neurosurgery
Oakland University William Beaumont School of Medicine
Royal Oak, Michigan, USA

George D. Picetti III, MD
Orthopedic Spine Surgeon
Sutter Neuroscience Institute
Sutter Medical Center Sacramento
Sacramento, California, USA

Jenna Rebelo, MD
Department of Surgery–Otolaryngology/Head and Neck
  Surgery Division
McMaster University Medical Centre
Hamilton, Ontario, Canada

Kesava (Kesh) Reddy, MBBS, FRCSC, FACS, FAANS, DABNS
Clinical Professor, McMaster University Degroot School of
  Medicine
Chief of Surgery
Hamilton General Site
Hamilton Health Sciences
Hamilton, Ontario, Canada

Alissa Redko, BA
Department of Neurosurgery
University of Texas Health Science Center at Houston
Houston, Texas, USA

Josh Ryan, MD
Department of Neurosurgery
Medstar Georgetown University Hospital
Washington, DC, USA

Shrinivas M. Rohidas, MD
Neurosurgeon
Dr. Rohidas's Centre for Minimally Invasive Spine and
  Neurosurgery
Prakruti Clinic
Maharashtra State, India

Faheem Sandhu, MD, PhD
Professor of Neurosurgery
Director of Spine Surgery
Co-Director, Center for Minimally Invasive Spine Surgery
Medstar Georgetown University Hospital
Washington, DC, USA

Meic H. Schmidt, MD, MBA, FAANS, FACS
Director, WMC Brain and Spine Institute
Professor and Department Chair of Neurosurgery
New York Medical College
Director of Neurosurgery
Westchester Medical Center and Health Network
Valhalla, New York, USA

Rudolph J. Schrot, MD, MAS
Neurosurgeon
Sutter Neuroscience Institute
Sutter Medical Center Sacramento
Sacramento, California

Jonathan S. Schuldt, MD
Universidad Catolica Santiago de Guayaquil,
Guayaquil, Ecuador
Clínica Kennedy of Endoscopic Spine Surgery
Santiago, Chile

Ji-Hoon Seong, MD
Clinical Instructor
Department of Neurosurgery
Seoul St. Mary's Hospital
The Catholic University of Korea
Seoul, South Korea

Zachary A. Smith, MD
Department of Neurosurgery
Northwestern University Feinberg School of Medicine
Chicago, Illinois, USA

Doron Sommer, MD, FRCSC
Clinical Professor
Rhinology and Endoscopic Surgery of the Skull Base
Department of Surgery–Otolaryngology/Head and Neck
  Surgery Division
McMaster University Medical Centre
Hamilton, Ontario, Canada

Sang Kyu Son
Suwon, South Korea

James H. Stephen, MD, MSE
Department of Neurosurgery
University of Pennsylvania
Philadelphia, Pennsylvania, USA

Brian Vinh, BS
Research Coordinator
Division of Neurosurgery
McMaster University Medical Centre
Hamilton, Ontario, Canada

Albert P. Wong, MD
Department of Neurological Surgery
Stanford University
Stanford, California, USA

Hee-Kit Wong, MD
University Spine Centre
University Orthopaedics
Hand and Reconstructive Microsurgery Cluster
National University Hospital
Singapore

Mengqiao Alan Xi, BS
Department of Neurosurgery
Oakland University William Beaumont School of Medicine
Rochester, Michigan, USA

1 Applied Anatomy and Percutaneous Approaches to the Lumbar Spine

Alfonso García, Akarawit Asawasaksakul, and Gun Choi

1.1 Introduction

After careful review of the anatomy of the spine in humans and in various primates, Putz and Müller-Gerbl concluded that the lumbar portion of the vertebral column has the ideal structure to simultaneously optimize the functions of mobility and stability.[1] However, low back pain is patients' predominant reason for seeking medical advice in the modern era, and it is necessary for a spine surgeon to have a thorough knowledge of clinical and surgical anatomy of this region. Because the present text focuses on percutaneous endoscopic disk surgeries, the discussion is restricted to the anatomy relevant to endoscopic spine surgery.

1.2 Surface Anatomy

- Although identifying the appropriate vertebral level for a percutaneous procedure can be easily accomplished by fluoroscopy, knowledge of the surface anatomy is necessary for a better topographic orientation for surgery.
- The most prominent and possibly the only palpable landmarks of the lower back are the lumbar spinous processes. In comparison to thoracic spinous processes, they present a flatter surface at the posterior tip.
- The L4 and L5 spinous processes are shorter than other lumbar segments and are sometimes difficult to palpate, especially the L5 spinous process. The L4 spinous process is the last spinous process that shows movement on palpation during flexion–extension range of motion (ROM).
- Generally, the L4 spinous process is in a horizontal plane with the superior boundary of the iliac crest; in 20% of the population, however, the iliac crest is in line with the L5 spinous process.[2]
- The tips of the transverse processes are located ~ 5 cm from the midline and are not palpable.
- The level of the superior border of the iliac crest in relation to the corresponding disk space is important in the surgeon's decision-making process.

1.3 Osseous Anatomy

1.3.1 Vertebral Bodies

- When viewed from above, the vertebral bodies of the lumbar spine are large and kidney-shaped.
- They are larger in males than in females.

1.3.2 Pedicles

- The pedicles of the lumbar vertebrae are short and stout.
- The superior vertebral notch is less distinct than in the cervical region, but the deep inferior vertebral notch forms the roof of the neural foramen.

1.3.3 Transverse Processes

- The transverse processes project posterolaterally after originating from the junction of the lamina and pedicle on the same side.
- They lie anterior to the articular process but posterior to the intervertebral foramen (IVF).
- The lumbar transverse processes are quite long, with those of L3 being the longest.
- The intertransverse distance at L4–L5 is much smaller than at L3–L4 and is even smaller at L5–S1.
- The accessory process projects from the posteroinferior part of the transverse process with the corresponding lamina.

1.3.4 Articular Processes

Superior Articular Processes

- Two superior articular processes are found for each lumbar vertebra, with a hyaline cartilage–covered facet at the end of each process.
- The facets are oriented in a vertical plane. Each lumbar articular facet faces posteromedially.
- The orientation of the superior articular facet varies with different vertebral levels; for example, the L4 superior facets (L3–L4 joint) are more sagittally oriented than the L5 facets (L4–L5 joint). Also the L5–S1 joint is more coronally oriented than the L5 facet (L4–L5 joint).

Inferior Articular Processes

- There are two inferior articular processes, each with a facet that exactly conforms to the superior facet of the vertebral body below.

Facet Joints

- The facets of the superior and inferior articular processes of a vertebra form a zygapophyseal joint.
- The facet joint is a synovial type of joint, with a surrounding joint capsule (**Fig. 1.1**).

1.4 Anatomy of the Intervertebral Foramen

The IVF is an area of great importance for percutaneous endoscopic procedures, both because it harbors the exiting nerve root and other vascular structures and because it is the area of entry for endoscopic spinal access (**Fig. 1.2**).

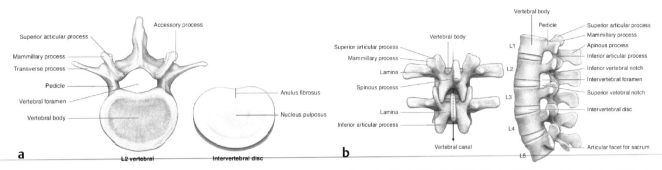

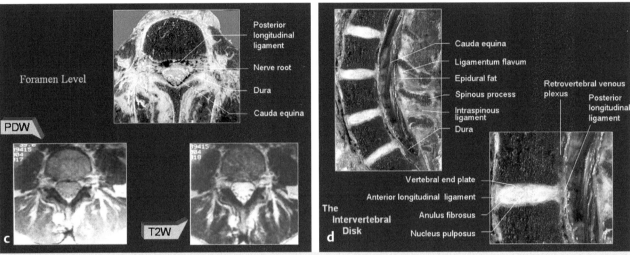

Fig. 1.1 (a–d) General anatomy of the spine. (From Laser Anatomy videodisc series Clinical and Imaging Anatomy of the Lumbar Spine and Sacrum by Wolfgang Rauschning, MD, PhD.)

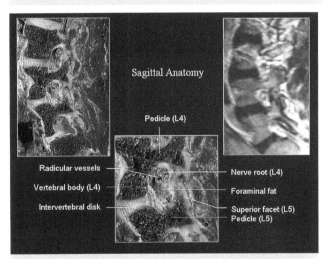

Fig. 1.2 Anatomy of the intervertebral foramen and its boundary. (From Laser Anatomy videodisc series Clinical and Imaging Anatomy of the Lumbar Spine and Sacrum by Wolfgang Rauschning, MD, PhD.)

1.4.1 Boundaries of the Foramen

The boundaries of the foramen contain two mobile joints—intervertebral disk (IVD) and zygapophyseal joints. Because of the mobility of these joints, the dimensions of the foramen change dynamically. The boundaries are:

- Roof: inferior vertebral notch of the pedicle of the superior vertebra, and ligamentum flavum at its outer free edge
- Floor: superior vertebral notch of the pedicle of the inferior vertebra, and posterosuperior margin of the inferior vertebral body
- Anterior wall: the posterior aspect of the adjacent vertebral bodies, the IVD, lateral expansion of the posterior longitudinal ligament, and the anterior longitudinal venous sinus
- Posterior wall: posteriorly bounded by the superior and inferior articular process of the facet joint at the same level as the foramen, and the lateral prolongation of the ligamentum flavum
- Medial wall: dural sleeve
- Lateral wall: a fascial sheet and overlying psoas muscle

1.4.2 Structures in the Intervertebral Foramen

- Spinal nerves (combined ventral and dorsal root in the root sheath)
- Dural root sleeve, which becomes continuous with the epineurium of the spinal nerve at the distal end of the foramen
- Lymphatic channels
- The spinal branch of a segmental artery, which, after entering the foramen, divides into three branches to supply the posterior arch, neural and intracanal structures, and posterior part of the vertebral bodies
- Communicating veins between internal and external vertebral venous plexuses
- Two to four recurrent meningeal (sinuvertebral) nerves
- Adipose tissue surrounding all the structures

1.4.3 Characteristics of the Intervertebral Foramen

- The greatest superoinferior dimension of the IVF is at L2–L3, and the dimension decreases from superior to inferior, which means it is smallest at L5–S1.
- The anteroposterior dimension remains more or less constant at all levels in the lumbar spine and is less than the superoinferior dimensions (at L5–S1, however, the anteroposterior dimension is greater than the superoinferior dimension).
- From L1 to L4, the IVF has a shape similar to an inverted pear, whereas at L5 the foramen is more oval.
- IVF dimensions in the male are slightly larger than in the female.
- With aging and degeneration, the foraminal dimensions change.

1.4.4 Accessory Ligaments of the Intervertebral Foramen

- More recent knowledge of the ligaments suggests that ligaments are found mainly at three locations in the foramen: the internal, intraforaminal, and external zones.
- Internal ligaments are found in the inferior aspect of the medial portion of the foramen, attaching the posterolateral aspect of the disk to the anterior surface of the superior articular process, bridging the superior vertebral notch of the inferior vertebra, and converting the notch into a compartment through which veins commonly course.
- The intraforaminal ligaments have three basic types:
  - The first type runs from the base of the pedicle to the inferior border of the same vertebral body. The recurrent meningeal nerve and a branch of the spinal artery are commonly found in the compartment formed by this ligament.
  - The second type of ligament attaches to the angle formed by the posterior end of the pedicle with the base of the transverse process and extends to the posterolateral part of the same vertebral body. A large branch of segmental artery travels through this anterosuperior compartment.
  - The third type of ligament originates from the upper anterior portion of the superior articular facet, extending to the posterolateral body of the vertebra above. The exiting root lies directly over this ligament.
- External ligaments have a common attachment to the base of the transverse process. From this they fan out in three different directions: superior, inferior, and transverse, attaching to the vertebral body of the same or a lower vertebra. They also form many small compartments through which neurovascular elements pass to or from the spinal canal.
- During percutaneous endoscopic lumbar diskectomy, the ligaments are not distinguished separately, because they have a minimal effect on the success of the operation.

1.5 Vascular Anatomy of the Foraminal Region

1.5.1 Venous Supply

External Venous Plexus

- The plexus of veins surrounding the external aspect of the vertebral column is called the external venous plexus.
- The veins can be divided into anterior and posterior, depending on their location in relation to the vertebral body.
- They communicate with segmental veins and also with the internal venous plexus through the IVF and transosseous channels.

Internal Venous Plexus

- The internal venous plexus is composed of veins located beneath the bony elements of the vertebral foramina (e.g., laminae, spinous processes, pedicles, and bodies) and embedded in a layer of loose adipose tissue.
- The veins contain many interconnected longitudinal channels coursing anteriorly and posteriorly to the canal, forming the Batson plexus.
- The peculiarity of this plexus is that it is a valveless plexus.
- Most surgical bleeding is from the venous plexus around the foraminal area. This can be a potential hazard in the foraminal adipose tissue, requiring careful attention during dissection in the area. For successful surgery, it is essential to avoid or to control bleeding.

1.5.2 Arterial Supply

External

- External arterial supply to the lumbar spine is from the lumbar segmental arteries.
- The lumbar segmental arteries send spinal branches to the vertebral canal through the IVF.

Internal

- On entering the IVF, each spinal branch divides into three further branches.
- One branch courses posteriorly to supply the laminae, ligamentum flavum, spinous processes, articular processes, posterior epidural tissue, and dura.
- The anterior branch supplies the posterior aspect of the vertebral body.
- A third branch (neural branch) courses to the spinal nerve and supplies the ventral and dorsal roots.
- It is important to review the foraminal sagittal MRI for any abnormal arteries in the lower part of the foramen at the entry site for the procedure. An abnormal artery can be a surgical contraindication.

1.6 Nerves of the Lumbar Spine in Relation to the Intervertebral Foramen

The neural structures important to percutaneous procedures are described here.

1.6.1 Dorsal and Ventral Roots and Spinal Nerves

- The spinal cord generally ends at or around the lower level of the L1 lumbar vertebra, due to differential growth of the spinal cord and vertebral somites.
- Dorsal and ventral roots, originating around the level of the thoracolumbar junction, travel through the lumbar cistern as the cauda equina before entering the dural sheath.
- The lumbar nerve root has to travel a considerable distance into the nerve root canal (the region in which the nerve splits from the dura to the lateral boundary of the relevant IVF) with a more oblique course before reaching the destined IVF.

1.6.2 Dorsal Root Ganglia

- The enlargement at the end of the dorsal root just proximal to the point at which it joins the ventral root is called the dorsal root ganglion (DRG).
- The DRG increases in diameter from L1 to L5.
- Because the S1 root canal is short, the DRG for S1 mostly lies intraspinally.
- Hasegawa et al (1996) categorized the ganglia topographically as intraspinal (within the canal), foraminal (within the IVF), and extraforaminal.[3]
- The DRG of the L1–L5 root lies mostly inside the IVF, with the upper ganglia lying more laterally and lower ganglia more medially in the IVF.
- As mentioned, the S1 root ganglion is mostly intraspinal.
- Care must be taken to prevent manipulation or heat injury to the DRG, because the most frequent complication is a postoperative dysesthesia.

1.6.3 Recurrent Meningeal Nerves

- The recurrent meningeal nerves are also called the sinuvertebral nerves of von Luschka.
- These nerves originate from the proximal portion of the ventral ramus, and they also receive a branch from the nearest gray communicating ramus of the sympathetic chain before traversing the IVF.
- These nerves also provide sensory innervation to the posterior periosteum of the vertebral body, posterior annulus, posterior longitudinal ligament, and anterior aspect of the spinal dura.

1.6.4 Anatomy of the Triangular Safe Zone

- The triangular safe zone is a zone for safe endoscopic access to pathology (e.g., disk herniation; **Fig. 1.3**).
- This safe area was described in 1991 by Dr. Parviz Kambin[4] as a triangular annular zone bordered anteriorly by the exiting root, inferiorly by the end plate of the lower lumbar segment, posteriorly by the superior articular process of the inferior vertebra, and medially by the traversing nerve root.
- The maximum safe area for insertion of the endoscopic sleeve is the medial end of the triangle.
- The surface of the annulus in this region is covered mostly by adipose tissue.
- The annular area is rich in nerves and vascular supply. This feature is clinically significant during an annulotomy (**Fig. 1.4**).
- The exiting nerve root forms the anterior boundary of the working zone, whereas the inferior boundary is the end plate of the lower vertebra, and medially the boundary extends to the traversing nerve root and the dural sac, which is overshadowed by the facet joint. In reality, the pedicle and the disk space are chosen as the reference points, because they are accepted radiographic landmarks during percutaneous procedures.
- The point of insertion is always referenced between the vertical lines drawn along the medial, mid-, and lateral pedicular lines and the horizontal lines drawn parallel to the end plates. With these reference points, the medial extent of the safe working zone is the medial pedicular line.
- Knowledge of the dimensions of the safe working zone is crucial in selecting the dimensions of the instruments to be used and the diameter of the working cannula to be inserted.
- Mirkovic et al[5] investigated the intervertebral foraminal anatomy of the L2 to S1 vertebrae to determine the dimensions of

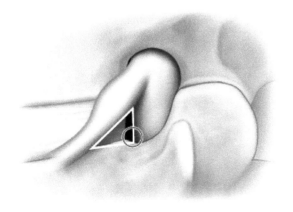

Fig. 1.3 Triangular safe zone (Kambin triangle): a zone for safe access to the pathology (disk herniation) via endoscopic instruments.

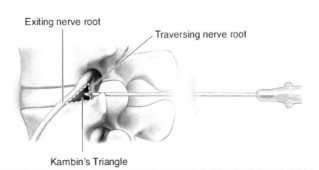

Exiting nerve root

Traversing nerve root

Kambin's Triangle

Fig. 1.4 Kambin triangle.

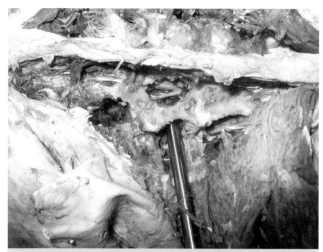

Fig. 1.5 The beveled cannula placed eccentrically within the safe zone and inside the disk.

the safe working zone and the largest working cannula that can be used. They reported the average dimensions of the triangular safe zone to be a width of 18.9 mm, a height of 12.3 mm, and a hypotenuse of 23 mm. A cannula with a diameter of 6.3 mm placed in the midpedicular line and slightly cephalad to the disk midline appears to be safe. Shifting the point of insertion medially to the medial third of the pedicle and slightly cephalad to the disk midline enables safe placement of a larger-diameter (7.5 mm) working cannula.

- In a cadaveric dissection study to determine safe zone dimensions, Wimmer and Maurer[6] concluded that the maximum safe canal diameter was 8 mm, on average, from the L1–L2 through the L3–L4 levels. From L4–L5 through L5–S1, the optimal diameter appeared to decrease to 7 mm. The authors attributed the decrease to the presence of a greater degree of disk degeneration at these levels. They also concluded that a smaller working cannula diameter is to be used if additional limiting circumstances need to be considered.

- In both of these studies, the impact of facet morphology on the three-dimensional space available for the passage of the cannula was not considered.

- Accordingly, hypertrophic facet joints with ligamentum flavum thickening may further limit the actual dimensions of the safe working zone.

- It is also worth mentioning that the actual diameter of the working cannula can be greater than the disk height because one can place the beveled cannula eccentrically within the safe zone and inside the disk. The cannula also helps to dilate the disk space (**Fig. 1.5**).

- Min et al, in cadaveric dissection of the exit zone of the IVF for analyzing the working zone of endoscopic diskectomy, showed that the mean distance from the nerve root to the lateral edge of the superior articular process of the lower vertebra was 11.6 mm ± 4.6 mm (range, 4.1–24.3 mm).[7] The mean angle between the nerve root and the disk was 79.6 degrees ± 7.6 degrees (range, 56.0–90.0 degrees). The authors stated that the actual working zone is not a triangle, but a trapezoidal space bound by the superior articular process and the exiting nerve root on the sides and completed by imaginary lines parallel to the inferior and superior end plates of the vertebra. The study was one of

the few that studied the nerve root anatomy in three dimensions without removing the facet joint and thus analyzing its relationship with the nerve rather than with the dural sac. The angle of the oblique side decreases, and the dimensions of the base increase, as one proceeds from the upper lumbar to the lower lumbar levels. This is very important for instrument positioning and size. In conclusion, the authors recommended avoiding blind puncture of the annulus and instead advised direct viewing of the annulus by endoscopy before annulotomy. If the preoperative imaging studies have been carefully examined, then it may be possible to avoid this step. For the beginner, the recommendation is very useful if there is any doubt about the positioning of the instrument. It is also recommended that the cannula be positioned as close as possible to, and scraping, the facet joint so as to gain more space (**Fig. 1.6**).[8]

- Osman and Marsolais studied the anatomical relationships of the diskectomy site (disk puncture) at the posterolateral corner of the disk in a single cadaveric specimen having a height of 6 feet. Diskectomy was performed with a 3-mm trephine within a cannula.[9] The distance from the medial edge of the diskectomy portal to the lateral edge of the dura was 11.5 mm, and the average distance from the midinterpedicular line to the dura was 9.8 mm. The average distance of the ventral rami from the diskectomy was 2.3 mm (range, 2–3 mm). Thus the dural sac is never at risk of direct injury during the placement of the working tools, but the exiting nerve root is very close to the entry portal. The authors also stated that, with portals made 7.5 to 10 cm from the midline, diskoscopy could be performed safely in the triangular zone in the angular range of 38 to 60 degrees at T12–L3 and in the angular range of 40 to 65 degrees at L3–S1.

- Because of the anatomical variations in the working zone, the percutaneous diskectomy procedure is done under local anesthesia. This allows close monitoring and assessment of the pain response to inserted instruments.

- It is also necessary preoperatively to view the patient's imaging studies to identify any congenital anomaly in the nerve root distorting the normal anatomy and thus the safe working zone. This may endanger the anomalous nerve root during the transforaminal approach.

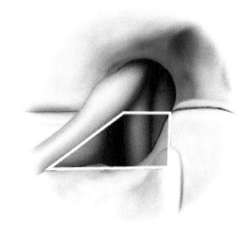

Fig. 1.6 Diagram showing the actual working zone.

1.7 Safe Needle Passage and Applied Anatomy

- During the passage of the needle posterolaterally toward the disk, one should decide the correct distance from the midline and also the correct angulations for the type of pathology being treated.
- Needle targeting is easier at all other lumbar levels except the L5–S1 disk level, which needs special consideration.
- The structures at risk of injury during the passage of the needle should be known and thus avoided.
- If the needle is targeted too vertically, there is a chance of penetration of the peritoneal contents, especially the sigmoid colon on the left side.
- This is of great concern if the same needle that has penetrated the colon by mistake is used for penetrating the disk. This incurs a very high chance of contamination of the avascular disk space and thus postoperative infection.
- The exiting nerve root is very close to the path of the instruments. Extreme horizontal passage of the needle can cause dural injury if one tries to penetrate the disk beyond the midpedicular line.

1.8 Anatomy of the Neural Foramen

- The IVF (**Fig. 1.7**) is oval, auricular, or inverted-teardrop shaped, depending on the length of the pedicle, height of the disk, and prominence of the facet and the intervertebral disk.
- It is an osteofibrous canal rather than a foramen.
- The lower portion of the neural foramen is used for the entrance of the working channel.
- It was observed that the upper part of the foramen was occupied by more than 50% neural tissue.[10] The average dimensions of the foramen were: height 13 to 16 mm (more at L1–L2 than at L5 and S1), width 7 to 9 mm, and area 83 to 103 mm². Direct cadaveric measurements of lumbar foraminal heights have varied from 11 to 19 mm.[8,9,10,11]
- Magnusson also reported on lumbar foraminal width. The average measurement from the front to the back of the foramen was 7 mm.[11]

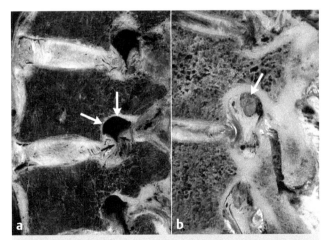

Fig. 1.7 (a,b) Anatomy of the neural foramen. The intervertebral foramen is oval, auricular, or inverted-teardrop in shape, depending on the length of the pedicle, height of the disk, and prominence of the facet and the intervertebral disk.

- Magnetic resonance imaging has also been performed in healthy subjects to measure normal values for the height of the IVF. The mean heights of the foramen were reported as: 17.1 ± 2 mm at L1–L2, 18.4 ± 1.7 mm at L2–L3, 18.1 ± 1.5 mm at L3–L4, and 17.1 ± 3.6 mm at L4–L5. As the nerve root slides under the medial edge of the pedicle, it takes an inferior and oblique direction away from the pedicle.
- The DRG location with respect to the foramen can be quite variable. However, some general trends are consistently reproduced in anatomical studies.
- The majority of lumbar DRGs are located within the anatomical boundaries of the IVF. Most commonly, the DRG is located directly beneath the foramen. Only at the S1 level is this rule not applicable. Studies have reported that the S1 DRG is within the spinal canal ~ 80% of the time (**Fig. 1.8**).[3,12]

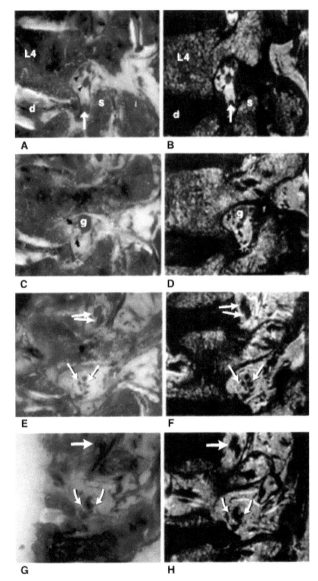

Fig. 1.8 (a–h) Position of dorsal root ganglia (DRGs) in the neural foramen. Most DRGs in the lumbar levels are located within the anatomical boundaries of the intervertebral foramen. Most commonly, DRGs within the foramen are located directly beneath the foramen. d, intervertebral disk; s, superior articular process; i, inferior articular process; g, dorsal root ganglion. (From Kostelic et al 1991.)

- As the spinal nerve reaches the foraminal outlet, it curves anterolaterally around the base of the subjacent pedicle and transverse process. Around this exit zone of the foramen, the spinal nerve divides into primary anterior and posterior rami.
- There is also condensation of the connective tissue within the foramen, which forms the transforaminal ligaments. They are a consistent finding in every neural foramen but vary in appearance from one disk to another. They are not easily isolated on gross cadaveric dissection, and they divide the foramen into so-called compartments, separating the neural structures from the vascular structures (**Fig. 1.9**).
- In addition to observing the endoscopic appearance of the tissues in the foramen within the disk and outside the disk, one has to correlate the appearance with the response to palpation in order to confirm the nature of the tissue.
- It is crucial to identify both the traversing nerve as well as the exiting nerve root while performing the procedure.
- In being more cautious, the beginner usually presumes that the dorsal structure visible in the endoscope is the traversing nerve and tends to shy away from it. This presumption naturally has an effect on the decompression achieved.
- Endoscopic diskectomy is a visual procedure, and one should identify the free decompressed nerve root clearly, whether it is the traversing nerve root or the exiting nerve root.
- Hence it is essential to know the endoscopic appearance of the local anatomy.

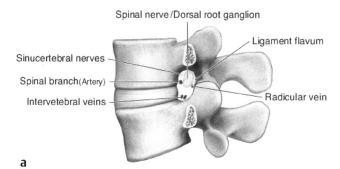

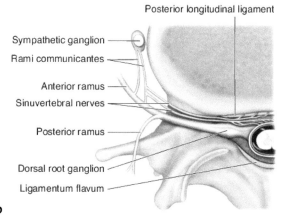

Fig. 1.9 (a,b) Anatomical relationship among the nerves, arteries, and veins in the neural foramen. There is condensation of the connective tissue within the foramen, which forms the transforaminal ligaments. These are not easily isolated on gross cadaveric dissection and divide the foramen into so-called compartments, separating neural from vascular structures.

- Be careful when using laser and cauterizing. Any severe pain response may be due to contact with neural tissues.
- Once inside the disk, there is no point of reference within the disk space to guide the endoscope and instruments to the site of the herniation.
- It is only with close preoperative planning and then intraoperative referencing with the image intensifier picture that one is guided to the herniation.

1.9 Endoscopic Anatomy

- With arthroscopy of joints (knee, ankle, etc.), there is a well-defined cavity within which to work. In endoscopic disk surgery, there is no well-defined cavity, and one has to create space so as to dissect one's way to the pathology.
- Endoscopic appearance changes with the degree of scope angulation selected and the distance from the tip of the cannula. A 20° spine endoscope is best suited for work in the foraminal and intradiskal area.
- With a 20° spine endoscope, the field of view that can be obtained shows the view straight ahead as well as a significant cone of view on one side.
- There is no blind spot straight ahead.
- With a spine endoscope that is 30 degrees or more, there is a blind spot ahead, especially when one is working with the endoscope very close to the tissues.
- Endoscopic anatomy can be learned from the start of the procedure through illustrative figures.
- Before annulotomy, one can visualize the periannular structures so as to be sure that the spinal nerve is not in the way of the trephine.
- The periannular structures consist of loosely woven fibrous tissue with some fatty tissue overlying it (**Fig. 1.10**).
- Once the fatty tissue is cleared off with the help of the radiofrequency bipolar cautery, one sees the superficial layer of the annular fibers and the lateral expanse of the posterior longitudinal ligament. These structures cannot be very well differentiated at this level in the foramen. If one examines the same structures with an open-bevel-shaped cannula, one will

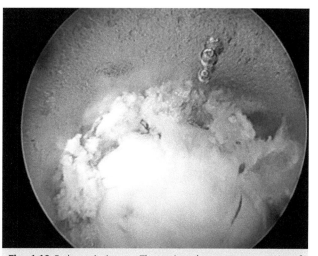

Fig. 1.10 Endoscopic image. The periannular structures consist of loosely woven fibrous tissue with some overlying fatty tissue.

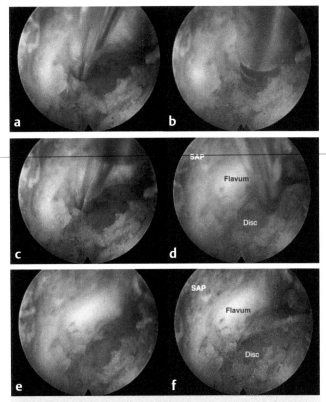

Fig. 1.11 (a–f) Once the fatty tissue is cleared off, the superficial layer of the annular fibers and the lateral part of the posterior longitudinal ligament are exposed. The overlying undersurface of the facet joint and the lateral extent of the ligamentum flavum that merge with the facet joint capsule are exposed as well. (In the figures, the superior articular process is also partially removed.)

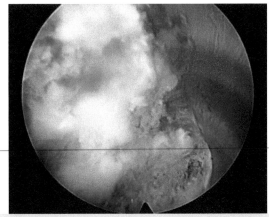

Fig. 1.12 Within the nucleus, the endoscope shows nuclear tissue with the appearance of fluffy cotton.

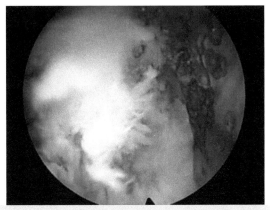

Fig. 1.13 Herniated fragment. The tail of the herniated fragment may be visible within the annular tear.

see the overlying undersurface of the facet joint and below that the lateral extent of the ligamentum flavum that transforms as the facet joint capsule as well (**Fig. 1.11**).

- There is no visible space between the ligamentum flavum and the annular structures in most individuals at this depth in the foramen, so usually one cannot see the epidural structures.
- Visualizing the exiting nerve root at this stage is neither routinely necessary nor advisable. Still, the nerve root can be seen after turning the scope cephalad and posteriorly along with the beveled working cannula.
- The nerve root is seen to be covered with fatty tissue and overlying blood vessels that are very sensitive to pressure.
- The visibility of the nerve root is hampered because of the presence of transforaminal ligaments extending from the surface of the disk to the facet joint and the base of the transverse process.
- In a routine case, the annular fibers are dilated with a blunt-ended dilator over the guidewire. Then the cannula is anchored in the disk over the dilator. A trephine may be indicated if the annulus is hard and the passage of the dilator is difficult.
- With the inside-out technique, one enters the posterior part of the disk completely with the cannula and then makes a space within the disk, which helps in proceeding toward the posterior part of the nuclear annular junction and thus to the herniated part.

- The main differentiating feature between the intradiskal and extradiskal endoscopic views is the absence of bleeding vessels within the disk. Only occasionally does one encounter neovascularization within the disk because of inflammation.
- In sequestration and transligamentous extrusion specimens, granulation tissue containing macrophages was commonly observed.[13]
- Within the nucleus, the endoscope shows nuclear tissue resembling fluffy cotton (**Fig. 1.12**).
- When stained with indigo carmine, degenerated acidic nuclear tissue stains blue and thus can be easily differentiated from the normal white nuclear tissue.
- Part of the degenerated nuclear tissue is also fragmented and lying loose.
- The annular tissue, on the other hand, is very tough and is in layers of fibers.
- The bipolar probe melts the nuclear tissue.
- In contrast, the annular fibers shrink to some extent, but they don't disintegrate.
- With most degenerated disks, the junction of the annulus and the nucleus is indistinct and thus not definable through the endoscope. Therefore, one removes the nuclear material in the posterior third of the disk in order to create space for clear visualization of the annulus.

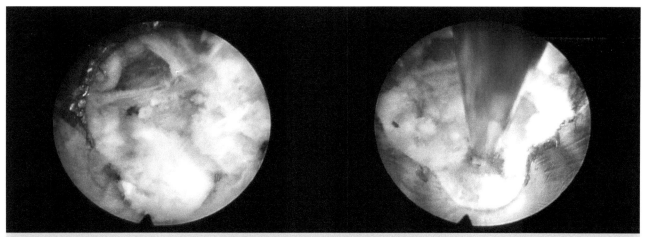

Fig. 1.14 Nuclear fragments trapped within the annular fibers are also seen in many cases. In these patients, it is necessary to dissect the annular fibers with the help of the Ho:YAG laser.

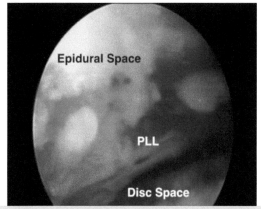

Fig. 1.15 The epidural adipose tissue has a tendency to move in and out of the working cannula as the patient inhales and exhales or with application of suction.

- If there is a big annular tear posteriorly that has led to the herniation, it is visualized as a big black hole, with discontinuity of the annular fibers.
- The tail of the herniated fragment may be visible within the annular tear (**Fig. 1.13**).
- Nuclear fragments trapped within the annular fibers are also seen in many cases, and in these patients it is necessary to dissect the annular fibers, with the help of the holmium:yttrium-aluminum-garnet (Ho:YAG) laser, from their attachment to the vertebral body. This separates the nuclear material more distinctly (**Fig. 1.14**).
- The majority of arthroscopic diskectomy and fragmentectomy is performed via a subligamentous approach to the intervertebral disk.
- Therefore, the operating surgeon must be familiar with visual diagnosis and be able to differentiate between epidural fat and periannular adipose tissue.
- Generally, the globs of epidural adipose tissue are larger than the periannular fat; in addition, whereas the periannular fatty tissue is stationary, the epidural adipose tissue has a tendency to move in and out of the working cannula as the patient inhales and exhales or with application of suction (**Fig. 1.15**).

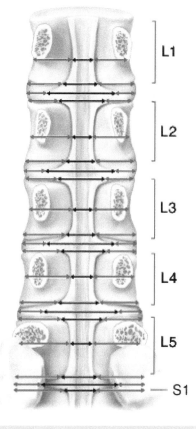

Fig. 1.16 The fibers of the posterior longitudinal ligament at the level of the intervertebral disk.

- In the lumbar region the posterior longitudinal ligament is a narrow, tough, fibrous band, detached and mobile at the level of the vertebral bodies.
- However, at the level of the intervertebral disk, the fibers of the posterior longitudinal ligament get interwoven with the superficial layer of the annulus, and this extends as an expansion laterally over the dorsolateral annulus (**Fig. 1.16**).

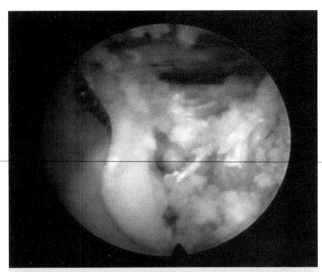

Fig. 1.17 A case of extruded transligamentous disk herniation. There is a large defect, and the epidural structures are visualized easily.

1.10 Special Considerations for L5–S1 Disk Transforaminal Access

- In contrast to other lumbar vertebral levels, L5–S1 has unique anatomical limitations: the high iliac crest, the presence of ala, the large facet joint, and the narrow foramen make a percutaneous transforaminal approach difficult.

- Ebraheim et al[14] analyzed the location of the extraforaminal lumbar nerve roots in relation to the intertransverse space by performing cadaveric dissection. They reported that the L5–S1 level presents difficulty in reaching the L5 nerve root and removing the extraforaminal disk herniation via the narrow intertransverse space due to lordotic curvature and the high iliac crest. Because the extraforaminal lumbar nerve root passes across the disk, one cannot be too careful in attempting to avoid nerve root injury. Ebraheim et al's study showed increases in the extraforaminal nerve root angle and diameter and the distance between the superior facet and lateral limit of the nerve root from cephalad to caudal. The height and width of the intertransverse space were greatest at the L3–L4 level and smallest at the L5–S1 level.

References

1   Putz RL, Müller-Gerbl M. The vertebral column—a phylogenetic failure? A theory explaining the function and vulnerability of the human spine. *Clin Anat* 1996;9(3):205–212
2   Oliver J, Middleditch A. *Functional Anatomy of the Spine.* 2nd ed. Philadelphia, PA: Elsevier; 2005
3   Hasegawa T, Mikawa Y, Watanabe R, An HS. Morphometric analysis of the lumbosacral nerve roots and dorsal root ganglia by magnetic resonance imaging. *Spine* 1996;21(9):1005–1009
4   Kambin P. Arthroscopic microdiskectomy. *Mt Sinai J Med* 1991;58(2):159–164
5   Mirkovic SR, Schwartz DG, Glazier KD. Anatomic considerations in lumbar posterolateral percutaneous procedures. *Spine* 1995;20(18):1965–1971
6   Wimmer C, Maurer H. Anatomic consideration for lumbar percutaneous interbody fusion. *Clin Orthop Relat Res* 2000; Oct;(379):236–241
7   Min JH, Jang JS, Jung Bj, et al. The clinical characteristics and risk factors for the adjacent segment degeneration in instrumented lumbar fusion. *J Spinal Disord Tech* 2008;21(5):305–309
8   Epstein BS, Epstein JA, Lavine L. The effect of anatomic variations in the lumbar vertebrae and spinal canal on cauda equina and nerve root syndromes. *Am J Roentgenol Radium Ther Nucl Med* 1964;91:1055–1063
9   Osman SG, Marsolais EB. Posterolateral arthroscopic discectomies of the thoracic and lumbar spine. *Clin Orthop Relat Res* 1994; Jul;(304):122–129
10 McPhee SJ, Papadakis MA, Tierney LM. *Current Medical Diagnosis and Treatment.* 44th ed. New York, NY: McGraw-Hill; 2005
11 Magnuson PB. Differential diagnosis of causes of pain in the lower back accompanied by sciatic pain. *Ann Surg* 1944;119(6):878–891
12 Hasue M, Kunogi J, Konno S, Kikuchi S. Classification by position of dorsal root ganglia in the lumbosacral region. *Spine* 1989;14(11):1261–1264
13 Harada A, Okuizumi H, Miyagi N, Genda E. Correlation between bone mineral density and intervertebral disc degeneration. *Spine* 1998;23(8):857–861
14 Ebraheim NA, Xu R, Huntoon M, Yeasting RA. Location of the extraforaminal lumbar nerve roots. An anatomic study. *Clin Orthop Relat Res* 1997; Jul;(340):230–235

- This expansion is richly innervated; thus, if one has not used sufficient topical local anesthesia, stimulation can result in severe pain during manipulation.

- The endoscopic appearance of the posterior longitudinal ligament is that of fibrous strands that run perpendicular to the end plates, as opposed to the oblique orientation of the annular lamellae.

- The posterior longitudinal ligament on the undersurface is avascular but may show neovascularization in certain cases of disk herniation.

- In extruded disk herniations that are transligamentous, there is a large defect and the epidural structures are thus easily visualized (**Fig. 1.17**).

- One can also encounter small, narrow, almost threadlike ligamentous structures connecting the lateral aspect of the dural radicular sleeve at the beginning of the traversing root to the posterior longitudinal ligament. These ligaments have been described as lateral Hoffman ligaments. These are clearly seen through the endoscope (**Fig. 1.18**).

- Once the fragment has been removed, the traversing root can also be visualized if the foramen is wide enough and there has been a big annular tear through which the herniation occurred. (**Video 15.1.**)

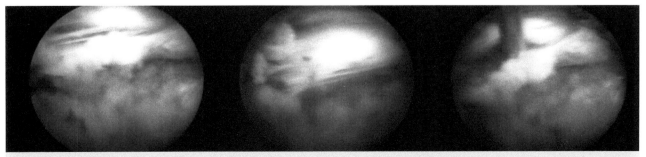

Fig. 1.18 Threadlike ligamentous structures connecting the lateral aspect of the dural radicular sleeve at the beginning of the traversing root to the posterior longitudinal ligament.

2 Percutaneous Endoscopic Lumbar Diskectomy: Transforaminal Approach

Akarawit Asawasaksakul, Ketan Deshpande, Gun Choi, and Alfonso García

2.1 Introduction

Kambin and Sampson in 1986[1] and Hijikata[2] in 1989 performed nonvisualizing nucleotomy via a posterolateral approach. Since then, due to advancements in technology and development of the visualizing endoscopic system, along with the irrigation channel and working portal, as well as specific endoscopic instruments, endoscopic spine surgery has become popular and yields better outcomes than ever before.[3,4,5,6,7,8]

In addition to the interlaminar approach described by Choi et al in 2006,[9] the transforaminal posterolateral approach is an endoscopic approach that can be used for several types of disk pathology.[6,10,11,12] This chapter describes the surgical technique and outlines crucial points in the procedure (**Video 2.1** and **Video 2.2**).

2.2 Step 1: Position and Anesthesia

- Percutaneous endoscopic lumbar diskectomy (PELD) by the transforaminal approach is performed under conscious sedation with the patient in the prone position on a radiolucent operating table.
- The patient's hips and knees should be in flexion to avoid stretching the lumbosacral plexus (**Fig. 2.1**).
- Lumbar lordosis should be obliterated using a Wilson's frame or sponge bolsters; this helps to increase the anteroposterior dimensions of the foramen, which facilitates the passage of the working cannula (**Fig. 2.2**).
- Level marking is done before scrubbing/draping to facilitate changes in position if needed (**Fig. 2.3**).

- Conscious sedation provides adequate analgesia and simultaneously allows continuous feedback from the patient, which helps avoid damage to neural structures.
- Midazolam (0.05 mg/kg IM) is administered half an hour before surgery, followed by 50 µg of fentanyl or remifentanil intraoperatively as necessary for pain.

2.3 Step 2: Skin Entry Point

- Axial MRI or CT is used to get an approximate idea of the distance of the skin entry point from the midline (**Fig. 2.4**). The needle trajectory is planned to target the ruptured fragment while avoiding the contents of the peritoneal sac.

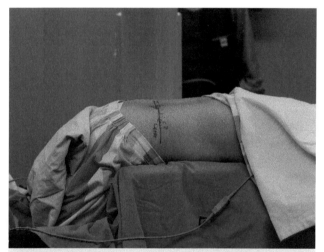

Fig. 2.1 Patient positioning.

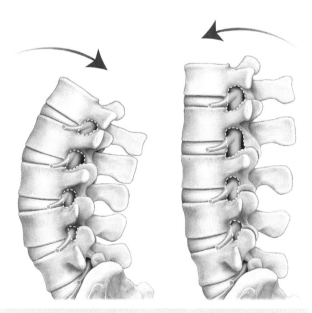

Fig. 2.2 Diagram illustrating the increase in foraminal dimensions with obliteration of lumbar lordosis.

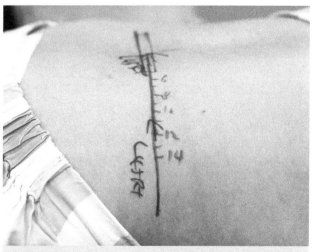

Fig. 2.3 Level marking.

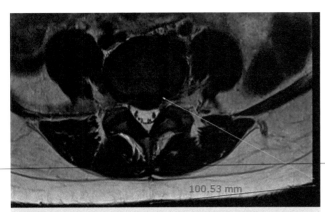

Fig. 2.4 Needle entry point estimation on preoperative MRI.

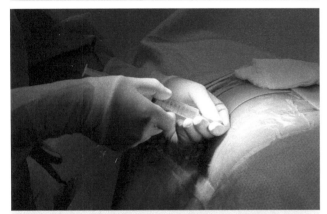

Fig. 2.5 Skin infiltration with local anesthetic.

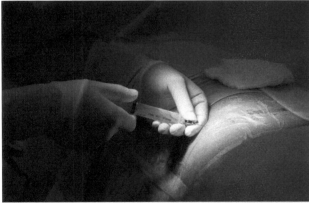
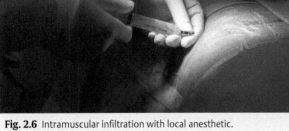

Fig. 2.6 Intramuscular infiltration with local anesthetic.

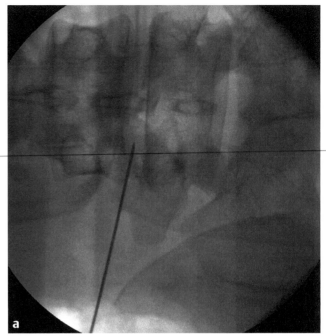

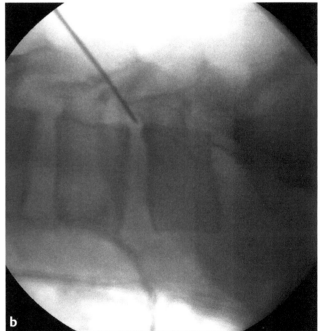

Fig. 2.7 (a,b) Needle tip location on AP and LAT views.

2.4 Step 3: Needle Insertion

- The skin is infiltrated with 1% lidocaine (~ 2–3 mL), and the intramuscular plane is infiltrated with 3 to 4 mL of 1% lidocaine using a 23 G spinal needle (**Fig. 2.5**, **Fig. 2.6**)
- The inclination of the needle trajectory is highly subjective and varies from patient to patient, depending on the location of the pathology, but usually the needle is directed from cranial to caudal, toward the inferior end plate at an angle of 10 to 15 degrees.
- The first bony resistance encountered is the superior facet; at this stage, one should confirm the needle location on both anteroposterior (AP) and lateral (LAT) views on C-arm fluoroscopy.
- The beveled end of the needle can be used to pass ventral to the facet. When the bevel of the needle is facing dorsally, the needle will tend to move ventrally; this helps the needle tip to skive off the undersurface of the facet.
- The location of the needle tip is again confirmed in both AP and LAT planes (**Fig. 2.7**).
- Epidural anesthesia: liberal use of lidocaine 1% solution (~ 5–6 mL) around the epidural region is recommended before puncturing the annulus; this step helps reduce the pain generated during the entry of the dilator into the annulus.

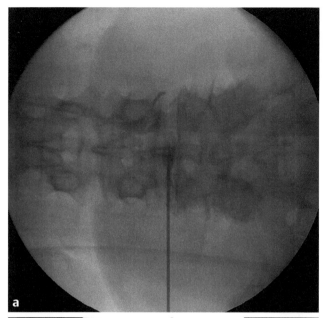

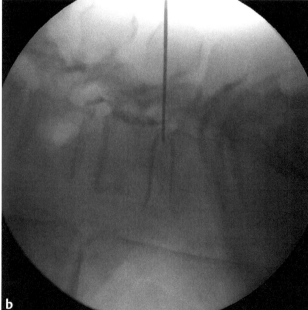

Fig. 2.8 (a,b) Diskography.

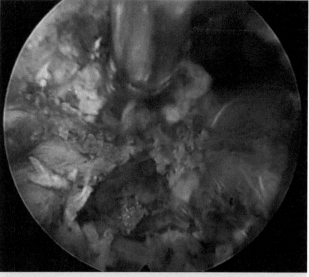

Fig. 2.9 Indigo-carmine-stained blue disk.

2.5 Step 4: Diskography

- Diskography is done using indigo carmine, radiopaque dye, and normal saline in a 2:1:2 ratio. The dye will be seen to leak through the annular tear into the epidural space concordant with the direction of the fragment herniation (**Fig. 2.8**).
- Indigo carmine, a pH indicator, selectively stains degenerated acidic nucleus and turns it blue, which aids easy identification of the pathologic disk in endoscopic views (**Fig. 2.9**).

2.6 Step 5: Instrument Placement

- The needle is replaced with a 0.9-mm blunt-tip guidewire and a blunt tapering dilator is passed over the guidewire in semi-circular motions until the tip of the dilator is firmly anchored in the annulus.
- The dilator has two channels, and the second channel can be used to supplement epidural anesthesia if the patient complains of pain during penetration of the annulus.
- During this step some patients may complain of localized back pain that does not need special attention, but if the patient complains of pain radiating down the thigh or leg, then the location of the dilator should be reconfirmed. Usually, changing the angulation of the dilator to more caudal helps move the dilator away from the exiting root and reduces the pain.
- In case of persistent pain, one may consider using sequential dilators (1 mm, 2 mm, 4 mm, 5 mm), which help to push the exiting root away from the target trajectory without significant pain, or sometimes the dilator and the guidewire may have to be removed and the direction changed from the first step.
- Radicular pain arising out of a traversing root is rare, as the traversing root is usually pushed more dorsally and is protected by the ruptured disk fragment itself. Still, if proximity to traversing root is suspected, then the dilator can be angled more ventrally to move away from the traversing root.
- After the dilator is anchored in the annulus, the guidewire is removed and the dilator is pushed into the disk until it reaches the spinous process on C-arm fluoroscopic AP view (**Fig. 2.10**). This is followed by passage of a 7.5-mm beveled working cannula over the dilator in circular motions, clockwise on the right side and anticlockwise on the left side.
- The beveled end should be facing the exiting root and later is rotated to face dorsally while crossing the facet, which helps to protect the exiting root and to slide the cannula easily under the facet.
- Finally, the working cannula should be facing dorsoinferiorly on the AP view (**Fig. 2.11**).

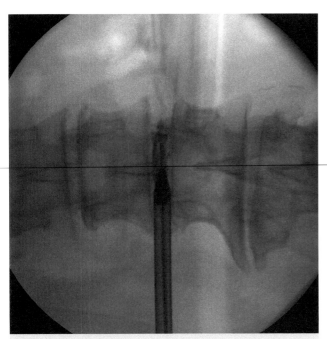

Fig. 2.10 Dilator insertion.

- The patient's feedback regarding leg pain is most important in preventing exiting or traversing root injury.

2.7 Step 6: Targeted Fragmentectomy

- The basic principle of PELD is to excise the constrained or unconstrained disk herniation, which sometimes requires widening of the annular opening to free the ruptured disk.
- It is recommended to keep the angle of the endoscope parallel to the bevel of the working cannula. This maximizes the surface area of the endoscopic view.
- The first step after passage of the endoscope inside the disk is to achieve a clear field, which is done using radiofrequency (RF) cautery for soft tissue clearance and hemostasis (**Fig. 2.12**).
- In the majority of the cases, if needle placement is accurate, the blue-stained disk is easily visualized in the center of the field and can be easily pulled out using endoforceps.
- The decompression extends from medial to lateral. After free movement of the posterior annulus and the PLL is confirmed, the cannula can be slowly retracted until it reaches the medial pedicular line and the foramen on AP view.
- The adequacy of decompression can be assessed by visual inspection of mobility of the dural sac along with the traversing root (**Fig. 2.13**). A blunt probe is further used to palpate and search for any remnant disk tissue, which can be removed with forceps. Visual confirmation and matching of the amount of disk removed to the MRI picture can also confirm the adequacy of decompression.

2.8 Complication Avoidance

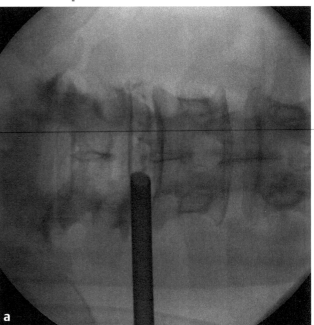

a

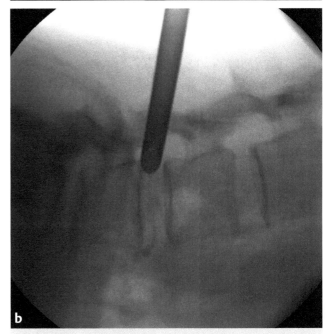

b

Fig. 2.11 (a,b) Cannula insertion.

- The two most painful sites in transforaminal PELD are skin and annulus entry; copious anesthetic infiltration at both these sites can easily prevent pain during the procedure.
- The entire procedure is performed under constant irrigation with antibiotic-infused cold normal saline solution. An Arthropump (Karl Storz GmbH & Co) controls the rate of irrigation. The recommended pressure for PELD is 20 to 40 mm Hg with 100% flow rate. Pressures can be adjusted depending on the clarity of the visual field, but keep in mind that prolonged excessive pressures may lead to postoperative headaches and, rarely, seizures.

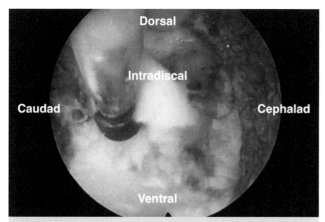

Fig. 2.12 Radiofrequency probe on endoscopic view.

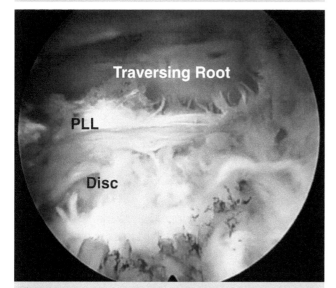

Fig. 2.13 Free traversing root.

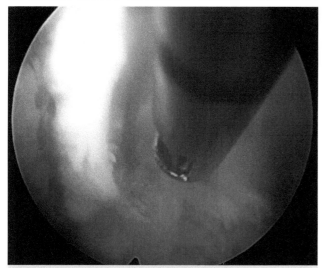

Fig. 2.14 Side-firing laser probe on endoscopic view.

- The advantages of irrigation are:
  - The field is cleared by washing off small blood clots.
  - Cold normal saline helps achieve hemostasis.

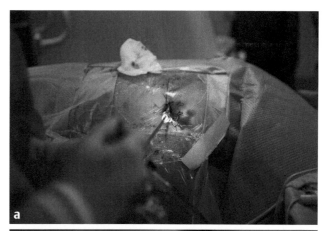

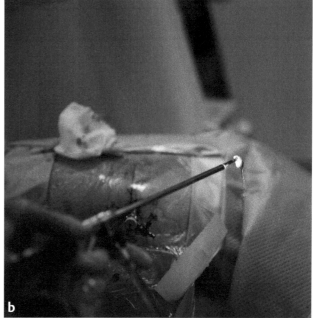

Fig. 2.15 (a,b) Removal of large disk fragment by pulling out the scope and forceps together.

- Thermal damage to the surrounding tissues is prevented by heat distribution during use of bipolar radiofrequency and laser.
  - Antibiotic-infused saline helps prevent bacterial infection.
- A side-firing laser (Ho:YAG) with penetration depth of 0.3 to 0.5 mm (**Fig. 2.14**) provides accuracy and prevents collateral damage. The preferred setting is pulsed mode, to allow time for heat to dissipate, and energy of 1.5 to 2 J per second at the frequency of 20 Hz, giving total laser energy of 30 to 40 W.
- Lasers must be used under strict endoscopic visualization, and all important structures must be visualized and identified before the actual use of lasers.
- Avoid direct lasering of end plates to prevent thermal necrosis.
- Adequate distance should be maintained between the endoscope lens and the laser tip to avoid damaging the lens.
- Removal of a large disk fragment may be difficult through the working channel of the endoscope. Under such circumstances, one can grab the fragment with a forceps and remove the endoscope and the forceps together, keeping the working cannula in place (**Fig. 2.15**).

2.9 Conclusion

Percutaneous endoscopic lumbar diskectomy (PELD) is one of the safest options to offer patients, since it can be performed under local anesthesia and the surgeon is able to communicate with, and monitor the patient at every step of the procedure. Apart from the surgeon-dependent procedure, an accurate diagnosis is of the utmost importance to arrive at the best outcome. Continual learning and working under an experienced endoscopic surgeon are recommended for the beginner.

References

1. Kambin P, Sampson S. Posterolateral percutaneous suction-excision of herniated lumbar intervertebral discs. Report of interim results. *Clin Orthop Relat Res* 1986; Jun;(207):37–43

2. Hijikata S. Percutaneous nucleotomy. A new concept technique and 12 years' experience. *Clin Orthop Relat Res* 1989; Jan;(238):9–23

3. Onik G, Helms CA, Ginsburg L, Hoaglund FT, Morris J. Percutaneous lumbar diskectomy using a new aspiration probe. *AJR Am J Roentgenol* 1985;*144*(6):1137–1140

4. Mathews HH. Transforaminal endoscopic microdiscectomy. *Neurosurg Clin N Am* 1996;*7*(1):59–63

5. Lee SH, Chung SE, Ahn Y, Kim TH, Park JY, Shin SW. Comparative radiologic evaluation of percutaneous endoscopic lumbar discectomy and open microdiscectomy: a matched cohort analysis. *Mt Sinai J Med* 2006;*73*(5):795–801

6. Choi G, Lee SH, Lokhande P, et al. Percutaneous endoscopic approach for highly migrated intracanal disc herniations by foraminoplastic technique using rigid working channel endoscope. *Spine* 2008;*33*(15):E508–E515

7. Osman SG, Marsolais EB. Posterolateral arthroscopic discectomies of the thoracic and lumbar spine. *Clin Orthop Relat Res* 1994; Jul;(304):122–129

8. Ahn Y, Lee SH, Lee JH, Kim JU, Liu WC. Transforaminal percutaneous endoscopic lumbar discectomy for upper lumbar disc herniation: clinical outcome, prognostic factors, and technical consideration. *Acta Neurochir (Wien)* 2009;*151*(3):199–206

9. Choi G, Lee SH, Raiturker PP, Lee S, Chae YS. Percutaneous endoscopic interlaminar discectomy for intracanalicular disc herniations at L5-S1 using a rigid working channel endoscope. *Neurosurgery* 2006;*58*(1, Suppl)

10. Choi G, Lee SH, Bhanot A, Raiturker PP, Chae YS. Percutaneous endoscopic discectomy for extraforaminal lumbar disc herniations: extraforaminal targeted fragmentectomy technique using working channel endoscope. *Spine* 2007;*32*(2):E93–E99

11. Ruetten S, Komp M, Godolias G. An extreme lateral access for the surgery of lumbar disc herniations inside the spinal canal using the full-endoscopic uniportal transforaminal approach—technique and prospective results of 463 patients. *Spine* 2005;*30*(22):2570–2578

12. Mayer HM, Brock M. Percutaneous endoscopic discectomy: surgical technique and preliminary results compared to microsurgical discectomy. *J Neurosurg* 1993;*78*(2):216–225

3 Percutaneous Endoscopic Lumbar Diskectomy: Extraforaminal Approach

Akarawit Asawasaksakul, Alfonso García, and Gun Choi

3.1 Introduction

Extraforaminal disk herniations, or "the hidden zone," as described by Macnab, extend out from the far lateral reaches of the spinal canal. These regions of the canal have only recently been understood, because the myelographic contrast material used to delineate the pathology was unable to reach the far lateral region. McCulloch and Young also described how patients who underwent an exploratory surgery awoke with leg pain because the disk was located outside the spinal canal, lateral to the pars.[1] The clinical syndrome became clear only after Abdullah,[2] in 1974, described extreme lateral disk herniation.

The diagnosis of extraforaminal disk herniation (EFDH) became more frequent owing to the availability of modern imaging methods like CT and MRI. But the surgical procedure still involved either removal of a significant portion of the facet joint or pars articularis resection, leading to instability and back pain.[3,4,5,6,7] The introduction of the paraspinal muscle-splitting (Wiltse's) approach changed the outcome, and success rates of 71 to 88% were reported.[2,3,4]

The development of surgical techniques and tools, such as the endoscope, the laser with a side-firing probe, and the steerable radiofrequency probe, made the percutaneous approach possible and helps to avoid postoperative instability.[8,9,10,11,12] Choi et al have reported an endoscopic extraforaminal approach called the *targeted fragmentectomy approach*.[13] This approach has some distinct features in comparison to the regular transforaminal approach:

- More medial entry point
- Steep needle angle
- Target fragmentectomy with very little or no removal of intradiskal contents

3.2 Clinical Presentation

The clinical presentation of an EFDH differs from canalicular disk herniation in many distinct ways:

- More common in young patients (average age 40 ± 2 years)
- Radicular pain is frightfully more severe
- Less significant back pain
- Valsalva maneuvers (coughing or sneezing) do not increase the pain
- Referred groin pain, from irritation of the psoas muscle

3.3 Surgical Technique

3.3.1 Position and Anesthesia

- Percutaneous endoscopic lumbar diskectomy (PELD) by the extraforaminal approach is performed with the patient under conscious sedation in the prone position on a radiolucent operating table.
- Patient's hips and knees should be in flexion to avoid stretching the lumbosacral plexus.
- Level marking is done before scrubbing/draping to facilitate changes in position if needed.
- Conscious sedation provides adequate analgesia and simultaneously allows continuous feedback from the patient, which helps avoid damage to neural structures.
- Midazolam is administered in a dose of 0.05 mg/kg IM half an hour before surgery, followed by 50 µg of fentanyl or remifentanil intraoperatively as necessary for pain.

3.3.2 Skin Entry Point

- Preoperative axial MRI or CT is used to approximate the distance from the skin entry point to the midline, and the needle trajectory is aimed to target the ruptured fragment while avoiding the contents of the peritoneal sac (**Fig. 3.1**).

3.3.3 Needle Insertion

- Target-level disk spaces are marked under the image intensifier, and they should be made parallel to each other by tilting the image intensifier in a cranial to caudal angulation.
- The spinous process and the iliac crest are marked in similar fashion.
- The point of entry, as calculated on preoperative CT or MRI axial images, is marked from the spinous process on the symptomatic side.
- The target point is the midpedicular line close to the superior end plate of the caudal vertebra on AP view and the posterior vertebral body margin on LAT view (**Fig. 3.2**).
- After skin infiltration with 1% lidocaine, an 18 G spinal needle is navigated under fluoroscopic guidance toward the target point.

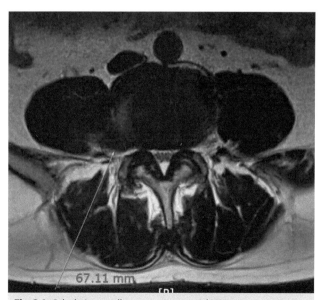

Fig. 3.1 Calculating needle entry point on axial MRI.

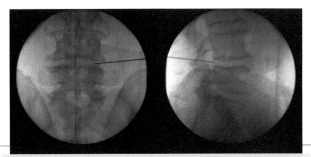

Fig. 3.2 Needle target point—midpedicular line on AP view and posterior body margin on LAT view.

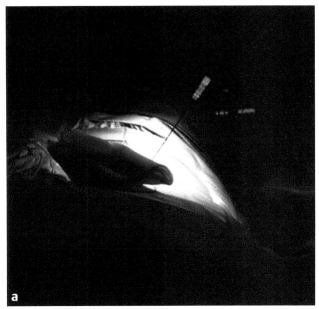

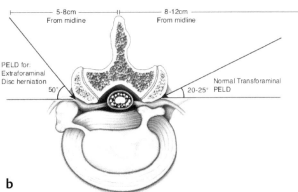

Fig. 3.3 (a,b) Needle insertion, demonstrating the difference between normal transforaminal PELD and extraforaminal PELD.

- The angle of needle entry is very steep compared with that for a routine transforaminal approach, varying between 10 and 50 degrees, as per the location of the pathology (**Fig. 3.3**).
- Additional local infiltration is done when the needle reaches the target point, to facilitate the entry of the obturator into the annulus.
- The needle is then advanced into the disk, and diskography is done using 2 to 3 mL of a mixture of radiopaque dye, indigo carmine, and normal saline in a 2:1:2 ratio (**Fig. 3.4**).

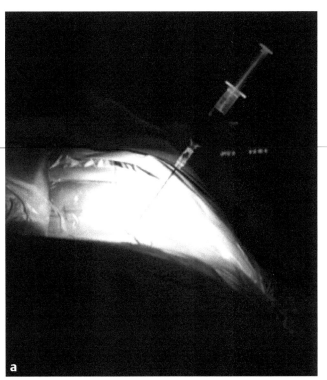

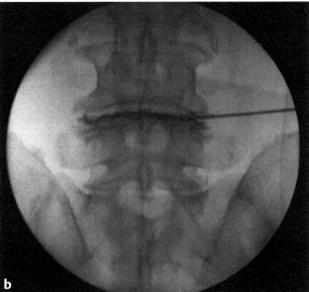

Fig. 3.4 (a,b) Diskography.

3.3.4 Dilator and Cannula Insertion

- The needle is replaced with a 0.8-mm blunt-tip guidewire and the tract is dilated using a blunt-tip obturator. At this point, some patients may complain of radicular leg pain, which is caused by irritation of the exiting nerve root.
- If patients complain of pain, it is recommended to use serial dilators from 1 to 5 mm in slow semicircular motions. These dilators can push the exiting root cranially, away from the surgical field.

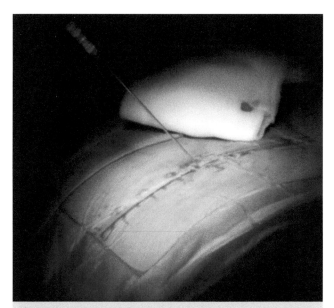

Fig. 3.5 Working cannula insertion.

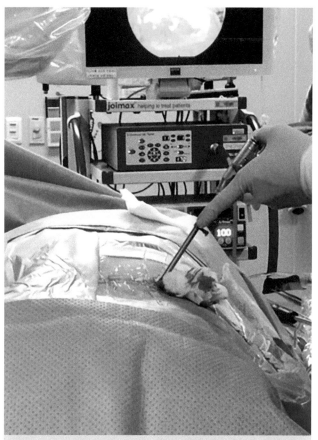

Fig. 3.7 Operating surgeon handling an endoscope in a high angulation position.

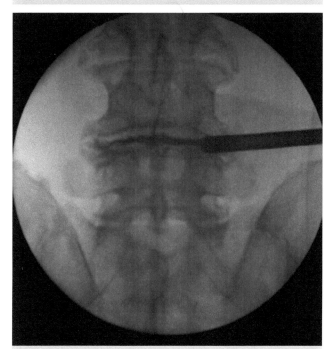

Fig. 3.6 Cannula location at midpedicular line on AP view.

- After withdrawal of the dilators, the regular blunt-tip obturator is passed over the guidewire and its tip is anchored in the annulus.
- Now a circular working cannula is passed over the obturator, with its tip resting over the outer surface of the disk (**Fig. 3.5**, **Fig. 3.6**). Although the circular cannula offers compromised visibility compared with the beveled cannula, its major advantage is protection of the exiting root so that the rest of the procedure can be safely performed.
- A 25° working channel endoscope is then passed through the cannula (**Fig. 3.7**).

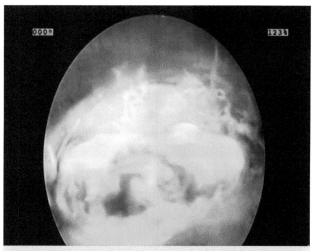

Fig. 3.8 Intervertebral disk stained blue by indigo carmine.

3.3.5 Endoscopic View

- Soft tissue clearance is done with flexible-tip bipolar radiofrequency.
- Blue-stained herniated disk is directly seen in the center of the cannula (**Fig. 3.8**).
- Annulus is penetrated using RF cautery and the opening is sufficiently widened using either RF or side-firing laser.

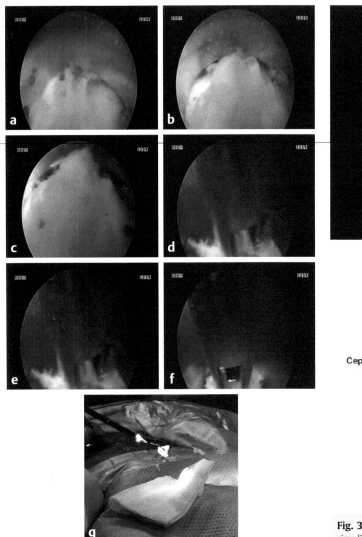

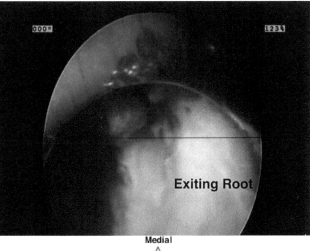

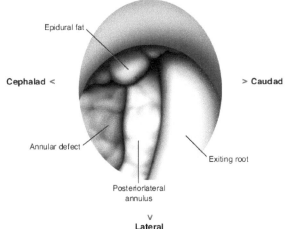

Fig. 3.10 (a,b) Exiting nerve root and annular defect. (**Fig. 3.10b** is a simplified illustration of **Fig. 3.10a**).

Fig. 3.9 (a,b,c) Disk fragment popping out of an annular defect and that can be easily removed by forceps. (**d,e,f,g**) Disk fragments can be easily removed using forceps and grasping their tail.

- The herniated fragment usually starts popping out through the annular opening. Further removal of the pathologic disk can be achieved using endoscopic forceps (**Fig. 3.9a–c**).
- The fragment can also be delivered into the field using the blunt probe. Grasping the tail of fragment and applying gentle traction is usually sufficient for its removal (**Fig. 3.9d–g**).
- Once the major fragment is removed, a blunt-tip probe is used to palpate for any remaining disk.
- The adequacy of decompression is confirmed by visual inspection of the exiting root. This can be done by slowly rotating the cannula backward, which allows the exiting root to fall in the center of the field (**Fig. 3.10**).
- Similarly, the shoulder of the exiting root should be inspected for any retained disk material.
- Hemostasis should be achieved using bipolar coagulation, and a suction drain can be inserted if necessary.
- Skin can be closed using a single nonabsorbable suture.

3.4 Complication Avoidance

- First, needle insertion is crucial to success of the procedure, since it determines the anchoring point. Preoperative calculation is absolutely required.
- Second, doing the procedure without indigo carmine is possible, but we recommend doing diskography with it, because the blue staining of acidic disk fragments is very helpful for distinguishing disk material from neural structures or normal disk.
- Targeted fragmentectomy is preferred to minimize the instability that is created by central debulking.
- Continuous irrigation with antibiotic-infused normal saline solution is also important; it flushes out blood, increasing visualization and lessening the infection rate.
- Always make sure that the irrigation pressure is not too high, and if the patient complains of neck pain during the procedure, halt the procedure and decrease the irrigation pressure immediately.
- A vacuum drain is preferable for preventing postoperative hematoma in cases of inadequate bleeding control before the end of the procedure.

3.5 Conclusion

The extraforaminal approach for percutaneous endoscopic lumbar diskectomy (PELD) is a bit different from regular PELD since the angle of the needle insertion is steeper, allowing one to go directly to the herniated fragment, not into the foramen. Because the procedure carries a risk of injuring the exiting root, local anesthesia with conscious sedation is recommended to perform the procedure safely. Under endoscopic view, differentiation of the herniation and nerve root can be troublesome, so staining the disk first with indigo carmine is a good option to make the procedure safer.

References

1   McCulloch JA, Young PH. Foraminal and extraforaminal lumbar disc herniations. In: McCulloch JA, Young PH, eds. *Essentials of Spinal Microsurgery*. Philadelphia, PA: Lippincott-Raven; 1998:383–428

2   Abdullah AF, Ditto EW III, Byrd EB, Williams R. Extreme-lateral lumbar disc herniations. Clinical syndrome and special problems of diagnosis. *J Neurosurg* 1974;*41*(2):229–234

3   Epstein NE. Different surgical approaches to far lateral lumbar disc herniations. *J Spinal Disord* 1995;*8*(5):383–394

4   Epstein NE. Evaluation of varied surgical approaches used in the management of 170 far-lateral lumbar disc herniations: indications and results. *J Neurosurg* 1995;*83*(4):648–656

5   Tessitore E, de Tribolet N. Far-lateral lumbar disc herniation: the microsurgical transmuscular approach. *Neurosurgery* 2004;*54*(4):939–942

6   Garrido E, Connaughton PN. Unilateral facetectomy approach for lateral lumbar disc herniation. *J Neurosurg* 1991;*74*(5):754–756

7   Jackson RP, Glah JJ. Foraminal and extraforaminal lumbar disc herniation: diagnosis and treatment. *Spine* 1987;*12*(6):577–585

8   Choi G, Lee SH, Raiturker PP, Lee S, Chae YS. Percutaneous endoscopic interlaminar discectomy for intracanalicular disc herniations at L5–S1 using a rigid working channel endoscope. *Neurosurgery* 2006;*58*

9   Yeung AT, Tsou PM. Posterolateral endoscopic excision for lumbar disc herniation: surgical technique, outcome, and complications in 307 consecutive cases. *Spine* 2002;*27*(7):722–731

10 Lew SM, Mehalic TF, Fagone KL. Transforaminal percutaneous endoscopic discectomy in the treatment of far-lateral and foraminal lumbar disc herniations. *J Neurosurg* 2001;*94*(2, Suppl):216–220

11 Jang JS, An SH, Lee SH. Transforaminal percutaneous endoscopic discectomy in the treatment of foraminal and extraforaminal lumbar disc herniations. *J Spinal Disord Tech* 2006;*19*(5):338–343

12 Lübbers T, Abuamona R, Elsharkawy AE. Percutaneous endoscopic treatment of foraminal and extraforaminal disc herniation at the L5–S1 level. *Acta Neurochir (Wien)* 2012;*154*(10):1789–1795

13 Choi G, Lee SH, Bhanot A, Raiturker PP, Chae YS. Percutaneous endoscopic discectomy for extraforaminal lumbar disc herniations: extraforaminal targeted fragmentectomy technique using working channel endoscope. *Spine (Phila PA 1976)* 2007;*32*(2):E93–E99

4 Percutaneous Endoscopic Lumbar Diskectomy for Migrated Lumbar Disk Herniation

Akarawit Asawasaksakul, Gun Choi, and Ketan Deshpande

4.1 Introduction

In the years since the introduction of the concept of percutaneous posterolateral nucleotomy by Kambin in 1973, percutaneous endoscopic lumbar diskectomy (PELD) has evolved.[1,2,3,4,5,6,7] PELD is increasingly the preferred treatment for lumbar disk herniation. The transforaminal approach offers several advantages: First, it provides protection of the posterior ligamentous and bony structures, with a lower incidence of postoperative instability,[8,9,10] facet joint arthropathy, and disk space narrowing.[2,3,4,5,11,12,13,14,15,16,17,18,19,20,21] Second, there is no interference with the epidural venous system that could lead to chronic neural edema and fibrosis.[2,14,15,16,22] Last, epidural scarring, a common sequel to open diskectomy, and which leads to clinical symptoms in more than 10% of patients, is rare with PELD.[23,24,25]

The narrow transforaminal window provides limited access that proves adequate for the removal of nonmigrated or low-grade migrated disk herniation, but the limited access may render the PELD procedure ineffective in cases of high-grade migrations.[6,7,25] Migrated intracanalicular disk herniation, especially high-grade migration, poses a greater challenge, even for an experienced endoscopic surgeon. The success of the PELD procedure depends considerably on appropriate placement of the working instruments in an optimal trajectory to directly visualize and access the migrated ruptured fragment.[19,26,27] Improper trajectory is an important cause of failure of the procedure, and the biggest difficulty encountered during retrieval of high-grade migrated disk herniation is obtaining the optimal trajectory,[26] because it is significantly hindered by the natural obstacles of the normal anatomy and is worsened by the degenerative changes.

Because of these limitations, foraminoplasty helps in addressing this issue. We define foraminoplasty as widening of the foramen by undercutting a ventral (nonarticular) part of the superior facet and sometimes the upper part of the inferior pedicle, along with ablation of the foraminal ligament to visualize the anterior epidural space and its contents. This can be achieved with the help of bone trephines or reamers, an endoscopic drill, endoscopic chisels, and side-firing holmium:yttrium-aluminum-garnet (Ho:YAG) laser (**Video 4.1**, **Video 4.2**, and **Video 4.3**).

4.2 Anatomical Considerations

Foraminoplasty is needed, especially to access high-grade migrated intracanalicular disk herniation, because of the following:
- Lumbar disk herniation is common at the lower levels, where the diameter of the intervertebral foramen is small in comparison to the diameter at the higher levels.[28]
- Degenerative changes leading to hypertrophy, overriding of facets, and thickening of the foraminal ligament may cause additional narrowing of the transforaminal window.

Table 4.1 Obstacle structures

1	Superior articular process (SAP)
2	Cranial part of the lower pedicle
3	Osteophyte from posterior vertebral body
4	Inferior articular process (IAP)

- High-grade migrated disk herniation lies in the region of the spinal canal that is hidden from the endoscopic view by natural anatomical barriers.
- The barriers prevent direct access to the migrated fragment (**Table 4.1**).
- Min et al[29] have demonstrated that the dimensions of the working zone in the sagittal plane, specifically the base dimension, are of clinical importance in the current practice of endoscopic surgery.
- Foraminoplasty provides adequate working space for excision of the ruptured fragment under direct endoscopic vision through the enlarged foramen.

4.3 Migrated Disk Herniation

- Whether extruded or not, herniation displaced either above or below the end plate level is called migrated disk herniation.
- Migrated disk herniation is classified into two grades depending on the extent of migration.
- If the extent of migration is greater than the measured height of the posterior marginal disk space on T2-weighted sagittal MRI, it is called a high-grade migration.[26,27,30,31]
- Migration smaller than the height of the disk space is classified as a low-grade migration (**Fig. 4.1**).[32]

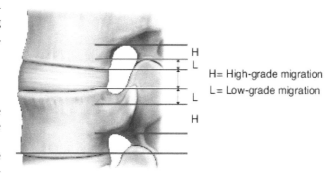

Fig. 4.1 The degree of migration of the herniated fragment in relation to the posterior height of the disk space.

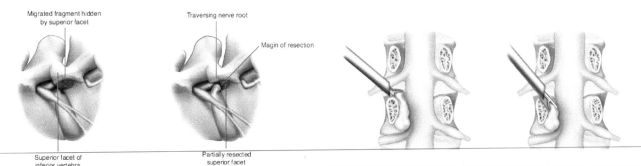

Fig. 4.2 Anatomical change of the neural foramen (a) before and (b) after foraminoplasty.

Fig. 4.3 Partial pediculectomy. Removal of the upper and medial walls of the pedicle (a), along with the undercutting of the superior facet (b), can aid visualization of, and access to, the ruptured fragment.

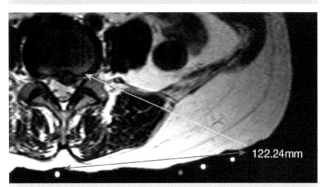

Fig. 4.4 Preoperative planning. Axial MRI or CT is used to calculate the distance of the skin entry point of the needle from the midline, and the needle trajectory is aimed to target the ruptured fragment while avoiding the contents of the peritoneal sac.

4.4 Types of Foraminoplasty

Foraminoplasty is classified into two types depending on the extent of bony resection.

4.4.1 Conventional Foraminoplasty

- Conventional foraminoplasty essentially involves undercutting of the nonarticular part of the superior facet and removal of the lateral edge of the ligamentum flavum in cases of downward-migrated disk herniation.
- It involves the release of the superior foraminal ligament and the ligamentum flavum in cases of upward-migrated disk herniation.
- The need for undercutting of the facet may diminish at lumbar levels above L3–L4.
- Because the upper part of the foramen is wider than the lower part and there is no superior facet to obstruct visualization of the anterior epidural space, bone cutting is not needed in cases of upward-migrated disks (**Fig. 4.2**).

4.4.2 Extended Foraminoplasty (Foraminoplasty with Partial Pediculectomy)

- In severely downward-migrated disk herniation where the ruptured fragment lies in close contact with the medial wall

of the pedicle, the upper part of the inferior pedicle may prevent its direct visualization.

- Removal of the upper and medial wall of the pedicle along with undercutting of the superior facet can help in visualizing and accessing the ruptured fragment (**Fig. 4.3**).
- The downward inclination of the endoscopic trajectory enables oblique cutting of the upper part of the pedicle.

4.5 Surgical Technique

4.5.1 Position and Anesthesia

- PELD is performed under local anesthesia with the patient in the prone position on a radiolucent table under the guidance of C-arm fluoroscopy.
- Conscious sedation with midazolam and fentanyl allows continuous feedback from the patient during the entire procedure to avoid causing damage to the neural structures.
- Midazolam is administered in the dose of 0.05 mg/kg IM 30 minutes before surgery, followed by another dose intravenously during surgery if required.
- Fentanyl dosage is 0.8 µg/kg intravenously 10 minutes before surgery, followed by additional doses intraoperatively if required.

4.5.2 Preoperative Planning

- Axial MRI or CT is used to calculate the distance of the needle's skin entry point from the midline.
- The scans are also used to calculate the needle trajectory, targeting the ruptured fragment while avoiding the contents of the peritoneal sac (**Fig. 4.4**).

4.5.3 Needle Insertion Technique

- It is imperative to achieve proper placement of the needle, which is facilitated by following these guidelines:
  - The site of annular puncture by the needle tip should be at a medial pedicular line in the anteroposterior view and at a posterior vertebral line in the lateral view on fluoroscopic imaging (**Fig. 4.5**). This corresponds to the Kambin safe triangle between exiting and traversing nerve roots.
  - The midpedicular line should be considered for upper lumbar disk herniation (L3, L4, and above) to avoid neural

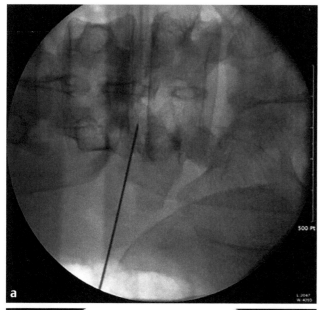

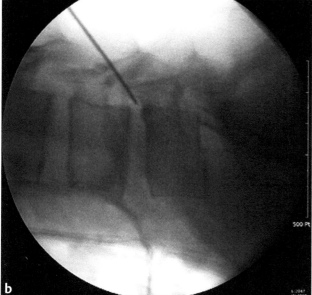

Fig. 4.5 Fluoroscopic views showing the position of the needle tip **(a)** at the medial pedicle line in the AP view and **(b)** at the posterior vertebral line in the lateral view. Note the downward inclination of the needle trajectory on the AP view.

the needle tip directed downward at a 30° angle to the lower end plate, reaching the lower part of the disk at the medial pedicular line (**Fig. 4.5**).

- The downward direction allows easy access to the downward-migrated fragment.
- Similarly, for an upward-migrated disk, the skin entry point is placed below the level of the disk.

4.5.5 Diskography

- Diskography is done by injecting 2 to 3 mL of a solution of radiopaque dye, indigo carmine, and normal saline mixed in a 2:1:2 ratio.
- The dye leaks through the annular tear into the epidural space, the direction being concordant with the anatomical location of the ruptured fragment.
- Indigo carmine, being a base, selectively stains the degenerated acidic nucleus blue, which helps in identification of the herniated fragment during endoscopic visualization.[37]
- The needle is replaced with a guidewire over which the blunt tapered obturator is passed.
- A 7-mm working cannula then replaces the obturator.
- A beveled cannula is used for a downward-migrated herniation and a round cannula for an upward-migrated herniation.

4.6 Downward-Migrated Herniations

- Undercutting of the superior facet is usually needed to access downward-migrated herniations.
- Foraminoplasty can be performed using bone trephines or an endoscopic drill, with the slight technique differences accordingly.

4.6.1 Foraminoplasty Using Bone Trephines

- The entire procedure is performed under strict fluoroscopic control, because it is not performed under endoscopic visualization.
- The beveled cannula is inserted until it touches the superior facet.
- Its position is confirmed on anteroposterior and lateral views on fluoroscopy.
- A 5- or 7-mm bone trephine is then inserted through the working cannula, depending on the amount of bone to be removed.
- Bone cutting is done with a twisting motion involving a moderate amount of force and under constant fluoroscopic control, confirming that it is not damaging the facet joint.
- Cautious intermittent tapping of the trephine with a mallet can speed up the procedure.
- The serrated end of the reamer must not pass beyond the medial border of the facet joint, to avoid neural injury.
- The bone chunk usually becomes impacted inside the trephine and comes out along with it.

injury, because the dural sac is bigger, with more nerve tissue, and lies more laterally due to the narrow width of the pedicles at the upper levels.[33,34,35,36]

4.5.4 Inclination of the Needle Trajectory

- The needle is directed either downward or upward depending on whether there is a downward-migrated or upward-migrated disk.
- The needle is inclined to make an angle corresponding to the herniation site.
- In the case of a downward-migrated herniation, skin entry of the needle starts slightly above the level of the disk, with

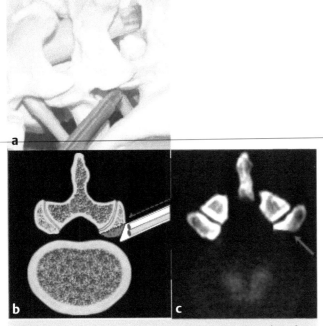

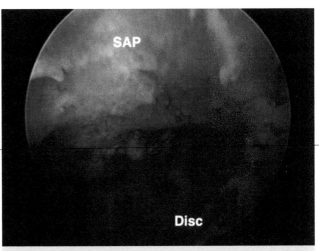

Fig. 4.7 Endoscopic view and illustration showing the large superior facet.

Fig. 4.6 (a,b) The position of the endoscopic reamer on the undersurface of the superior facet. It is not violating the facet joint. **(c)** Axial CT scan showing the undercut superior facet without violation of the facet joint.

- If it does not, it can be removed with a forceps under fluoroscopic control.
- There is not much bleeding if the procedure is done carefully (**Fig. 4.6**).

4.6.2 Foraminoplasty Using an Endoscopic Drill

- The entire procedure is done under direct endoscopic visualization.
- A 6.9 × 6.5-mm endoscope with a working channel of 3.7 mm is inserted through the beveled working cannula.
- The principal anatomical structure that obstructs proper visualization of the ruptured fragment is the large superior facet, covered with the capsular ligament (**Fig. 4.7**).
- The undersurface of the superior facet (the nonarticular part) is removed with an endoscopic drill (**Fig. 4.8**).
- A round bur with a 3.0- or 3.5-mm diamond tip is used.
- A diamond bur, owing to its fine and delicate drilling capabilities, is less likely to cause injury to the neural structures.
- The hemostatic function of the powdery, fine bone dust formed while drilling is an added advantage.
- Intermittent drilling with continuous cold saline irrigation minimizes temperature elevation and its substantial effect on nerves and other structures.
- Because the bone-cutting procedure is done under endoscopic visualization, direct injury to the nerve root is a rarity.
- The lateral edge of the ligamentum flavum, which prevents direct contact of the rotating bur with the nerve root, offers additional protection.
- In cases of extreme migration, the ruptured fragment may lie in close proximity to the medial wall of the pedicle of the inferior vertebra, hidden from endoscopic view.

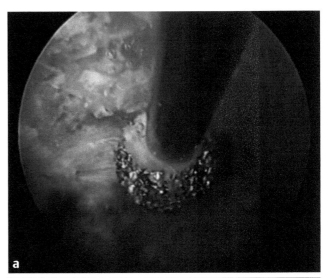

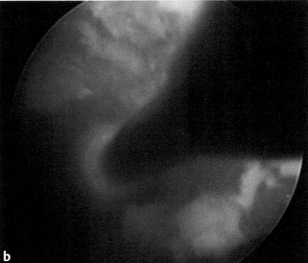

Fig. 4.8 (a,b) Endoscopic view and illustration showing the undercutting of the superior facet with the endoscopic drill.

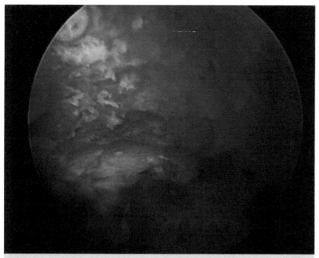

Fig. 4.9 Endoscopic view and illustration showing the undercut superior facet and the exposed ligamentum flavum.

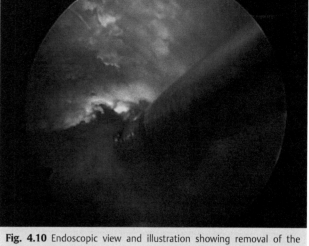

Fig. 4.10 Endoscopic view and illustration showing removal of the ligamentum flavum with laser.

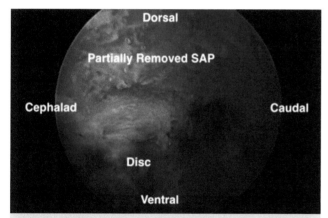

Fig. 4.11 Endoscopic view and illustration showing exposed ruptured fragment.

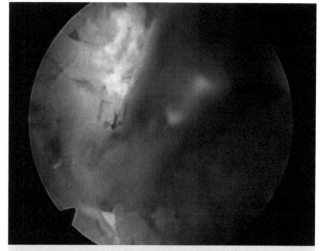

Fig. 4.12 Endoscopic view and illustration showing forceps grasping the ruptured fragment.

- A partial pediculectomy involving removal of the upper border and part of the medial border of the pedicle can help to gain access to the fragment.

4.6.3 Diskectomy Procedure

- After undercutting of the superior facet, the lateral edge of the ligamentum flavum is exposed (**Fig. 4.9**).
- It covers the ruptured fragment and prevents it from being seen.
- The ligamentum flavum is removed with a side-firing Ho:YAG laser (**Fig. 4.10**).
- Additional maneuvers, such as levering the cannula to make it more horizontal and downward tilting, can assist in localizing the fragment.
- Removal of some fibrotic bands along with part of the annulus exposes the fragment completely (**Fig. 4.11**).
- After removal of the ligamentum flavum and adequate release of the annulus, the blue-stained ruptured fragment can be clearly seen.

- The exposed fragment is then removed with forceps under direct visualization (**Fig. 4.12**, **Fig. 4.13**).
- After retrieval of the ruptured fragment, the traversing root with the posterior longitudinal ligament can easily be seen.
- Bleeding is controlled with the help of a flexible bipolar radiofrequency probe.
- The tip of the probe, being curved, is used to palpate for any remaining fragments (**Fig. 4.14**).
- Pressure control by intermittently blocking the irrigation fluid outflow with the thumb allows the traversing nerve root to move freely, which confirms complete decompression (**Fig. 4.14**).[2,3,4,5,13,15,16,38] This is similar to the Valsalva maneuver.

4.7 Upward-Migrated Herniations

- In upward-migrated disk herniation, the approach needle is targeted at the lower part of the disk space to protect the posteriorly displaced exiting nerve root (**Fig. 4.15**, **Fig. 4.16**).

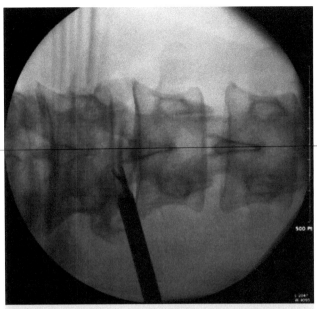

Fig.4.13 Fluoroscopic image showing the position of the forceps while grasping the fragment.

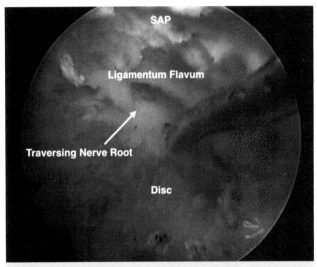

Fig. 4.14 Endoscopic picture and illustration showing the tip of the bipolar probe palpating for remaining fragments. SAP: superior articular process.

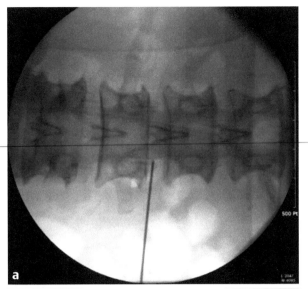

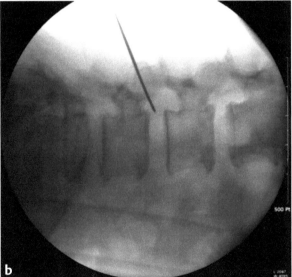

Fig. 4.15 Positions of the needle shown in (**a**) AP and (**b**) lateral views.

- If the herniation is migrated upward completely without any intradiskal component, the procedure is done following the principle of targeted fragmentectomy.
- Target fragmentectomy means removal of only the ruptured fragment without damaging the normal central disk.
- For this purpose, the obturator should not be inserted too deep inside the disk.
- A round-end working cannula is used instead of a beveled cannula to avoid penetration of the annulus.
- The round cannula is initially placed on the surface of the annulus at the level of the disk space (**Fig. 4.17**).
- After initial exploration of the epidural space, the cannula is gradually moved upward, retracting the exiting root and surrounding the soft tissues with its edges.

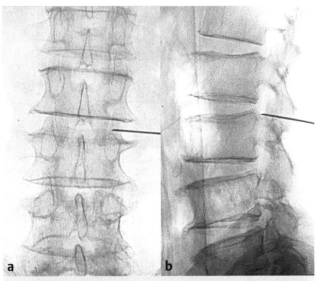

Fig. 4.16 The stained ruptured fragment (*arrows*) during diskography on (**a**) AP and (**b**) lateral views.

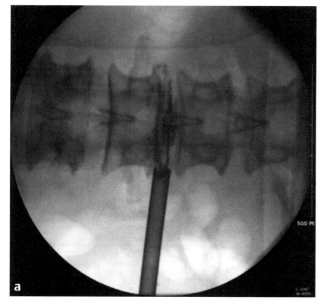

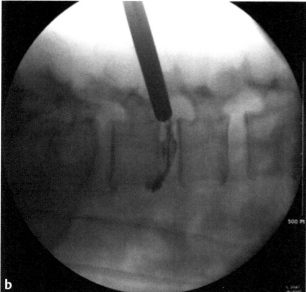

Fig. 4.17 Initial position of the round cannula on the surface of the annulus shown in (**a**) AP and (**b**) lateral views.

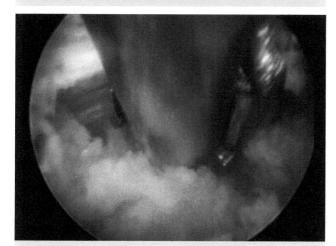

Fig. 4.20 Endoscopic view of the forceps grasping the ruptured fragment.

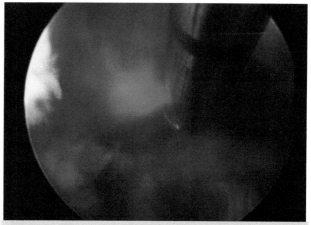

Fig. 4.18 Endoscopic view of the laser beam pointed to the foraminal ligament (at the 10 o'clock position). The foraminal ligament is released with the help of a laser.

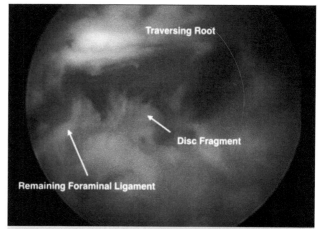

Fig. 4.19 Endoscopic view of the exposed ruptured fragment after the release of the foraminal ligament.

- At this point, the ruptured fragment can be seen lying in the axilla between the exiting and the traversing root, partly covered by the superior foraminal ligament and ligamentum flavum on the other side.
- Release of the ligaments with the Ho:YAG laser exposes the ruptured fragment (**Fig. 4.18**, **Fig. 4.19**).
- The ruptured fragment is then removed manually with forceps (**Fig. 4.20**, **Fig. 4.21**).
- If there is a migrated fragment without any intradiskal component, the cannula remains in the epidural space without penetrating the annulus, allowing the performance of targeted fragmentectomy.
- In the case of an intradiskal component, the migrated fragment is retrieved first, followed by removal of the intradiskal component.

4.8 Complication Avoidance

1. The most important part of the procedure is to determine where the disk is and how to reach the herniation site. Do not allow inappropriate needle placement, because it will make the procedure more difficult.

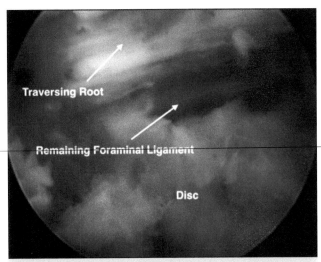

Fig. 4.21 Endoscopic view of the decompressed traversing nerve root after removal of the ruptured fragment.

2. We recommend using a diamond-tip bur for foraminoplasty, since it can be directly visualized under the endoscope, and there is minimal risk of injury to the nerve root.

3. Diskography with indigo carmine is strongly recommended, since the blue-stained disk is easily identified and distinguished from other structures.

4. Grasp the disk at its tail and pull gently, being careful not to break it, to avoid the necessity to do more bone work to remove the remainder.

5. When grasping the disk, rotate the endoscope a bit to visualize the mouth of forceps and to give better exposure of what you are grasping.

4.9 Conclusion

With migrated herniation, getting to the fragments can be difficult, so the trajectory of the needle insertion is crucial for a successful outcome. For downward-migrated herniation, a cephalad to caudal direction is correct, and for upward-migrated herniation, a caudal to cephalad direction should be attempted. If the fragments still cannot be reached (especially with high-grade migrated herniation), foraminoplasty via removal of the superior articular process and partial pediculectomy using a bur are useful. Finally, the surgeon should be aware of the difficulties and should master regular PELD before attempting to address more extensive indications.

References

1 Hijikata S, Yamagishi M, Nakayma T. Percutaneous discectomy: a new treatment method for lumbar disc herniation. *J Tokyo Denryoku Hosp* 1975;5:39–44

2 Kambin P, O'Brien E, Zhou L, Schaffer JL. Arthroscopic microdiscectomy and selective fragmentectomy. *Clin Orthop Relat Res* 1998; Feb;(347):150–167

3 Yeung AT, Tsou PM. Posterolateral endoscopic excision for lumbar disc herniation: surgical technique, outcome, and complications in 307 consecutive cases. *Spine* 2002;27(7):722–731

4 Yeung AT. Minimally invasive disc surgery with the Yeung endoscopic spine system (YESS). *Surg Technol Int* 1999;8:267–277

5 Yeung AT. The evolution of percutaneous spinal endoscopy and discectomy: state of the art. *Mt Sinai J Med* 2000;67(4):327–332

6 Mayer HM, Brock M. Percutaneous endoscopic lumbar discectomy (PELD). *Neurosurg Rev* 1993;16(2):115–120

7 Mayer HM, Brock M. Percutaneous endoscopic discectomy: surgical technique and preliminary results compared to microsurgical discectomy. *J Neurosurg* 1993;78(2):216–225

8 Macnab I. Negative disc exploration. An analysis of the causes of nerve-root involvement in sixty-eight patients. *J Bone Joint Surg Am* 1971;53(5):891–903

9 McCulloch JA, Young PH. Microsurgery for lumbar disc herniation. In: McCulloch JA, Young PH, eds. *Essentials of Spinal Microsurgery*. Philadelphia, PA: Lippincott-Raven; 1998:329–382

10 Osman SG, Nibu K, Panjabi MM, Marsolais EB, Chaudhary R. Transforaminal and posterior decompressions of the lumbar spine. A comparative study of stability and intervertebral foramen area. *Spine* 1997;22(15):1690–1695

11 Iida Y, Kataoka O, Sho T, et al. Postoperative lumbar spinal instability occurring or progressing secondary to laminectomy. *Spine* 1990;15(11):1186–1189

12 Kambin P, Cohen LF, Brooks M, Schaffer JL. Development of degenerative spondylosis of the lumbar spine after partial discectomy. Comparison of laminotomy, discectomy, and posterolateral discectomy. *Spine* 1995;20(5):599–607

13 Kambin P, Casey K, O'Brien E, Zhou L. Transforaminal arthroscopic decompression of lateral recess stenosis. *J Neurosurg* 1996;84(3):462–467

14 Kambin P, Sampson S. Posterolateral percutaneous suction-excision of herniated lumbar intervertebral discs. Report of interim results. *Clin Orthop Relat Res* 1986; Jun;(207):37–43

15 Kambin P, Gellman H. Percutaneous lateral discectomy of the lumbar spine: a preliminary report. *Clin Orthop Relat Res* 1983;174:127–132

16 Kambin P. Posterolateral percutaneous lumbar discectomy and decompression. In: Kambin P, ed. *Arthroscopic Microdiscectomy: Minimal Intervention in Spinal Surgery*. Baltimore, MD: Urban & Schwarzenberg; 1991:67–100

17 Mochida J, Toh E, Nomura T, Nishimura K. The risks and benefits of percutaneous nucleotomy for lumbar disc herniation. A 10-year longitudinal study. *J Bone Joint Surg Br* 2001;83(4):501–505

18 Natarajan RN, Andersson GB, Patwardhan AG, Andriacchi TP. Study on effect of graded facetectomy on change in lumbar motion segment torsional flexibility using three-dimensional continuum contact representation for facet joints. *J Biomech Eng* 1999;121(2):215–221

19 Schaffer JL, Kambin P. Percutaneous posterolateral lumbar discectomy and decompression with a 6.9-millimeter cannula. Analysis of operative failures and complications. *J Bone Joint Surg Am* 1991;73(6):822–831

20 Weber BR, Grob D, Dvořák J, Müntener M. Posterior surgical approach to the lumbar spine and its effect on the multifidus muscle. *Spine* 1997;22(15):1765–1772

21 Zander T, Rohlmann A, Klöckner C, Bergmann G. Influence of graded facetectomy and laminectomy on spinal biomechanics. *Eur Spine J* 2003;12(4):427–434

22 Parke WW. The significance of venous return impairment in ischemic radiculopathy and myelopathy. *Orthop Clin North Am* 1991;22(2):213–221

23 Cooper RG, Mitchell WS, Illingworth KJ, Forbes WS, Gillespie JE, Jayson MI. The role of epidural fibrosis and defective fibrinolysis in the persistence of postlaminectomy back pain. *Spine* 1991;16(9):1044–1048

24 Ross JS, Robertson JT, Frederickson RC, et al; ADCON-L European Study Group. Association between peridural scar and recurrent radicular pain after lumbar discectomy: magnetic resonance evaluation. *Neurosurgery* 1996;38(4):855–861

25 Hermantin FU, Peters T, Quartararo L, Kambin P. A prospective, randomized study comparing the results of open discectomy with those of video-assisted arthroscopic microdiscectomy. *J Bone Joint Surg Am* 1999;81(7):958–965

26 Lee SH, Kang BU, Ahn Y, et al. Operative failure of percutaneous endoscopic lumbar discectomy: a radiologic analysis of 55 cases. *Spine* 2006;31(10):E285–E290

27 Lee S, Kim SK, Lee SH, et al. Percutaneous endoscopic lumbar discectomy for migrated disc herniation: classification of disc migration and surgical approaches. *Eur Spine J* 2007;16(3):431–437

28 Ditsworth DA. Endoscopic transforaminal lumbar discectomy and reconfiguration: a postero-lateral approach into the spinal canal. *Surg Neurol* 1998;49(6):588–597

29 Min JH, Kang SH, Lee JB, Cho TH, Suh JK, Rhyu IJ. Morphometric analysis of the working zone for endoscopic lumbar discectomy. *J Spinal Disord Tech* 2005;18(2):132–135

30 Ahn Y, Lee SH, Park WM, Lee HY. Posterolateral percutaneous endoscopic lumbar foraminotomy for L5–S1 foraminal or lateral exit zone stenosis. Technical note. *J Neurosurg* 2003;99(3, Suppl):320–323

31 Fardon DF, Milette PC; Combined Task Forces of the North American Spine Society, American Society of Spine Radiology, and American Society of Neuroradiology. Nomenclature and classification of lumbar disc pathology. Recommendations of the Combined Task Forces of the North American Spine Society, American Society of Spine Radiology, and American Society of Neuroradiology. *Spine* 2001;26(5):E93–E113

32 Choi G, Lee SH, Raiturker PP, Lee S, Chae YS. Percutaneous endoscopic interlaminar discectomy for intracanalicular disc herniations at L5–S1 using a rigid working channel endoscope. *Neurosurgery* 2006;58

33 Attar A, Ugur HC, Uz A, Tekdemir I, Egemen N, Genc Y. Lumbar pedicle: surgical anatomic evaluation and relationships. *Eur Spine J* 2001;10(1):10–15

34 Kim NH, Lee HM, Chung IH, Kim HJ, Kim SJ. Morphometric study of the pedicles of thoracic and lumbar vertebrae in Koreans. *Spine* 1994;19(12):1390–1394

35 Söyüncü Y, Yildirim FB, Sekban H, Ozdemir H, Akyildiz F, Sindel M. Anatomic evaluation and relationship between the lumbar pedicle and adjacent neural structures: an anatomic study. *J Spinal Disord Tech* 2005;18(3):243–246

36 Zindrick MR, Wiltse LL, Doornik A, et al. Analysis of the morphometric characteristics of the thoracic and lumbar pedicles. *Spine* 1987;12(2):160–166

37 Lew SM, Mehalic TF, Fagone KL. Transforaminal percutaneous endoscopic discectomy in the treatment of far-lateral and foraminal lumbar disc herniations. *J Neurosurg* 2001;94(2, Suppl):216–220

38 Yeung AT, Yeung CA. Advances in endoscopic disc and spine surgery: foraminal approach. *Surg Technol Int* 2003;11:255–263

5 Percutaneous Endoscopic Lumbar Diskectomy with Foraminotomy

Akarawit Asawasaksakul, Gun Choi, and Alfonso García

5.1 Introduction

Herniated nucleus pulposus is one of the most common spine problems in the modern world, and it can be treated endoscopically, but there are some challenges in the endoscopic technique for treating difficult or complicated herniations, such as in the case of highly downward-migrated or upward-migrated disks or in patients with a narrow foraminal diameter. The main challenge is the space limitation that prevents tilting the scope and visualizing all the related structures and that limits the trajectory of the endoscopic instruments. In this situation, foraminoplasty is a great help, because it enlarges the foraminal diameter to accommodate the need for space (**Video 5.1**).

5.2 Foraminal Anatomy

5.2.1 Normal Arrangement

Before attempting foraminoplasty, knowledge of normal foraminal anatomy is crucial for surgical planning and preparing for unexpected situations. See Chapter 1 for a complete discussion of the anatomy.

Because the exiting nerve root courses underneath the cephalad pedicle, the exiting root can be visualized on the surgeon's left in the left transforaminal approach. Vascular structures usually run along the nerve root and are rarely encountered in normal situations. Lateral extension of the ligamentum flavum can also be clearly visualized through the endoscope.

5.2.2 Possible Obstacle

Foraminal cut MRI is very helpful in determining what to expect during the procedure and which wall of the foramen will need to be partially removed. The considerations include disk position, the size of the foramen, and whether any bony part of the foraminal wall impinges on the nerve root. For example, if the disk is highly downward-migrated, partial caudad pediculectomy should be considered to allow better angulation for the endoscopic procedure, or, if are there any bony spurs from the posterior vertebral body, if the ventral part of the superior articular process impinges on exiting nerve root, or if the foramen is too small to accommodate the endoscope, removal of the impingement together with enlargement of the foraminal diameter is important.

Foraminal vessels, especially arteries, should also be kept in mind for potential bleeding. An artery that is situated in the inferior third of the foramen is the most at risk.

5.3 Migrated Disk Herniation

We usually use posterior marginal disk height to determine the extent of migration. If the disk has migrated more than the posterior marginal disk height as measured from the adjacent end

plate level, it is considered a high-grade migrated herniation; if it has migrated less, it is called low-grade migration.[1,2,3]

Most of the time that foraminoplasty is considered, the disk has gone beyond low-grade migration (**Fig. 5.1**).

5.4 Patient Selection

Possible indications for the procedure include:[4]

1. Predominant unilateral leg pain with or without associated back pain
2. Positive nerve root tension sign
3. Corresponding findings on CT and MRI
4. Soft disk herniation
5. Failure of conservative treatment for more than 6 weeks

Possible contraindications include:

1. Associated bony spinal stenosis
2. Calcified disk
3. Spinal instability
4. Herniation at the L5–S1 level with high iliac crest and thick transverse process

5.5 Surgical Technique

Most cases that need foraminoplasty involve downward-migrated herniation, especially highly migrated cases. With upward-migrated herniation, because the working site is in the upper, larger part of the foramen, foraminoplasty is usually not necessary.

5.5.1 Step 1: Patient Position and Preoperative Planning

- The patient is placed in the prone position with hips and knees flexed.
- Local anesthesia plus conscious sedation is preferable.
- The skin entry point can be calculated using axial MRI.

5.5.2 Step 2: Needle Insertion

- Needle insertion depends on the location of the migrated fragments, but usually the inclination of the trajectory is at an angle of ~ 30 degrees to the end plate.
- For caudal migration, the trajectory of the needle should be cephalocaudal.
  - Thus, the skin entry point should be cephalad to the level of the disk.
- When inserting the needle, try to aim toward the disk fragments.
- The final position of the needle should be at the medial pedicular line on the anteroposterior (AP) view for L4–L5 and below; for the upper lumbar spine (L3–L4 and above),

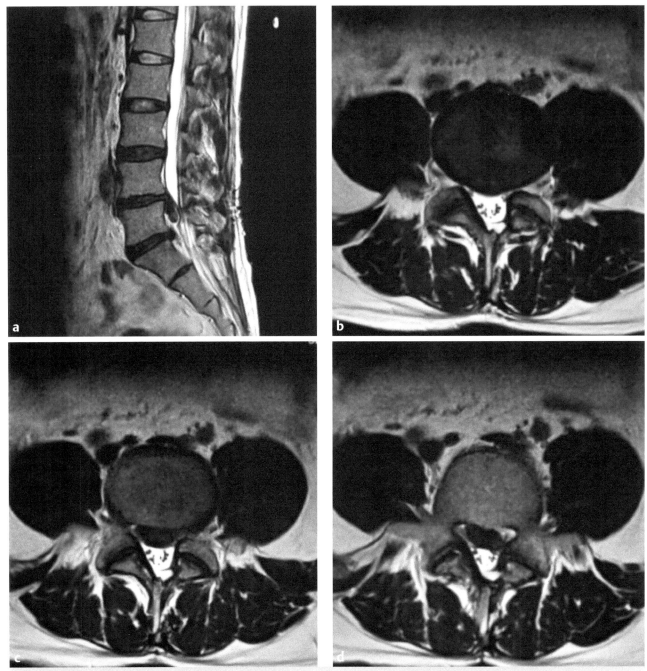

Fig. 5.1 (**a**) MRI sagittal view shows highly downward-migrated disk at the L4–L5 level. (**b–d**) Axial views of downward-migrated fragments.

the midpedicular line is safer to avoid neural injury, because the dural sac is larger, with more nerve tissue.[5,6,7,8] On lateral view, the tip of the needle should be on the posterior vertebral line[9,10,11,12,13,14,15,16] (**Fig. 5.2**).

5.5.3 Step 3: Diskography

- Diskography (**Fig. 5.3**) uses 2 to 3 mL of a solution of opaque dye, indigo carmine, and normal saline (in a 2:1:2 ratio).
- Dye leakage into the epidural space should be in the same direction as fragment herniation.

5.5.4 Step 4: Guidewire Insertion and Skin Incision

- Same as normal PELD.

5.5.5 Step 5: Dilator and Working Cannula Insertion

- Same as normal PELD.

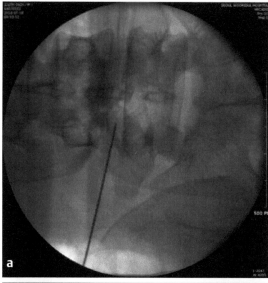

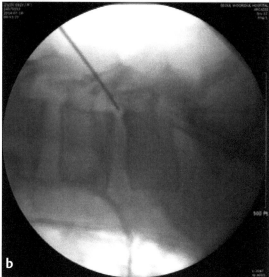

Fig. 5.2 (a) Needle position in anteroposterior (AP) view. **(b)** Needle position in lateral view.

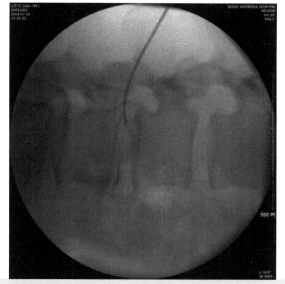

Fig. 5.3 Dye leakage into the epidural space after diskography.

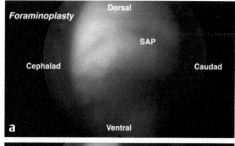

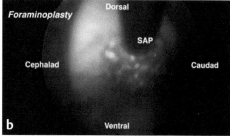

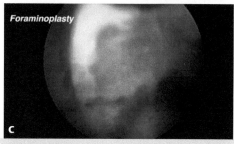

Fig. 5.4 (a,b,c) Removal of the superior facet using the endoscopic ball-tipped diamond bur.

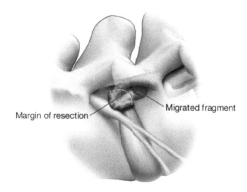

Fig. 5.5 Removal of the bony part of the foramen, including the superior wall of the pedicle, to accommodate direction of the scope.

5.5.6 Step 6: Endoscopic Procedures

- After proper placement of the working cannula, the endoscope is introduced and foraminoplasty is initiated.
  - In downward-migrated herniation, the superior articular process of the caudad vertebra usually prevents visualization of the migrated fragment; therefore, removal of the undersurface of this bony part widens the foramen and gives better exposure of the disk (**Fig. 5.4**).[17,18]
  - In some cases of high-grade migration, partial pediculectomy is a great help in accommodating the trajectory of the scope and in giving better visualization of the fragments behind the pedicle (**Fig. 5.5**).

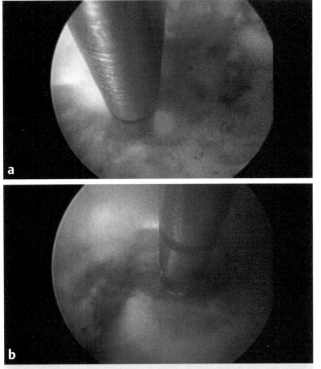

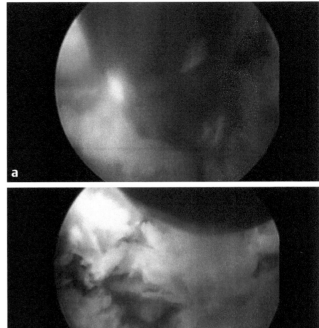

Fig. 5.6 (a,b) Removal of the ligamentum flavum and foraminal ligaments using the Ho:YAG laser with a side-firing probe.

Fig. 5.8 (a,b) Removal of fragment using endoscopic forceps.

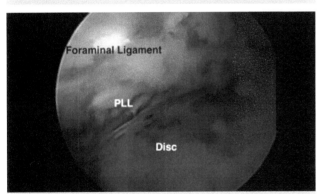

Fig. 5.7 Exposure of the disk after foraminal ligament removal.

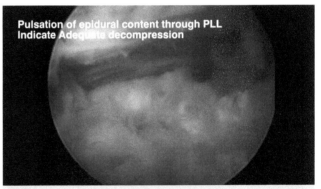

Fig. 5.9 Full decompression of the nerve root after removal of the migrated fragment.

○ A diamond bur is recommended for the procedure, because it helps control bleeding through creation of bone dust.

○ Extension of the ligamentum flavum and other foraminal ligaments are removed using the Ho:YAG laser with a side-firing probe (**Fig. 5.6**).

○ During the procedure, levering of the scope horizontally sometime helps to get a better view of the fragments (**Fig. 5.7**).

○ In situations where only the tail of the fragment can be seen, grasping the tail with the endoscopic forceps and gently pulling the fragment out is usually sufficient (**Fig. 5.8**).

5.5.7 Step 7: Check for Adequacy of Decompression

• The RF bipolar probe is useful in checking for any remaining fragment.

• After decompression, the fully decompressed nerve root and pulsating epidural content should be seen (**Fig. 5.9**).

• The amount of disk fragments removed should be correlated with the MRI findings. If they don't match, further search for the remnants should be conducted.

5.6 Complication Avoidance

The complications of this procedure begin with needle insertion. If the needle is inserted into a position that does not correlate with the herniated fragment that needs to removed, the surgeon will end up doing more foraminoplasty and thus increasing the risk of bleeding. Partial pediculectomy is another cause of bleeding if pedicle removal is excessive. The ball-tip diamond bur is helpful in decreasing bleeding. For patients who undergo foraminoplasty, we recommend that a vacuum drain be placed to reduce postoperative hematoma.

Preoperative planning using MRI and CT is very important. Determining the fragments' size and quantity and the trajectory of the scope for the procedure is a great help in preventing unexpected events that affect the outcome and in allowing the surgeon to plan how to cope with corresponding developments.

Adequacy of the decompression can be determined by comparing the disk removed with the imaging investigation, by observing pulsatile epidural contents, by observing bleeding after removal of the main fragments (due to release of venous congestion), and by directly visualizing of the decompressed nerve root.

5.7 Conclusion

Foraminoplasty is a useful method for reaching the herniation site in downward-migrated herniation, by burring out the superior articular process together with the superior aspect of the pedicle. Use of the diamond bur is recommended, because it has an advantage over the regular endoscopic shaver in terms of bleeding control. Foraminoplasty allows retrieval of the herniated fragments in difficult cases, and it is helpful in foraminal stenosis as well.

References

1 Lee SH, Kang BU, Ahn Y, et al. Operative failure of percutaneous endoscopic lumbar discectomy: a radiologic analysis of 55 cases. *Spine* 2006;*31*(10):E285–E290
2 Lee S, Kim SK, Lee SH, et al. Percutaneous endoscopic lumbar discectomy for migrated disc herniation: classification of disc migration and surgical approaches. *Eur Spine J* 2007;*16*(3):431–437
3 Fardon DF, Milette PC; Combined Task Forces of the North American Spine Society, American Society of Spine Radiology, and American Society of Neuroradiology. Nomenclature and classification of lumbar disc pathology recommendations of the Combined Task Forces of the North American Spine Society, American Society of Spine Radiology, and American Society of Neuroradiology. *Spine* 2001;*26*(5):E93–E113
4 Choi G, Lee SH, Lokhande P, et al. Percutaneous endoscopic approach for highly migrated intracanal disc herniations by foraminoplastic technique using rigid working channel endoscope. *Spine* 2008;*33*(15):E508–E515
5 Attar A, Ugur HC, Uz A, Tekdemir I, Egemen N, Genc Y. Lumbar pedicle: surgical anatomic evaluation and relationships. *Eur Spine J* 2001;*10*(1):10–15
6 Kim NH, Lee HM, Chung IH, Kim HJ, Kim SJ. Morphometric study of the pedicles of thoracic and lumbar vertebrae in Koreans. *Spine* 1994;*19*(12):1390–1394
7 Söyüncü Y, Yildirim FB, Sekban H, Ozdemir H, Akyildiz F, Sindel M. Anatomic evaluation and relationship between the lumbar pedicle and adjacent neural structures: an anatomic study. *J Spinal Disord Tech* 2005;*18*(3):243–246
8 Zindrick MR, Wiltse LL, Doornik A, et al. Analysis of the morphometric characteristics of the thoracic and lumbar pedicles. *Spine* 1987;*12*(2):160–166
9 Kambin P, O'Brien E, Zhou L, Schaffer JL. Arthroscopic microdiscectomy and selective fragmentectomy. *Clin Orthop Relat Res* 1998; Feb;(347):150–167
10 Kambin P, Casey K, O'Brien E, Zhou L. Transforaminal arthroscopic decompression of lateral recess stenosis. *J Neurosurg* 1996;*84*(3):462–467
11 Kambin P, Gellman H. Percutaneous lateral discectomy of the lumbar spine. A preliminary report. *Clin Orthop Relat Res* 1983;*174*:127–132
12 Kambin P. Posterolateral percutaneous lumbar discectomy and decompression. In: Kambin P, ed. *Arthroscopic Microdiscectomy: Minimal Intervention in Spinal Surgery*. Baltimore, MD: Urban & Schwarzenberg; 1991:67–100
13 Yeung AT, Tsou PM. Posterolateral endoscopic excision for lumbar disc herniation: Surgical technique, outcome, and complications in 307 consecutive cases. *Spine* 2002;*27*(7):722–731
14 Yeung AT. Minimally invasive disc surgery with the Yeung endoscopic spine system (YESS). *Surg Technol Int* 1999;*8*:267–277
15 Yeung AT. The evolution of percutaneous spinal endoscopy and discectomy: state of the art. *Mt Sinai J Med* 2000;*67*(4):327–332
16 Yeung AT, Yeung CA. Advances in endoscopic disc and spine surgery: foraminal approach. *Surg Technol Int* 2003;*11*:255–263
17 Min JH, Kang SH, Lee JB, Cho TH, Suh JK, Rhyu IJ. Morphometric analysis of the working zone for endoscopic lumbar discectomy. *J Spinal Disord Tech* 2005;*18*(2):132–135
18 Hijikata S, Yamagishi M, Nakayma T. Percutaneous discectomy: a new treatment method for lumbar disc herniation. *J Tokyo Den-ryoku Hosp* 1975;*5*:39–44

6 Surgical Technique for Percutaneous Endoscopic Laser Annuloplasty/Nucleoplasty

Akarawit Asawasaksakul and Gun Choi

6.1 Introduction

Diskogenic pain is one of the most difficult back pains to distinguish by clinical symptoms. The pathophysiology of diskogenic back pain involves granulation tissue ingrowth into the disk space via an annular defect (fissure, tear, or cleft) resulting from either degenerative disease or trauma. The granulation tissue results in angiogenesis, free nerve ingrowth, and a chronic intradisk inflammatory process that irritates free nerve endings in the area.[1,2] There are many procedures for coping with diskogenic pain, such as fusion surgery or total disk replacement, but since the advent of minimally invasive techniques, there are more options.

The era of intradiskal treatment began in 1975 when Hijikata et al reported on percutaneous posterolateral intradiskal nucleotomy for indirect nerve root decompression[3] and advanced again in 1983 with Kambin et al's report on the outcome of percutaneous lateral diskectomy of the lumbar spine.[4] The nonvisualized methods continued to be developed by many surgeons,[5,6,7,8] but after the introduction of the endoscope, many spine surgeons applied and developed the use of endoscopic spinal treatment, including Kambin et al, who used the arthroscope for microdiskectomy in 1997;[9] Yeung et al, who introduced transforaminal endoscopic decompression in 2002;[10,11] and Choi et al, who introduced percutaneous endoscopic diskectomy via the interlaminar approach in 2005.[12] This led to the concept of using endoscopic procedures to treat diskogenic back pain by direct visualization of the inflammation and annular defect, nucleoplasty to manage inflammation, and annuloplasty to narrow the annular defect.

In 2002, Yeung et al introduced thermal discoplasty and annuloplasty using the YESS endoscope via a transforaminal approach;[11] they were followed in the same year by Tsou et al's description of the surgical technique for posterolateral transforaminal diskectomy and annuloplasty for chronic lumbar diskogenic back pain[10] and in 2010 by Lee's introduction of the use of laser for nucleoplasty and annuloplasty (**Video 6.1**).[13]

6.2 Diagnosis

There are many causes of low back pain, such as mechanical instability, intervertebral disk pathology, facet joint pain, neurogenic pain, and miscellaneous causes,[13] but usually 40% of low back pain is diskogenic.[14] The clinical challenges with diskogenic back pain start with how to make the most accurate diagnosis with the least invasive method. As is well known, the characteristics of diskogenic back pain include sitting intolerance, difficulty in lifting heavy objects, extension catch, increased pain after a hard working day, and loss of ability to maintain a posture for 30 minutes, but all of these symptoms are mostly nonspecific. Because of this, MRI and provocative diskography are very helpful diagnostic tests for diskogenic back pain.

MRI can show an annular defect on both T1 and T2, and it can show thickening of the posterior portion of the annulus

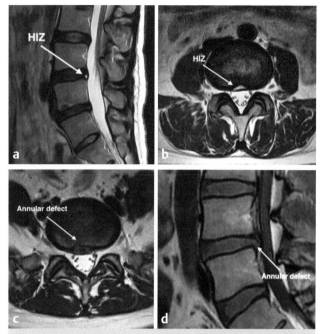

Fig. 6.1 (**a,b**) High intensity zone (HIZ), annular defect. (**c,d**) Annular defect.

and the disk trapped inside the defect. The HIZ (high intensity zone) is also a helpful finding in T2 MRI (**Fig. 6.1**). If the characteristics of the pain and the MRI findings correlate, the diagnosis can be confirmed using provocative diskography.[15] During diskography, a sharp, shooting pain is present upon injection at the pathologic level due to the increase in intradiskal pressure that stimulates the nerve endings. Furthermore, dye leakage from the annular defect can be found. If the symptoms of the back pain are clearly established, diskography can be done in the same setting with the percutaneous endoscopic laser annuloplasty/nucleoplasty. The important thing about provocative diskography is that the examiner also obtains a normal reference from a normal disk level (**Table 6.1**).

Table 6.1 Summary of investigation findings

Diagnostic Tool	Positive Finding
Clinical symptoms	Sitting intolerance Difficulty lifting heavy objects Extension catch Increased pain after hard working day Loss of ability to maintain posture for 30 minutes
MRI	Annular defect with both T1 and T2 imaging Thickening of posterior annulus HIZ (high intensity zone) on T2 imaging
Provocative diskography	Positive with sharp, shooting pain

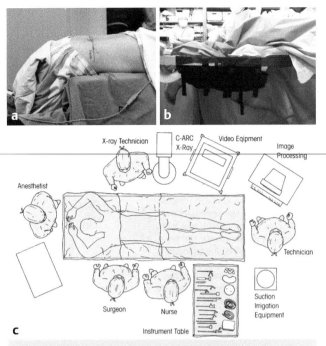

Fig. 6.2 (a,b) Patient positioning. (c) Equipment set-up.

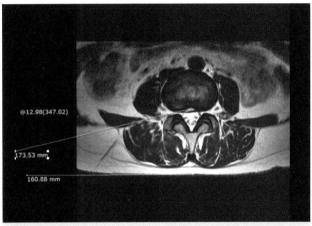

Fig. 6.3 Skin entry point calculated using MRI.

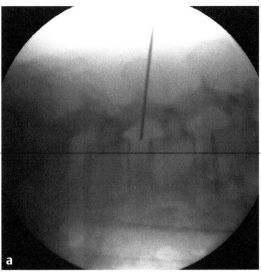

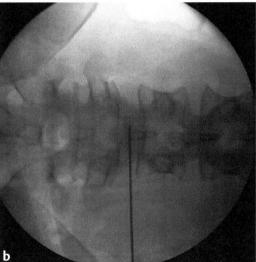

Fig. 6.4 Needle insertion: trajectory and angulation. (a) Lateral view. (b) AP view.

6.3 Etiology and Indications for Surgery

Since diskogenic low back pain has many causes, such as internal disk disruption (IDD), degenerative disk disease (DDD), herniated nucleus pulposus (HNP), and damage to the annulus, there still some controversies about which procedure is better for treating diskogenic pain, but common relative indications for surgery are:

- Disabling diskogenic back pain that has been confirmed by provocative diskography
- Failed conservative treatment (such as medication, exercise, and physical therapy) lasting more than 6 months

6.4 Surgical Technique

6.4.1 Position and Setting

For the posterolateral transforaminal approach, the patient is placed in the prone position, with bolster padding at the pelvis and abdomen, on a spinal operating table. The hips and knees are flexed (**Fig. 6.2a,b**). The operating surgeon should always stand on the symptomatic side, and the intraoperative image intensifier should be located on the opposite side (**Fig. 6.2c**). Level marking and draping are done. A tip for draping is to leave the ankles and both feet exposed, so that, when asked, the patient can move the ankles and the surgeon can observe the movement to ensure the safety of neurologic status.

6.4.2 Anesthesia and Conscious Sedation

We recommend conscious sedation using remifentanil plus propofol and local anesthesia with skin infiltration by 2 to 3 mL of 1% lidocaine and paraspinal muscle infiltration by 6 to 8 mL; wait 1 minute for full effect. The most painful points in the

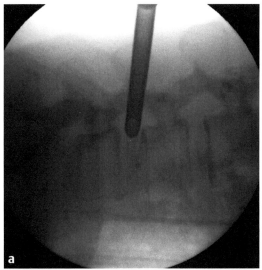

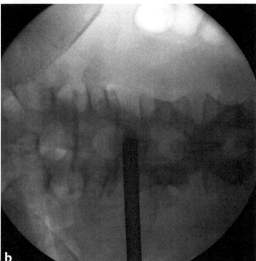

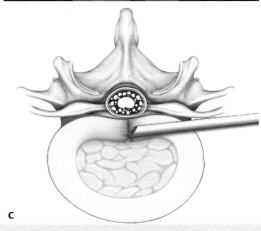

Fig. 6.5 Obturator insertion. (**a**) Lateral view. (**b**) AP view. (**c**) Diagram of obturator position.

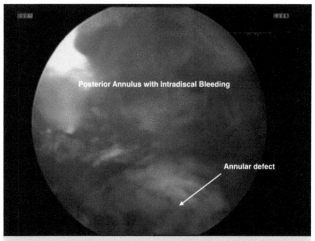

Fig. 6.6 Endoscopic view of posterior annular defect with label.

6.4.3 Needle Insertion and Working Channel Establishment

Needle insertion is considered the most important step for establishing the working channel and for optimal visualization. Our recommendation is use of the 18 G spinal needle introduced under fluoroscopic guidance according to the location of pathology. The entry point is calculated preoperatively using MRI (**Fig. 6.3**). Usually, the entry point is 8 to 12 cm from the midline. In comparison to PELD, the angle of the needle should be a bit more horizontal and the final position of the needle tip should be at the posterior vertebral body line in the lateral view and just at the medial pedicular border in the anteroposterior (AP) view. Unlike in PELD, the insertion is more posterior. Diskography using a solution indigo carmine, contrast, and normal saline solution in a 2:1:2 ratio is done after needle insertion,[12,16] followed by guidewire insertion through the needle (**Fig. 6.4**).

Skin incision is needed before putting in the dilator. The dilator is inserted to establish a working portal for the endoscope under intraoperative image guidance. After the dilator passes the medial pedicular border, gentle hammering is possible to reach the point just past midline. During beveled obturator insertion, make sure the bevel is facing dorsally (**Fig. 6.5**).

6.4.4 Annuloplasty/Nucleoplasty Procedure

After the proper working channel is established, the posterior-most disc has been reached. A 20° angled endoscope and the beveled cannula make visualization of the inner part of the posterior annulus possible. The annular defect can be located, and some trapped nucleus pulposus stained by indigo carmine can be visualized inside the defect (**Fig. 6.6**). At this point, because diskogenic back pain is the result of inflammation and granulation tissue ingrowth, intradiskal bleeding can be seen. This sign confirms the diagnosis and indicates that the outcome of the procedure will be beneficial to the patient (**Fig. 6.6**).

procedure are skin entry and annulus penetration; therefore, we also recommend infiltration with another 2 to 3 mL of 1% lidocaine just before penetrating the annulus; this will be enough to minimize the pain. A stronger concentration (e.g., 2%) may paralyze motor function as well and could compromise the protection against iatrogenic neural injury.

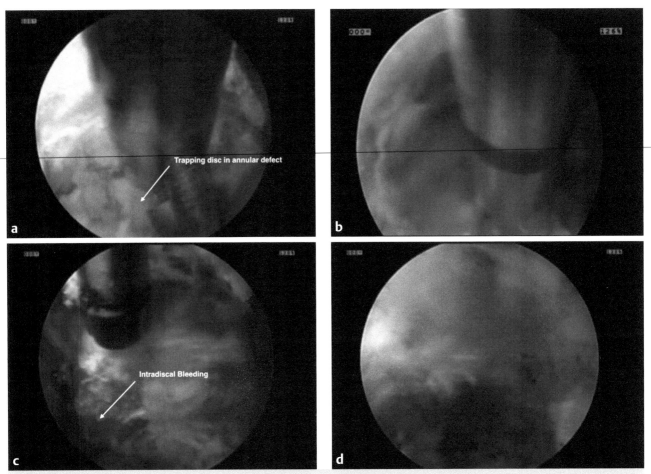

Fig. 6.7 (**a**) Removal of disk using endoscopic forceps. (**b**) Annuloplasty using side-firing laser. Coagulation of the bleeding and inflammation tissue using radiofrequency (RF) bipolar cautery, (**c**) before coagulation and (**d**) after coagulation and finished annuloplasty.

After identification of the annular defect and trapped disk material, the disk is removed using endoscopic forceps. If the trapped disk is too large, the opening of the defect can be widened using a side-firing holmium:yttrium-aluminum-garnet (Ho:YAG) laser to accommodate the removal. After the disk is removed, annuloplasty is done using the side-firing Ho:YAG laser. Inflamed tissue and bleeding are managed using both the side-firing Ho:YAG laser and endoscopic radiofrequency (RF) bipolar cautery (**Fig. 6.7**).

Finally, if needed, the traversing root and epidural space can be visualized by gradually withdrawing the obturator and endoscope.

6.5 Complication Avoidance

During the procedure, because the patient remains conscious, the operating surgeon can continuously evaluate the patient's neurologic function and avoid complications. Complications are rarely seen, but they are possible and should be prevented.

- Neural injury due to careless needle insertion occurs rarely, because patients themselves are the best neuromonitoring system.
- Dural tear is possible but is rarely seen in this procedure, because the tip of the cannula is anchored in the annulus and epidural content does not need to be visualized.

- Neck pain is caused by an increase in intracranial pressure due to inflow of irrigation fluid. We recommend adjusting the flow according to bleeding and lowering the pressure after hemostatic control is achieved with the RF bipolar cautery.
- In our experience so far, postoperative infection is unknown because of use of continuous intraoperative irrigation with antibiotic-infused saline.
- Persistent symptoms after surgery are avoided by strictly selecting only patients who have diskogenic back pain. We strongly recommend the use of provocative diskography for diagnosis of diskogenic back pain. If inflammation and intradiskal bleeding are observed intraoperatively, we can confirm that the patient will improve after the procedure.

6.6 Conclusion

Percutaneous endoscopic laser annuloplasty/nucleoplasty has the benefit of visualization of intradiskal pathology and removal of the entrapped fragment that is the main cause of chronic inflammation leading to diskogenic back pain. The clear visualization and the use of the Ho:YAG laser with a side-firing probe allow the surgeon to accomplish both annuloplasty and nucleoplasty in the same procedure.

References

1 Kauppila LI. Ingrowth of blood vessels in disc degeneration. Angiographic and histological studies of cadaveric spines. *J Bone Joint Surg Am* 1995;77(1):26–31

2 Tsou PM, Alan Yeung C, Yeung AT. Posterolateral transforaminal selective endoscopic discectomy and thermal annuloplasty for chronic lumbar discogenic pain: a minimal access visualized intradiscal surgical procedure. *Spine J* 2004;4(5):564–573

3 Hijikata S, Yamagishi M, Nakayma T. Percutaneous discectomy: a new treatment method for lumbar disc herniation. *J Tokyo Den-ryoku Hosp* 1975;5:39–44

4 Kambin P, Gellman H. Percutaneous lateral discectomy of the lumbar spine. A preliminary report. *Clin Orthop Relat Res* 1983; 174:127–132

5 Onik G, Helms CA, Ginsberg L, Hoaglund FT, Morris J. Percutaneous lumbar diskectomy using a new aspiration probe: porcine and cadaver model. *Radiology* 1985;155(1):251–252

6 Hayashi K, Thabit G III, Bogdanske JJ, Mascio LN, Markel MD. The effect of nonablative laser energy on the ultrastructure of joint capsular collagen. *Arthroscopy* 1996;12(4):474–481

7 Saal JA, Saal JS. Intradiscal electrothermal treatment for chronic discogenic low back pain: prospective outcome study with a minimum 2-year follow-up. *Spine* 2002;27(9):966–973

8 Hermantin FU, Peters T, Quartararo L, Kambin P. A prospective, randomized study comparing the results of open discectomy with those of video-assisted arthroscopic microdiscectomy. *J Bone Joint Surg Am* 1999;81(7):958–965

9 Kambin P. Arthroscopic microdiscectomy. In: Frymoyer JW, ed. *The Adult Spine: Principle and Practice.* 2nd ed. Philadelphia: Lippincott-Raven Publishers; 1997:2023–2036

10 Tsou PM, Yeung AT. Transforaminal endoscopic decompression for radiculopathy secondary to non-contained intracanal lumbar disc herniation. *Spine J* 2002;2:41–48

11 Yeung AT, Tsou PM. Posterolateral endoscopic excision for lumbar disc herniation: Surgical technique, outcome, and complications in 307 consecutive cases. *Spine* 2002;27(7):722–731

12 Choi G, Lee SH, Raiturker PP, Lee S, Chae YS. Percutaneous endoscopic interlaminar discectomy for intracanalicular disc herniations at L5–S1 using a rigid working channel endoscope. *Neurosurgery* 2006;58

13 Lee SH, Kang HS. Percutaneous endoscopic laser annuloplasty for discogenic low back pain. *World Neurosurg* 2010;73(3):198–206

14 Schwarzer AC, Aprill CN, Derby R, Fortin J, Kine G, Bogduk N. The prevalence and clinical features of internal disc disruption in patients with chronic low back pain. *Spine* 1995;20(17):1878–1883

15 Guyer RD, Ohnmeiss DD. Lumbar discography. Position statement from the North American Spine Society Diagnostic and Therapeutic Committee. *Spine* 1995;20(18):2048–2059

16 Choi G, Lee SH, Deshpande K, Choi H. Working channel endoscope in lumbar spine surgery. *J Neurosurg Sci* 2014;58(2):77–85

7 Interlaminar Surgical Approach for Percutaneous Endoscopic Laser Annuloplasty/Nucleoplasty

Akarawit Asawasaksakul, Alfonso García, Ketan Deshpande, and Gun Choi

7.1 Introduction

Apart from the transforaminal approach for percutaneous endoscopic laser annuloplasty/nucleoplasty, currently the interlaminar approach is one of the most popular approaches for percutaneous decompression procedures. In 2006, Choi et al[1] first reported the successful endoscopic removal of an L5–S1 disk herniation using this approach. In 2008, Ruetten et al[2] compared endoscopic diskectomy with microdiskectomy and found comparable clinical results but less tissue trauma with the endoscopic technique. Recently, many authors have also reported the application of this approach and successful outcomes.[3,4,5,6]

7.2 Anatomical Considerations

Thorough knowledge of anatomy is an essential requirement in every surgical specialty.

- Endoscopic spine surgery is a target-oriented surgery that relies on a precise mental projection of a pathologic lesion and its relations to surrounding bony landmarks.
- Unlike in microsurgery, in endoscopic surgery the surgeon does not have the liberty of visually identifying the bony landmarks and then going through them to find the neurologic structures.
- The surgeon must know the relation of the various neural structures to the surrounding bone and must rely heavily on fluoroscopic guidance to insert the needle at the exact target point identified on the preoperative plan while avoiding all the important anatomical structures lying in between.
- Another important aspect of endoscopic spine surgery is familiarity with the endoscopic appearance of the various anatomical structures.

This chapter describes percutaneous interlaminar endoscopic diskectomy at the L5–S1 level in three sections:

- Discussion of the unique anatomical features of the L5–S1 segment that make it amenable to the interlaminar approach.
- Description of the methods used to project various important anatomical structures (as defined on CT and MRI) onto the radiographs and to make the preoperative plan.
- Description of the endoscopic appearances of various anatomical structures seen during the procedure so the reader can have a fair idea of what to expect before embarking upon the procedure.

The interlaminar approach applies not only to the L5–S1 level, but also to other levels.

7.3 Unique Features of the L5–S1 Anatomy

The L5–S1 level has unique anatomical features that apply to interlaminar endoscopic diskectomy:

- Most of the lumbar disks have a laminar overhang, meaning that the lamina of the upper vertebra extends inferiorly so that the disk space lies at a level relatively superior to the lower margin of the lamina. However, the laminar overhang over the disk space decreases from the upper lumbar to the lower lumbar levels. At the L5–S1 level, the cephalocaudal distance between the lower margin of the L5 lamina and the upper margin of the L5–S1 disk space varies from 3.0 to 8.5 mm. This is the smallest laminar overhang of the lumbar levels.
- The small laminar overhang at the L5–S1 level creates a relatively larger interlaminar space.
- The inferior margins of the upper lamina lie at a level relatively posterior to that of the superior margins of the lower lamina in the whole of the lumbar spine. This difference is seen more clearly at the L5–S1 level than at the other levels.
- In combination with a wider interlaminar space and a negligible laminar overhang, this arrangement creates a trapezoidal configuration that allows more working space for the outer cannula and its manipulation during the procedure, especially if the initial needle trajectory is kept at a 5 to 10° caudocranial angle.
- The maximum interlaminar width, as defined by the distance measured between the most inferomedial aspects of the inferior facets, is also greater at the L5–S1 space than at the upper levels (**Fig. 7.1**).
- The average interlaminar width at L5–S1 is 31 mm (range 21 to 40 mm), as compared to an average width of 23.5 mm at the L4–L5 level, due to the relatively wider laminae of L5.[7]
- The wider interlaminar width provides for easy passage of the working cannula (**Fig. 7.1**).
- The S1 nerve root has a relatively cephalad exit from the thecal sac compared with the upper lumbar levels. The S1 nerve root exits from the thecal sac at the level of the L5–S1 disk space or above it. In their cadaver analysis of the origin of lumbar spinal roots in relation to the intervertebral disk, Suh et al reported that the S1 nerve root originated above the level of the L5–S1 disc in 75% of the subjects and at the level of the disk in 25%, but never below the level of the disk.[8,9,10,11]

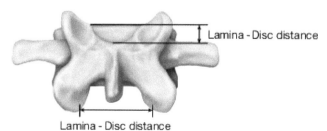

Posterior view

Lamina - Disc distance

Lamina - Disc distance

Fig. 7.1 Illustration of the maximum interlaminar width at the L5–S1 level.

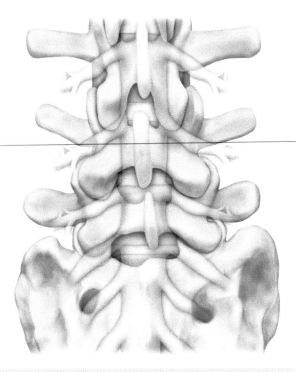

Fig. 7.2 Illustration of the S1 nerve root, which takes off at a relatively smaller angle from the thecal sac.

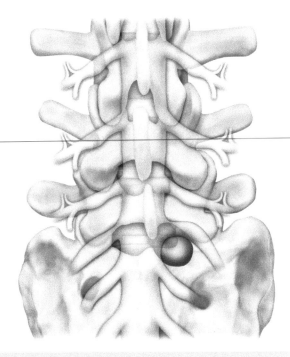

Fig. 7.3 Illustration of an axillary disk herniation, which can displace the S1 nerve root far into the subarticular region, creating a potential space between the thecal sac and the nerve root.

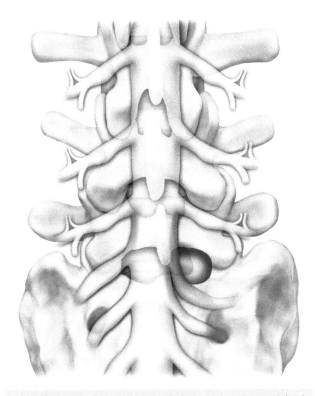

Fig. 7.4 Illustration of a shoulder disk herniation at the L5–S1 level, which pushes the S1 nerve root medially, toward the thecal sac.

- The S1 nerve root average take-off angle from the thecal sac is 17.9 ± 5.8 degrees. Although this angle is relatively less than that at the upper lumbar levels, an L5–S1 disk herniation is more likely to be axillary because of the cephalad exit of the S1 nerve root in front of the L5–S1 disk space (**Fig. 7.2**).[10,11]

- Axillary disk herniation can also displace the S1 nerve root far into the subarticular region, creating a potential space between the thecal sac and the nerve root. This artificial space created by the pathologic lesion can be gainfully exploited for carrying out a safe interlaminar endoscopic diskectomy (**Fig. 7.3**).

- Shoulder disk herniation at the L5–S1 level is relatively uncommon; in this case, the herniated disk pushes the S1 nerve root medially, toward the thecal sac, and the needle can be targeted directly over the hernia mass lying over the supermodel aspect of the pedicle (**Fig. 7.4**).

- The ligamentum flavum is a 2- to 6-mm thick, yellow structure that spans the interlaminar space. It is an active ligament that has an essential biomechanical role. It also acts as a protective barrier for the thecal sac, and any injury to it is probably not without consequences.[12]

- Peridural fibrosis is the direct consequence of intrusion into the spinal canal with a break in the ligamentum flavum because peridural fibrosis occurs due to fibroblasts derived from overlying detached muscle that have gained access to the spinal canal.[12,13,14]

- Although the ligamentum flavum is thinnest at the L5–S1 level, it is the only major protective barrier for the neural structures at this level because of the minimal laminar overhang. Therefore, preservation of the integrity and continuity of the ligamentum flavum at the L5–S1 level is most important.

- During L5–S1 percutaneous interlaminar endoscopic diskectomy, splitting the fibers of the ligamentum flavum longitudinally and then widening the hole by the passage of sequential

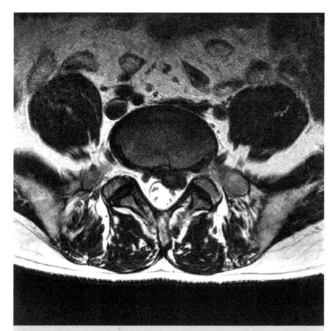

Fig. 7.5 Sagittal T2-weighted MRI showing slight downward migration of the herniated L5–S1 disc.

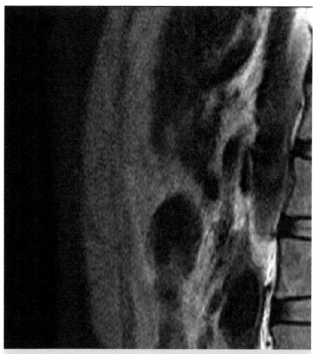

Fig. 7.6 Axial T2-weighted MRI showing sequestrated herniation of the L5–S1 disk at the left side.

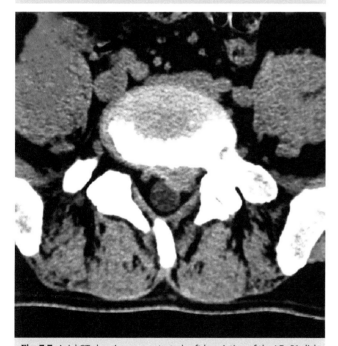

Fig. 7.7 Axial CT showing sequestrated soft herniation of the L5–S1 disk at the left side.

dilators creates an opening. Upon withdrawal of the working cannula and endoscope, the opening in the ligamentum flavum closes spontaneously and restores the continuity of the protective barrier.

- As the S1 nerve root exits the thecal sac at the level of the L5–S1 disk space and lies directly opposite the disk, the initial needle target is identified inferior to the disk space in the axilla of the S1 root. This anatomy helps to avoid any damage to the S1 nerve root by the advancing needle.
- Once the needle tip is located at the level of the superior end plate of the S1 vertebra in the lateral C-arm view, the

guidewire is passed. Then, passing sequential dilators over the guidewire creates the working space. These steps help to push the S1 nerve root further away from the working area and to protect it.

7.4 Preoperative Planning

The correlation of various anatomical structures and the pathologic lesion as identified by CT and MRI scans and their projection on the X-rays are vital to preoperative planning (**Fig. 7.5**).

- On sagittal MRI, the extent of downward or upward migration of the herniated disk is noted (**Fig. 7.5**, **Fig. 7.6**, **Fig. 7.7**).
- On axial MRI and CT, the location of the herniated disk and its relation to the nerve root, along with any deviation of the concerned nerve root and indentation of the thecal sac by the herniated disk, are identified.
- Axial CT is also used to calculate the site of the skin entry point with reference to the medial pedicular line and the midspinal line (**Fig. 7.8**).
- Next, all of these findings are projected onto anteroposterior (AP) X-rays to create the preoperative plan that will guide the surgeon during the procedure.
  - First, the pedicles of the L5 and S1 vertebrae are identified and marked on the X-ray film.
  - Next, imaginary lines are drawn to represent the thecal sac and the exit of various nerve roots from it, along with their relation to the surrounding bony landmarks. From the CT and MRI findings, the displaced S1 nerve root, along with the thecal sac that has been indented by the herniated disk fragment, can be drawn (**Fig. 7.9**). The intended target point for initial needle positioning can also be drawn.

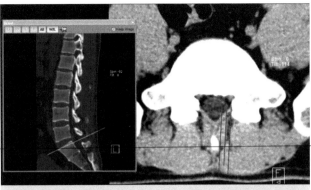

Fig. 7.8 Topogram on the left shows the level of the axial image (at the level of the superior end plate of S1) to be used for preoperative planning.

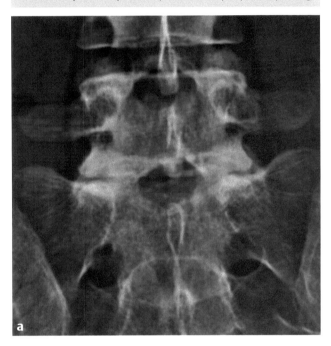

a

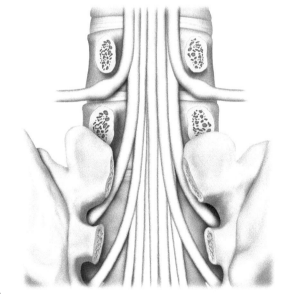

b

Fig. 7.9 (a,b) Imaginary lines of the root drawn using closed axial CT or MRI.

○ It is not always easy to identify the S1 nerve root on CT or MRI, but attempts must be made to see and imagine the root by using closed axial CT or MRI slices (**Fig. 7.9**).

7.5 Identification of Anatomical Structures on the Endoscopic View

There are two methods for gaining entry into the epidural space:

7.5.1 First Method

- In the first method, which is considered safer than the second, the needle tip is advanced to penetrate the ligamentum flavum, and then serial dilators are inserted over the guidewire to create a working path.

- At this stage, the circular-tip working cannula is introduced, and its tip is anchored over the spinolaminar junction and the position is confirmed with lateral C-arm fluoroscopy (**Fig. 7.10a**). The working channel endoscope is introduced, and the ligamentum flavum is identified by its pale yellow fibrils running vertically, in a cephalocaudal direction.

- The ligamentum flavum is a two-layered structure consisting of a superficial posterior layer and a deep anterior layer. The two layers of the ligamentum flavum can be split longitudinally with the help of a blunt dissecting probe to gain entry into the epidural space (**Fig. 7.10b**).

- If the ligamentum flavum is thick, an endoscopic scissor can also be used to cut it, but this will create a postoperative defect.

- After the fibers of the ligamentum flavum are split, the working cannula, along with the endoscope, is advanced further anteriorly. The next structure to be visualized is usually the epidural fat, which can be identified as small, shiny yellow globules interspersed with small-caliber blood vessels, giving it a reddish tint (**Fig. 7.11**).

- After coagulation of the vessels and of the epidural fat with the help of a bipolar radiofrequency probe, the working cannula is advanced further, and the next structure to be seen could be neural tissue, blue-stained herniated disk tissue, or the posterior longitudinal ligament (PLL), depending on the nature of the pathology. Most commonly, either the herniated disk tissue stained blue by indigo carmine injected for diskography or the PLL is visualized first, along with some anterior epidural fat tissue (**Fig. 7.12**).

- If neural tissue is seen first, it means there is still little working space available.

- In such a case, the guidewire is introduced again under endoscopic vision, avoiding any damage to the surrounding neural tissue.

- The tip of the guidewire is advanced up to the posterior surface of the S1 vertebral body just below the superior end plate of the S1 vertebra. Now the endoscope is withdrawn, and a working space is created in the epidural space by the insertion of sequential dilators over the guidewire.

- Then the working cannula is changed to a beveled tip. The beveled-tip cannula can confer an advantage in guarding nerve root by rotating the bevel under endoscopic view. This

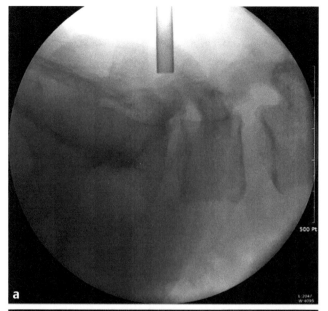

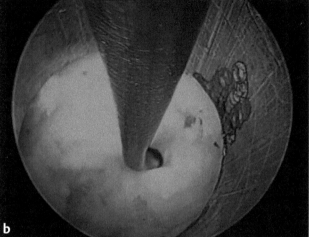

Fig. 7.10 (a) Fluoroscopic view of the circular-tip working cannula anchored at the dorsal cortex of the L5 lamina. **(b)** Endoscopic view of the two layers of the ligamentum flavum that can be split longitudinally with the help of a blunt dissecting probe to gain entry into the epidural space.

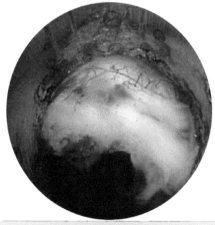

Fig. 7.13 Endoscopic view of part of the posterior longitudinal ligament, which can take up the blue color of indigo carmine.

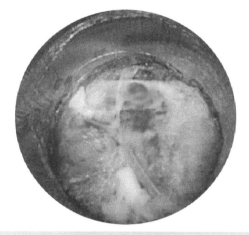

Fig. 7.11 Endoscopic view after splitting of the fibers of the ligamentum flavum shows the epidural fat, which can be identified by its small, shiny yellow globules interspersed with small-caliber blood vessels coursing through it, giving it a reddish tint.

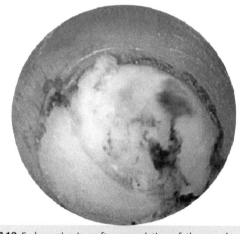

Fig. 7.12 Endoscopic view after coagulation of the vessels and the epidural fat. The working cannula is advanced further, and the next structure to be seen could be neural tissue, blue-stained herniated disk tissue, or the posterior longitudinal ligament.

helps to gradually push away the S1 nerve root and widen the axillary or shoulder space.

- On introduction of the endoscope at this stage, usually the blue-stained herniated disk tissue, along with some epidural fat, can be visualized (**Fig. 7.12**).
- After removal of the extruded herniated disk tissue, one can visualize the remnants of the PLL, which can be identified by the presence of an arcade of multiple small-caliber vessels coursing irregularly along its shiny white surface.
- Some part of the PLL can also take up the blue color of indigo carmine due to the long-standing presence of very small nuclear fragments inside it (**Fig. 7.13**).

7.5.2 Second Method

- For the second method, if the herniation is large enough to push the traversing root medially or laterally on the MRI, we can directly insert the needle into the herniated disk.
- At this point, after the working channel is established and the scope is inserted, the blue-stained disk is easily seen.

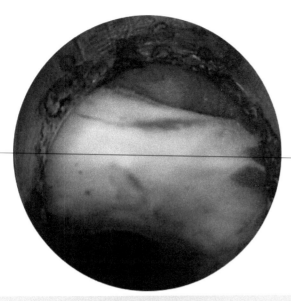

Fig. 7.14 Endoscopic view of the nerve root and dura, which are pinkish and usually have one or two blood vessels coursing longitudinally along their posterior surface with minimal branching.

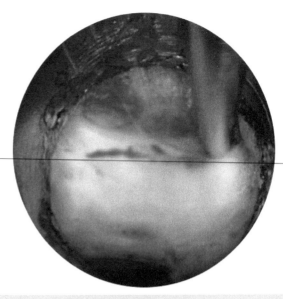

Fig. 7.15 Endoscopic view of the S1 nerve root, which can be seen as fully decompressed. The adequacy of decompression can be verified by palpating with a probe along the shoulder region.

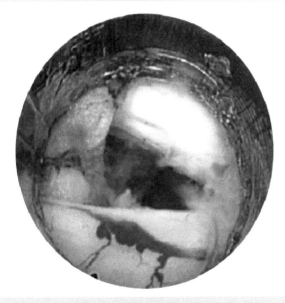

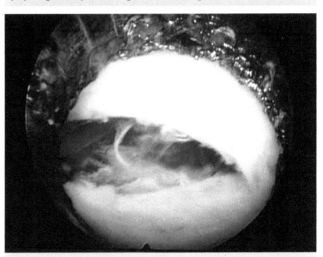

Fig. 7.17 Endoscopic view of the free course of the S1 nerve root and thecal sac.

Fig. 7.16 Endoscopic view of the S1 nerve root, which can be seen coursing from the 11 to the 3 o'clock position. The thecal sac is seen coursing from the 4 to the 7 o'clock position. The black hole in the center represents the hollow space left after removal of the herniated fragment. (The 9 o'clock position is caudal and 3 o'clock is cephalic; the 12 o'clock position is lateral and 6 o'clock is medial.)

- Sometimes it is difficult to differentiate the PLL from the neural tissue, especially at the level of the vertebral body, because it has vertically running superficial fibers that are not very strongly attached to the underlying bone, thus making them relatively mobile.[15]
- However, the two structures can be differentiated by the presence of several small-caliber vessels over the white surface of the PLL, whereas the nerve root and dura are pinkish and usually have one or two blood vessels coursing longitudinally along their posterior surface with minimal branching (**Fig. 7.14**).

- After removal of the herniated disk tissue, the S1 nerve root can be seen as fully decompressed, and the adequacy of decompression can be verified by palpating with a probe along the shoulder region (**Fig. 7.15**).
- The endoscope and the working cannula are gradually withdrawn by making gentle, circular, twisting motions, and the thecal sac and the S1 nerve root can be visualized.
- The adequacy of decompression is further confirmed by the free course of the S1 nerve root (**Fig. 7.16**).

After confirming the free course of the S1 nerve root and thecal sac, the endoscope and the working cannula are withdrawn further, and the opening created in the ligamentum flavum can be seen to close spontaneously (**Fig. 7.17**, **Fig. 7.18**).

- On further withdrawal of the cannula, the working path created through the muscle fibers by serial dilatation can be seen to close spontaneously without creating any dead space (**Fig. 7.19**).

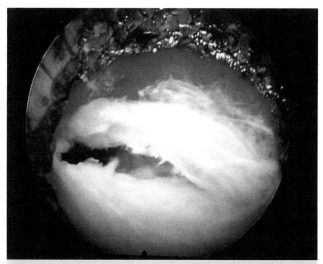

Fig. 7.18 The endoscope and the working cannula are withdrawn further, and the opening created in the ligamentum flavum can be seen to close spontaneously.

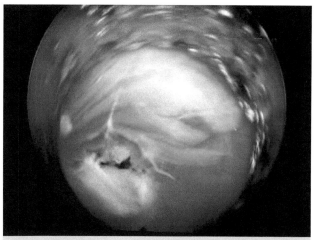

Fig. 7.19 Upon further withdrawal of the cannula, the working path created through the muscle fibers by serial dilatation closes spontaneously without creating any dead space.

- In the second method, the spinal needle tip is initially positioned over the posterior surface of the S1 vertebral body just below its lateral C-arm view.

- In such cases, the first structure to be visualized upon insertion of the endoscope should be either the epidural fat, along with the small-caliber blood vessels coursing through it (**Fig. 7.11**), or the herniated disk tissue, which will appear blue because of the earlier injection of indigo carmine into the disk (**Fig. 7.12**). The other structures are identified as described for the first method.

7.6 Conclusion

For procedures at the L5–S1 level, the interlaminar technique is very useful in both normal patients and patients with a high iliac crest. Compared with the transiliac technique, the interlaminar technique makes it easier to obtain a good exposure of the fragments. Communication with the patient before and during the operation is very important, since during rotation of the working cannula, the patient will have radiating pain from stretching of the nerve root, and thus periannular infiltration or conversion to general anesthesia may be considered.

References

1   Choi G, Lee SH, Raiturker PP, Lee S, Chae YS. Percutaneous endoscopic interlaminar discectomy for intracanalicular disc herniations at L5–S1 using a rigid working channel endoscope. *Neurosurgery* 2006;*58*

2   Ruetten S, Komp M, Merk H, Godolias G. Full-endoscopic interlaminar and transforaminal lumbar discectomy versus conventional microsurgical technique: a prospective, randomized, controlled study. *Spine* 2008;*33*(9):931–939

3   Choi G, Prada N, Modi HN, Vasavada NB, Kim JS, Lee SH. Percutaneous endoscopic lumbar herniectomy for high-grade down-migrated L4–L5 disc through an L5–S1 interlaminar approach: a technical note. *Minim Invasive Neurosurg* 2010;*53*(3):147–152

4   Dezawa A, Sairyo K. New minimally invasive discectomy technique through the interlaminar space using a percutaneous endoscope. *Asian J Endosc Surg* 2011;*4*(2):94–98

5   Sencer A, Yorukoglu AG, Akcakaya MO, et al. Fully endoscopic interlaminar and transforaminal lumbar discectomy: short-term clinical results of 163 surgically treated patients. *World Neurosurg* 2014;*82*(5):884–890

6   Ahn Y. Percutaneous endoscopic decompression for lumbar spinal stenosis. *Expert Rev Med Devices* 2014;*11*(6):605–616

7   Ebraheim NA, Miller RM, Xu R, Yeasting RA. The location of the intervertebral lumbar disc on the posterior aspect of the spine. *Surg Neurol* 1997;*48*(3):232–236

8   Hasegawa T, Mikawa Y, Watanabe R, An HS. Morphometric analysis of the lumbosacral nerve roots and dorsal root ganglia by magnetic resonance imaging. *Spine* 1996;*21*(9):1005–1009

9   Cohen MS, Wall EJ, Brown RA, Rydevik B, Garfin SR. 1990 AcroMed Award in basic science. Cauda equina anatomy. II: Extrathecal nerve roots and dorsal root ganglia. *Spine* 1990;*15*(12):1248–1251

10 McCulloch JA, Young PH. Musculoskeletal and neuroanatomy of the lumbar spine. In: McCulloch JA, Young PH, eds. *Essentials of Spinal Microsurgery*. Philadelphia, PA: Lippincott-Raven; 1998:249–292

11 Suh SW, Shingade VU, Lee SH, Bae JH, Park CE, Song JY. Origin of lumbar spinal roots and their relationship to intervertebral discs: a cadaver and radiological study. *J Bone Joint Surg Br* 2005;*87*(4):518–522

12 Askar Z, Wardlaw D, Choudhary S, Rege A. A ligamentum flavum-preserving approach to the lumbar spinal canal. *Spine* 2003;*28*(19):E385–E390

13 Aydin Y, Ziyal IM, Duman H, Türkmen CS, Başak M, Sahin Y. Clinical and radiological results of lumbar microdiskectomy technique with preserving of ligamentum flavum comparing to the standard microdiskectomy technique. *Surg Neurol* 2002;*57*(1):5–13

14 Boeree N. The reduction of peridural fibrosis. In: Gunzburg R, ed. *Lumbar Disc Herniation*. Philadelphia, PA: Lippincott Williams & Wilkins; 2002:185–196

15 Loughenbury PR, Wadhwani S, Soames RW. The posterior longitudinal ligament and peridural (epidural) membrane. *Clin Anat* 2006;*19*(6):487–492

8 Percutaneous Endoscopic Interlaminar Lumbar Diskectomy: Structural Preservation Technique for L5–S1 Herniated Nucleus Pulposus

Hyeun Sung Kim, Ji Soo Jang, Il Tae Jang, Sung Hoon Oh, and Chang Il Ju

8.1 Introduction

Microscopic lumbar diskectomy has been the standard operation in lumbar disk surgery for herniated nucleus pulposus (HNP), but recently, percutaneous endoscopic lumbar diskectomy (PELD) has developed significantly.[1,2,3,4,5] PELD can be classified into transforaminal PELD (PETLD)[1,6,7,8,9,10,11,12,13,14,15] and interlaminar PELD (PEILD)[1,16,17,18,19,20,21] according to the approach. Each method has its own advantages and disadvantages. The indications and anatomical and surgical tips for the two kinds of PELD are discussed in this chapter.[6,17,18,19,20,21,31]

8.2 Anatomical Considerations

8.2.1 Classification

See **Table 8.1**, **Table 8.2**, and **Fig. 8.1**.

8.2.2 Anatomical Limitations of PETLD and Rationale for PEILD

The condition of the foramen and the iliac crest should be checked before using the transforaminal approach, because in cases associated with a narrow foramen, a shallow suprapedicular area, or a high iliac crest, it will be difficult to approach the target point (**Fig. 8.2**).[22,23,24,25] The rationale for PEILD in L5–S1 HNP is shown in **Fig. 8.3**. Anatomical features of the interlaminar space are shown in **Fig. 8.4**.

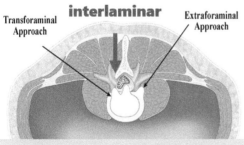

Fig. 8.1 Classification of percutaneous endoscopic lumbar diskectomy.

Table 8.1 Advantages and disadvantages of PELD procedures for L5–S1 HNP

	Posterolateral	Interlaminar
Approach	Transforaminal	Trans-shoulder
	Transiliac	Trans-axilla
Ligamentum flavum	Spare	Resection or Spare
Annulus repair	Impossible	Possible
Indications	Limited	Wide
Adhesion	Weak	Weak or Strong

Table 8.2 Advantages and disadvantages of two different percutaneous interlaminar approaches

	Shoulder Approach	Axilla Approach
Learning curve	Short	Moderate
Downward migration	Difficult	Easy
Upward migration	Easy	Difficult
Nerve root retraction	Hard	Weak
Annulus sealing	Difficult	Easy

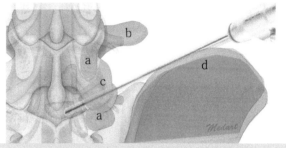

Fig. 8.2 Anatomical limitations of percutaneous endoscopic transforaminal lumbar diskectomy of L5–S1 HNP. a: pedicle; b: transverse process; c: facet joint; d: iliac crest.

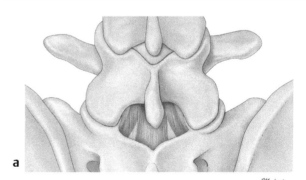

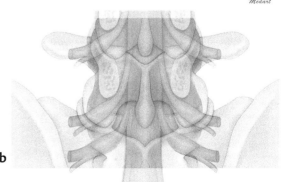

Fig. 8.3 General anatomy of the interlaminar space. (**a**) The L5–S1 level has a wide interlaminar and shoulder space. (**b**) The axillary area is located more cranially than the upper level.

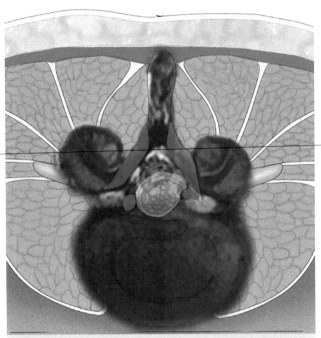

Fig. 8.4 Anatomical features of the interlaminar space. a: facet joint; b: ligamentum flavum; c: dura; d: nerve root; e: herniated nucleus pulposus.

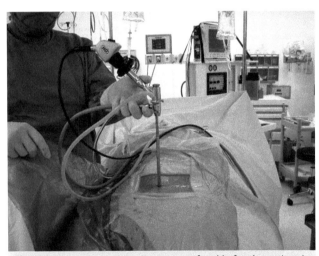

Fig. 8.6 The prone position is more comfortable for the patient in percutaneous endoscopic lumbar diskectomy work.

8.3 Indications and Applications

Recently, the techniques and devices used in PELD have developed significantly. Therefore, nearly all kinds of lumbar disk disease can be treated using PELD, but PELD is not easy to perform due to the steep learning curve, especially in difficult and complicated cases.

PEILD requires a wide interlaminar space. PEILD is especially indicated at the L5–S1 level.

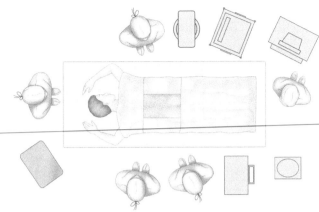

Fig. 8.5 Standard operating room set-up. A: surgeon; B: nurse; C: anesthetist; D: X-ray technician; E: technician; F: instrument table; G: C-arm X-ray; H: video equipment; J: image processing; K: suction irrigation equipment.

8.4 Surgical Procedures

8.4.1 Operating Room Setup

Fig. 8.5 shows the standard set-up for the operating room, including the positions of the surgeon, nurse, and instrument table, as well as the positions of the X-ray machine and the video and image-processing equipment.

8.4.2 Anesthesia

For the interlaminar approach, an epidural block or general anesthesia is an appropriate choice, because the nerve roots are directly retracted, which causes severe pain. General anesthesia reduces the patient's anxiety and intraoperative pain, but it lacks the benefit of neural monitoring.

8.4.3 Positioning and Skin Marking

The patient is placed in the prone position for PELD (**Fig. 8.6**). Planning the entry point of the working channel is important in PEILD for successful disk removal and for avoiding structural damage, including neural damage (**Video 8.1**).

The entry point for PEILD is the "V" point:

- The V point is the intersection of the ligamentum flavum, inferior articular process, and superior articular process.
- Approximately 1 cm from midline of spinous process
- The deepest portion lies between the ligamentum flavum and lamina.
- Most lateral part of ligamentum flavum
- The beveled-tip working channel can tightly insert into the V point (**Fig. 8.7**).

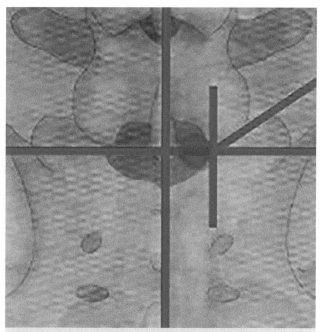

Fig. 8.7 V point (pink spot): the intersection of the ligamentum flavum, inferior articular process, and superior articular process.

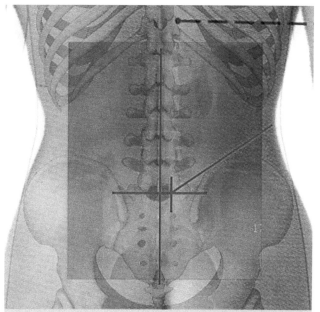

Fig. 8.8 Illustration of percutaneous endoscopic interlaminar lumbar diskectomy. a, spinal column midline; b, transverse line on the widest part of the interspinous space; c, V point; d, indigo carmine insertion line into Kambin's transforaminal triangle.

with the safe bony structures of the superior articular process, the needle is repositioned in Kambin's triangle (**Fig. 8.8**, **Fig. 8.9**).

After guide needle insertion, indigo carmine dye is injected into the disk space to identify the degenerated or pathologic disk (**Video 8.2**).

8.4.5 Skin Incision and Working Channel Insertion

After injection of indigo carmine into the operative area, a skin incision is made at the point estimated preoperatively. After skin incision, subdermal fascia should be dissected to allow insertion of the working channel. Then the obturator is inserted into the target point. The working channel is inserted through the obturator. After optimal positioning of the working channel on the target point, the percutaneous endoscope is inserted into the working channel. Insertion of a round-tip working channel is shown in **Fig. 8.10**, and insertion of a beveled-tip working channel is shown in **Fig. 8.11**. The anatomical approach point for PEILD is shown in **Fig. 8.12** (**Video 8.3a,b**).

8.4.6 Ligamentum Flavum Approach

Ligamentum Flavum Resection Technique[19]
- Cut the ligamentum flavum using the punch.
- The procedure is similar to conventional microscopic lumbar diskectomy.
- This technique is especially indicated in the shoulder approach.

Indirect Ligamentum Flavum Splitting Technique[18,26]
- Insert the 18 G needle into the axilla.
- Check the free axilla area after the dye injection.

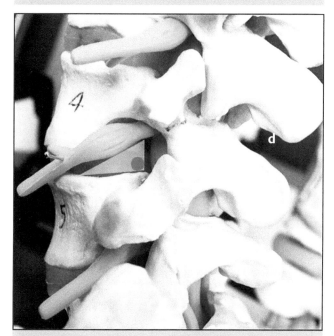

Fig. 8.9 An 18 G needle is inserted into Kambin's triangle. Needle insertion into the orange circled area provides the best targeting.

8.4.4 Evocative Chromodiskography: Transforaminal Approach

To achieve good results with targeted fragmentectomy, evocative chromodiskography can be performed to assess the degenerated or pathologic disk using indigo carmine dye. Fluoroscopic imaging is used to determine the placement of the needle tip, and the needle tip is advanced toward the more caudal and dorsal part of Kambin's triangle. To reduce the occurrence of neural injury, the needle should be positioned on the ventral part of the facet joint (superior articular process) in the first step. After making contact

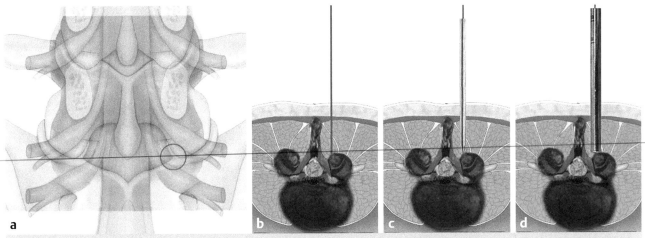

Fig. 8.10 Insertion of the round working channel. The round working channel is more familiar and safe; however, it requires more muscle work, and sometimes it is difficult to find the target point on the ligamentum flavum. (**a**) Target point for the round working channel. (**b**) The first step is insertion of the guide needle on the bony structures near the V point. (**c**) The second step is insertion of the obturator through the guide needle. (**d**) The third step is insertion of the round working channel through the obturator.

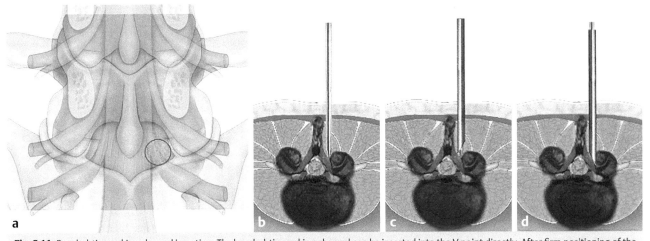

Fig. 8.11 Beveled-tip working channel insertion. The beveled-tip working channel can be inserted into the V point directly. After firm positioning of the beveled working channel in the V point, muscle work can decrease more sufficiently and the exposure of ligamentum flavum is also easier. (**a**) Target point of the beveled working channel. (**b**) The first step is insertion of the obturator into the V point. (**c**) The second step is insertion of the beveled working channel using the counter side beveled to avoid the bony obstacle of beveled working channel insertion. (**d**) The third step is rotational insertion of the beveled working channel toward the V point after contact with the ligamentum flavum.

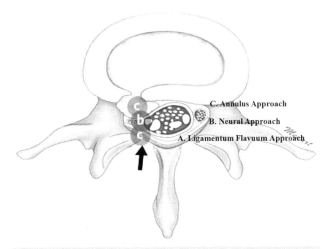

Fig. 8.12 Three anatomical approach points for percutaneous endoscopic interlaminar lumbar diskectomy: a, ligamentum flavum; b, neural structures; c, annulus pulposus.

- Insert the needle into the free axilla area and change to a guidewire.
- Insert the working channel, following the guidewire through the ligamentum flavum.

Direct Ligamentum Flavum Splitting Technique[17,30,31]

- A clear surgical view can be secured by splitting the ligamentum flavum with the probe or other surgical instruments to insert the working channel into the pathologic area.
- Place the working channel in contact with the ligamentum flavum.
- Split the ligamentum flavum using the probe.
- Introduce the working channel through the split ligament.
- Preserve the anatomical structures, especially the ligamentum flavum and facet joint (**Fig. 8.13**, **Fig. 8.14**, **Fig. 8.15**, **Video 8.4**).

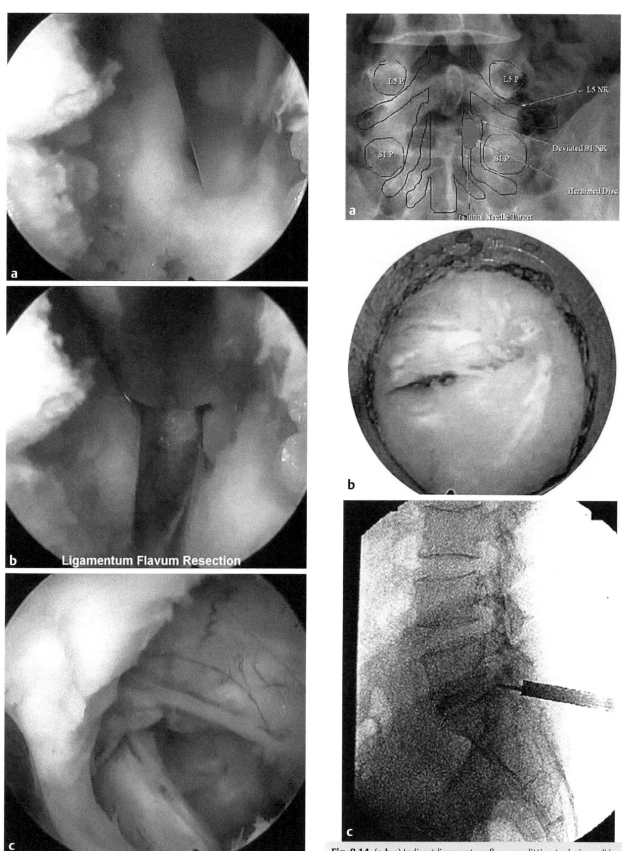

Fig. 8.13 Ligamentum flavum resection technique. (**a**) Splitting of the ligamentum flavum using the probe. (**b**) Resection of the ligamentum flavum close to the target point using the punch. (**c**) Exposure of the target point after resection of the ligamentum flavum.

Fig. 8.14 (**a,b,c**) Indirect ligamentum flavum splitting technique. (Used with permission from Choi G, Lee SH, Raiturker PP, Lee S, Chae YS. Percutaneous endoscopic interlaminar diskectomy for intracanalicular disc herniations at L5–S1 using a rigid working channel endoscope. *Neurosurgery*. 2006 Feb;58(1 Suppl):59–68.)

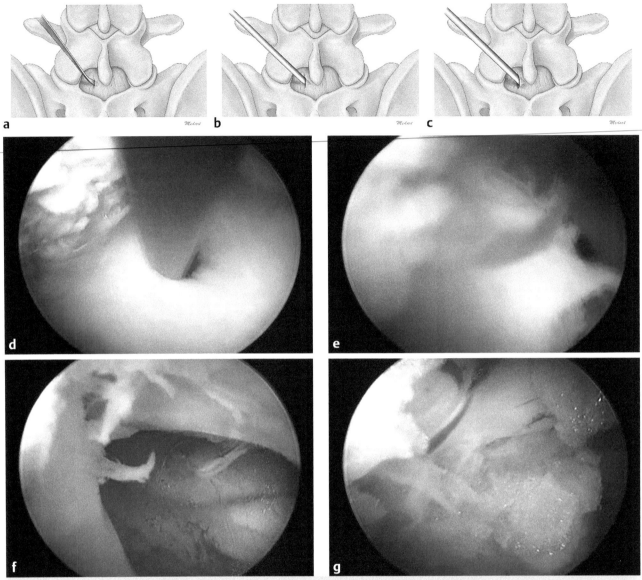

Fig. 8.15 Direct ligamentum flavum splitting technique. **(a,b,c)** Anatomical sequence of the direct ligamentum flavum splitting technique. **(d,e,f,g)** Video sequence of the direct ligamentum flavum splitting technique: splitting of the ligamentum flavum using the probe, insertion of the beveled working channel into the split ligament, and rotational insertion of the beveled working channel into the target point. (Used with permission from Kim CH, Chung CK. Endoscopic interlaminar lumbar diskectomy with splitting of the ligament flavum under visual control. *J Spinal Disord Tech*. June 2012;25(4):210–217.)

8.4.7 Neural Approach

Shoulder Approach[19,30]

- Approach between the laminar and shoulder area of the S1 nerve root.
- The approach is familiar, because it is similar to the conventional approach.
- Advantages: Useful for upward-migrated HNP.
- Disadvantages: In extreme cases of downward migration or central location, it can be difficult to use the shoulder approach.

Axilla Approach[17,18,27,28,29,30]

- Approach between the S1 nerve root and dura.
- Has a learning curve.

- Advantages: Useful for downward-migrated HNP.
- Disadvantages: Difficult with upward-migrated HNP.

See **Fig. 8.16**.

8.4.8 Annulus Approach: Decompression/Diskectomy

Annulus Resection Approach (Fig. 8.17)

- Resect the annulus around the protruded area to expose the pathologic disk.
- The approach is familiar, because it is similar to the conventional approach.
- Use of this approach is associated with a high risk of recurrence.

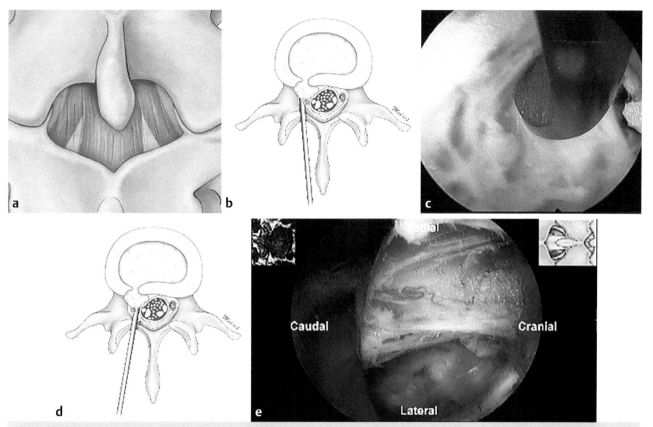

Fig. 8.16 Rigid percutaneous endoscopic interlaminar lumbar approach for nerve root retraction. (**a,b,c**) Shoulder approach. (**d,e**) Axilla approach. (Used with permission from Choi G, Lee SH, Raiturker PP, Lee S, Chae YS. Percutaneous endoscopic interlaminar diskectomy for intracanalicular disc herniations at L5–S1 using a rigid working channel endoscope. *Neurosurgery*. 2006 Feb;58(1 Suppl):59–68.)

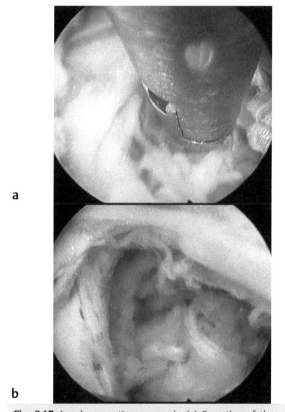

Fig. 8.17 Annulus resection approach. (**a**) Resection of the annulus using the punch or forceps. (**b**) Appearance after resection of the annulus.

Fissure Fragmentectomy and Annular Sealing Technique[19]

- Make a fissure with a punch or a probe; the probe is preferred because it is less likely to cause an injury to the annulus.
- Sometimes, in cases with a huge ruptured disk, a fissure is already formed. Thus, it is preferable to try to find an existing fissure instead of creating a new one.
- Always attempt to perform the diskectomy through the fissure unless it is impossible. Remove the pathologic disk sufficiently to make certain that there is no disk remnant left.
- If the bulging annulus is swept with the radiofrequency probe from the distal to the proximal end of the fissure, the size of the bulging disk decreases, as does the size of the fissure.
- As the final step, perform coagulation around the fissure and make certain it is sealed tight (**Fig. 8.18**, **Fig. 8.19**, **Fig. 8.20**).

8.5 Structural Preservation

Surgical procedures for structural preservation PEILD include:
- Ligamentum flavum splitting technique combined with the annular sealing technique.
- Sufficient annular sealing around the fissure using radiofrequency coagulation.

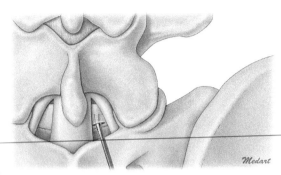

a

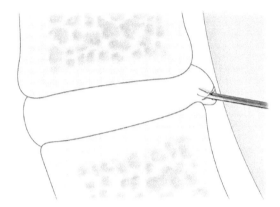

b

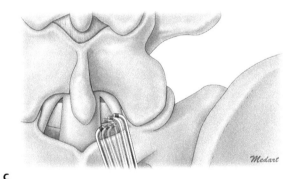

c

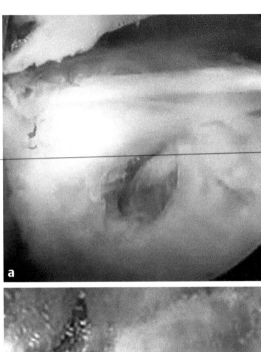

a

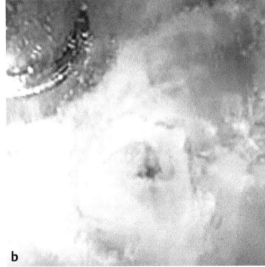

b

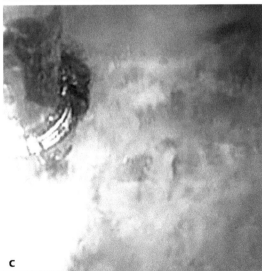

c

Fig. 8.18 Fissure fragmentectomy and annular sealing technique. (**a,b**) Fissure fragmentectomy. (**c**) Annular sealing technique. (Used with permission from Kim HS, Park JY. Comparative assessment of different percutaneous endoscopic interlaminar lumbar diskectomy (PEID) techniques. *Pain Physician* 2013;16(4):359–367.)

Benefits of structural preservation PEILD are:
- Anatomical structures, especially the ligamentum flavum, facet joint, and annulus, are preserved.
- The weakened annulus pulposus is strengthened.
- Early relapse is reduced after annular sealing.
- Postoperative adhesions are reduced.
- See **Fig. 8.21** and **Fig. 8.22** (**Video 8.5 and Video 8.6**).

Fig. 8.19 Video sequence of the annular sealing technique. (**a**) Fissure construction for pathologic disk removal. (**b**) Annular sealing should be performed from outside to inside. (**c**) Appearance after annular sealing technique. (Used with permission from Kim HS, Park JY. Comparative assessment of different percutaneous endoscopic interlaminar lumbar diskectomy (PEID) techniques. *Pain Physician* 2013;16(4): 359–367.)

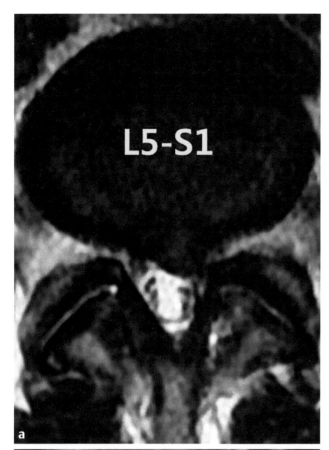

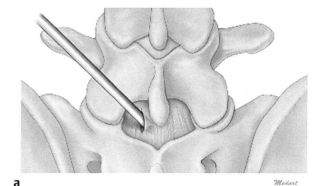

a

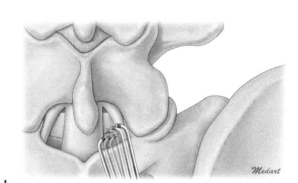

b

Fig. 8.21 Structural preservation percutaneous endoscopic interlaminar lumbar diskectomy for L5–S1 HNP using the combination of (**a**) ligamentum flavum splitting technique and (**b**) annular sealing technique.

8.6 Advancements in Percutaneous Endoscopic Interlaminar Lumbar Diskectomy

8.6.1 Structural Preservation PEILD for Severe Canal Compromise with L5–S1 HNP (Fig. 8.23)

- Carefully split the ligamentum flavum.
- The axilla approach is beneficial for severe canal compromise with L5–S1 HNP.
- Check the contralateral side between the protruded annulus and the ventral part of the dura (**Video 8.7, Video 8.8, and Video 8.9**).

8.6.2 Structural Preservation PEILD for High-Grade Downward-Migrated L5–S1 HNP (Fig. 8.24)

- The axilla approach is beneficial with PEILD for a downward-migrated disk.
- Split the inferior part of the ligamentum flavum.
- Check the inferior area sufficiently.
- Manipulation of the working channel toward the inferior area is sometimes blocked by the superior part of the S1 lamina. It may require percutaneous endoscopic drilling.

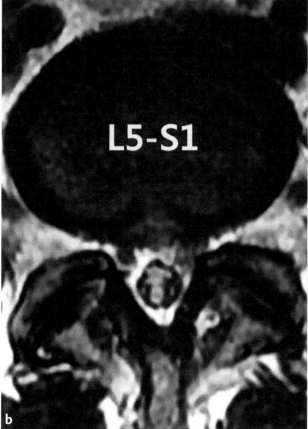

Fig. 8.20 MRI of annular sealing technique. (**a**) Preoperative image. (**b**) Postoperative image.

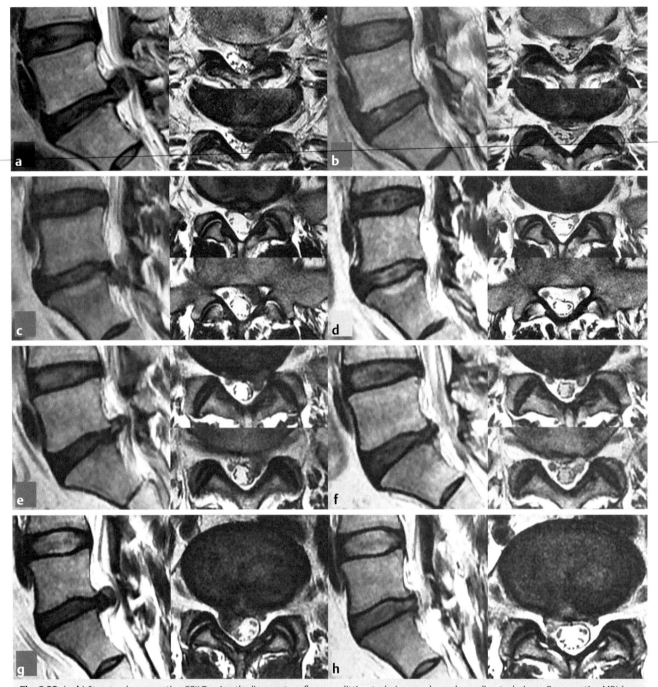

Fig. 8.22 (a–h) Structural preservation PEILD using the ligamentum flavum splitting technique and annular sealing technique. Preoperative MRI (**a, c, e, g**). Postoperative MRI (**b, d, f, h**) checked immediately after the operation.

8.6.3 Structural Preservation PEILD for Upward-Migrated L5–S1 HNP (Fig. 8.25)

- The shoulder approach is beneficial with PEILD for an upward-migrated disk.
- Split the superior part of the ligamentum flavum.
- Check the superior area sufficiently.
- Manipulation of the working channel toward the superior area is sometimes blocked by the inferior part of the L5 lamina. It may require percutaneous endoscopic drilling (**Video 8.10**).

8.6.4 Structural Preservation PEILD for Foraminal to Upward-Migrated L5–S1 HNP: Contralateral PEILD (Fig. 8.26)

- The contralateral interlaminar approach is applicable when an ipsilateral transforaminal or interlaminar approach is not easy due to the anatomical limitation posed by the iliac crest, facet joint, and L5 lamina.

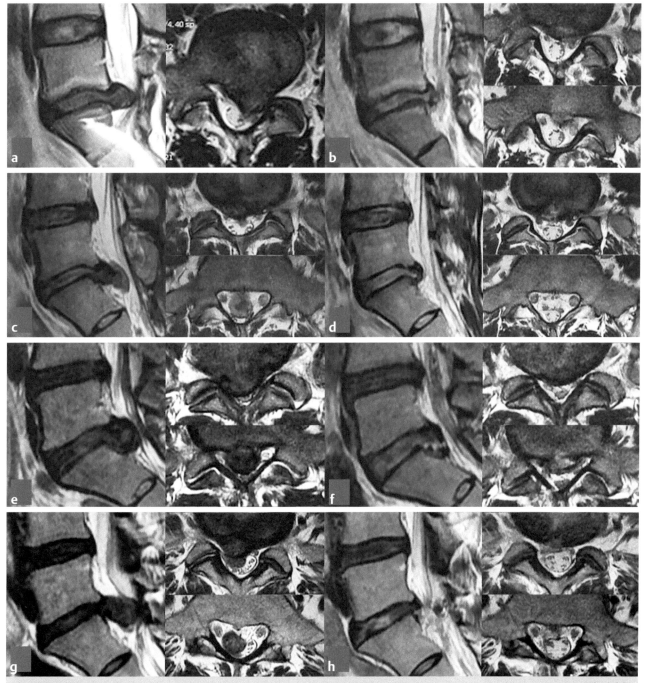

Fig. 8.23 (a–h) Structural preservation PEILD for severe canal compromise with L5–S1 HNP. Preoperative MRI (**a, c, e, g**). Postoperative MRI (**b, d, f, h**) checked immediately after the operation.

- The contralateral interlaminar approach provides sufficient access from the foraminal to the superior part of the L5–S1 level.
- The shoulder approach is beneficial with contralateral PEILD for a foraminal to upward-migrated disk.
- The superior part of the ligamentum flavum is split.
- Check the foraminal to superior area sufficiently.
- Manipulation of the working channel toward the foraminal to superior area is sometimes blocked by the inferior part of the L5 lamina and superior articular process of S1. It may require percutaneous endoscopic drilling (**Fig. 8.27**, **Video 8.11**).

8.6.5 Structural Preservation Revision PEILD for Recurrent HNP after Open Lumbar Diskectomy (Fig. 8.28, Fig. 8.29)

- First, find the bony structures close to the adherent tissue.
- Find the safe route close to the preserved laminae.
- Dissect the adherent tissue from the bony structures using the probe.
- The procedure incurs a risk of dural tear or root injury (**Video 8.12**).

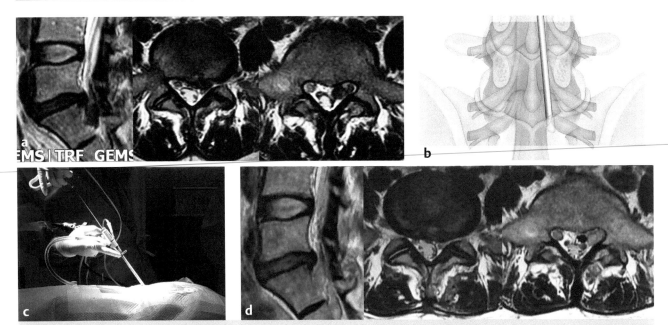

Fig. 8.24 Structural preservation PEILD for high-grade downward-migrated L5–S1 HNP. Axilla approach provides easier access to the downward-migrated disk. (**a**) Preoperative MRI. (**b**) High-grade downward-migrated L5–S1 HNP in the axilla. (**c**) Manipulation of the working channel toward the inferior area. (**d**) Postoperative MRI checked immediately after the operation.

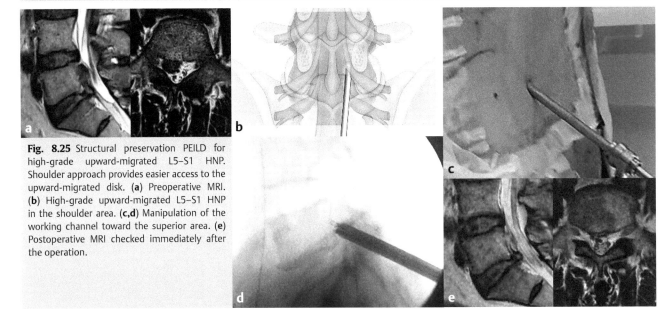

Fig. 8.25 Structural preservation PEILD for high-grade upward-migrated L5–S1 HNP. Shoulder approach provides easier access to the upward-migrated disk. (**a**) Preoperative MRI. (**b**) High-grade upward-migrated L5–S1 HNP in the shoulder area. (**c,d**) Manipulation of the working channel toward the superior area. (**e**) Postoperative MRI checked immediately after the operation.

8.6.6 Structural Preservation Revision PEILD after a Previous Structural Preservation PEILD (Fig. 8.30)

- Approach using the same route is possible.
- Find the free epidural space.
- Carefully dissect the previously operated area (**Video 8.13**).

8.6.7 Symptomatic Partial Calcified L5–S1 HNP: Calcification Floating Technique

- See **Fig. 8.31** and **Fig. 8.32** (**Video 8.14**).

8.7 Complications

8.7.1 Early Relapse

- Early relapse after the surgery can be reduced by annulus sealing.

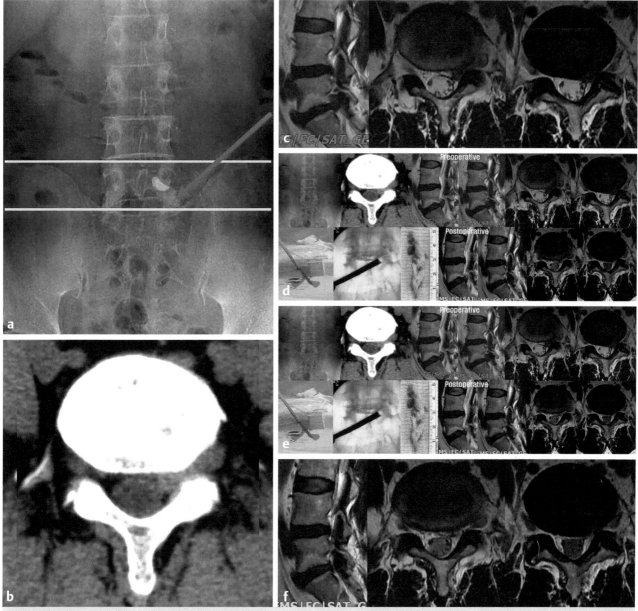

Fig. 8.26 Structural preservation contralateral interlaminar approach for foraminal to upward-migrated L5–S1 HNP. (**a**) Preoperative X-ray. (**b**) Preoperative CT. (**c**) Preoperative MRI. (**d**) Contralateral interlaminar approach. (**e**) Removed huge ruptured disk. (**f**) Postoperative MRI checked immediately after the operation.

- Sufficient bed rest to allow healing of the surgical field helps to reduce early relapse.

8.7.2 Vascular Injury

- Do not perform the diskectomy too deeply, to avoid causing a vascular injury.
- Caution must be used to avoid prevertebral aortic injury.

8.7.3 Nerve Injury

- Nerve injuries can be successfully prevented by gentle retraction of the nerve root.
- When dural tearing occurs during surgery, it is better not to proceed with the surgery and to stop.

8.7.4 Infection

- To reduce the chance of postoperative infection, clear surgical fields and infection control procedures should be needed.

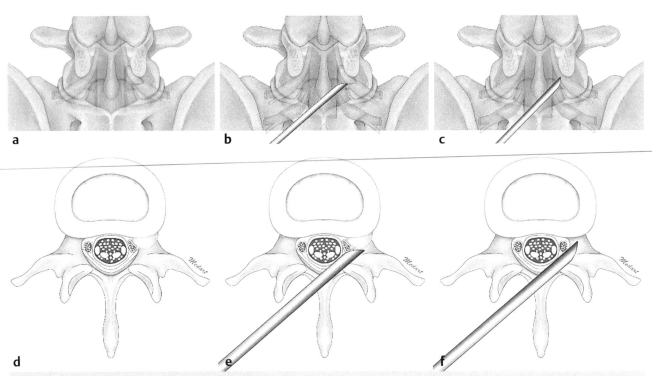

Fig. 8.27 Structural preservation contralateral interlaminar approach for foraminal to upward-migrated L5–S1 HNP. (**a,d**) Contralateral interlaminar approach provides sufficient access. (**b,e**) Exposure of the contralateral target point after splitting of the ligamentum flavum using the beveled working channel. (**c,f**) After removal of the pathologic disk, check the free foraminal space.

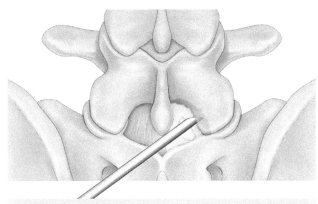

Fig. 8.28 Structural preservation revision PEILD for recurrent HNP after open lumbar diskectomy. Dissection of the adherent tissue from the bony structure. (Used with permission from Kim CH, Chung CK, Jahng TA, Yang HJ, Son YJ. Surgical outcome of percutaneous endoscopic interlaminar lumbar diskectomy for recurrent disk herniation after open diskectomy. *J Spinal Disord Tech*. 2012;25(5):125–133.)

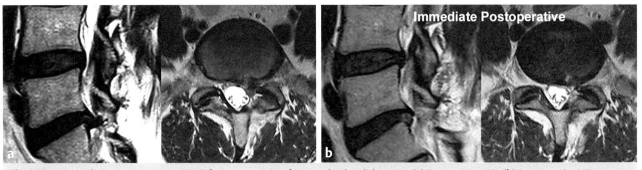

Fig. 8.29 Structural preservation revision PEILD for recurrent HNP after open lumbar diskectomy. (**a**) Preoperative MRI. (**b**) Postoperative MRI.

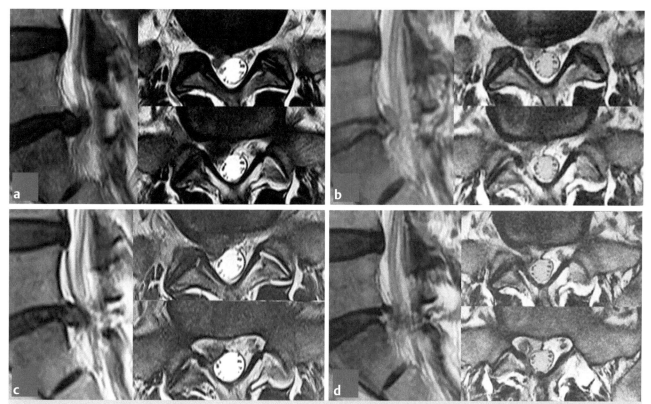

Fig. 8.30 Structural preservation revision PEILD after previous structural preservation PEILD. (**a**). Initial MRI. (**b**) Postoperative MRI after first PEILD. (**c**) MRI taken 2 years later due to abrupt onset of symptoms similar to the initial symptoms. (**d**) Postoperative MRI after second PEILD. The postoperative MRI was checked immediately after the operation.

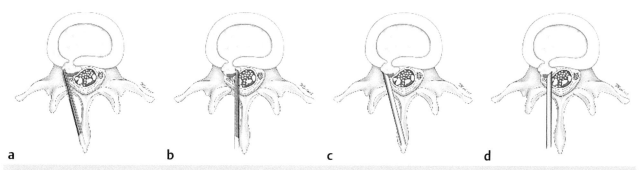

Fig. 8.31 Percutaneous endoscopic interlaminar calcification floating technique. (**a,b**) Resection of the annulus around the calcified HNP. (**c,d**) Rotation of the beveled working channel after wrapping the working channel into the calcified HNP.

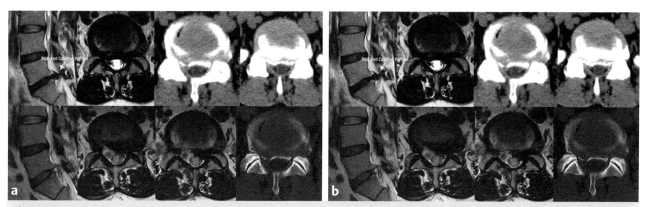

Fig. 8.32 Symptomatic partial calcified L5–S1 HNP: Calcification floating technique. (**a**) Preoperative MRIs. (**b**) Postoperative MRIs checked immediately after the operation.

References

1. Kim DH, Choi G, Lee SH. *Endoscopic Spine Procedures*. Thieme Medical Publishers; 2011:11
2. Abdullah AF, Wolber PG, Warfield JR, Gunadi IK. Surgical management of extreme lateral lumbar disc herniations: review of 138 cases. *Neurosurgery* 1988;*22*(4):648–653
3. Ahn Y, Lee SH, Park WM, Lee HY, Shin SW, Kang HY. Percutaneous endoscopic lumbar discectomy for recurrent disc herniation: surgical technique, outcome, and prognostic factors of 43 consecutive cases. *Spine* 2004;*29*(16):E326–E332
4. McCulloch JA. Principles of Microsurgery for Lumbar Disc Diseases. New York: Raven Press, 1989.
5. Mekhail N, Kapural L. Intradiscal thermal annuloplasty for discogenic pain: an outcome study. *Pain Pract* 2004;*4*(2):84–90
6. Ditsworth DA. Endoscopic transforaminal lumbar discectomy and reconfiguration: a postero-lateral approach into the spinal canal. *Surg Neurol* 1998;*49*(6):588–597
7. Tsou PM, Yeung AT. Transforaminal endoscopic decompression for radiculopathy secondary to intracanal noncontained lumbar disc herniations: outcome and technique. *Spine J* 2002;*2*(1):41–48
8. Tsou PM, Alan Yeung C, Yeung AT. Posterolateral transforaminal selective endoscopic discectomy and thermal annuloplasty for chronic lumbar discogenic pain: a minimal access visualized intradiscal surgical procedure. *Spine J* 2004;*4*(5):564–573
9. Ruetten S, Komp M, Godolias G. An extreme lateral access for the surgery of lumbar disc herniations inside the spinal canal using the full-endoscopic uniportal transforaminal approach—technique and prospective results of 463 patients. *Spine* 2005;*30*(22):2570–2578
10. Jasper GP, Francisco GM, Telfeian AE. Endoscopic transforaminal discectomy for an extruded lumbar disc herniation. *Pain Physician* 2013;*16*(1):E31–E35
11. Eustacchio S, Flaschka G, Trummer M, Fuchs I, Unger F. Endoscopic percutaneous transforaminal treatment for herniated lumbar discs. *Acta Neurochir (Wien)* 2002;*144*(10):997–1004
12. Gibson JN, Cowie JG, Iprenburg M. Transforaminal endoscopic spinal surgery: the future 'gold standard' for discectomy?—A review. *Surgeon* 2012;*10*(5):290–296
13. Yeung AT, Tsou PM. Posterolateral endoscopic excision for lumbar disc herniation: surgical technique, outcome, and complications in 307 consecutive cases. *Spine* 2002;*27*(7):722–731
14. Yeung AT, Yeung CA. Advances in endoscopic disc and spine surgery: foraminal approach. *Surg Technol Int* 2003;*11*:255–263
15. Yeung AT. The evolution of percutaneous spinal endoscopy and discectomy: state of the art. *Mt Sinai J Med* 2000;*67*(4):327–332
16. Maroon JC. Current concepts in minimally invasive discectomy. *Neurosurgery* 2002;*51*(5, Suppl)S137–S145
17. Kim HS, Park JY. Comparative assessment of different percutaneous endoscopic interlaminar lumbar discectomy (PEID) techniques. *Pain Physician* 2013;*16*(4):359–367
18. Choi G, Lee SH, Raiturker PP, Lee S, Chae YS. Percutaneous endoscopic interlaminar discectomy for intracanalicular disc herniations at L5–S1 using a rigid working channel endoscope. *Neurosurgery* 2006;*58*
19. Ruetten S, Komp M, Godolias G. A new full-endoscopic technique for the interlaminar operation of lumbar disc herniations using 6-mm endoscopes: prospective 2-year results of 331 patients. *Minim Invasive Neurosurg* 2006;*49*(2):80–87
20. Ruetten S, Komp M, Merk H, Godolias G. Use of newly developed instruments and endoscopes: full-endoscopic resection of lumbar disc herniations via the interlaminar and lateral transforaminal approach. *J Neurosurg Spine* 2007;*6*(6):521–530
21. Ruetten S, Komp M, Merk H, Godolias G. Full-endoscopic interlaminar and transforaminal lumbar discectomy versus conventional microsurgical technique: a prospective, randomized, controlled study. *Spine* 2008;*33*(9):931–939
22. Min JH, Kang SH, Lee JB, Cho TH, Suh JK, Rhyu IJ. Morphometric analysis of the working zone for endoscopic lumbar discectomy. *J Spinal Disord Tech* 2005;*18*(2):132–135
23. Kim HS, Ju CI, Kim SW, Kim JG. Endoscopic transforaminal suprapedicular approach in high grade inferior migrated lumbar disc herniation. *J Korean Neurosurg Soc* 2009;*45*(2):67–73
24. Chae KH, Ju CI, Lee SM, Kim BW, Kim SY, Kim HS. Strategies for noncontained lumbar disc herniation by an endoscopic approach: transforaminal suprapedicular approach, semi-rigid flexible curved probe, and 3-dimensional reconstruction CT with discogram. *J Korean Neurosurg Soc* 2009;*46*(4):312–316
25. Ahn Y. Transforaminal percutaneous endoscopic lumbar discectomy: technical tips to prevent complications. *Expert Rev Med Devices* 2012;*9*(4):361–366
26. Choi G, Prada N, Modi HN, Vasavada NB, Kim JS, Lee SH. Percutaneous endoscopic lumbar herniectomy for high-grade down-migrated L4–L5 disc through an L5–S1 interlaminar approach: a technical note. *Minim Invasive Neurosurg* 2010;*53*(3):147–152
27. Kim JS, Choi G, Lee SH. Percutaneous endoscopic lumbar discectomy via contralateral approach: a technical case report. *Spine* 2011;*36*(17):E1173–E1178
28. Kim CH, Chung CK, Jahng TA, Yang HJ, Son YJ. Surgical outcome of percutaneous endoscopic interlaminar lumbar diskectomy for recurrent disk herniation after open diskectomy. *J Spinal Disord Tech* 2012;*25*(5):E125–E133
29. Kim CH, Chung CK, Woo JW. Surgical outcome of percutaneous endoscopic interlaminar lumbar discectomy for highly migrated disc herniation. *J Spinal Disord Tech* 2012;:15
30. Kim CH, Chung CK. Endoscopic interlaminar lumbar discectomy with splitting of the ligament flavum under visual control. *J Spinal Disord Tech* 2012;*25*(4):210–217
31. Lee JS, Kim HS, Jang JS, Jang IT. Structural preservation percutaneous endoscopic lumbar interlaminar discectomy for L5–S1 herniated nucleus pulposus. *BioMed Res Int* 2016;*2016*:6250247

9 Percutaneous Endoscopic Decompressive Laminectomy and Foraminotomy

Gun Choi, Ketan Deshpande, and Akarawit Asawasaksakul

9.1 Introduction

Technical advances in endoscopic instruments are allowing spine surgeons to take on the challenge of lumbar decompression by the most minimally invasive approach possible. But the procedure is still in developmental phases, with indications limited to selective cases. We wish to present a brief discussion about the current application of endoscopy in lumbar canal stenosis (**Video 9.1**).[1,2,3,4]

9.2 Choice of Patient

Indications:
- Lower limb radiculopathy or claudication from neurologic origin with or without back pain not responding to conservative treatment
- Evidence of stenosis on magnetic resonance imaging and/or computed tomography correlating with clinical presentation

Contraindications:
- Degenerative spondylolisthesis (grade 2 or more)
- Profound neurological deficit
- Cauda equina syndrome

9.2.1 Classification

For all practical purposes, canal stenosis can be divided based on location:
- Central stenosis
- Lateral recess stenosis
- Foraminal stenosis

9.3 Central Stenosis

9.3.1 Technique

Step 1: Position and Anesthesia

- Conscious sedation (with propofol and remifentanil) supplemented with a caudal block with patient prone, with hips and knees in flexion and abdomen supported over bolsters.
- Level marking—target level end plates and the interlaminar window are roughly marked under fluoroscopic guidance.
- Entry point—approximately midway between the spinous process and the lateral extension of the interlaminar window (**Fig. 9.1**).
- Skin and intended tract infiltration—with 1% lidocaine ~ 2 to 3 mL.

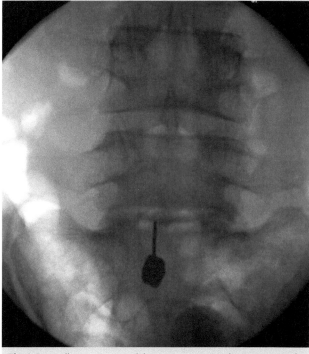

Fig. 9.1 Needle entry in central decompression—interlaminar approach.

Step 2: Skin Entry

- Target point—base of spinous process of proximal vertebra in antero-posterior (AP) view and posterior to the lamina in lateral (LAT) view

Step 3: Needle Insertion and Dilation

- Needle insertion—from the mentioned entry point an 18G 90-mm spinal needle is directed toward the base of the spinous process in slightly medial and cranial direction till it reaches the desired point in both AP and LAT views.
- Serial dilation—needle is replaced by a blunt tip guide wire and after a skin incision of ~ 9 to 10 mm, the tract is serially dilated until the 4th dilator (**Fig. 9.2**, **Fig. 9.3**) under fluoroscopic guidance, a circular working cannula, is passed over the final dilator and the scope is passed through it.
- This complete procedure is performed under continuous pressure irrigation using cold, antibiotic instilled normal saline. RF is used initially to clear the fat and paraspinal soft tissue and to enhance visibility.

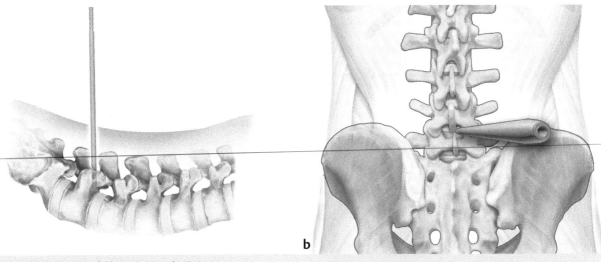

Fig. 9.2 (a,b) Showing serial dilation in AP and LAT views.

Step 4: Decompression

- Decompression is begun by locating the junction of the superior lamina and the base of the spinous process (SP) (**Fig. 9.4**; **Fig. 9.5**).
- One should always keep the ligamentum flavum intact till the end of bony decompression, as it acts to shield the thecal sac and protect it from any inadvertent injury.
- The next step is to make an opening in the flavum, which can be done either with a blunt tip probe or endoscopic scissors and further widened using an endo punch or a side-firing laser.
- Central stenosis cases do not require diskectomy as post-operatively the thecal sac along with its contents will fall posteriorly away from the disc, so we can keep the disk intact.
- Also in the majority of the cases visualization of the traversing root is not essential but can be easily visualized, if need arises, by tilting the scope laterally.
- At this stage, one can replace the circular cannula with a beveled cannula and use the beveled end as a root retractor to get a visual confirmation of the adequacy of decompression (**Fig. 9.6**).
- Hemostasis is achieved using the RF cautery, and a hemo-vac drain can be inserted with a single stay suture at the skin.

9.4 Lateral Recess Stenosis

Depending on the etiology and the target level, the choice of approach may vary (**Table 9.1**).

9.4.1 Interlaminar Technique

There are two aspects of choosing an interlaminar approach to perform lateral recess decompression, ipsilateral interlaminar and contralateral interlaminar, with both the techniques having their own advantages and limitations (**Table 9.2**).

Ipsilateral Interlaminar

- *Step 1: Position and Anesthesia*

- General anesthesia is preferred with patient in prone position with hips and knees in flexion and abdomen supported over bolsters.

- Level marking—target level end plates and the interlaminar window are roughly marked under fluoroscopic guidance
- *Step 2: Skin Entry Point*

- Lateralmost point of the interlaminar window (**Fig. 9.7**)
- Target point—lateral end of the proximal lamina in AP and posterior to the lamina in LAT view C-arm

- *Step 3: Needle Insertion and Dilation*

- From the mentioned entry point an 18-gauge 90-mm spinal needle is directed toward the junction of the lamina with the facet till it reaches the desired point in both AP and LAT views.

Table 9.1 Brief summary of the classification and the choice of approach for various stenotic pathologies

Location	Type	Etiology	Level	Choice of Approach
Central	Either	Either	Any	Interlaminar
Lateral Recess	Bony	Superior facet	L1–L5	Transforaminal
			L5–S1	Interlaminar > Transforaminal
		Inferior facet	any	Interlaminar
	Soft tissue	either	any	Interlaminar
	Combined	either	any	Interlaminar
Foraminal	Either	either	any	Transforaminal

Table 9.2 The pros and cons of both interlaminar approaches in lateral recess decompression

Contralateral interlaminar	Ipsilateral interlaminar
- Ease of access to lateral recess - Maximum facet can be preserved - Good even for central decompression, as base of spinous process and superior lamina can be accessed	- Maximum soft tissue preservation - Familiar approach - Retraction of root may be difficult/painful - Needs more facetal decompression

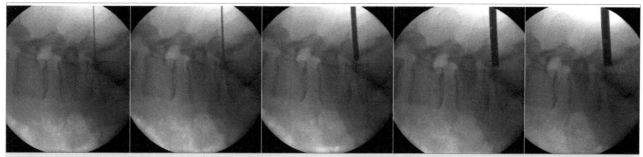

Fig. 9.3 Serial dilators on C-arm lateral view.

- Serial dilation—a blunt-tip guidewire is inserted and after a skin incision of ~ 9 to 10 mm, the tract is serially dilated until the 4th dilator under fluoroscopic guidance (**Fig. 9.3**); a circular working cannula is passed over the final dilator and the scope is passed through it.

- *Step 4: Decompression*

- After soft tissue clearance with RF cautery, the lamino-facetal junction is identified and endo-drill is used to bur out the hypertrophied facet and the lateral lamina. An arthroscopic shaver also comes in handy, as it comes with an anterior protective sleeve (**Fig. 9.8**).

- The ligamentum flavum is cut in similar fashion and the opening widened.

- The next critical step is to identify and isolate the traversing root. If sufficient bony decompression is already achieved, then the traversing root can be easily located, but if not, then further bony decompression has to be undertaken with a shaver until the root is sufficiently visualized.

- Once the traversing root is identified, a beveled cannula is used to isolate the root medially away from the surgical field. Further decompression can be safely continued using a shaver (**Fig. 9.9**), or a diamond bur and diskectomy can be performed if needed.

- The end point of procedure is the visual confirmation of the free traversing root. Wound is closed with a single skin suture over hemo-vac drain. **Fig. 9.10** demonstrates animations to summarize this approach.

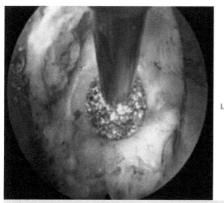

Fig. 9.4 The drilling of spinous process and superior lamina.

Cranial

Superior lamina

Lateral

Medial

Drill

Lig. Flavum

Caudal

Fig. 9.5 Endoscopic view of drilling of lamina in the interlaminar approach.

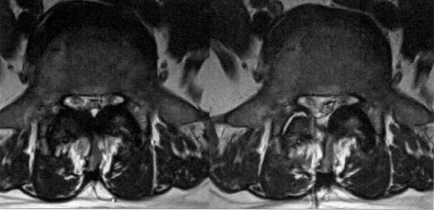

Fig. 9.6 Pre- and postoperative axial views in the central stenosis interlaminar approach.

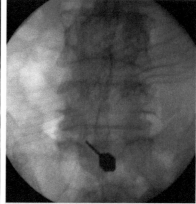

Fig. 9.7 Interlaminar ipsilateral lateral recess approach—needle entry.

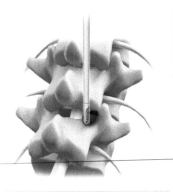

Fig. 9.8 Use of an arthroscopic shaver in lateral recess.

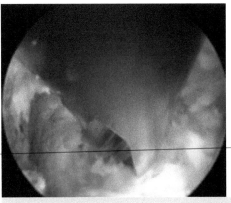

Fig. 9.9 Endoscopic view of shaver in lateral recess.

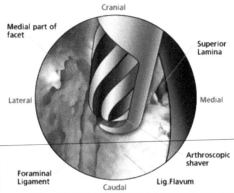

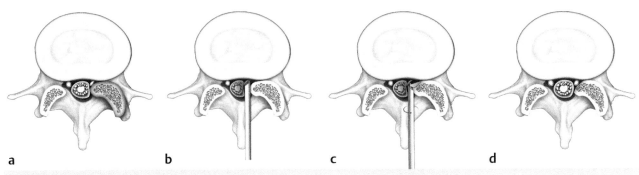

Fig. 9.10 (**a**) Lateral recess stenosis. (**b**) Insertion of beveled cannula. (**c**) Rotating the beveled cannula to protect the traversing root and decompression of the lateral recess. (**d**) Decompressed lateral recess with free traversing root.

Contralateral Interlaminar

- *Step 1: Position and Anesthesia*

- General anesthesia is preferred with the patient in prone position with hips and knees in flexion and abdomen supported over bolsters

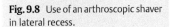

Fig. 9.11 Interlaminar contralateral lateral recess approach—needle entry.

- Level marking—target level end plates and the interlaminar window are roughly marked under fluoroscopic guidance

- *Step 2: Skin Entry Point*

- Approximately midway between spinous process and the lateral extension of the interlaminar window on the asymptomatic (contralateral) side (**Fig. 9.11**)

- Target point—base of spinous process of proximal vertebra in AP view and posterior to the lamina in LAT view

- *Step 3: Needle Insertion and Dilation*

- From the mentioned entry point, an 18-gauge 90-mm spinal needle is directed toward the base of the spinous process in slightly medial and cranial direction till it reaches the desired target point in both AP and LAT views.

- Serial dilation—a blunt tip guide wire is inserted and after a skin incision of ~ 9 to 10 mm, the tract is serially dilated till the final dilator under fluoroscopic guidance (**Fig. 9.3**), a circular working cannula, is passed over the final dilator and the scope is passed through it.

- *Step 4: Decompression*

- The initial part of the procedure is similar to interlaminar for central stenosis, in which the lamina and spinous junction is identified and the base of spinous process is burred to create space to pass the cannula on the contralateral side.

- After this the cannula is progressed further toward the contralateral facet by drilling the way across the lamina (**Fig. 9.12**).

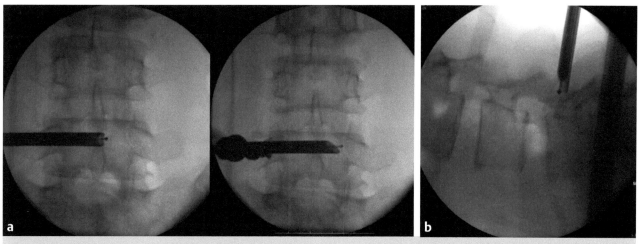

Fig. 9.12 **(a)** Showing progression of the cannula toward contralateral lamina **(b)** Showing location of the cannula and bur for lateral recess decompression in lateral view C-arm.

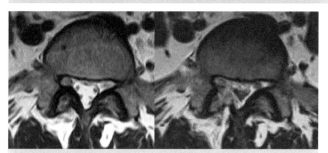

Fig. 9.13 Lateral recess stenosis, pre- and post-operative, interlaminar approach.

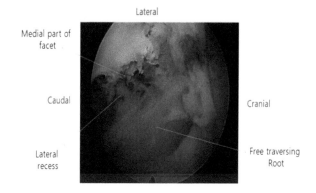

- Flavum needs to be kept intact so as to avoid damaging the thecal sac. On reaching the facet, the bony decompression is performed in similar fashion using a drill or a shaver. The rest of the procedure is similar to the interlaminar ipsilateral approach (already mentioned).

The contralateral approach provides the angulation with which we can approach the facet joint, helping the surgeon to slide the cannula underneath it. This way, we can perform targeted decompression of the most pathological portion of the facet—i.e., ventral and medial portion of superior articular process (SAP)—and preserve the rest of the facet. Second, in our experience, the isolation of the root is also fairly easy and pain-free if the procedure is done under conscious sedation (**Fig. 9.13**; **Fig. 9.14**).

9.5 Foraminal Stenosis

The spinal nerve roots exit through the intervertebral foramina, and the proportion between the size of the foramen and the relative space occupied by the root determines the chance of root compression in the intervertebral foramen. The intervertebral foramen has, as part of its boundaries, two movable joints—the intervertebral joint anteriorly and the zygapophyseal joint posteriorly. The compact bone of the deep arches of the inferior vertebral notch of the vertebra above and the shallow superior vertebral notch of the vertebra below form the superior and inferior boundaries, respectively.[5] The etiology of the foraminal stenosis includes SAP hypertrophy, or flavum hypertrophy, or the combination of both with or without a ruptured disc.

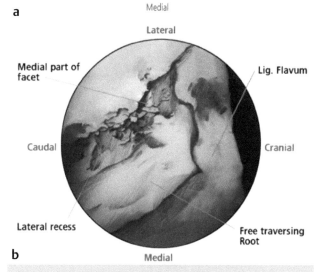

Fig. 9.14 **(a,b)** Endoscopic view of decompressed traversing root after lateral recess decompression.

9.5.1 Foraminoplasty Technique

Step 1: Position and Anesthesia

- Conscious sedation with patient prone, with hips and knees in flexion and abdomen supported over bolsters, with the surgeon standing on the symptomatic side

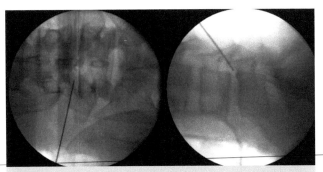

Fig. 9.15 Target point for needle in foraminoplasty in AP and LAT view.

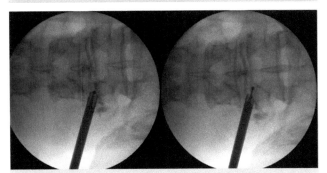

Fig. 9.17 Progression of drill in foraminoplasty.

- Level marking—target level end plates are marked and a line is drawn extending laterally from the SP at the level of the target disk.

Step 2: Skin Entry Point

- Calculated on pre-op MR or CT axial images targeting the foramen and avoiding the contents of the peritoneum
- Target point—base of SAP in AP and anterior margin of facet joint in LAT view (**Fig. 9.15**)
- Skin and intermuscular infiltration—1% lidocaine is used ~ 3 mL for skin with 24-gauge needle and 6 to 7 mL for intermuscular plane delivered using a 23-gauge spinal needle

Step 3: Needle Insertion and Dilation

- Needle entry—an 18-gauge 120-mm spinal needle is directed toward the target point under fluoroscopic AP and LAT views and in slightly cranial to caudal angulation.
- An alternative method is to use the tunnel view on C-arm; in this method, the C-arm is tilted along the medial-lateral plane to open out the facet joint on the symptomatic side, which usually is around 35 to 40 degrees. The needle is directed toward the SAP, keeping the long axis of the needle parallel to the C-arm angulation. The needle is usually progressed further to anchor it within the disc.
- A blunt-tip guidewire is passed through it.
- The tract is dilated using a single blunt dilator with tapering mouth, and a beveled cannula is passed over it up to the foramen.

Step 4: Decompression

- After soft tissue clearance, the facet joint is identified.

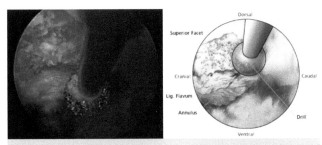

Fig. 9.16 Endoscopic view of use of diamond bur in foraminoplasty.

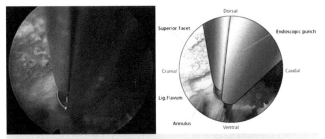

Fig. 9.18 Endoscopic view of use of punch in foraminoplasty.

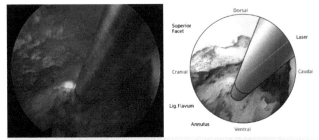

Fig. 9.19 Endoscopic view of use of laser in foraminoplasty.

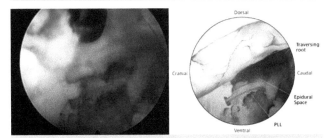

Fig. 9.20 Endoscopic view of free traversing root after foraminoplasty.

- The lateral capsule of the joint is cleared using the RF cautery, and the superior facet is drilled using the endo-drill (**Fig. 9.16**; **Fig. 9.17**).
- Bony bleeding usually encountered at this stage and can be controlled by regulating the flow of the irrigation fluid.
- The drill is moved along the cranial to caudal axis to decompress the foramen. The position of the drill tip can be confirmed in between with reference to the lower pedicle on AP view.
- The superior and medial portion of the pedicle can also be included in the decompression zone depending on the amount of stenosis.
- After bony decompression, medial foraminal ligaments and flavum are visualized. This soft tissue decompression can be performed using a punch or a laser (**Fig. 9.18**; **Fig. 9.19**).

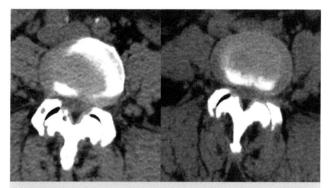

Fig. 9.21 Pre- and postoperative CT images in transforaminal foraminoplasty.

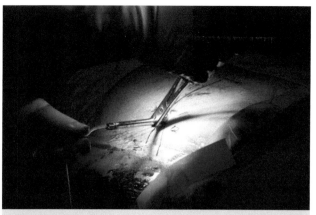

Fig. 9.22 Drain insertion.

- Beyond the flavum lies the traversing root surrounded by epidural fat and blood vessels. Free disc fragments, if any, can be seen and easily removed at this stage.
- Free movement of the traversing root and thecal sac marks the end point of decompression (**Fig. 9.20**; **Fig. 9.21**). The wound is closed with a single skin suture with or without hemo-vac drain (**Fig. 9.22**).
- If hemo-vac drain is used, then it can be removed after 4 to 6 hours.

References

1   Lee SH, Lee SJ, Park KH, et al. [Comparison of percutaneous manual and endoscopic laser diskectomy with chemonucleolysis and automated nucleotomy]. *Orthopade* 1996;*25*(1):49–55
2   Knight MT, Goswami A, Patko JT, Buxton N. Endoscopic foraminoplasty: a prospective study on 250 consecutive patients with independent evaluation. *J Clin Laser Med Surg* 2001;*19*(2):73–81
3   Choi G, Prada N, Modi HN, Vasavada NB, Kim JS, Lee SH. Percutaneous endoscopic lumbar herniectomy for high-grade down-migrated L4-L5 disc through an L5-S1 interlaminar approach: a technical note. *Minim Invasive Neurosurg* 2010;*53*(3):147–152
4   Choi G, Lee SH, Deshpande K, Choi H. Working channel endoscope in lumbar spine surgery. *J Neurosurg Sci* 2014;*58*(2):77–85
5   Devi R, Rajagopalan N. Morphometry of lumbar intervertebral foramen. *Indian J Orthop* 2005;*39*(3):145–147

10 Unilateral Biportal Endoscopic Decompression for Lumbar Spinal Stenosis

Jin Hwa Eum, Sang Kyu Son, Ketan Deshpande, and Alfonso García

10.1 Introduction

Traditionally, lumbar stenosis is treated with an open decompressive laminectomy, a foraminotomy, or fusion surgeries.[1,2,3,4] Recently, minimally invasive spinal surgical methods have developed to improve muscle preservation and other surrounding normal anatomical structures.[3,5,6] Microscopic bilateral decompression via a unilateral approach has been used in the treatment of lumbar spinal stenosis.[3,5] Percutaneous endoscopic interlaminar decompression for lumbar stenosis remains a challenging procedure even for an experienced endoscopic surgeon.[7] Additionally, vision is restricted and technical difficulties can arise in spite of using a microscope or uniportal spinal endoscope. Our technique of unilateral biportal endoscopy (UBE) is a modification of percutaneous uniportal interlaminar epidural endoscopic surgery. The UBE decompression method is based on the same operative technique as other surgical procedures, such as ipsilateral microscopic laminotomy and bilateral decompression, with patients in the prone position. Compared with open microscopic spinal surgery, the UBE technique can reduce muscle injury and allow excellent visualization of the contralateral traversing root. This chapter introduces and describes the technique for UBE decompression in the treatment of lumbar spinal stenosis (**Video 10.1**).[8,9]

10.2 Equipment

Equipment used in the unilateral biportal endoscopic procedure is as follows. During the procedure, we use a 3.5-mm spherical bur (Conmed Linvatec, Utica, NY), a 0°, 4-mm diameter arthroscope (Conmed Linvatec, Utica, NY), a bipolar flexible radiofrequency probe (Ellman), serial dilators, a specially designed dissector, a pressure pump irrigation system (Smith & Nephew Inc., Memphis, TN), and standard laminectomy instruments, such as hook dissectors, Kerrison punches, and pituitary forceps.

10.3 Surgical Procedure

The UBE procedure is similar to knee arthroscopy. Two portals are used: one portal is used for continuous irrigation and endoscopic viewing and the other portal is used for insertion and manipulation of the instruments used in decompression (e.g., in laminotomy and flavectomy). See **Fig. 10.1** for a right-sided UBE procedure.

10.3.1 Position and Anesthesia

The procedures are performed with the patient under general or epidural anesthesia on a radiolucent operating table over a Wilson frame. The patient is placed in the prone position to minimize abdominal pressure. A waterproof surgical drape is applied after induction of anesthesia.

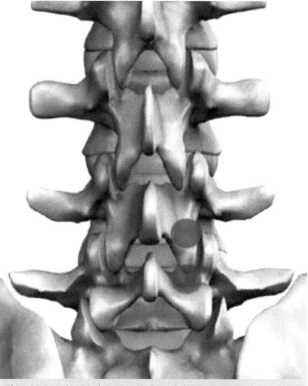

Fig. 10.1 Right-sided L4–L5 unilateral biportal endoscopy (UBE). Anteroposterior diagram of the working portal, represented by the red dot, and the scope portal, represented by the blue dot.

10.3.2 Target Point

The target pathologic stenotic level is identified under fluoroscopic guidance. The exact target point is the intersection between the lower lamina margin and 1 cm lateral to the spinous process ipsilaterally, as determined through the associated lateralizing symptoms. In the absence of lateralizing signs or symptoms, a left-sided approach is preferred for a right-handed surgeon.

10.3.3 Working Channel Portal

To establish the working channel portal, a 1.5-cm skin incision is made slightly obliquely above the target point, following the direction of the multifidus muscle fibers. Serial dilators are then inserted toward the lower lamina. Following removal of the dilators, a specially designed dissector is used on the lower lamina. Interlaminar soft tissue is dissected medially to laterally toward the medial margin of the facet joint capsule (**Fig. 10.2**, **Fig. 10.3**, **Fig. 10.4**).

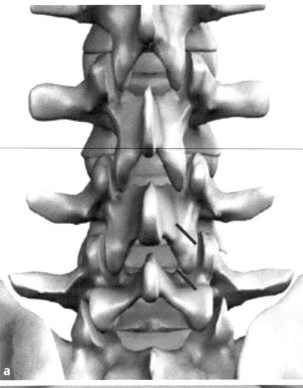

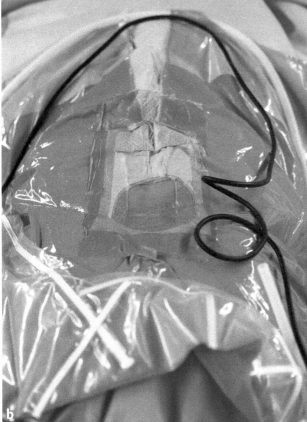

Fig. 10.2 (a,b) For a right-sided L4–L5 approach, first the target point is localized under C-arm fluoroscopy. A slightly oblique 1.5-cm skin incision is made above the lower margin of the L4 lamina, following the direction of the multifidus muscle. After proper dilation and muscle dissection, a second, oblique incision is made just 1.5 cm distal to the first incision.

10.3.4 Endoscopic Portal

The endoscopic portal is always made to the left of the working channel portal; that is, if a right-sided approach is needed, then this portal will be made distal to the working channel (for a right-handed surgeon), and if a left-sided approach is needed, then the endoscopic portal will be made proximal to

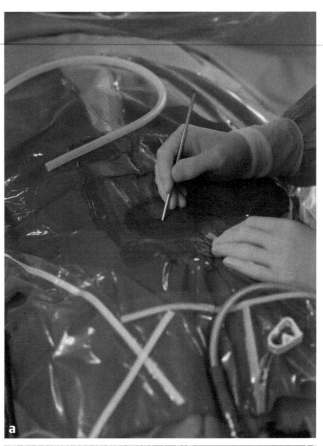

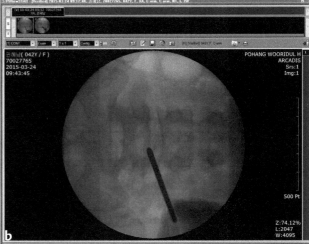

Fig. 10.3 (a) Right-sided L4–L5 unilateral biportal endoscopy (UBE). Anteroposterior C-arm view of the initial dilator introduced through the working channel portal and aimed to the inferior margin of the L4 lamina, close to the base of the corresponding spinous process. **(b)** After the working portal incision is made, the surgeon introduces a dilator and checks, using C-arm fluoroscopy, for the target point.

the working channel. An easy way to remember this is that a right-handed surgeon will hold the scope with the left hand and the instruments with the right hand.

The second portal is made through a 1.0-cm skin incision ~ 2 to 3 cm above the upper edge of the first caudal port skin incision; the second portal serves to accommodate the insertion of a

6-mm diameter cannula and scope. A 0°, endoscope is inserted through the cranial portal after insertion of the cannula.

A saline irrigation pump is connected to the endoscope and is set to a pressure of 20 to 30 mm Hg during the procedure; a continuous, controlled flow of saline solution irrigation is essential to prevent excessive elevation of the epidural pressure. Surgical instruments are inserted through the caudal working portal (**Fig. 10.1**, **Fig. 10.5**).

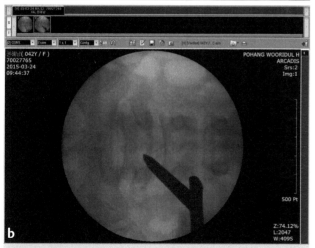

Fig. 10.4 (a) Right-sided L4–L5 unilateral biportal endoscopy (UBE). Anteroposterior C-arm view of the muscle dissector introduced through the working channel portal and aimed to the inferior margin of the L4 lamina, close to the base of the corresponding spinous process. **(b)** Corresponding to **Fig. 10.4a**. After initial dilation of a dissector is introduced to partially detach muscle from the base of the spinous process, and the position is verified with C-arm fluoroscopy.

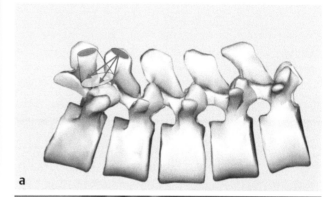

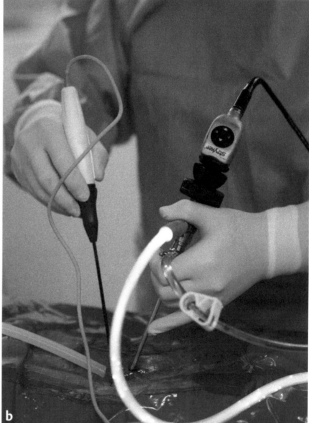

Fig. 10.5 (a) Right-sided L4–L5 unilateral biportal endoscopy (UBE). Lateral diagram of the working portal (represented by the red dot) and the scope portal (blue dot). The translucent oval and the blue arrows represent the viewing field and instrument working angles, respectively. **(b)** Surgeon's frontal view of a left-sided UBE approach. Notice that a right-handed surgeon will hold the endoscope and camera with the left hand and the instruments with the right hand.

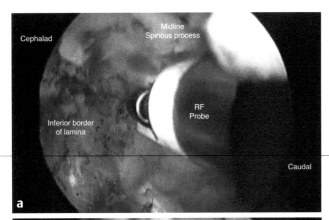

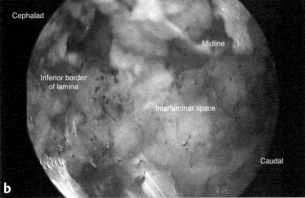

Fig. 10.6 **(a)** Endoscopic view after triangulation. The radiofrequency probe is used to create a working space by tissue ablation and coagulation. **(b)** After using the RF probe, we can identify the interlaminar space, the inferior border of the lamina above, and the spinous process in the midline still covered by soft tissue.

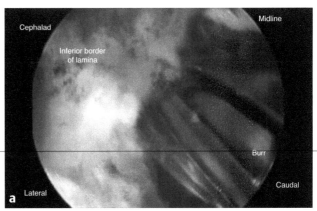

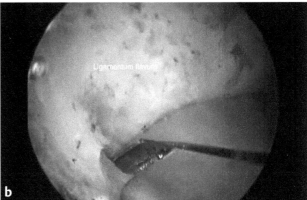

Fig. 10.7 **(a)** Endoscopic view of the use of the bone bur for initial laminectomy. **(b)** Use of Kerrison rongeurs to augment the laminectomy. Notice that the ligamentum flavum is still intact.

10.4 Decompression Procedure

It is important to mention that since a 0°, endoscope is used, the tips of the working instruments are in a deeper plane than the scope. After triangulation with the endoscope and instruments, minor bleeding control is accomplished, and the radiofrequency probes are used for debridement of soft tissue remnants overlying the lamina and ligamentum flavum (**Fig. 10.6**).

Following complete exposure of the lower lamina, bony decompression is performed under magnified endoscopic vision, with the 3.5-mm soft tissue protected drill and Kerrison punches (**Fig. 10.7**).

The ligamentum flavum is left intact to act as a protective shield for neural structures. The upper border of the lower lamina is removed for the ipsilateral foraminotomy as needed. The endoscopic anatomic view is very similar to the microscopic view of a posterior midline unilateral laminotomy.

In the case in **Fig. 10.8**, the ipsilateral ligamentum flavum was removed until full mobilization of the lateral border of the nerve root could be achieved.

After this step, the fully mobile nerve root can be retracted and the ruptured disk is exposed and carefully removed (**Fig. 10.9**, **Fig. 10.10**).

Contralateral decompression can be performed at high magnification and with a good endoscopic field of vision. Contralateral flavectomy and sublaminar decompression are performed with a Kerrison punch and curet. The endoscope can be moved to

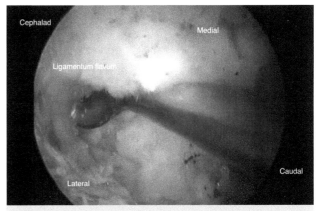

Fig. 10.8 Detachment of the ligamentum flavum with curet.

the contralateral side by taking advantage of muscle and skin elasticity, rather than adjusting the patient's position or making additional skin incisions. Contralateral decompression is then performed until the descending nerve root can be clearly identified and decompressed. In the case of a symptomatic patient with ipsilateral disk herniation, the surgeon can perform the diskectomy under endoscopic view, without needing to make extra incisions. The level of neural decompression can be assessed by normal respiratory-induced dural pulsation confirmed with endoscopic direct view and the use of a blunt probe.

Epidural bleeding is controlled by adjusting the pump pressure and by coagulation with flexible radiofrequency probes.

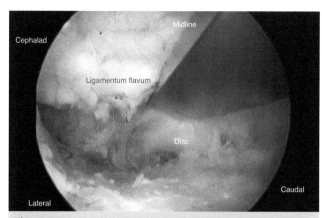

Fig. 10.9 Exposure of the herniated disk using a regular nerve retractor through the instrument portal.

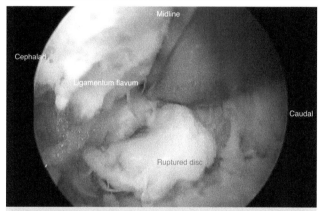

Fig. 10.10 Ruptured disk.

The skin incisions are closed after removal of the instruments and endoscope.

10.5 Tips and Pearls

- This technique gives better and easier visualization of the contralateral structures and assessment of foraminal decompressed areas.
- The anatomy and approach are familiar, similar to those in microscopic diskectomy.
- Working ease: Mostly standard instruments can be used through the caudal portal.
- Reduced bleeding: Continuous infusion of cold irrigation allows better bleeding control.
- The fluid from continuous-pressure irrigation enables slight compression of the dura mater and widening of the contralateral epidural space during procedures. Therefore, the authors suggest that contralateral decompression may be easier to perform, with a lower risk of dural tears.

10.6 Complications

Possible complications of the UBE technique are classified into immediate and delayed.

10.6.1 Immediate Complications

- Dural tears: In the authors' experience, the incidence of dural tears is very low, because the technique provides a familiar approach to the spine and therefore a shorter learning curve.
- If a dural tear is encountered during the procedure, it should be assessed immediately following the surgery, and it should be sutured in the same setting using an open approach.
- Injury to neural structures: Improved visualization with the endoscope and a clear visual field with continuous-pressure irrigation reduce the incidence of neural injury.
- Increased epidural pressure is a serious complication leading to postoperative neck pain and possible seizures, but because the UBE is a biportal procedure, it allows free outflow of the irrigation fluid via the second working channel.

10.6.2 Delayed Complications

- Infection: Continuous flow of antibiotic-instilled normal saline largely prevents accumulation and inoculation of microbes.
- Recurrence of disk herniation: UBE allows a targeted approach to the annular rupture site without violation of the normal annulus. Annuloplasty can be done in all cases, reducing the risk of recurrence. Even if recurrent disk herniation occurs, one can easily approach the target with the same UBE technique. Careful patient selection and assessment for high risk for recurrence are encouraged.

10.7 Discussion

Microdiskectomy and minimally invasive diskectomy decrease surgical exposure and trauma and have success rates of ~ 90%.[10,11] It is a well-recognized fact that *less invasive* means *muscle preserving*, and therefore less damage to other normal structures. Hence, these techniques reduce postoperative morbidity and the incidence of perineural and intraneural fibrosis and enhance the preservation of the epidural venous system.[12]

Open, decompressive laminectomies have been proven to be both safe and effective in treating lumbar stenosis but may also cause disruption of, and damage to, normal anatomical structures, such as the supraspinous ligament, interspinous ligament, spinous process, lamina, facet joints, ligamentum flavum, and paraspinal musculature, leading to severe muscle atrophy.[13,14,15,16,17] Because the surgeon's view is located outside of the spinal canal in open microsurgery and the range of motion of instruments is limited in microendoscopic tubular surgery, extensive laminectomy and changing the patient's position intraoperatively may be necessary to reach proper decompression of the contralateral exiting or traversing nerve root. For these reasons, and because of the need to preserve normal muscle attachments and other important spine stabilizers, minimally invasive surgical approaches have been rapidly evolving. Although endoscopic spinal decompression for lumbar stenosis is recommended, some surgeons are still not familiar with the technique. UBE combines the advantages of standard open surgery and endoscopic spine surgery.

When UBE is performed, an endoscope and a high-definition camera are used to put the surgeon's view inside the spinal canal; therefore, laminectomy and facetectomy may be minimized under excellent visualization without changing the patient's position. Technical advantages of UBE and its differences from microendoscopic tubular decompression and percutaneous endoscopic lumbar decompression are:

1. 360° vision without straight, restricted, tubular vision
2. Free range of motion of instruments, not tubular restricted motion
3. Easy bilateral decompression
4. Less bleeding because of continuous-pressure saline irrigation

The UBE technique is a modification of translaminar epidural endoscopy, using standard arthroscopic instruments.[18,19] This concept is different from spinal endoscopic approaches through one portal. Two skin incisions are made, one for the endoscope and the other for working instruments. Thus, the endoscopic system is similar to joint arthroscopy, where triangulation of scope and instruments is essential. The two portals are ipsilateral, and when the endoscope is introduced, it meets the instruments at the interlaminar area. C-arm fluoroscopy aids in localizing the precise skin entry point for reaching the disk and foramen. Inflow of irrigating saline goes through the endoscopic cannula, and outflow comes out through the working portal. Ordinary laminectomy instruments are used through the working channel. Therefore, this endoscopic operating procedure has the same steps and "feeling" as an open surgery, but without retraction of muscle and an improved view, as mentioned earlier. Since UBE decompression for lumbar central stenosis is done with the patient in the prone position, it allows excellent visualization of ipsilateral and contralateral spinal canal anatomy, and multilevel decompression is fairly easy and possible.

10.8 Conclusion

UBE is a video-assisted procedure that enables the surgeon to use an endoscope to enlarge the field of view while improving the identification of vital landmarks. The anatomical view presented to the surgeon is very similar to that of conventional open surgery, and it allows for an exceptional and extraordinary navigation experience to the contralateral, sublaminar, and foraminal areas, which makes the procedure safer by enhancing the view of neural and vascular structures. Therefore, decompression using UBE may be an attractive and minimally invasive technique that is safe for treatment of degenerative lumbar stenosis.

References

1   Costa F, Sassi M, Cardia A, et al. Degenerative lumbar spinal stenosis: analysis of results in a series of 374 patients treated with unilateral laminotomy for bilateral microdecompression. *J Neurosurg Spine* 2007;7(6):579–586 PubMed
2   Martin BI, Mirza SK, Comstock BA, Gray DT, Kreuter W, Deyo RA. Reoperation rates following lumbar spine surgery and the influence of spinal fusion procedures. *Spine* 2007;32(3):382–387 PubMed
3   Mobbs RJ, Li J, Sivabalan P, Raley D, Rao PJ. Outcomes after decompressive laminectomy for lumbar spinal stenosis: comparison between minimally invasive unilateral laminectomy for bilateral decompression and open laminectomy: clinical article. *J Neurosurg Spine* 2014;21(2):179–186 PubMed
4   Javid MJ, Hadar EJ. Long-term follow-up review of patients who underwent laminectomy for lumbar stenosis: a prospective study. *J Neurosurg* 1998;89(1):1–7 PubMed
5   Poletti CE. Central lumbar stenosis caused by ligamentum flavum: unilateral laminotomy for bilateral ligamentectomy: preliminary report of two cases. *Neurosurgery* 1995;37(2):343–347 PubMed
6   Ikuta K, Tono O, Tanaka T, et al. Surgical complications of microendoscopic procedures for lumbar spinal stenosis. *Minim Invasive Neurosurg* 2007;50(3):145–149 PubMed
7   Sairyo K, Sakai T, Higashino K, Inoue M, Yasui N, Dezawa A. Complications of endoscopic lumbar decompression surgery. *Minim Invasive Neurosurg* 2010;53(4):175–178 PubMed
8   Hu ZJ, Fang XQ, Zhou ZJ, Wang JY, Zhao FD, Fan SW. Effect and possible mechanism of muscle-splitting approach on multifidus muscle injury and atrophy after posterior lumbar spine surgery. *J Bone Joint Surg Am* 2013;95(24):e192–e199(1–9) PubMed
9   Podichetty VK, Spears J, Isaacs RE, Booher J, Biscup RS. Complications associated with minimally invasive decompression for lumbar spinal stenosis. *J Spinal Disord Tech* 2006;19(3):161–166 PubMed
10 Kahanovitz N, Viola K, Muculloch J. Limited surgical discectomy and microdiscectomy. A clinical comparison. *Spine* 1989;14(1):79–81 PubMed
11 Spengler DM. Lumbar discectomy. Results with limited disc excision and selective foraminotomy. *Spine* 1982;7(6):604–607 PubMed
12 Garg B, Nagraja UB, Jayaswal A. Microendoscopic versus open discectomy for lumbar disc herniation: a prospective randomised study. *J Orthop Surg (Hong Kong)* 2011;19(1):30–34 PubMed
13 Adams MA, Hutton WC. The mechanical function of the lumbar apophyseal joints. *Spine* 1983;8(3):327–330 PubMed
14 Adams MA, Hutton WC, Stott JR. The resistance to flexion of the lumbar intervertebral joint. *Spine* 1980;5(3):245–253 PubMed
15 Cusick JF, Yoganandan N, Pintar FA, Reinartz JM. Biomechanics of sequential posterior lumbar surgical alterations. *J Neurosurg* 1992;76(5):805–811 PubMed
16 Onik G, Mooney V, Maroon JC, et al. Automated percutaneous discectomy: a prospective multi-institutional study. *Neurosurgery* 1990;26(2):228–232
17 Foley KT, Smith MM. Microendoscopic discectomy. *Tech Neurosurg* 1997;3:301–307
18 De Antony DJ, Claro ML. Argentina: translaminar epidural lumbar endoscopy in hernias occupying over 50% of the radicular canal and decompression in lateral spinal stenosis. *Arthroskopie* 1999;12(2):79–84
19 De Antoni DJ, Claro ML, Poehling GG, Hughes SS. Translaminar lumbar epidural endoscopy: anatomy, technique, and indications. *Arthroscopy* 1996;12(3):330–334

11 Percutaneous Unilateral Biportal Endoscopic Diskectomy and Decompression for Lumbar Degenerative Disease

Dong Hwa Heo, Jin Hwa Eum, and Sang Kyu Son

11.1 Introduction

Traditionally, spinal endoscopic surgery was performed using a monoportal technique via one channel.[1,2,3,4] One-portal spinal endoscopic surgery needs specially optimized devices, and there are surgical limitations, especially with the interlaminar approach. Recently, percutaneous endoscopic surgery has been attempted for decompression and fusion.[5,6] Although instruments for one-portal endoscopic systems have been vigorously developed, endoscopic surgical treatments for migrated disk herniation and spinal stenosis still may be difficult and have a steep learning curve.[3,4] Moreover, there are complications with endoscopic surgery.[6] The percutaneous unilateral biportal endoscopic (UBE) approach combines the advantages of microscopic spinal surgery and endoscopic spinal surgery.[7,8] The technique is a modification and fusion of translaminar endoscopic surgery and conventional microscopic surgery.[5,7,8,9,10] The surgical procedure is similar to that for thoracoscopic or arthroscope surgery. We have used the UBE approach for the treatment of lumbar degenerative disease, such as lumbar disk herniation (including upward- and downward-migrated ruptured disks), extraforaminal ruptured disk, foraminal stenosis, and central stenosis.[8] This chapter introduces and describes our surgical technique.

11.2 Indications

Indications for UBE surgery are similar to those for conventional open surgery and more:

- Lumbar spinal stenosis without significant instability, such as spondylolisthesis
- Central lumbar herniated disk: Upward migration, downward migration, calcified disk
- Extraforaminal and foraminal lumbar disk herniation
- Recurrent lumbar disk herniation
- Foraminal stenosis

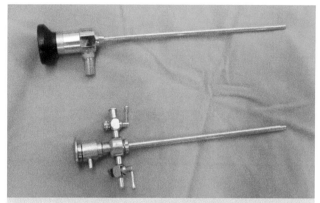

Fig. 11.1 Biportal endoscopic spine surgery uses a 0° arthroscope.

11.3 Equipment

All standard devices for open spinal surgery are available for UBE surgery. The 0° endoscope is an arthroscopic system that is used in knee or shoulder arthroscopic surgeries (**Fig. 11.1**). For exposing the laminar and interlaminar space, a specially designed periosteal dissector and serial dilators are used (**Fig. 11.2**). However, the specialized instruments can be replaced with other serial dilators and a small periosteal dissector or elevator. For the dissection of soft tissue and bleeding control, we use radiofrequency probes that are already used in arthroscopic surgery or single-portal spinal endoscopic surgery. For removal of bony structures, such as in laminectomy and foraminotomy, we prefer the one-sided protected drill (**Fig. 11.3**). All types of arthroscopic and endoscopic drill systems are available for biportal endoscopic surgery. For the continuous saline irrigation, we prefer a pressure-pump irrigation system. Simple water-pressure control using the height of the saline bag on the fluid stand is also possible.

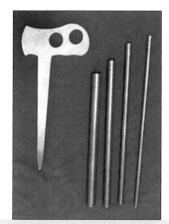

Fig. 11.2 Periosteal dissector and serial dilator for biportal endoscopic surgery.

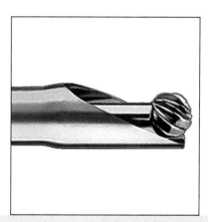

Fig. 11.3 A one-side protected drill is used for laminotomy and facetectomy.

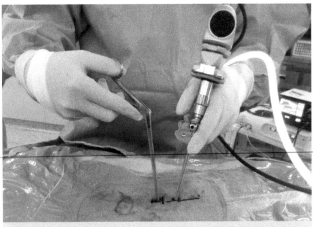

Fig. 11.4 Intraoperative view of percutaneous unilateral biportal endoscopic surgery for the lumbar spine.

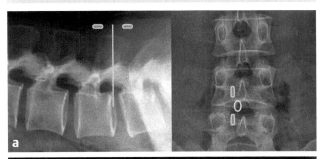

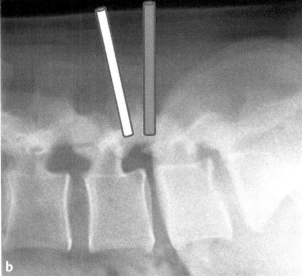

Fig. 11.5 (a) Incision points of two portals for central stenosis or herniated disk. **(b)** The cranial portal is the endoscopic channel, and the caudal portal is the working channel.

- Arthroscope
- Periosteal dissector
- Serial dilators
- Standard laminectomy instruments, such as hook dissectors, double-ended dissector, Kerrison punches, and pituitary forceps
- 3.5-mm spherical bur (ConmedLinvatec, Utica, NY), 0° 4-mm diameter arthroscope (ConmedLinvatec, Utica, NY)

- Bipolar flexible radiofrequency probe (Ellman Trigger-Flex Probe, Ellman International, NY)
- VAPR radiofrequency electrode (DePuy Mitec, Warsaw, IN)
- Pressure-pump irrigation system (Smith & Nephew, Inc., Memphis, Tennessee)

11.4 Surgical Procedure

UBE surgery is similar to an arthroscopic or a thoracoscopic operation (**Fig. 11.4**). The procedure is performed under general or epidural anesthesia. The patient is placed on a radiolucent operating table for fluoroscopic guidance. We prefer a Wilson frame or a Jackson operating table to minimize abdominal pressure in the prone position. A waterproof surgical drape is applied due to continuous saline irrigation.

11.4.1 Percutaneous Unilateral Biportal Endoscopic Diskectomy for Lumbar Disk Herniation (Video 11.1 and Video 11.2)

Two portals are made: one portal is used for continuous irrigation and endoscopic viewing, and the other portal is used for insertion and manipulation of the instruments used in diskectomy and decompression procedures (e.g., laminotomy and removal of ligamentum flavum; **Fig. 11.4**).[8]

The operation level is identified under C-arm fluoroscopic guidance. The exact target point is the intersection of the lower lamina margin and a line 1 cm lateral to the spinous process. Endoscopic and working portals are made ipsilaterally with the ruptured disk. A 1- to 1.5-cm skin incision (caudal portal) is made vertically above the target point (**Fig. 11.5**). We try to make the two portals into loose connective tissue between

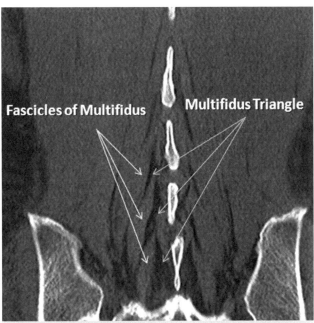

Fig. 11.6 The multifidus triangle is an area of loose connective tissue between fascicles of the multifidus muscle. Two portals are made in the triangle.

fascicles of the multifidus muscle (multifidus triangle, **Fig. 11.6**). A K-wire is introduced through the skin incision in the direction of the target point. Serial dilators are inserted toward the lower lamina.

Following removal of the dilators, a specially designed dissector (**Fig. 11.2**) is moved to the lower lamina. Interlaminar soft tissue is dissected laterally to the medial margin of the facet capsule. A second 0.5- to 1-cm incision for the endoscope (cranial portal) is made, ~ 2 to 3 cm above the upper edge of the first caudal skin incision (**Fig. 11.5**). A 0° endoscope is inserted through the cranial portal after insertion of the cannula. A saline irrigation pump is connected to the endoscope and set to a pressure of 20 to 30 mm Hg (height pressure control: 150–170 cm) during the procedure; the continuous flow of saline irrigation should clear the endoscopic surgical view and prevent bleeding in the operative field. The irrigation fluid flows from the scope portal to the working portal. Surgical instruments are inserted through the caudal working portal.

After triangulation of the endoscope and instruments (**Fig. 11.7**), radiofrequency probes are used for debridement of the soft tissue overlying the lamina and ligamentum flavum. If lower laminar and interlaminar spaces are completely exposed, the surgical endoscopic view is clearer due to expansion of holding space for irrigation fluid. Following complete exposure of the lower lamina and ligamentum flavum in the target interlaminar space, ipsilateral partial laminotomy is performed under magnified endoscopic vision, with a 3.5-mm soft tissue protected drill

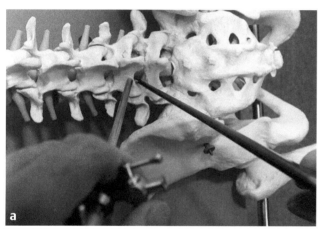

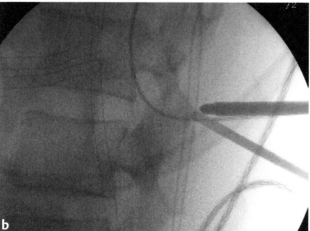

Fig. 11.7 (a,b) Triangulation with endoscope and instrument.

and Kerrison punches (**Video 11.1**). The endoscopic anatomical view is very similar to the microscopic view in posterior laminotomy and diskectomy. The ipsilateral ligamentum flavum is removed until full identification of the lateral border of the nerve root. The upper border of the lower lamina and medial border of the facet are removed (medial facetectomy) for the ipsilateral foraminotomy as needed. If there are particles from an upward- or downward-migrated ruptured disk, a more extended unilateral laminectomy of the upper or lower lamina is achieved for complete removal of the particles. According to the surgeon's preference, an additional annular incision and diskectomy can be performed after removal of the ruptured disk particles. Percutaneous unilateral biportal endoscopic diskectomy (UBED) is similar to conventional micro-diskectomy.

Case 1 (Video 11.1)

A 38-year-old female complained of severe radiating pain in the left leg refractory to conservative management. Lumbar plain radiography showed narrowing of the interlaminar space at L5 second area (**Fig. 11.8a**). Preoperative MRI showed a ruptured disk with stenosis of L5 second (**Fig. 11.8b**). We performed UBED (left-side unilateral laminotomy, medial foraminotomy, and removal of ruptured disk particles). Postoperative MRI shows complete removal of the disk particles (**Fig. 11.8c**).

Case 2 (Video 11.2)

A 48-year-old male presented with left leg pain. Preoperative MRI showed that ruptured disk particles had migrated to the L4 pedicle area (**Fig. 11.9a,b**). We performed UBED successfully. Migrated disk was completely removed (**Fig. 11.9c**). Postoperative MRI shows removal of the disk particles.

11.4.2 Percutaneous Unilateral Biportal Endoscopic Bilateral Decompression via Unilateral Approach for Lumbar Central Stenosis (Video 11.3)

Portal sites are determined by the associated lateralizing symptoms and site of disk herniation. If there are no lateralizing symptoms or disk herniation, a left-side approach is preferred for a right-handed surgeon. UBED is performed in the ipsilateral area (ipsilateral laminotomy with medial foraminotomy). Then contralateral decompression can be performed at high magnification and with a good endoscopic field of vision (**Fig. 11.10a,b**). If the endoscope is tilted to the contralateral sublaminar area, contralateral sublaminar and foraminal areas are clearly demonstrated (**Fig. 11.10a**).

Removal of contralateral ligamentum flavum and sublaminar decompression are performed with a Kerrison punch and curet. If there is thickened contralateral lamina, the ventral portion of the lamina is removed with the drill and punch. The endoscope is moved to the contralateral side by taking advantage of muscle and skin elasticity rather than by adjusting the patient's position or by making additional skin incisions. Contralateral decompression is performed until the contralateral descending nerve root has been identified and decompressed. If a patient is symptomatic and has ipsilateral disk herniation, it is possible

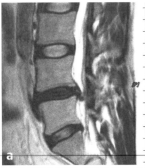
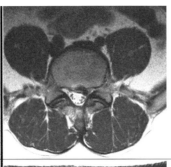
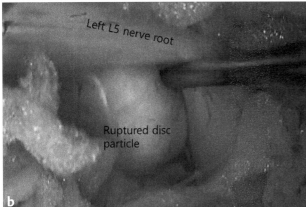
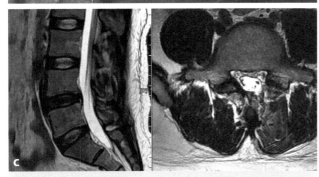

Fig. 11.8 Images of a 38-year-old woman with severe left leg pain. (**a**) Preoperative MRI shows the ruptured disk at L4–L5. (**b**) Intraoperative endoscopic image show ruptured disk particle compressed left L5 nerve root. (**c**) After percutaneous UBE discectomy, ruptured disk particles have been removed.

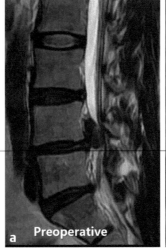
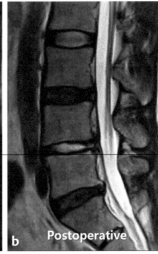
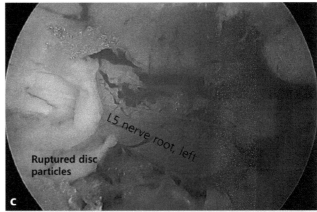

Fig. 11.9 Images of a 42-year-old man with radicular pain in the left leg. (**a**) Preoperative MRI shows that ruptured disk particles have migrated to the L4 pedicle area. (**b**) After percutaneous UBE diskectomy, migrated disk particles were completely removed. (**c**) endoscopic images shows ruptured disk particles compressed dura mater.

for the surgeon to perform a diskectomy under endoscopic view. Epidural bleeding is controlled by adjusting the pump pressure and by coagulation with flexible radiofrequency probes. The blood drainage catheter is inserted on a case-by-case basis. The skin incisions are closed after removal of the instruments and endoscope.

Case 3 (Video 11.3)

An 73-year-old man presented with pain in both legs with claudication refractory to conservative management. Severe central canal stenosis at L3–L4 was revealed at preoperative MRI (**Fig. 11.11a,b**). We performed bilateral decompression via the left-side unilateral approach using biportal endoscopic surgery. Postoperatively, the spinal canal was well decompressed, and the patient's symptoms were improved (**Fig. 11.11c,d**).

11.4.3 Percutaneous Unilateral Biportal Endoscopic Surgery for Lumbar Foraminal Stenosis and Extraforaminal Disk Herniation (Video 11.4)

Two portals are made in the paraspinal area. The target point is the midportion of the foramen in the lateral X-ray view. The first, caudal, working portal is made at the intersection of a point 1 cm lateral to the lateral border of the pedicle and the lower end plate. The second, cranial, endoscopic portal is made on the lower margin of the transverse process of the upper vertebral body under C-arm fluoroscopic guidance (**Fig. 11.12**).

A K-wire is introduced through the skin incision in the direction of the target point. Serial dilators are inserted toward the transverse process. Following removal of the dilators, a dissector is moved to the transverse process. Soft tissue is dissected at the isthmus and lateral border of the facet capsule. A 0° endoscope is inserted through the cranial portal after insertion of the

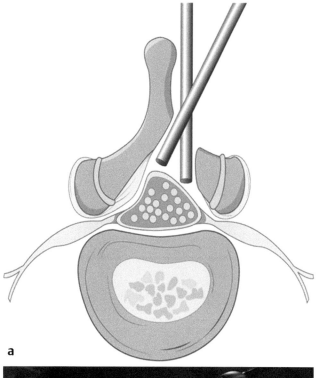

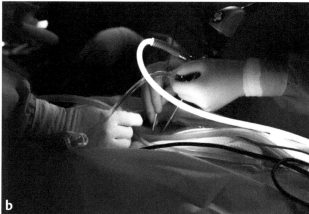

Fig. 11.10 (**a**) An endoscope is tilted to the contralateral sublaminar space for contralateral decompression. (**b**) Intraoperative picture of contralateral decompression.

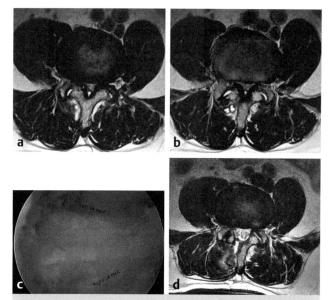

Fig. 11.11 A 73-year-old man presented with severe pain in both legs with claudication. (**a**,**b**) Preoperative MR images show spinal stenosis at L4–L5. (**c**) After UBE surgery, central canal is fully decompressed. (**d**) Postoperative MR images show good decompression status of the spinal canal.

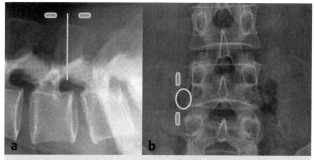

Fig. 11.12 Two points for making portals in treating foraminal stenosis or extraforaminal disk herniation. (**a**, lateral view; **b**, anteroposterior view). Triangulation target point is the midportion of the foramen.

cannula. After triangulation with the endoscope and instrument, radiofrequency probes are used for debridement of the soft tissue overlying the cranial transverse process, isthmus, and superior articular process. If there is foraminal stenosis due to hypertrophied bony structures, we remove the lower portion of the cranial transverse process, isthmus, and lateral border of the superior articular process as needed using the drill and Kerrison punch. The sacral alar portion is removed in cases of L5 second foraminal stenosis as needed. After the intertransverse ligament is carefully removed, we explore the exiting root. If there are ruptured disk particles or a protruded disk, diskectomy is performed under endoscopic view. The endoscopic anatomical view is very similar to the microscopic view in the posterior paramedian Wiltse approach.

Case 4 (Video 11.4)

A 31-year-old man complained of radicular pain in his left leg. His past history included endoscopic diskectomy for left extraforaminal disk herniation of L4–L5. MRI showed recurrent disk herniation at the left extraforaminal area of L4–L5 (**Fig. 11.13a,b**). The patient's symptoms improved after biportal endoscopic diskectomy (**Fig. 11.13c,d**)

11.5 Benefits

- Easy handling
- Familiar surgical anatomy
- Minimal muscle injury
- Use of the same surgical devices as in conventional open spinal surgery
- Easy pressure control of continuous saline irrigation due to biportal system

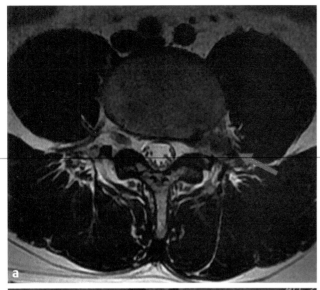

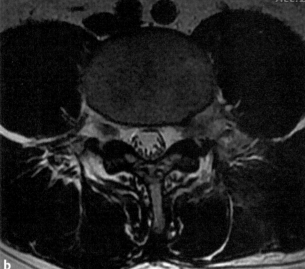

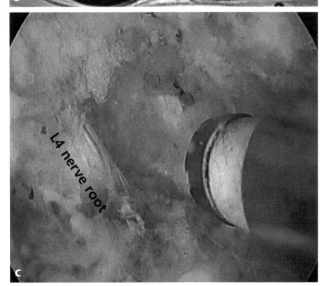

Fig. 11.13 A-31 year old man presented with left leg pain. (**a,b**) Preoperative MRI shows disk herniation in the left side extraforaminal area at L4–L5 (red arrow). (**c**) Postoperative MRI and intraoperative endoscopic image show complete removal of the ruptured disk.

- Wider surgical view than in one-portal endoscopy
- Migrated ruptured disk can be addressed
- Short learning curve

This approach uses two channels: one portal is used for the endoscope, and the other permits entry of the surgical instruments.[8,11] Therefore, the endoscopic system is similar to that used for joint arthroscopy and uses a triangulation approach. The two portals are ipsilateral, and the endoscope meets the surgical instruments at the interlaminar and epidural area. Consequently, handling of the instruments is easy and unrestricted, as in microscopic surgery. Standard laminectomy and diskectomy instruments can be inserted and used through the working portal.

This biportal endoscopic approach combines the advantages of standard open surgery and endoscopic spinal surgery. The technique is a modification and fusion of translaminar endoscopic surgery and microscopic surgery. UBE is similar to a microendoscopic tubular decompression approach.[10,12] The UBE method is based on the same operative technique as microscopic surgical procedures, such as microdiskectomy and ipsilateral microscopic laminotomy and bilateral decompression. Therefore, the surgical anatomy and endoscopic view are similar to those in conventional microscopic surgery. Furthermore, because the endoscopic surgical view is familiar to the surgeon, it may help in reducing the learning curve. The conventional one-portal endoscopic approach has surgical limitations in cases of migrated disk herniation and herniated disk with concomitant spinal stenosis. In contrast, the biportal approach safely permits extended laminectomy. Migrated disk is also an indication for biportal endoscopic surgery.

The contralateral sublaminar space can be easily viewed by shifting the endoscope without changing the patient's position. The biportal endoscopic approach allows the surgical area to be viewed at high magnification and enables a good field of vision of the contralateral, sublaminar, and foraminal areas.

Minimally invasive surgical techniques have been developed to reduce the damage to surrounding tissues,[9,13,14,15] and the UBE approach minimizes soft tissue damage. Minimizing damage to surrounding tissues can prevent postoperative back pain and muscle atrophy.[14,16]

11.6 Complications

Accidental dural tearing can occur during surgery. The dural tear site can be directly repaired by clipping under endoscopic view. A small amount epidural hematoma can develop; in our experience, it spontaneously resolves under conservative management without additional surgical intervention. Although the continuous saline irrigation system enables good visualization and reduces intraoperative bleeding, excessive irrigation may induce meningeal irritation.[17,18] The symptoms are easily controlled with conservative management, including bed rest with analgesic medication. (Some of the first patients who underwent biportal endoscopic surgery complained of meningeal irritation headache and neck pain. Because at that time the learning curve was steep, the operative time was relatively long, and the amount of saline irrigation was much greater than in more recent procedures. Fortunately, postoperative headaches did not occur in patients who were operated on more recently and who had a shortened operative time.)

11.7 Conclusion

The anatomic view in UBE surgery is very similar to that in conventional open surgery, and allows for good visualization of the contralateral, sublaminar, and foraminal areas. UBED may be an alternative and minimally invasive procedure for treatment of degenerative lumbar stenosis.

References

1   Yeung AT. The evolution and advancement of endoscopic foraminal surgery: one surgeon's experience incorporating adjunctive technologies. *SAS J* 2007;*1*(3):108–117 PubMed

2   Ahn Y. Percutaneous endoscopic decompression for lumbar spinal stenosis. *Expert Rev Med Devices* 2014;*11*(6):605–616 PubMed

3   Lee S, Kim SK, Lee SH, et al. Percutaneous endoscopic lumbar discectomy for migrated disc herniation: classification of disc migration and surgical approaches. *Eur Spine J* 2007;*16*(3):431–437 PubMed

4   Lee SH, Kang BU, Ahn Y, et al. Operative failure of percutaneous endoscopic lumbar discectomy: a radiologic analysis of 55 cases. *Spine* 2006;*31*(10):E285–E290 PubMed

5   Komp M, Hahn P, Oezdemir S, et al. Bilateral spinal decompression of lumbar central stenosis with the full-endoscopic interlaminar versus microsurgical laminotomy technique: a prospective, randomized, controlled study. *Pain Physician* 2015;*18*(1):61–70 PubMed

6   Sairyo K, Sakai T, Higashino K, Inoue M, Yasui N, Dezawa A. Complications of endoscopic lumbar decompression surgery. *Minim Invasive Neurosurg* 2010;*53*(4):175–178 PubMed

7   De Antoni DJ, Claro ML, Poehling GG, Hughes SS. Translaminar lumbar epidural endoscopy: anatomy, technique, and indications. *Arthroscopy* 1996;*12*(3):330–334 PubMed

8   Hwa Eum J, Hwa Heo D, Son SK, Park CK. Percutaneous biportal endoscopic decompression for lumbar spinal stenosis: a technical note and preliminary clinical results. *J Neurosurg Spine* 2016;*24*(4):602–607 PubMed

9   Costa F, Sassi M, Cardia A, et al. Degenerative lumbar spinal stenosis: analysis of results in a series of 374 patients treated with unilateral laminotomy for bilateral microdecompression. *J Neurosurg Spine* 2007;*7*(6):579–586 PubMed

10   Minamide A, Yoshida M, Yamada H, et al. Endoscope-assisted spinal decompression surgery for lumbar spinal stenosis. *J Neurosurg Spine* 2013;*19*(6):664–671 PubMed

11   Osman SG, Schwartz JA, Marsolais EB. Arthroscopic discectomy and interbody fusion of the thoracic spine: A report of ipsilateral 2-portal approach. *Int J Spine Surg* 2012;*6*:103–109 PubMed

12   Yoshimoto M, Miyakawa T, Takebayashi T, et al. Microendoscopy-assisted muscle-preserving interlaminar decompression for lumbar spinal stenosis: clinical results of consecutive 105 cases with more than 3-year follow-up. *Spine* 2014;*39*(5):E318–E325 PubMed

13   Poletti CE. Central lumbar stenosis caused by ligamentum flavum: unilateral laminotomy for bilateral ligamentectomy: preliminary report of two cases. *Neurosurgery* 1995;*37*(2):343–347 PubMed

14   Mobbs RJ, Li J, Sivabalan P, Raley D, Rao PJ. Outcomes after decompressive laminectomy for lumbar spinal stenosis: comparison between minimally invasive unilateral laminectomy for bilateral decompression and open laminectomy: clinical article. *J Neurosurg Spine* 2014;*21*(2):179–186 PubMed

15   Podichetty VK, Spears J, Isaacs RE, Booher J, Biscup RS. Complications associated with minimally invasive decompression for lumbar spinal stenosis. *J Spinal Disord Tech* 2006;*19*(3):161–166 PubMed

16   Hu ZJ, Fang XQ, Zhou ZJ, Wang JY, Zhao FD, Fan SW. Effect and possible mechanism of muscle-splitting approach on multifidus muscle injury and atrophy after posterior lumbar spine surgery. *J Bone Joint Surg Am* 2013;*95*(24):e192 (1–9) PubMed

17   Choi G, Kang HY, Modi HN, et al. Risk of developing seizure after percutaneous endoscopic lumbar discectomy. *J Spinal Disord Tech* 2011;*24*(2):83–92 PubMed

18   Joh JY, Choi G, Kong BJ, Park HS, Lee SH, Chang SH. Comparative study of neck pain in relation to increase of cervical epidural pressure during percutaneous endoscopic lumbar discectomy. *Spine* 2009;*34*(19):2033–2038 PubMed

12 Transforaminal Epiduroscopic Laser Annuloplasty for Diskogenic Pain

Victor Lo, Jongsun Lee, Ashley E. Brown, Alissa Redko, and Daniel H. Kim

12.1 Introduction

Low back pain can affect up to 85% of the population at some point in life.[1] In most cases, low back pain is self-limiting; however, it can become chronic and disabling in 5% of patients.[2] The precise anatomical cause can often be difficult to identify. It has been estimated that ~ 40% of chronic low back pain originates from the intervertebral disk.[3] Histologic analysis of intervertebral disk revealed significant sensory innervation in the posterolateral aspect of the annulus fibrosus.[4] Direct stimulation of the outer annulus fibrosus in vivo demonstrated concordant pain.[5]

Treatment of chronic diskogenic low back pain has been challenging. Conservative measures often fail to reduce the pain or to improve function. Lumbar arthrodesis for diskogenic pain reported only a 46% satisfactory clinical outcome rate.[6] Successful fusion by elimination of a painful motion segment has not demonstrated a significant improvement in pain and functional status.[7] In addition, the surgery is associated with its complication risks, morbidity, and prolonged recovery. This has led to the development of minimally invasive intradiskal therapeutic approaches to open surgical procedures, including intradiskal electrothermal therapy (IDET), radiofrequency ablation (RFA), cryotherapy, percutaneous endoscopic laser diskectomy (PELD), and percutaneous endoscopic laser annuloplasty (PELA).[8,9] The proposed mechanism of action of intradiskal therapy is a combination of destruction of the annular nociceptors and shrinkage of the intervertebral disk.[10,11,12]

Given that the pain-generating regions of diskogenic pain are located in the posterolateral aspect of the annulus, an extradiskal epidural approach can also be utilized for assessment and treatment. An extradiskal epidural approach has the added benefit of direct visualization with a flexible endoscope (epiduroscopy) of the epidural space and its structures. In addition, the epidural structure can be assessed to determine whether it is concordant with the patient's clinical symptoms. Lumbosacral epiduroscopy has been demonstrated to be more accurate in identifying vertebral level pathology than clinical assessment or MRI.[13] In addition, epiduroscopic findings were noted to be predictive of treatment outcomes.[14] The epiduroscopic approach has been previously reported to treat lumbar stenosis and back-leg pain syndrome.[15,16,17,18,19,20,21] However, the traditional approach for epiduroscopy, with its entry site through the sacral hiatus, may be limited by bony stenosis of the hiatus, lumbar stenosis, or epidural scarring from previous surgery.[22]

In combination with epiduroscopy, the use of a laser can enhance the treatment efficacy for diskogenic pain. Systematic review of the literature for use of laser in lumbar disk decompression demonstrated positive results, with 75% of patients reporting significant pain relief for 12 or more months.[23] Laser disk decompression has also been demonstrated to be comparable to diskectomy.[24] Various types of lasers have been used in managing spinal disorders.[25,26,27] One, the neodymium:yttrium-aluminum-garnet (Nd:YAG) laser, has

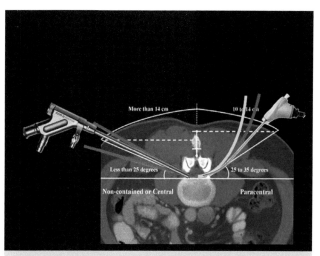

Fig. 12.1 The standard endoscope (*left*) has a fixed trajectory to the neural foramen from the skin entry site. A curved endoscope (*right*) has a similar skin entry site and can navigate into the neural foramen with a less steep trajectory, thus bypassing potential anatomical barriers.

been demonstrated to be effective in managing spine disorders in several clinical studies.[28,29,30,31]

This chapter describes an approach for the management of diskogenic pain utilizing a novel curved spinal endoscope and introduction technique in combination with a Nd:YAG laser. The curved endoscope provides transforaminal access where rigid spinal endoscopes or anatomical barriers may limit passage (**Fig. 12.1**). Transforaminal epiduroscopic laser annuloplasty (TELA) provides a minimally invasive and direct approach to the evaluation and treatment of diskogenic pain.

12.2 Indications for TELA

- Internal disk disruption (IDD)
- Herniated nucleus pulposus (HNP) with predominately axial back pain
- Annular tear
- Adhesions secondary to failed back surgery syndrome
- Diskal cyst
- Mild to moderate neuroforaminal stenosis

12.3 Contraindications to TELA

- Large HNP with radiculopathy
- Severe neuroforaminal stenosis
- Spinal instability
- Modic changes
- Patients with high iliac crest and L5–S1 level pathology

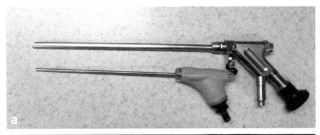

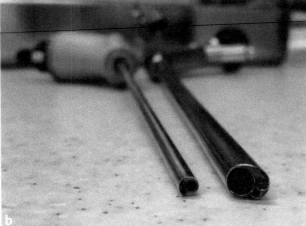

Fig. 12.2 (a,b) NeedleView CH (NeedleView CH, BioVision Technologies, Golden, Corolado) micro-endoscope compared with a Vertebris endoscope (PANOVIEW PLUS Spine Endoscope; Richard Wolf, Vernon Hills, Illinois). NeedleView CH has an outer diameter of 3.4 mm with a 1.85 mm working channel and a 160 mm working length. Vertebris has an outer diameter of 6.9 mm × 5.6 mm with a 4.1 mm working channel and a 205 mm working length.

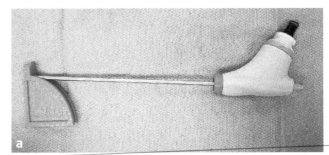

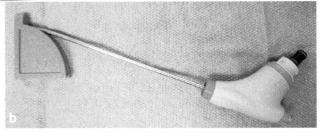

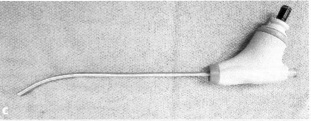

Fig. 12.3 The endoscope is bent to the desired entry angle. (a) The endoscope is placed on the molding frame. (b) A curve in the distal end is made to the desired angle. (c) The final configuration of the bent endoscope.

12.4 NeedleView HD Endoscope System

- The endoscopic system is a disposable semirigid fiberoptic-based micro-endoscope with a single working channel (NeedleView CH; BioVision Technologies, Golden, CO). The endoscope has a 160-mm working length with a 3.4-mm outer diameter. There is a 1.85-mm diameter working channel and a built-in 0.7-mm fiberoptic channel with 17,000-pixel resolution (**Fig. 12.2**).
- The distal third of the endoscope can be bent to a desired angle to facilitate entry into the ventral epidural space from a transforaminal approach (**Fig. 12.3**).

12.5 NeedleCam HD Visualization System

- The NeedleCam HD system (NeedleCam HD; BioVision Technologies) incorporates a light-emitting diode (LED) light source and a high-resolution camera in a single compact unit.
- The light source and video images are transmitted through a single cable. The video output is connected to a high-definition display with 1920 × 1080 resolution.

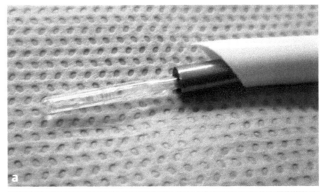

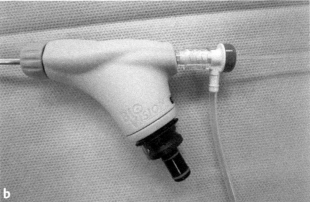

Fig. 12.4 (a) Side-firing Nd:YAG laser tip. (b) Insertion of laser fiber through the endoscope.

12.6 Laser Device

- A pulsed Nd:YAG laser with a wavelength of 1,414 nm is transmitted through 3 m fiber (Accuplasti; Lutronic, Goyang, South Korea).
- The laser is delivered through a 550 µm side-firing opening (**Fig. 12.4**).

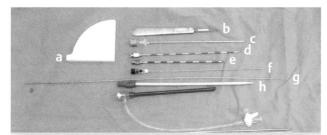

Fig. 12.5 Instruments required for introduction of the curved endoscope. **a**, Endoscope bender; **b**, No. 15 blade for skin incision; **c**, 18 G spinal needle; **d**, 18 G Tuohy needle; **e**, 14 G Tuohy needle; **f**, 21 G spinal needle; **g**, guidewire; and **h**, flexible dilator and sheath.

12.7 Equipment Required for Endoscope Introduction

See **Fig. 12.5**.

- 18 G spinal needle
- 21 G spinal needle
- 14 G × 127-mm Tuohy needle
- 18 G × 152-mm Tuohy needle
- 12 F cannula and 12 F dilator
- 70-cm guidewire
- Endoscope bender
- No. 15 blade

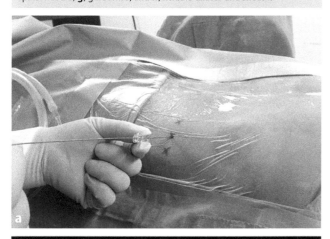

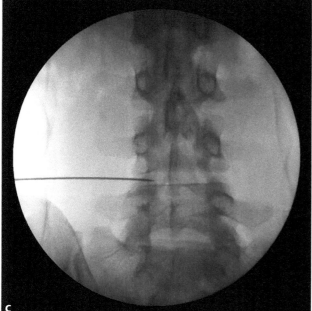

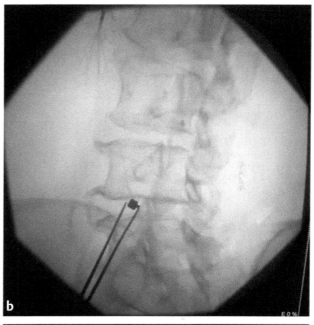

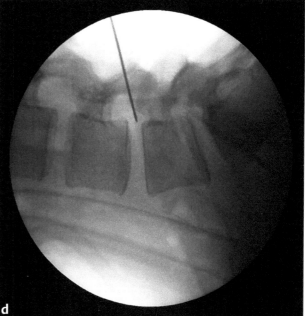

Fig. 12.6 (**a**) Insertion of spinal needle. (**b**) Oblique fluoroscopic projection to confirm trajectory to disk space. (**c**) AP fluoroscopic image to confirm needle position at neural foramen. (**d**) Lateral image to confirm needle position at the neural foramen.

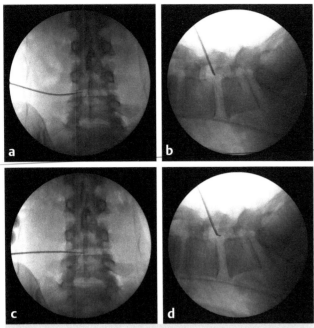

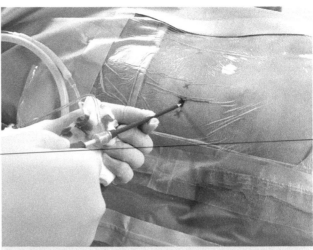

Fig. 12.8 Passage of dilator and sheath over the guidewire into the epidural space.

Fig. 12.7 (a) Fluoroscopic AP view of 14 G Tuohy needle with guidewire in lateral recess. (b) Fluoroscopic lateral view of 14 G Tuohy needle with guidewire through the foramen in lateral recess. (c) Fluoroscopic AP view after advancement of the guidewire into the ventral epidural space. (d) Fluoroscopic lateral view after advancement of guidewire into the ventral epidural space.

12.8 Anesthesia

- The procedure is performed under conscious sedation.
- Local anesthetic is administered at the skin entry site and along the trajectory of the endoscope.

12.9 Patient Positioning

- The patient is placed in the prone position on a Wilson frame and radiolucent operating table.
- The spine is flexed intraoperatively with the Wilson frame.
- The C-arm fluoroscopy unit is positioned for anteroposterior (AP) and lateral images.

12.10 Technique for TELA

- Axial MRI or CT is used to calculate the distance of the skin entry site from midline, with the trajectory to the neural foramen. The typical distance is 9 to 13 cm from midline.
- Inject the skin entry point with local anesthetic.
- The 18 G spinal needle is inserted until the epidural space is reached (Fig. 12.6a,b). This is confirmed with AP and lateral fluoroscopy (Fig. 12.6c,d).
- The stylet is then removed, and the guidewire is passed in the epidural space at the lateral recess (subarticular zone). The epidural location of the guidewire is confirmed with AP and lateral images.
- The spinal needle is then removed, and the 14 G Tuohy needle is inserted over the guidewire into the epidural space. The guidewire is then advanced into the ventral epidural space (Fig. 12.7).
- The 14 G needle is removed, and the location of the guidewire is confirmed on fluoroscopy.
- The 12 F dilator-sheath is slid over the guidewire (Fig. 12.8), and the ventral location in the epidural space is confirmed with contrast (Fig. 12.9a,b).

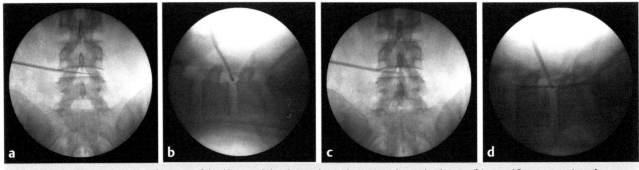

Fig. 12.9 (a) AP fluoroscopy view of passage of the dilator and sheath over the guidewire into the epidural space. (b) Lateral fluoroscopy view of passage of dilator and sheath in the epidural space. (c) Contrast injection through the sheath confirms ventral epidural location on AP fluoroscopy. (d) Contrast injection through the sheath confirms epidural position on lateral fluoroscopy.

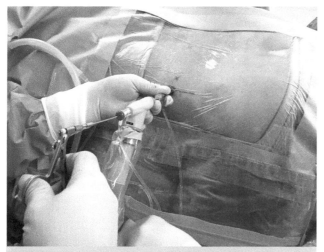

Fig. 12.10 Insertion of the endoscope into the epidural space.

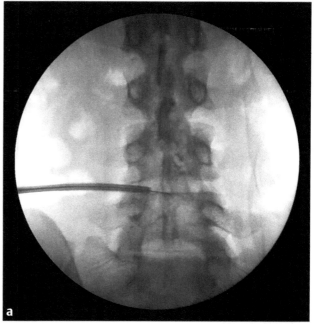

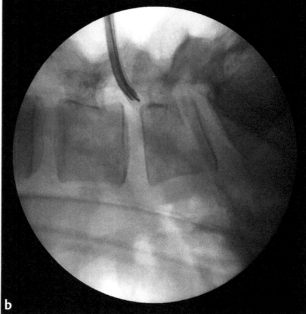

Fig. 12.11 **(a)** AP fluoroscopic confirmation of endoscope position. **(b)** Lateral fluoroscopic confirmation of endoscope position.

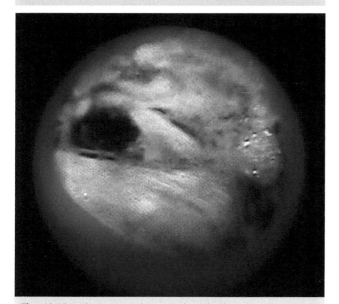

Fig. 12.12 Endoscope in the ventral epidural space: the annulus, epidural fat, and epidural space are visualized.

- After removal of the dilator, the ventral location of the sheath in the epidural space is confirmed with AP and lateral fluoroscopy, followed by contrast injection (**Fig. 12.9c,d**).
- The NeedleView micro-endoscopic camera is bent to the desired angle and is inserted into the sheath, into the epidural space (**Fig. 12.10**), and confirmed with fluoroscopy (**Fig. 12.11**). Ventral epidural anatomy is identified on endoscopy (**Fig. 12.12**).
- At this point, the epidural region can be probed (**Fig. 12.13a,b**) or diskography (**Fig. 12.13c,d**) can be performed. Endoscopic forceps can also be introduced for removal of free fragments (**Fig. 12.14**, **Fig. 12.15**).

12.11 Laser Annuloplasty

- The side-firing Nd:YAG laser is introduced through the working channel into the epidural space.

- The laser is applied (0.25 W, 150 mJ at 20 Hz, with 0.5–1.0 second pulses at intervals of 1–2 seconds) to a total energy delivery of ~ 500 J (**Fig. 12.16**).
- The laser setting can be adjusted for either thermal ablation of the nociceptive nerve endings or coagulation for annular shrinkage.

12.12 Potential Complications

- Dural or neural injury
- Annular damage
- Headaches from intracranial hypertension

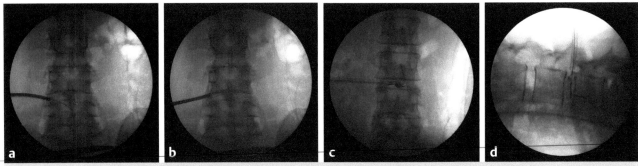

Fig. 12.13 (a) AP fluoroscopy of a probe maneuvered caudally in the ventral epidural space. (b) AP fluoroscopy of a probe maneuvered rostrally in the ventral epidural space. (c) AP fluoroscopy of diskogram. (d) Lateral fluoroscopy of a diskogram.

12.13 Illustrative Case Videos

Video 12.1 Transforaminal epiduroscopic laser annuloplasty for right L4–L5 herniated disk.

Video 12.2 Transforaminal epiduroscopic laser annuloplasty for right L3–L4 herniated disk.

12.14 Conclusion

One of the main mechanisms of diskogenic pain is damage to the posterior annulus.[32] Nociceptive free nerve endings in the annulus fibrosus represent the source of the pain-generating signals.[33,34] Initial management options include medications and physical therapy. A surgical procedure is considered after failure of conservative management. With the lack of demonstrated treatment efficacy for open surgical procedures for diskogenic

pain, minimally invasive techniques, such as IDET, RFA, PELD, and PELA, offer attractive options.[6,7,8,9]

Minimally invasive treatment options with an intradiskal approach, such as IDET, RFA, and PELA, require the creation of a new annular opening to allow entry of the treatment device. This can potentially lead to new diskogenic pain symptoms or disk herniation. An extradiskal epidural approach would eliminate the risk of further damaging the intervertebral disk during the treatment process. In addition, with intradiskal procedures, one cannot visualize the entire annular surface within the spinal canal to assess for other sites of pathology. To inspect the annular surface within the spinal canal, an endoscope can be used to visualize the epidural space. The standard spine endoscope, such as

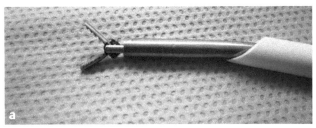

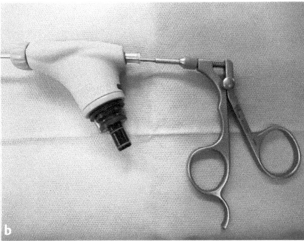

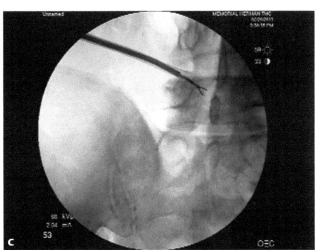

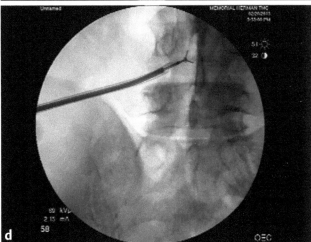

Fig. 12.14 (a) Endoscopic forceps, 1.5 mm. (b) Endoscopic forceps through the working channel. (c) AP fluoroscopy of endoscopic forceps in the ventral epidural space reaching caudally. (d) AP fluoroscopy of endoscopic forceps in the ventral epidural space reaching rostrally.

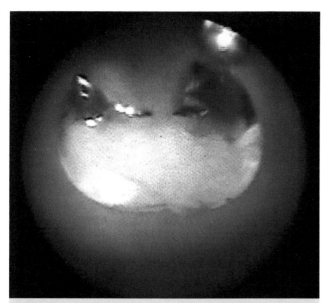

Fig. 12.15 Endoscopic forceps removing intervertebral disk material (*arrow*).

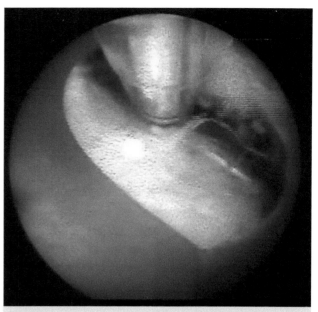

Fig. 12.16 Annuloplasty with side-firing Nd-YAG laser.

the one used in PELD, is effective for diskectomy, with less tissue disruption than in open surgery;[3] however, its rigid construction limits visualization of the entire disk surface. In addition, the position of the working channel is critical to the success of the procedure.[35] To see the entire annular portion of the disk, access into the ventral lumbar epidural space is required.

Epiduroscopy is an effective approach to access the epidural space. In addition, epiduroscopy has the benefit of direct visualization of structures within the epidural space and the ability to probe to assess whether symptoms can be reproduced. Epiduroscopy has been reported to treat lumbar stenosis and back-leg pain syndrome with an approach through the sacral hiatus.[15,16,17,18,19,20,21] Introduction of the epiduroscope through the sacral hiatus to lumbar disk pathology requires navigating the endoscope over a relatively long distance. In addition, bony stenosis of the sacral hiatus or lumbar epidural space may make passing the endoscope to the target impossible.

The chapter describes a novel approach to the ventral epidural space through the lumbar neural foramen and passage of a laser for treatment, transforaminal epiduroscopic laser annuloplasty (TELA). This is accomplished by passing a 3.4-mm outer diameter bendable endoscope in combination with a flexible sheath for a total outer diameter of 4 mm. In addition, the presence of a working channel allows the passage of endo-forceps or laser. The TELA technique uses a 1,414-nm side-firing Nd:YAG laser passed into the epidural space for thermal ablation of the free nerve endings in the annulus as well as annular shrinkage for decompression.

References

1. Andersson GB. Epidemiological features of chronic low-back pain. *Lancet* 1999;*354*(9178):581–585 PubMed
2. Andersson GB, Svensson HO, Odén A. The intensity of work recovery in low back pain. *Spine* 1983;*8*(8):880–884 PubMed
3. Schwarzer AC, Aprill CN, Derby R, Fortin J, Kine G, Bogduk N. The prevalence and clinical features of internal disc disruption in patients with chronic low back pain. *Spine* 1995;*20*(17):1878–1883 PubMed
4. Yoshizawa H, O'Brien JP, Smith WT, Trumper M. The neuropathology of intervertebral discs removed for low-back pain. *J Pathol* 1980;*132*(2):95–104 PubMed
5. Kushlich SD, Ulstrom CL, Michael CJ. The tissue origin of low back pain and sciatica: a report of pain response to tissue stimulation during operations on the lumbar spine using local anesthesia. *Orthop Clin North Am* 1991;*22*:181–187
6. Wetzel FT, LaRocca SH, Lowery GL, Aprill CN. The treatment of lumbar spinal pain syndromes diagnosed by discography. Lumbar arthrodesis. *Spine* 1994;*19*(7):792–800 PubMed
7. Mirza SK, Deyo RA. Systematic review of randomized trials comparing lumbar fusion surgery to nonoperative care for treatment of chronic back pain. *Spine* 2007;*32*(7):816–823 PubMed
8. Singh K, Ledet E, Carl A. Intradiscal therapy: a review of current treatment modalities. *Spine* 2005;*30*(17, Suppl)S20–S26 PubMed
9. Lee SH, Kang HS. Percutaneous endoscopic laser annuloplasty for discogenic low back pain. *World Neurosurg* 2010;*73*(3):198–206
10. Sachs BL, Vanharanta H, Spivey MA, et al. Dallas discogram description. A new classification of CT/discography in low-back disorders. *Spine* 1987;*12*(3):287–294 PubMed
11. Zhou Y, Abdi S. Diagnosis and minimally invasive treatment of lumbar discogenic pain—a review of the literature. *Clin J Pain* 2006;*22*(5):468–481 PubMed
12. Macnab I. Negative disc exploration. An analysis of the causes of nerve-root involvement in sixty-eight patients. *J Bone Joint Surg Am* 1971;*53*(5):891–903 PubMed
13. Bosscher HA, Heavner JE. Diagnosis of the vertebral level from which low back or leg pain originates. A comparison of clinical evaluation, MRI and epiduroscopy. *Pain Pract* 2012;*12*(7):506–512 PubMed
14. Bosscher HA, Heavner JE. Lumbosacral epiduroscopy findings predict treatment outcome. *Pain Pract* 2014;*14*(6):506–514 PubMed
15. Lee GW, Jang SJ, Kim JD. The efficacy of epiduroscopic neural decompression with Ho:YAG laser ablation in lumbar spinal stenosis. *Eur J Orthop Surg Traumatol* 2014;*24*(Suppl 1):S231–S237 PubMed
16. Ruetten S, Meyer O, Godolias G. Endoscopic surgery of the lumbar epidural space (epiduroscopy): results of therapeutic intervention in 93 patients. *Minim Invasive Neurosurg* 2003;*46*(1):1–4 PubMed
17. Jo DH, Kim ED, Oh HJ. The comparison of the result of epiduroscopic laser neural decompression between FBSS or not. *Korean J Pain* 2014;*27*(1):63–67 PubMed
18. Kallewaard JW, Vanelderen P, Richardson J, Van Zundert J, Heavner J, Groen GJ. Epiduroscopy for patients with lumbosacral radicular pain. *Pain Pract* 2014;*14*(4):365–377 PubMed
19. Igarashi T, Hirabayashi Y, Seo N, Saitoh K, Fukuda H, Suzuki H. Lysis of adhesions and epidural injection of steroid/local anaesthetic during epiduroscopy potentially alleviate low back and leg pain in elderly patients with lumbar spinal stenosis. *Br J Anaesth* 2004;*93*(2):181–187 PubMed
20. Avellanal M, Diaz-Reganon G. Interlaminar approach for epiduroscopy in patients with failed back surgery syndrome. *Br J Anaesth* 2008;*101*(2):244–249 PubMed
21. Sakai T, Aoki H, Hojo M, Takada M, Murata H, Sumikawa K. Adhesiolysis and targeted steroid/local anesthetic injection during epiduroscopy alleviates pain and reduces sensory nerve dysfunction in patients with chronic sciatica. *J Anesth* 2008;*22*(3):242–247 PubMed
22. Manchikanti L, Abdi S, Atluri S, et al. An update of comprehensive evidence-based guidelines for interventional techniques in chronic spinal pain. Part II: guidance and recommendations. *Pain Physician* 2013;*16*(2, Suppl)S49–S283 PubMed

23 Brouwer PA, Brand R, van den Akker-van Marle ME, et al. Percutaneous laser disc decompression versus conventional microdiscectomy in sciatica: a randomized controlled trial. *Spine J* 2015;*15*(5):857–865 PubMed

24 Gottlob C, Kopchok GE, Peng SK, Tabbara M, Cavaye D, White RA. Holmium:YAG laser ablation of human intervertebral disc: preliminary evaluation. *Lasers Surg Med* 1992;*12*(1):86–91 PubMed

25 Pan L, Zhang P, Yin Q. Comparison of tissue damages caused by endoscopic lumbar discectomy and traditional lumbar discectomy: a randomised controlled trial. *Int J Surg* 2014;*12*(5):534–537 PubMed

26 Quigley MR, Shih T, Elrifai A, Maroon JC, Lesiecki ML. Percutaneous laser discectomy with the Ho:YAG laser. *Lasers Surg Med* 1992;*12*(6):621–624 PubMed

27 Sato M, Ishihara M, Arai T, et al. Use of a new ICG-dye-enhanced diode laser for percutaneous laser disc decompression. *Lasers Surg Med* 2001;*29*(3):282–287 PubMed

28 Choy DS, Case RB, Fielding W, Hughes J, Liebler W, Ascher P. Percutaneous laser nucleolysis of lumbar disks. *N Engl J Med* 1987;*317*(12):771–772 PubMed

29 Choy DS, Ascher PW, Ranu HS, et al. Percutaneous laser disc decompression. A new therapeutic modality. *Spine* 1992;*17*(8):949–956 PubMed

30 Gangi A, Dietemann JL, Ide C, Brunner P, Klinkert A, Warter JM. Percutaneous laser disk decompression under CT and fluoroscopic guidance: indications, technique, and clinical experience. *Radiographics* 1996;*16*(1):89–96 PubMed

31 Yonezawa T, Onomura T, Kosaka R, et al. The system and procedures of percutaneous intradiscal laser nucleotomy. *Spine* 1990;*15*(11):1175–1185 PubMed

32 Moneta GB, Videman T, Kaivanto K, et al. Reported pain during lumbar discography as a function of anular ruptures and disc degeneration. A re-analysis of 833 discograms. *Spine* 1994;*19*(17):1968–1974 PubMed

33 Bogduk N, Tynan W, Wilson AS. The nerve supply to the human lumbar intervertebral discs. *J Anat* 1981;*132*(Pt 1):39–56 PubMed

34 Bogduk N, Windsor M, Inglis A. The innervation of the cervical intervertebral discs. *Spine* 1988;*13*(1):2–8 PubMed

35 Choi KC, Lee JH, Kim JS, et al. Unsuccessful percutaneous endoscopic lumbar discectomy: a single-center experience of 10,228 cases. *Neurosurgery* 2015;*76*(4):372–380

13 Tubular Endoscopic Lumbar Laminoforaminotomy and Diskectomy [1]

Mick Perez-Cruet and Alan Mengqiao Alan Xi

13.1 Introduction

Minimally invasive surgical (MIS) approaches to spine decompression were developed with the goal of preserving paraspinal soft tissues. A microscope is typically used in MIS procedures to provide a three-dimensional (3D) view of the regional anatomy.[1,2,3] However, endoscopic approaches have been described as well.[4,5] Muscle dilators of increasing diameters can be used to approach the spine while sparing the paraspinal musculature. However, recent developments in retractor systems allow an approach to the spine in a muscle-sparing fashion but reduce the risk of insertion of K-wire or muscle dilators into the spinal canal (**Fig. 13.1**). Additionally, we have tended away from the endoscopic system and toward use of the microscope, which provides excellent 3D visualization of the anatomy and helps to facilitate the procedure (**Video 13.1**).

The METRx System (Medtronic, Memphis, TN) was one of the earliest and is one of the most frequently used tool sets in minimally invasive microdiskectomy. Our group has substantial experience with this system. The assembly consists of serial muscle dilators and a tubular retractor available in 14-, 16-, 18-, and 20-mm stainless or 18-mm disposable. The bayoneted instruments are slender and therefore greatly minimize crowding within the working channel.[6,7] This chapter describes the use of the microscope for performing minimally invasive muscle-sparing lumbar microdiskectomy and foraminotomy.

13.2 Operating Room Setup and Patient Preparation

There should be sufficient space in the operating room to accommodate the microscope and C-arm fluoroscopy, while

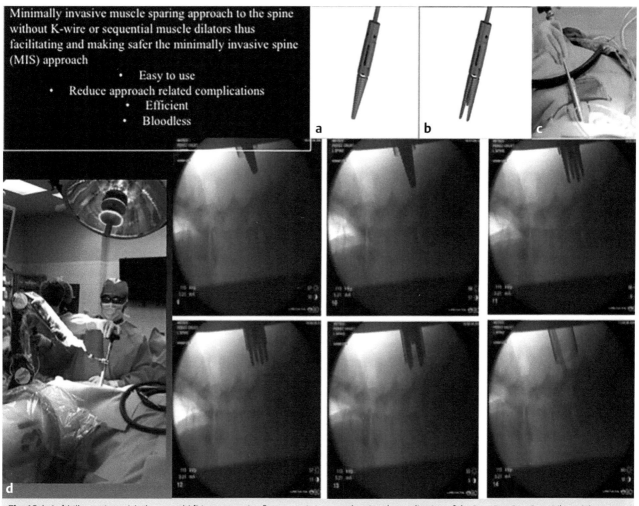

Fig. 13.1 (a,b) Illustrations, **(c)** photo, and **(d)** intraoperative fluoroscopic images showing the application of the BoneBac One-Step Dilator (Thompson MIS, Salem, NH) used in a muscle-splitting approach to the spine. The technique prevents muscle damage while approaching the spine in a bloodless fashion, and it eliminates the need for K-wire and sequential muscle dilators.

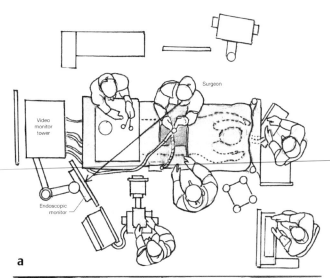

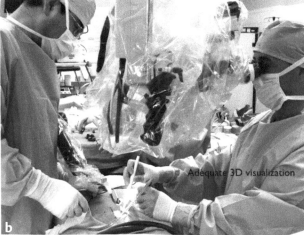

Fig. 13.2 (**a**) Operating room setup allowing the surgeon to visualize the workspace with minimal effort. (**b**) The microscope is balanced and surgically draped with a viewing port for the surgeon and assistant.

leaving abundant working area for the surgeon and operating room personnel. The patient is placed in a prone position under general anesthesia. The patient's abdomen is supported with rolls or frames to prevent excessive venous bleeding that may obscure the intraoperative view. The patient's back is sterilized and draped in a routine fashion (**Fig. 13.2**). The microscope is balanced and surgically draped with a viewing port for the surgeon and assistant (**Fig. 13.2**).

13.3 Muscle-Sparing Approach to the Spine

The level is identified using an 18 G spinal needle and lateral fluoroscopy. The needle is positioned 1.5 cm lateral to the midline and directly over the disk space of interest. Once the level is identified, the needle is removed and an incision is made 1.5 cm or a finger-breadth lateral to the midline over the disk space of interest. The lumbodorsal fascia is cut with Bovie cautery parallel to the spinous processes. The BoneBac One-Step Dilator (see Fig. 13.1) or K-wire and serial muscle dilators can be used

to approach the spine with the aid of lateral fluoroscopy to guide the approach (**Fig. 13.3**). The incision should be only as large as the diameter of the final tubular retractor (usually < 20 mm). Care is taken not to advance the K-wire or muscle dilators into the canal. We frequently dock above the spine, especially in a redo operation, and then approach the spine directly under microscope visualization. The One-Step Dilator or muscle dilators can be used to perform this portion of the procedure by docking directly on visualized laminar facet bone. Using this method, we have not experienced any dural tears or neural injury.

The first dilator is placed over the K-wire and is advanced through the soft tissue using a twisting motion. Once the dilator docks on the bony surface and its location is confirmed

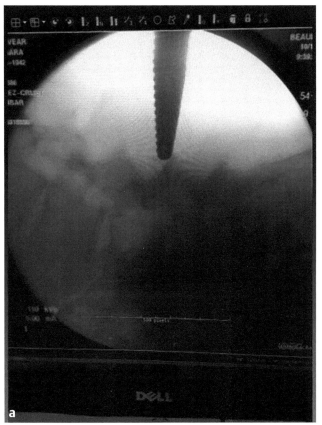

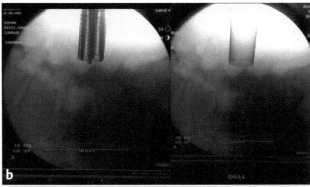

Fig. 13.3 (**a,b**) The One-Step Dilator (Thompson MIS) is introduced and deployed, allowing a cylindrical working channel to be established via the tubular retractor. This eliminates the need for K-wire and multistep dilators.

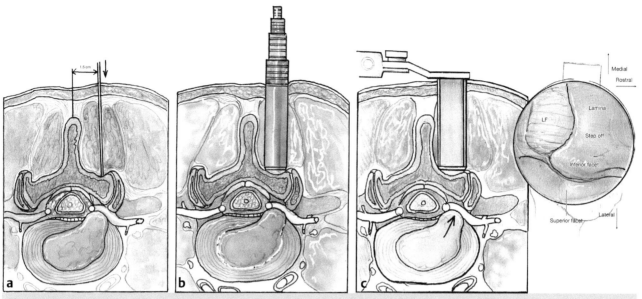

Fig. 13.4 Illustrations showing (**a**) K-wire and (**b**) sequential muscle dilators over which (**c**) a tubular retractor is placed.

on fluoroscopy, the K-wire is removed. Fluoroscopic guidance should be used for this process. It is important to pay attention to the depth of the dilator tip so that it does not enter the spinal canal. The second, third, and fourth dilators are telescoped over the initial dilator in sequence down the working trajectory onto the laminar surface (**Fig. 13.4**). The tubular retractor is then placed over the final dilator until it docks on the laminofacet junction. The distal end of the retractor features a 20° bevel tip shaped to the curvature of the bone, facilitating tight contact and preventing soft tissue from creeping under the tip and obstructing the view. Applying downward force on the retractor toward the lamina also prevents soft tissue creep. Next, the tubular retractor is secured to the flexible arm. The muscle dilators are removed, exposing a clear tubular corridor through which the procedure can be performed. A final lateral fluoroscopic image is used to confirm that the retractor is firmly in place and at the appropriate level. If repositioning is necessary, the tubular retractor is unlocked from the flexible arm, wanded toward the desired location, and locked again to the flexible arm. This maneuver enables the surgeon to place objects of interest in the center of the surgical field and facilitates the procedure.

13.4 Laminoforaminotomy and Removal of Ligamentum Flavum

From this point, the surgeon will encounter five anatomical layers, from superficial to deep: soft tissue, bony lamina and facet, ligamentum flavum, neural structures, and the intervertebral disk in question. The first three layers are removed sequentially. Note that each of the three layers should be cleared to a sufficiently large extent before pursuing a deeper layer. Otherwise, the opening becomes successively smaller at each deeper level, restricting the working space for the final diskectomy.

The bony facet and lamina can be palpated with a Bovie tip. The soft tissue is then circumferentially removed with Bovie

cautery to expose the lamina and medial facet complex. Care is taken not to disrupt the synovial capsule overlying the facet joint; however, we have encountered no adverse clinical event if this occurs.

Once the lamina and medial facet joint are exposed, an M8 cutting bur is used to perform the laminotomy. All drilled bone is collected using the BoneBac Press and is used to reconstruct the laminar defect at completion of the decompression (**Fig. 13.5**).

Once adequate laminotomy has been performed, a small curet is used to separate the ligamentum flavum from the ventral underside of the lamina. The ligament flavum is left intact to cover the underlying neural structures during bone removal. A hemilaminotomy and medial facetectomy are performed using either a Kerrison punch or drill. The ligamentum flavum is detached from the inferior cut edge of the superior lamina using a small up-going curet and by sweeping under the lamina to detach the ligament. Utmost care is taken to avoid accidental

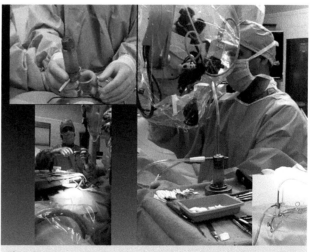

Fig. 13.5 Intraoperative photos showing use of BoneBac Press (Thompson MIS, Salem, NH) to collect the patient's drilled autograph bone for fusion material.

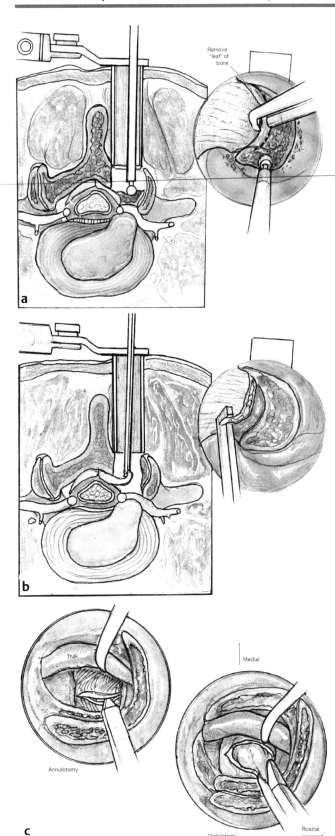

Fig. 13.6 Illustrations showing (**a**) laminotomy performed with drill and Kerrison punch while preserving the ligamentum flavum. (**b**) Exposure of rostral edge of ligamentum flavum and removal of ligament. (**c**) Exposure of traversing nerve root and preforming annulotomy with 11-blade scalpel.

dural tear. The ligamentum flavum is peeled back dorsally and caudally using a twisting motion and then is removed with a Kerrison punch (**Fig. 13.6**).

13.5 Diskectomy

Once the ligamentum flavum is sufficiently removed, the traversing nerve root may be readily visualized. Using a suction retractor, the nerve root is retracted medially for protection. The epidural space is explored. Bipolar cautery forceps or cotton patties with hemostatic agents are used to stop bleeding from epidural veins.

The disk herniation may be visualized at this point. If disk material is not already extruded, an annulotomy knife is used to introduce a puncture in the disk. The disk material is removed with a micro pituitary rongeur. Tightly packed disk material can be removed en bloc, whereas sequestrated disk material is relatively soft and is removed in a piecemeal fashion. The disk space is examined for residual fragments so that disk material is removed as much as possible. We do not scrape the adjacent vertebral body end plates, as this can devascularize the end plates and potentially lead to recurrent disk herniations. Finally, the nerve root is explored to confirm that adequate decompression has been achieved (**Fig. 13.6**).

13.6 Closure and Postoperative Care

The surgical site is irrigated generously before closure. Bipolar cautery is applied to stop any bleeding from the paraspinal muscles. The fascia is reapproximated with one or two interrupted sutures. The subcutaneous tissue is closed in an inverted manner. Mastisol skin adhesive (Ferndale Laboratories, Ferndale, MI) and Steri-Strips are applied to the surgical wound before covering it with a sterile adhesive dressing. Alternatively, Dermabond (Ethicon Endo-Surgery Inc., Somerville, NJ) is used to reapproximate the skin (**Fig. 13.7**).

The procedure is done on an outpatient basis. Postoperatively, the patient is sent to the ambulatory ward for observation and recovery. The patient is usually able to return home within one or two days, as soon as he or she is able to eat, ambulate, and void. The first follow-up is usually 2 weeks postoperatively. Some patients have reported immediate relief of symptoms, while others require a longer period of recuperation.

Furthermore, we have found that lamina reconstruction using autograft collected from the surgical site can potentially lead to reduced perineural scar formation by allowing for biological restoration of the laminar defect (**Fig. 13.8**).

13.7 Clinical Outcomes

An initial analysis of 150 consecutive patients yielded promising results.[7] The patients ranged from 18 to 76 years old (mean = 44) and consisted of 93 men and 57 women. The METRx MED system was used with the aim of reducing neural compression secondary to disk herniation. Surgery performed at different levels was as follows: three (2%) at L2–L3, 12 (8%) at L3–L4, 53 (35.3%) at L4–L5, and 82 (54.6%) at L5–S1. Outcomes were based on the modified MacNab criteria. Results of the study are shown

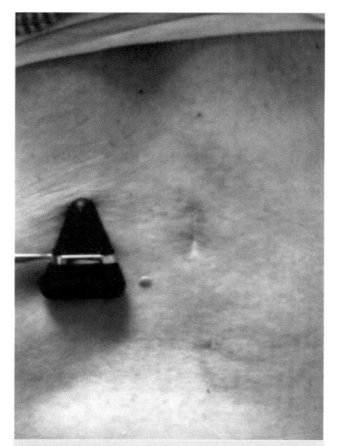

Fig. 13.7 Postoperative appearance of incision after lumbar microdiskectomy.

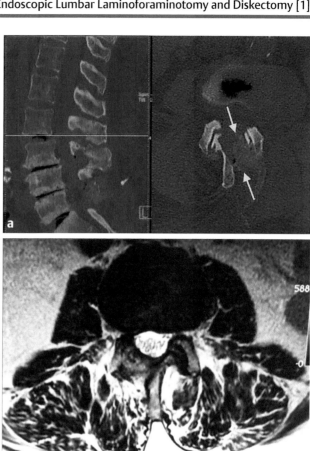

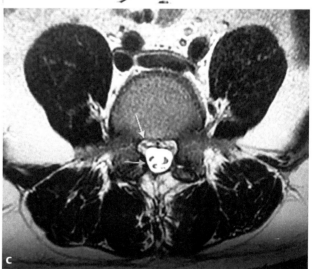

Fig. 13.8 (a) Immediate postoperative CT after minimally invasive laminectomy with biologic laminar reconstruction using autograft collected from the surgical site with the BoneBac Press. (b) Postoperative MRI taken 6 months postoperatively showing reconstructed laminar defect on the right side. (c) Comparative postoperative MRI after traditional lumbar laminectomy with noted perineural scar formation and absence of lamina and spinous process.

in **Table 13.1**. In addition, significant economic advantages were demonstrated with the MED technique, with short return-to-work time (mean 17 days), reduced hospital stays (mean 7.7 hours), and reduced operative time achieved through operative proficiency (75 minutes in the last 30 cases). A small number of patients developed complications, including eight (5.3%) with dural tears that were subsequently repaired, one (0.7%) with a superficial wound infection successfully controlled with oral antibiotics, and one (0.7%) with a delayed pseudomeningocele formation.

Table 13.1 Outcome results using the modified MacNab criteria

Outcome	Results	Definition
Excellent	77%	Complete pain and functional recovery
Good	17%	Occasional pain and return to modified work
Fair	3%	Some improved functional capacity without return to work
Poor	3%	No symptomatic or functional improvement requiring reoperation

Other teams have also investigated the effectiveness of the METRx microendoscopic system.[6,8,9,10] Their results mirrored the ones reported above. Specifically, the minimally invasive MED approach resulted in outcome scores statistically equivalent to those for the open approach, as determined by the validated visual analog scale (VAS) and Oswestry Disability Index (ODI) questionnaire systems. In addition, all authors reported reduced operative time, reduced blood loss, and decreased hospital stay.

13.8 Other Uses of the Microendoscopic Approach

As already stated, the MED approach to lumbar diskectomy requires a somewhat extended period learning period. As the surgeon develops proficiency in conducting the surgery safely and comfortably, it can be extended to address other degenerative diseases of the spine. The system can be used to perform bilateral decompression for stenosis from a single ipsilateral incision site.[11] Endoscopy enables the surgeon to achieve contralateral decompression due to its ability to visualize sublaminar contents beyond the confines of the tubular retractor. Outcomes associated with this approach are comparable to those in the open approach.[7,12,13,14] In treating cervical disk herniation using the microendoscopic posterior cervical laminoforaminotomy and diskectomy, Soliman reported 91% good to excellent postoperative improvement assessed by the Japanese Orthopaedic Association (JOA) score, the Odom criteria, and VAS score.[15] Microendoscopic transforaminal lumbar interbody fusion with instrumentation has also been used to treat lumbar spondylolisthesis.[16] All of these studies reported improved perioperative measurements, such as operative time, volume of blood loss, recovery time, and postsurgical pain.

13.9 Conclusion

Minimally invasive lumbar microdiskectomy is a safe and effective minimally invasive surgical approach for disk herniation and associated degenerative changes of the lumbar spine. The microscope provides several advantages over the use of the endoscope, including improved visualization. Although this approach can present an initial challenge to surgeons who are accustomed to traditional open procedures, the approach can be mastered with practice to improve perioperative and postoperative patient outcomes while performed on an outpatient basis.

References

1 Hellinger J. Technical aspects of the percutaneous cervical and lumbar laser-disc-decompression and -nucleotomy. *Neurol Res* 1999;21(1):99–102
2 Marks RA. Transcutaneous lumbar diskectomy for internal disk derangement: a new indication. *South Med J* 2000;93(9):885–890
3 Maroon JC, Onik G, Vidovich DV. Percutaneous discectomy for lumbar disc herniation. *Neurosurg Clin N Am* 1993;4(1):125–134
4 Foley KT, Smith MM. Microendoscopic discectomy. *Tech Neurosurg* 1997;3:301–30
5 Perez-Cruet MJ, Smith M, Foley K. Microendoscopic lumbar discectomy. In: Perez-Cruet MJ, Fessler RG, eds. *Outpatient Spinal Surgery*. St Louis, MO: Quality Medical Publishing; 2002:171–18
6 Casal-Moro R, Castro-Menéndez M, Hernández-Blanco M, Bravo-Ricoy JA, Jorge-Barreiro FJ. Long-term outcome after microendoscopic diskectomy for lumbar disk herniation: a prospective clinical study with a 5-year follow-up. *Neurosurgery* 2011;68(6):1568–1575
7 Perez-Cruet MJ, Foley KT, Isaacs RE, et al. Microendoscopic lumbar discectomy: technical note. *Neurosurgery* 2002;51(5, Suppl):S129–S136
8 Jhala A, Mistry M. Endoscopic lumbar discectomy: experience of first 100 cases. *Indian J Orthop* 2010;44(2):184–190
9 Kulkarni AG, Bassi A, Dhruv A. Microendoscopic lumbar discectomy: technique and results of 188 cases. *Indian J Orthop* 2014;48(1):81–87
10 Wu X, Zhuang S, Mao Z, Chen H. Microendoscopic discectomy for lumbar disc herniation: surgical technique and outcome in 873 consecutive cases. *Spine* 2006;31(23):2689–2694
11 Perez-Cruet MJ, Bean JR, Fessler RG. Microendoscopic lumbar discectomy. In: Perez-Cruet MJ, ed. *An Anatomic Approach to Minimally Invasive Spine Surgery*. London, U.K.: CRC Press Taylor & Francis Group; 2006:539–555
12 Castro-Menéndez M, Bravo-Ricoy JA, Casal-Moro R, Hernández-Blanco M, Jorge-Barreiro FJ. Midterm outcome after microendoscopic decompressive laminotomy for lumbar spinal stenosis: 4-year prospective study. *Neurosurgery* 2009;65(1):100–110
13 Mobbs RJ, Li J, Sivabalan P, Raley D, Rao PJ. Outcomes after decompressive laminectomy for lumbar spinal stenosis: comparison between minimally invasive unilateral laminectomy for bilateral decompression and open laminectomy: clinical article. *J Neurosurg Spine* 2014;21(2):179–186
14 Pao JL, Chen WC, Chen PQ. Clinical outcomes of microendoscopic decompressive laminotomy for degenerative lumbar spinal stenosis. *Eur Spine J* 2009;18(5):672–678
15 Soliman HM. Cervical microendoscopic discectomy and fusion: does it affect the postoperative course and the complication rate? A blinded randomized controlled trial. *Spine* 2013;38(24):2064–2070
16 Isaacs RE, Podichetty VK, Santiago P, et al. Minimally invasive microendoscopy-assisted transforaminal lumbar interbody fusion with instrumentation. *J Neurosurg Spine* 2005;3(2):98–105

14 Tubular Endoscopic Lumbar Laminoforaminotomy and Diskectomy [2]

Joachim M. Oertel and Benedikt W. Burkhardt

14.1 Introduction

Compression of neural structures in the lumbar spine is frequently caused by disk herniation. Lumbar radiculopathy is one of the most common symptoms that spine surgeons have to deal with. If conservative treatment is unsuccessful, surgery should be considered. Lumbar diskectomy and radicular decompression have been the most commonly performed surgical procedures for pathologies in this region for many decades.[1,2,3] While the traditional open approach resulted in damage to the paraspinal muscles, the technique was further refined by using an operating microscope, which offered better illumination and which allowed "mini-open" approaches in the 1970s. However, significant iatrogenic trauma was still associated with the technique.[2,3]

In the early 1990s, percutaneous dilation systems were introduced to lumbar spine surgery. The idea was to dilate the muscles instead of dissecting them from the osseous structures. In 1996, Foley and Smith introduced a system that enabled the surgeon to perform lumbar disk surgery in a standard open bimanual microsurgical technique via endoscopic visualization. Approaching the lumbar spine via dilation of the paraspinal muscles offers the advantage of less muscular damage, decreased postoperative pain, faster recovery, and shorter hospital stay.[4,5,6,7,8,9] Even recurrent disk prolapse can be successfully approached.[10] While the mid-term results are identical to the standard microdiskectomy, short-term benefits of the application of a tubular system are obvious. This chapter describes the technique for laminoforaminotomy and diskectomy using a tubular endoscopic system (EasyGO!, Karl Storz GmbH & Co. KG, Tuttlingen, Germany).

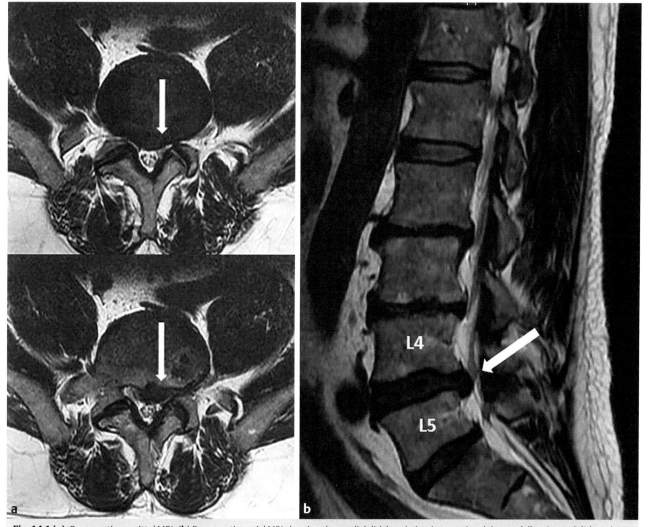

Fig. 14.1 (a) Preoperative sagittal MRI. **(b)** Preoperative axial MRI showing the medial disk herniation (**a**, *upper*) and the caudally migrated disk prolapse (**a**, *lower*).

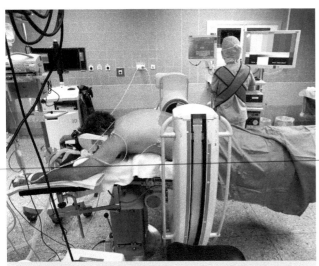

Fig. 14.2 Patient positioning and room setup.

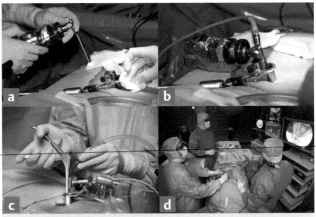

Fig. 14.3 (**a**) Skin incision, (**b,c**) insertion of the dilators, and (**d**) placement of working trocar.

14.2 Indications

- Lumbar disk herniation
- Lateral recess stenosis
- Central canal stenosis
- Lumbar synovial cyst

14.3 Exclusion Criteria

- Spinal instability

14.4 Case Presentation

- A 54-year-old man presented with a history of mild low back pain. For 8 weeks he had suffered from left sciatic pain. The leg pain was scored 8/10 on the VAS. Conservative treatment was unsuccessful.
- After heavy lifting, he developed foot drop (⅗ paresis) on the left side.

- MRI showed a central spinal stenosis with medial disk herniation and partial caudal migration in segment L4–L5 (**Fig. 14.1**).

14.5 Preoperative Plan

- Careful analysis of the ideal surgical approach is done based on preoperative imaging data (MRT, CT, myelogram, postmyelogram CT).
- If spinal instability cannot be ruled out, lateral, flexion, and extension X-rays are recommended.

14.6 Patient Positioning and Anesthesia (Video 14.1)

- The procedure is performed under general anesthesia. Perioperative antibiotics are administered.
- The patient is placed centered on the operating table in the prone position. The neck is in neutral position, and the abdomen is decompressed on a Wilson frame. Pressure points are padded, and a C-arm for lateral fluoroscopy is installed to identify the affected segment (**Fig. 14.2**).

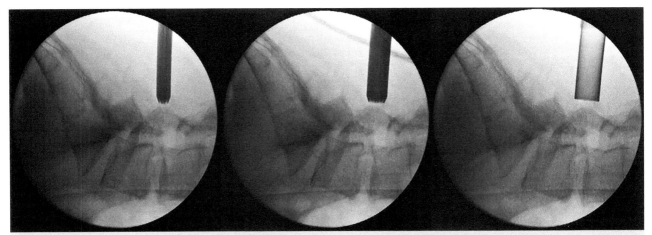

Fig. 14.4 Fluoroscopic control during application of the dilation system and positioning of the working trocar (*left to right*).

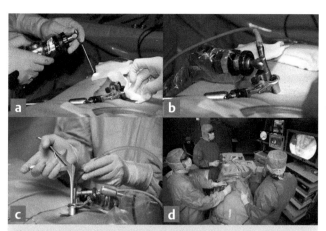

Fig. 14.5 (a,b) Insertion of the endoscope, (c) bimanual surgery, and (d) intraoperative room setup.

- Skin incision is ~ 2 cm paramedian of the spinous process on the affected side. A longitudinal incision ~ 1.0 to 2.5 cm long, depending on the selected trocar, is made (**Fig. 14.3**).

- The muscle fascia is opened. While some surgeons recommend application of a guidewire, the authors prefer to put the smallest dilator in direct contact with the bony surface of the upper vertebral lamina under lateral fluoroscopic control. Soft tissue and muscles are pushed away and dilated by sliding the various dilators one over the other. After tissue dilation, the working trocar is placed on the lamina-facet complex and fixed in position by connection to the endoscope holding arm (**Fig. 14.4**).

- The endoscope, which is connected to the three-chip high-definition (HD) camera head as well as the light cable, is introduced.

- The full-HD endoscopic unit is generally positioned contralateral to the surgeon so that the surgeon can assume a comfortable position while operating using the bimanual technique (**Fig. 14.5**).

14.7 Endoscopic Surgical Technique (Video 14.2)

- After insertion of the 30° endoscope (**Fig. 14.6**), bipolar cautery and grasper (*left and middle*) are used for removal of

remnant muscle tissue in order to display the osseous part of the spinous process (*right, white strips*), the lamina (*white stars*), and the interlaminar window (*small arrow*).

- In cases of hyperostosis and/or ossification of the ligament, a diamond drill should be used for partial laminectomy to expose the ligamentum flavum (**Fig. 14.7**). The authors recommend a diamond drill to reduce the risk of dural tear and the risk of injury to the nerve fascicles (*upper row*). When the interlaminar fenestration is large enough, a dissector or nerve hook (*lower row, middle picture*) is used to detach the ligamentum flavum from the undersurface of the lamina starting from medial to lateral.

- Once the ligamentum flavum is detached from the lamina, a Kerrison punch is used to remove the ligament and to continue with the laminotomy from medial to lateral and cranial to caudal.

- Subsequently, the interlaminar fenestration is enlarged and the decompression is directed laterally and caudally to the neuroforamen. The working channel may be need to be repositioned to achieve optimum view at the surgical field.

- If necessary, resection of the most medial part of the facet should be performed.

- Lateral fluoroscopy may be used intraoperatively to control the extent of the laminotomy or foraminotomy.

- After foraminotomy and decompression of the nerve root, a nerve hook should be passed into the neuroforamen to verify adequate decompression (**Fig. 14.8**).

- After exposure and decompression of the nerve root, a nerve hook is used to mobilize the nerve root medially and to expose the posterior longitudinal ligament (PLL) to visualize the subligamentous disk herniation.

- Scissors are used to open the PLL.

- Subsequently, the disk herniation is removed with a grasper, and diskectomy is performed (**Fig. 14.9**).

- After laminoforaminotomy and diskectomy, a nerve hook is used to verify adequate decompression.

- In cases of diffuse bleeding, a collagen sponge coated with the human coagulation factors fibrinogen and thrombin is helpful to control bleeding (**Fig. 14.10**).

- After laminoforaminotomy and diskectomy, it is recommended that the working trocar be removed under endoscopic control to detect and immediately treat bleeding sources in the paraspinal muscle. The thoracolumbar fascia can be

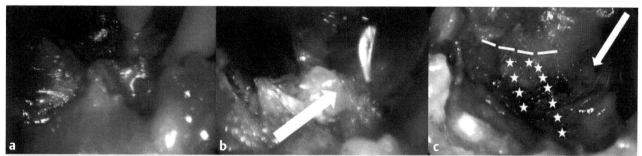

Fig. 14.6 (a,b) Removal of remnant muscle and soft tissue with bipolar cautery and grasper and**(c)** display of the spinous process and interlaminar window. *White strips*, part of the spinous process; *white stars*, lamina; *small arrow*, interlaminar window.

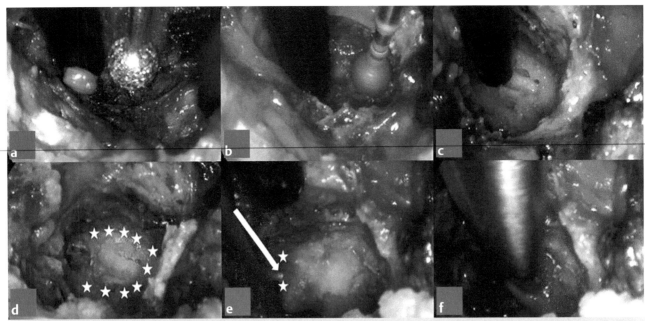

Fig. 14.7 *Upper row* (*left to right*): (**a,b**) Laminotomy with diamond drill and (**c**) exposure of the ligamentum flavum. (**d**) After identification of the ligamentum flavum (*white stars*), (**e**) the ligament (*white stars*) is mobilized with a hook (*white arrow*). (**f**) Resection of the ligament with the Kerrison punch. For orientation: the upper part of each image is medial, the lower part of each image is lateral. Left is cranial, right is caudal.

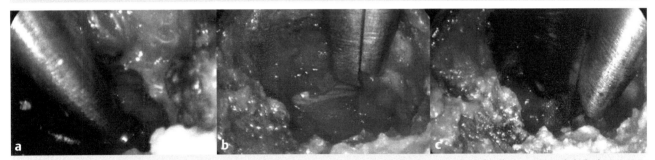

Fig. 14.8 (**a,b,c**) Exposure of the dura and foraminotomy with Kerrison punch. For orientation: the upper part of each image is medial, the lower part of each image lateral. Left is cranial, right caudal.

closed using 2.0 interrupted sutures in thin patients. In obese patients, it is advisable to coapt subcutaneous tissue, followed by use of subcuticular suture. Skin adhesive allows the patient to shower on the first postoperative day.

14.8 Tips

- The trajectory of the trocar should be perpendicular to the pathology. If a straight approach to the target point is not made, there is frequently difficulty with remnant connective and muscle tissue prolapsing into the surgical field underneath the working sheath. This can often cause significant delay in the surgical procedure.
- A skin incision that is too short makes insertion of the working sheath difficult. It also incurs a risk of skin ischemia if the sheath is inserted under too much tension.

- Application of the dilation system should be performed under fluoroscopic control to secure a perfect position of the working sheath at the lamina.
- If a very long working trocar has to be applied in very obese patients, use a larger diameter, due to the limited angulation of the instruments at depth.
- Always expose the dura and the roots from medial to lateral and from cranial to caudal to avoid dural tears and nerve root injuries.
- Tight closure of the fascia prevents subcutaneous hematoma.
- Even minimal postoperative hemorrhage might result in significant epidural hematoma, since the surgical wound is very small. Thus, do not hesitate to insert a drain if there is any doubt.
- Last, but most important:
  If you do not feel comfortable with the intraoperative situation, *then you should not hesitate to switch to an open microsurgical exposure.*

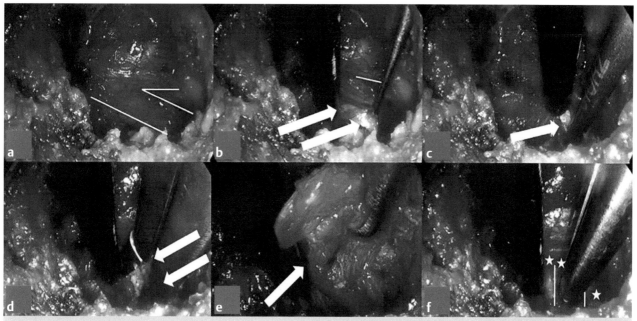

Fig. 14.9 (**a**) Exposure of dural sac and nerve root exiting laterally from the dura (*white strips*). (**b**) The disk herniation (*white arrows*) is exposed by mobilizing the nerve root medially with a nerve hook (nerve root axilla marked by *white strip*). (**c**) Incision of the PLL with endoscopic scissors (*white arrow*). (**d,e**) Removal of disk herniation (*white arrow*) with grasper (*white arrows*). (**f**) Subsequent diskectomy with grasper (*strips*) and retracted nerve root (*white stars*). For orientation: the upper part of each image is medial, the lower part of each image lateral. Left is cranial, right caudal.

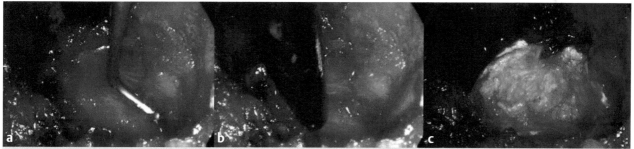

Fig. 14.10 (**a,b**) Verification of decompression with a nerve hook and (**c**) application of fibrin patch.

14.9 Postoperative Management

- Postoperative pain medication consists of a nonsteroidal anti-inflammatory drug (NSAID) in combination with a proton pump inhibitor.

- If necessary, low-potency oral narcotics may be used for postoperative management.

- Mobilization on the day of surgery should be the goal for all patients.

- Patients are encouraged to walk on the first postoperative day.

- Lifting heavy weights or excessive rotation of the lumbar spine should be avoided for 4 to 6 weeks postoperatively.

- Physical therapy for strengthening of the core muscles is recommended and can be extended to sport exercises at the time.

References

1   Mixter WJ. Rupture of the lumbar intervertebral disk: an etiologic factor for so-called "sciatic" pain. *Ann Surg* 1937;106(4):777–787
2   Caspar W. A new surgical procedure for lumbar disc herniation causing less tissue damage through a microsurgical approach. *Adv Neurosurg* 1977;4:74–80
3   Yasargil M. Microsurgical operation of herniated lumbar disc. *Adv Neurosurg* 1977;4:81
4   Khoo LT, Fessler RG. Microendoscopic decompressive laminotomy for the treatment of lumbar stenosis. *Neurosurgery* 2002;51(5, Suppl):S146–S154
5   Palmer S, Turner R, Palmer R. Bilateral decompression of lumbar spinal stenosis involving a unilateral approach with microscope and tubular retractor system. *J Neurosurg* 2002;97(2, Suppl):213–217
6   Rosen DS, O'Toole JE, Eichholz KM, et al. Minimally invasive lumbar spinal decompression in the elderly: outcomes of 50 patients aged 75 years and older. *Neurosurgery* 2007;60(3):503–509
7   O'Toole JE, Eichholz KM, Fessler RG. Surgical site infection rates after minimally invasive spinal surgery. *J Neurosurg Spine* 2009;11(4):471–476
8   Kim KT, Lee SH, Suk KS, Bae SC. The quantitative analysis of tissue injury markers after mini-open lumbar fusion. *Spine* 2006;31(6):712–716
9   Oertel JM, Mondorf Y, Gaab MR. A new endoscopic spine system: the first results with "Easy GO". *Acta Neurochir (Wien)* 2009;151(9):1027–1033
10 Smith JS, Ogden AT, Shafizadeh S, Fessler RG. Clinical outcomes after microendoscopic discectomy for recurrent lumbar disc herniation. *J Spinal Disord Tech* 2010;23(1):30–34

15 Tubular Lumbar Decompressive Laminectomy and Foraminotomy

Alan Mengqiao Alan Xi and Mick Perez-Cruet

15.1 Introduction

Lumbar spinal stenosis is one of the leading causes of low back pain, leg pain, physical disability, and reduced quality of life in the elderly population.[1] The aging intervertebral disk is prone to a series of biological changes that lead to its structural decline. As disk height is lost, the spinal canal and neural foramina can become constricted, resulting in spinal stenosis. This is further accentuated by the secondary hypertrophic changes in ligamentum flavum and facet joints.[2] Surgery represents a definitive treatment for the underlying pathology, directly addressing age-related deterioration in the structural integrity of the spine.[3] As our active population ages, an increasing number of patients have shown interest in seeking surgical intervention for spinal stenosis to maintain their quality of life.[4]

Diagnosis of lumbar spinal stenosis depends on both clinical and radiographic evidence. The typical presenting symptoms of lumbar spinal stenosis include unilateral or bilateral low back pain, leg pain, weakness, paresthesia, and neurogenic claudication. While the other symptoms are relatively obvious, neurogenic claudication may not be readily differentiated from vascular claudication. It is characterized by symptomatic relief when the lumbar spine is placed in flexion. A useful diagnostic tool is the bicycle test, where the patient is instructed to ride a stationary bicycle while leaning forward on the handles.[5] Alleviation of pain suggests neurogenic claudication, while aggravation of pain points to a vascular origin. Neurologic symptoms tend to remain benign until the very late stages of the disease, when foraminal dimensions become severely compromised. Impingement of the cauda equina can result from acute disk herniation at the level of preexisting stenosis, leading to autonomic disturbances, such as loss of bladder control.

If a constellation of these symptoms and signs are evident upon the initial visit, then plain films should be considered first to explore the existence of motion segment diseases. Once it is confirmed, the surgeon may proceed with MRI of the lumbar spine. The detailed soft tissue rendition on MRI is particularly useful in identifying disk abnormalities, facet and ligamentum flavum hypertrophy, and impinged neural structures (**Fig. 15.1**). Alternatively, myelography in conjunction with CT can be used in patients unsuitable for MRI or when the patient has had previous surgery and hardware placement. It is critical to understand, however, that a canal that appears stenotic on imaging may not be symptogenic. Surgery is indicated only in the presence of both radiographic and clinical evidence, to avoid complications associated with unnecessary decompression.

15.2 Surgical Options for Lumbar Decompression

Recently, minimally invasive spine surgery (MIS) has gained significant popularity among surgeons as an alternative to the traditional open approach. In open decompression, access to the lumbar spine is gained through a large incision, paraspinal muscles are stripped away, and the lamina is usually removed bilaterally, along with an en bloc resection of the spinous process and associated ligaments, including the ligamentum flavum. Although this method results in structurally complete decompression of the spinal canal, it imposes a large number

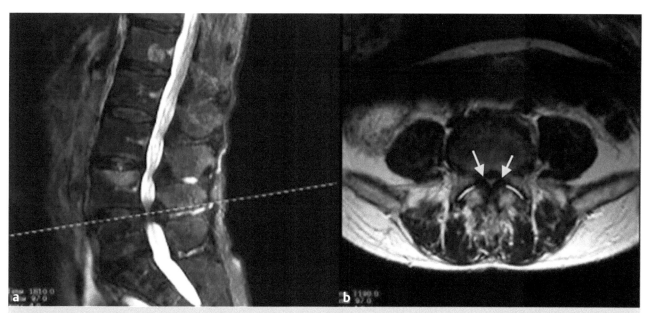

Fig. 15.1 (a) Sagittal and (b) axial T2-weighted MRI demonstrates severe spinal stenosis at the L4–L5 level and hypertrophy of the ligamentum flavum (*yellow arrows*).

of physical changes on the already degenerate spine, raising concern about too much decompression. Additionally, important structural elements of the spine are removed (i.e., spinous process and interspinous ligament) that are not part of the offending pathology. The surgical trauma and debris can lead to formation of extensive perineural scar, which may explain the suboptimal outcomes associated with open procedures (**Fig. 15.2**). Extensive paraspinal muscular retraction and injury often

lead to scar and injury of these important structural support muscles.

The minimally invasive laminectomy technique was designed as a more refined approach for the treatment of lumbar stenosis. In this method, microscopic or endoscopic visual access is achieved through a series of tubular muscle dilations, which preserve much of the musculature lining the spinal column.[6,7] Initially, a bilateral approach was used that involved paired

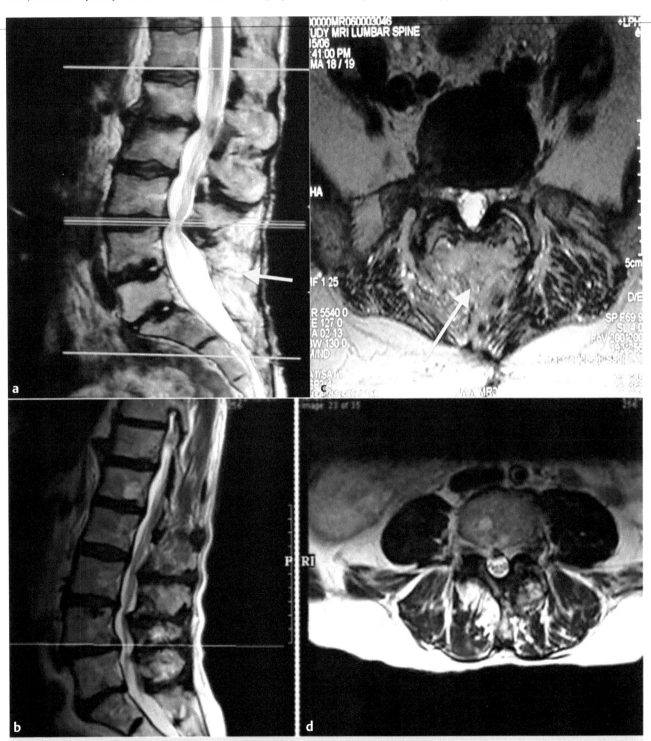

Fig. 15.2 (**a**) Sagittal and (**b**) axial T2-weighted MRIs showing open laminectomy (*top images*) versus (**c**) sagittal and (**d**) axial MRIs after minimally invasive laminectomy (*bottom images*). Note the extensive paraspinal scarring (*yellow arrow*) secondary to open decompression, while scarring is absent with the minimally invasive approach.

incisions on either side of the lumbar pathology. Later, a unilateral approach was developed to further reduce tissue damage and promote postoperative recovery.[8] This is achieved through a single paraspinal incision followed by muscle dilation to approach the spine. The ipsilateral lamina and lateral recess are first decompressed. Then the working channel is readjusted to establish a trajectory to the contralateral side, whereupon the spinous process and contralateral lamina are undercut and the contralateral neural foramen is decompressed. After bony decompression, the ligamentum flavum is removed and facet fusion is performed. The technique has been refined to ensure adequate neural decompression while achieving arthrodesis that will help to prevent recurrence of the stenosis.

The contralateral decompression procedure, however, can present a challenge to surgeons, because the line of sight is confined by the circumference of the working channel. The endoscopic camera captures images beyond the boundaries of the working channel and projects them onto a monitor. Instruments can then reach to territories not directly visible and can be manipulated with camera guidance. One of the disadvantages of using an endoscopic system, however, is that it produces two-dimensional video images rather than the stereoscopic, three-dimensional images seen with surgical microscopy. In addition, it takes a certain amount of practice to acquire the

hand-eye coordination for endoscopic maneuvers. It is therefore advisable to defer surgery on morbidly obese patients and same-level reoperation cases until considerable experience is attained, as these situations typically entail greater level of proficiency. Additionally, the camera tip of the endoscope tends to get dirty and frequently requires cleaning, which delays the procedure. For these reasons, we have moved away from the endoscope and developed a technique using the microscope. To facilitate contralateral decompression, the patient is tilted slightly away from the surgeon, the tubular retractor is wanded laterally, and the spinous process and contralateral lamina are undercut. In this manner, excellent microscopic visualization is used to achieve adequate decompression.

The METRx system (Medtronic, Memphis, TN) was one of the earliest instrument sets used for performing minimally invasive laminectomy. Our group has substantial experience with this system. The tubular retractor comes in different diameters, ranging from 14 mm to 26 mm in stainless material or 18 mm in disposable material. We typically use an 18-mm diameter tubular retractor for performing MIS laminectomy. Recently, newer systems have been developed that eliminate the K-wire and muscle dilators and allow for a safer approach to the spine (**Fig. 15.3**). Long, slender bayonetted instruments facilitate visualization through the working channel. The clinical safety

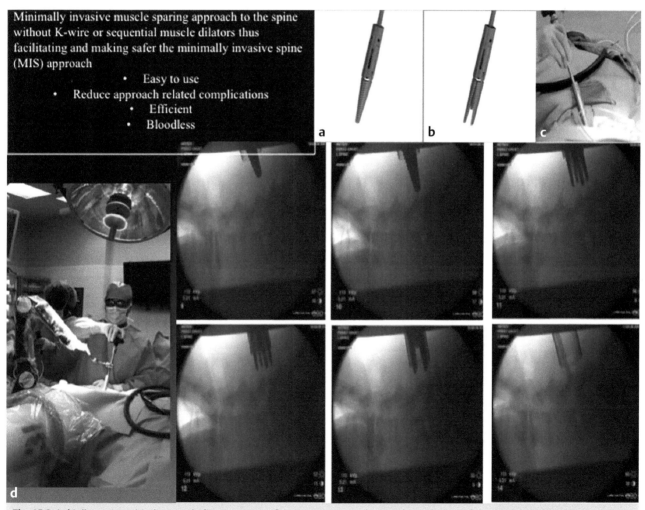

Fig. 15.3 (**a,b**) Illustrations, (**c**) photo, and (**d**) intraoperative fluoroscopic images showing the application of the One-Step Dilator (Thompson MIS, Salem, NH) to approach the spine in a muscle-splitting fashion. The technique prevents muscle damage while approaching the spine bloodlessly.

and effectiveness of this system have been investigated and confirmed by several studies.[9,10,11] This chapter describes the MIS laminectomy technique.

15.3 Preoperative Preparation

The operating room should be large enough to accommodate C-arm fluoroscopy and the microscope. The C-arm is set up for lateral imaging. The patient is prepared and draped in a standard surgical fashion under general anesthesia. The patient is positioned prone on a Wilson frame on a fluoroscopy-compatible operating table. The spine is flexed to increase the interlaminar and interspinous spaces, providing more room to accommodate instruments in the surgical site. The abdomen is allowed to hang free, to reduce intraoperative venous bleeding by decreasing abdominal back-pressure.

15.4 Establishment of Tubular Working Channel

With the appropriate surgical level identified, an 18 G spinal needle is inserted 1.5 cm lateral to the midline. Fluoroscopy is used to confirm the proper level, which should lie directly over the intervertebral disk space of interest. Spinal stenosis occurs at the disk space; thus, positioning the tubular retractor appropriately facilitates adequate and complete neural decompression. The needle is repositioned if necessary. An incision is made with scalpel and Bovie cautery parallel to the spinous process ~ 1.5 cm lateral to the midline overlying the disk space of interest. The lumbodorsal fascia is also cut parallel to the spinous process to facilitate passage of the muscle dilators through the muscles toward the spine. The incision should be only as large as the diameter of the final tubular retractor.

With the lumbodorsal fascia cut, the One-Step Dilator is advanced through the paraspinal muscles toward the facet complex (**Fig. 15.4**). Alternatively, the first and subsequent muscle dilators can be used to approach the spine, and a tubular retractor of the appropriate length is passed over the final dilator (**Fig. 15.5**) or the opened One-Step Dilator. Fluoroscopy is used to guide the approach and to confirm final docking of the tubular retractor. The tubular retractor is fastened onto a flexible arm, which in turn is anchored to the operating table. It is optimal to choose the shortest tubular retractor possible to reach the lamina so that the top of the tube sits flush on the patient's skin when locked in place.

15.5 Ipsilateral Decompression

The microscope is brought into the operative field and soft tissue is dissected and removed with electrocautery to expose the ipsilateral lamina and facet complex. If needed, lateral fluoroscopy can be used to reconfirm the proper operative level. Using a cutting M8 bur, the ipsilateral lamina is removed to expose the rostral edge of the ligamentum flavum (**Fig. 15.6**).

All drilled autograft is collected using the BoneBac Press (Thompson MIS, Salem, MA) and is used for performing bilateral facet fusion once the decompression is completed (**Fig. 15.7**).

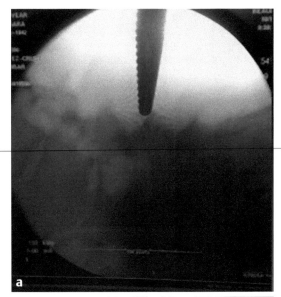
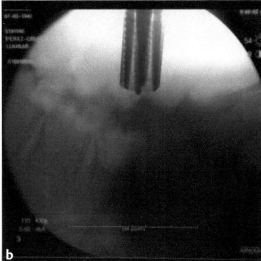
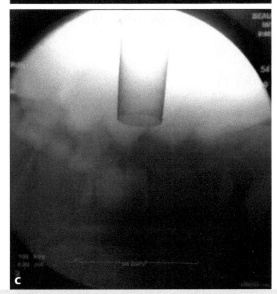

Fig. 15.4 (**a**) Intraoperative fluoroscopic images showing use of the One-Step Dilator to approach the spine. (**b**) Opening of the dilator and placement of the tubular retractor over it. (**c**) Removal of the dilator, leaving the tubular retractor in place.

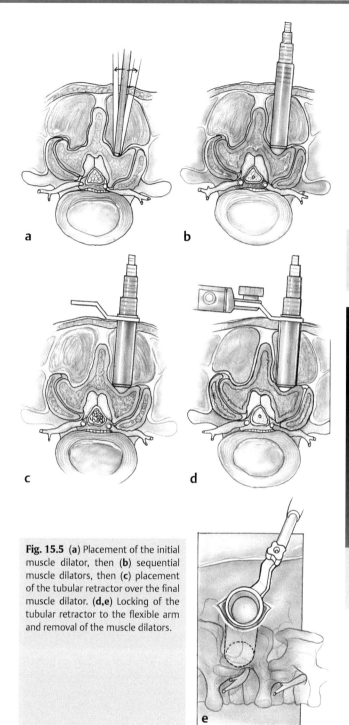

a b

c d

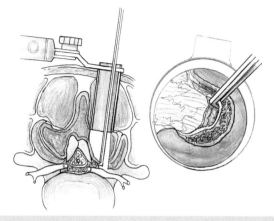

Fig. 15.6 Illustration showing ipsilateral laminectomy performed using a cutting bur on a high-speed drill. The ligamentum flavum is exposed but left in place to protect the underlying neural structure and dura during bony decompression.

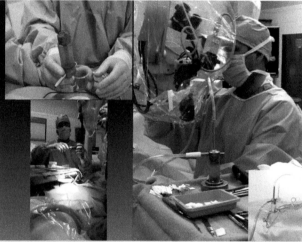

Fig. 15.7 Intraoperative photos showing use of BoneBac Press (Thompson MIS) to collect drilled autograft from the surgical site that is used for in situ bilateral posterior facet fusion after decompressive laminectomy.

Fig. 15.5 (**a**) Placement of the initial muscle dilator, then (**b**) sequential muscle dilators, then (**c**) placement of the tubular retractor over the final muscle dilator. (**d,e**) Locking of the tubular retractor to the flexible arm and removal of the muscle dilators.

e

15.6 Contralateral Decompression

Once the ipsilateral laminectomy is completed, the patient is tilted 5 to 10° away from the surgeon by slight tilting of the operating table. Care is taken not to over-tilt the table and risk movement of the patient. The tubular retractor is then angled laterally to medially to visualize the base of the spinous process on the contralateral side (**Fig. 15.8**). The key to optimal contralateral decompression is establishing a good line of sight without standing in an awkward posture. If needed, the operating table can be raised appropriately. The surgeon should maintain an ergonomically comfortable posture.

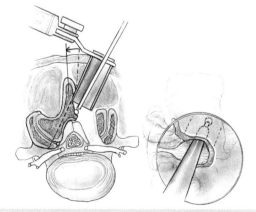

Fig. 15.8 Illustration showing tilting of the operating table away from the surgeon and movement of the tubular retractor laterally to view the base of the spinous process after ipsilateral laminectomy. Soft tissue is removed at the base of the spinous process with Bovie cautery, and the drill is used to undercut the spinous process, contralateral lamina, and medial aspect of the contralateral facet complex.

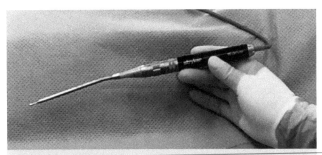

Fig. 15.9 A long tapered Stryker drill (Kalamazoo, MI) is used to perform the MIS laminectomy.

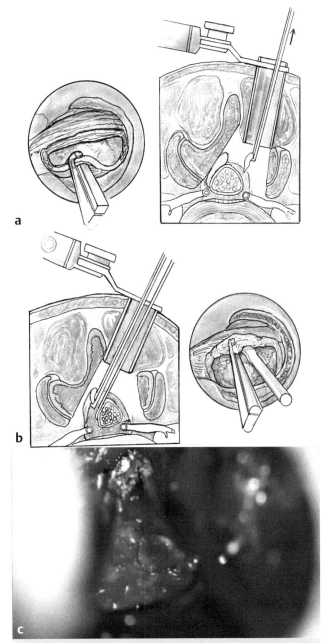

Fig. 15.10 (a) After bony decompression is achieved, the ligamentum flavum is first removed on the ipsilateral side. (b) Once ipsilateral decompression is achieved, the ligamentum flavum is removed on the contralateral side. (c) The contralateral ligamentum flavum can be shrunk with a CO_2 laser and then removed with a Kerrison punch.

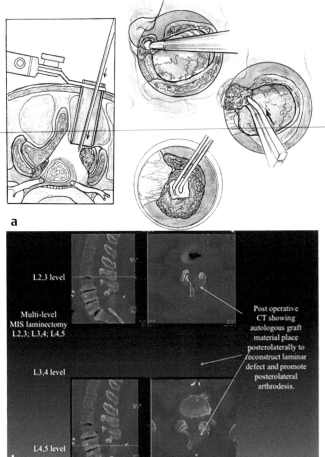

Fig. 15.11 (a) Illustrations showing placement of morselized autograft bone that was collected from the surgical site onto the decorticated ipsilateral and contralateral facet complexes to achieve a posterior arthrodesis. (b) Immediate postoperative CT showing MIS laminectomy and bone graft.

The ligamentum flavum is maintained to protect the dura during drilling. A long tapered drill is ideal for this procedure (**Fig. 15.9**).

The two sleeves of the ligamentum flavum are left in place and the midline is identified by the separation between the two sleeves. A bony shell can be left in place and removed with a Kerrison punch or further drilling after the ligamentum flavum is removed. Once bony decompression is achieved, the ligamentum flavum is removed first on the ipsilateral side and then on the contralateral side (**Fig. 15.10**). Shrinkage of the contralateral ligamentum flavum with a CO_2 laser allows easier and safer removal of the ligament with a Kerrison punch and can reduce the incidence of durotomy (**Fig. 15.10**).

After adequate decompression is achieved, morselized autograft collected using the BoneBac Press is packed into the decorticated facet joints bilaterally to achieve a posterolateral arthrodesis. This helps to stabilize the segment and to prevent recurrence of lumbar stenosis (**Fig. 15.11**). Typically, this also results in restoration of the laminectomy defect on the ipsilateral side and has been shown to potentially reduce perineural scar formation (**Fig. 15.12**, **Video 15.1**).

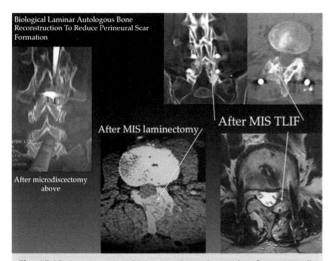

Fig. 15.12 Postoperative CT images 6 to 12 months after minimally invasive lumbar microdiskectomy, laminectomy, and transforaminal lumbar interbody fusion. Note posterior fusion and reconstruction of the laminar defect. Review of postoperative MRI images has shown reduction in perineural scar formation with this technique.

To decompress an adjacent level, the tubular retractor is removed and the spine is approached as previously described. The procedure is then repeated. Up to four adjacent levels of stenosis have been decompressed using this method.

15.7 Closure and Postoperative Care

Bovie cautery, bone wax, and thrombin-soaked Gelfoam are applied to establish complete hemostasis before closure. The tubular retractor is removed and the dilated muscles spring back to the normal anatomical position. The lumbodorsal fascia is reapproximated using interrupted 2–0 Vicryl sutures. Subcutaneous stitches and skin glue are applied to reapproximate the skin edges. The skin is typically closed with skin staples

or sutures in morbidly obese patients or patients undergoing a redo operation.

The relatively small incision and sparing of paraspinal anatomy result in faster postoperative recovery. After the surgery, the patient is sent to the ambulatory ward. Normal physical activities may be resumed as tolerated by the patient. Most patients are discharged within two days.

15.8 Conclusion

MIS laminectomy is an effective treatment for lumbar spinal stenosis. Despite the initial learning curve, the approach benefits patients by generating positive outcomes while minimizing tissue trauma, postoperative pain, and recovery time. Mastery of the technique can help a surgeon achieve excellent clinical outcomes in a cost-effective manner.

References

1   Deyo RA, Weinstein JN. Low back pain. *N Engl J Med* 2001;*344*(5):363–370
2   Benoist M. Natural history of the aging spine. *Eur Spine J* 2003;*12*(Suppl 2):S86–S89
3   Weinstein JN, Tosteson TD, Lurie JD, et al; SPORT Investigators. Surgical versus nonsurgical therapy for lumbar spinal stenosis. *N Engl J Med* 2008;*358*(8):794–810
4   Hofstetter CP, Hofer AS, Wang MY. Economic impact of minimally invasive lumbar surgery. *World J Orthop* 2015;*6*(2):190–201
5   Yukawa Y, Lenke LG, Tenhula J, Bridwell KH, Riew KD, Blanke K. A comprehensive study of patients with surgically treated lumbar spinal stenosis with neurogenic claudication. *J Bone Joint Surg Am* 2002;*84-A*(11):1954–1959
6   Aryanpur J, Ducker T. Multilevel lumbar laminotomies: an alternative to laminectomy in the treatment of lumbar stenosis. *Neurosurgery* 1990;*26*(3):429–432
7   Postacchini F, Cinotti G, Perugia D, Gumina S. The surgical treatment of central lumbar stenosis. Multiple laminotomy compared with total laminectomy. *J Bone Joint Surg Br* 1993;*75*(3):386–392
8   Young S, Veerapen R, O'Laoire SA. Relief of lumbar canal stenosis using multilevel subarticular fenestrations as an alternative to wide laminectomy: preliminary report. *Neurosurgery* 1988;*23*(5):628–633
9   Castro-Menéndez M, Bravo-Ricoy JA, Casal-Moro R, Hernández-Blanco M, Jorge-Barreiro FJ. Midterm outcome after microendoscopic decompressive laminotomy for lumbar spinal stenosis: 4-year prospective study. *Neurosurgery* 2009;*65*(1):100–110
10 Khoo LT, Fessler RG. Microendoscopic decompressive laminotomy for the treatment of lumbar stenosis. *Neurosurgery* 2002;*51*(5, Suppl):S146–S154
11 Mobbs RJ, Li J, Sivabalan P, Raley D, Rao PJ. Outcomes after decompressive laminectomy for lumbar spinal stenosis: comparison between minimally invasive unilateral laminectomy for bilateral decompression and open laminectomy. Clinical article. *J Neurosurg Spine* 2014;*21*(2):179–186

16 Tubular Endoscopic Lumbar Hemilaminectomy and Foraminotomy

Benedikt W. Burkhardt and Joachim M. Oertel

16.1 Introduction

Lumbar canal stenosis and lumbar disk herniation may cause claudication or lumbar radiopathy with pain radiating down the extremities in a dermatomal distribution, sensory deficits, and loss of motor strength. It represents one of the most common symptoms that spine surgeons have to deal with. If conservative treatment is unsuccessful, surgery should be considered for decompression of the neuronal structures. Lumbar diskectomy and laminoforaminotomy are the most commonly performed surgical approaches in surgery for pathologies in this region.[1] The traditional open approach results in damage to the paraspinal back muscles due to tissue dissection, as well as damage to the midline structures. The surgical approach was further developed by using an operating microscope, which offered better illumination of the surgical field, and consequently resulted in "mini-open" approaches in the 1970s. However, significant iatrogenic trauma was still associated with the technique.[2,3] In the early 1990s, tubular dilation systems were used for the first time in lumbar spine surgery. The idea was to dilate the muscle instead of dissecting it from the osseous structures.

Foley and Smith first introduced a system that enables the surgeon to perform lumbar disk surgery in standard open bimanual microsurgical technique via microscopic and/or additionally endoscopic visualization in 1997. This technique, using microsurgical instruments and additional endoscopic visualization, became known as microendoscopic diskectomy (MED). The technique offers the advantages of less muscle damage, decreased postoperative pain, faster postoperative recovery, and shorter in-hospital stay.[4,5,6,7,8] Furthermore, the clinical outcome after surgery via a tubular system is comparable to the standard microsurgical technique. The authors have demonstrated that several degenerative disorders of the cervical and lumbar spine can be treated effectively via microendoscopic technique.[9,10,11,12,13,14,15] This chapter describes the technique of endoscopic lumbar hemilaminectomy and foraminotomy using a tubular endoscopic system (EasyGO!, Karl Storz GmbH & Co. KG, Tuttlingen, Germany).[16,17]

16.2 Indications

- Ipsilateral mono- and bisegmental lumbar canal stenosis
- Bilateral mono- and bisegmental lumbar canal stenosis
- Lateral recess stenosis with or without subligamentous disk protrusion
- Hypertrophic facet joint with subsequent lumbar lateral recess or foraminal stenosis
- Bony foraminal stenosis and lumbar synovial cyst

16.3 Exclusion Criteria

- Spinal instability

16.4 Case Presentation

- A 65-year-old man presented with a history of mild low back pain. For 6 months he had suffered from spinal claudication with left-sided radiating leg pain. The leg pain was scored 7/10 on the visual analog scale. Walking distance had decreased to 50 to 100 m. Conservative treatment was unsuccessful.
- The preoperative examination showed foot drop (⅘ paresis) and quadriceps weakness (⅘ paresis) on the left side.
- Post-myelogram CT showed a central spinal stenosis due to hypertrophy of the ligamentum flavum in segments L3–L4 and L4–L5 (**Fig. 16.1**)

16.5 Preoperative Plan

- Careful analysis of the ideal surgical approach is done based on preoperative imaging data (MRI, CT, post-myelogram CT).

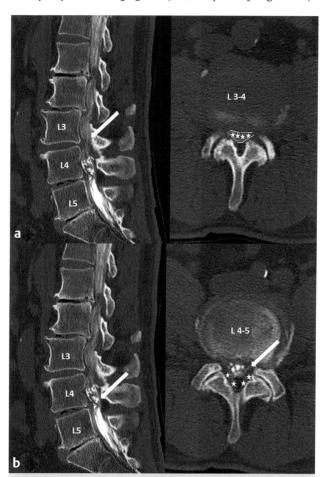

Fig. 16.1 (a) Preoperative sagittal and axial post-myelogram CT scans. The dural sac (*white stars*) is severely compressed and the contrast agent is blocked (*arrow*) in segment L3–L4 and upward. **(b)** Preoperative sagittal and axial post-myelogram CT scans shows the hypertrophied ligamentum flavum (*white stars*) and the compressed dural sac (*white arrow, right picture*).

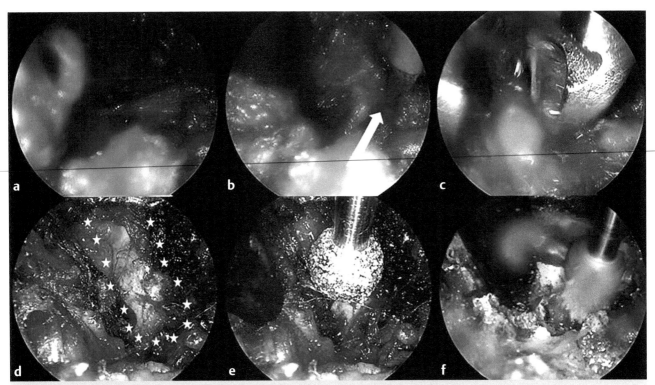

Fig. 16.2 (**a,b,c**) Removal of remnant connective tissue and display of lamina with grasping forceps and bipolar cautery. (**d**) Identification of the lamina (*white stars*). (**e,f**) Subsequent thinning out of the lamina by diamond drill. For orientation: the upper part of each image is medial, the lower part of each image lateral. Left is cranial, right caudal.

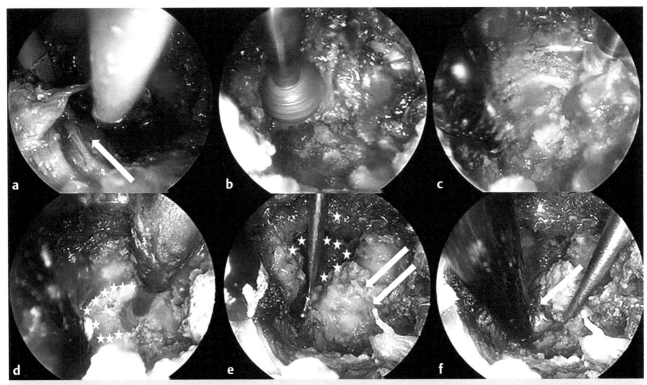

Fig. 16.3 (**a**) Bipolar cautery is used for hemostasis (*arrow*). (**b,c,d**) The hemilaminectomy is performed by subsequent thinning out of the lamina with the diamond drill and Kerrison punch. (**d**) The area of hemilaminectomy is marked with stars. (**e**) For a contralateral decompression by undercutting, the base of the spinous process has to be identified (*stars*). (**f**) Subsequently, the ligamentum flavum (*arrows*) is dissected from the dural sac with a microhook. For orientation: the upper part of each image is medial, the lower part of each image lateral. Left is cranial, right caudal.

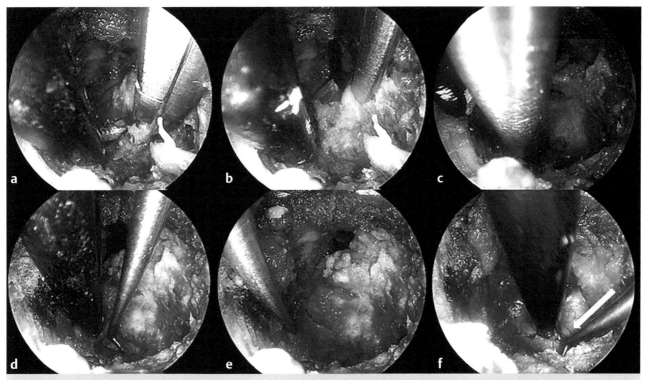

Fig. 16.4 **(a)** A grasping forceps is used for resection of the detached ligamentum flavum. **(b,c)** A 2-, 3-, and/or 4-mm Kerrison punch is used to resect the ligamentum flavum from cranial to caudal and medial to lateral. **(d)** If there are any adhesions, the microhook is applied to separate the dural sac and ligament and **(e)** to ensure sufficient decompression. **(f)** In foraminotomy, the hook (*arrow*) is used to secure sufficient nerve root decompression far into the foramen with preservation of facet joint integrity. For orientation: the upper part of each image is medial, the lower part of each image lateral. Left is cranial, right caudal.

- If spinal instability cannot be ruled out, lateral, flexion, and extension X-rays should be taken.

- Depending on the procedure and planned working trocar position, the skin incision may need to be adjusted.

16.6 Patient Position and Anesthesia (See Also Chapter 14)

- The procedure is performed under general anesthesia. Perioperative antibiotics are administered.
- The patient is centered on the operating table in the prone position, with decompression of the abdomen. Pressure points are padded, and a C-arm for lateral fluoroscopy is installed to identify the affected segment.
- Skin incision is ~ 2 cm paramedian of the spinous process for ipsilateral decompression. For bilateral decompression, the skin incision should be a little bit more lateral of the spinous process for better angulation while undercutting. The length of the skin incision is 1.1 to 2.3 cm, depending on the selected trocar.
- After the muscle fascia is dissected, the smallest dilator is put in direct contact with the bony surface of the upper vertebral lamina under lateral fluoroscopic control. Soft tissue and muscles are pushed aside and dilated by sliding the various dilators one over the other. After sequential tissue dilation, the working trocar is placed on the facet complex and is fixed in position by connection to the endoscope holding arm.
- For a monosegmental decompression, the working trocar should be placed perpendicular to the intervertebral space.
- For a bisegmental decompression, the trajectory of the working trocar should be perpendicular to the lamina.

16.7 Endoscopic Surgical Technique (Video 16.1)

- The 30° endoscope is inserted and remnant muscle and connective tissue (**Fig. 16.2a,b,c**) are removed with grasping forceps and bipolar cautery (arrow) to display the lamina (white stars, **Fig. 16.2d**).
- Subsequently, the lamina is thinned out with a diamond drill (**Fig. 16.2e,f**).
- If bleeding from the facet arteries occurs, bipolar cautery can be used to control it (**Fig. 16.3a**).
- After the ligamentum flavum is visualized, decompression is initiated by drilling the base (white stars) of the spinous process prior to undercutting (**Fig. 16.3b,c,d**).
- During the decompression, the working sheath can be repositioned to achieve a better view of the surgical field.
- For a contralateral decompression by undercutting, the base of the spinous process has to be identified (**Fig. 16.3e**).
- Once the ligamentum flavum is displayed, a nerve hook can be used to detach it from the dural sac (**Fig. 16.3e,f**; white arrow).
- A grasper can be used to remove the ligamentum flavum to further decompress the dural sac (**Fig. 16.4a,b**).
- Then a 2-, 3-, and/or 4-mm Kerrison punch can be used to remove the ligament and to continue with the decompression from medial to lateral and cranial to caudal (**Fig. 16.4b-f**).

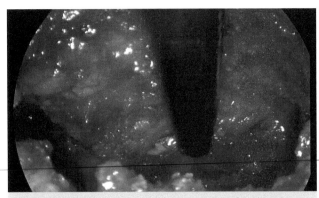

Fig. 16.5 Ipsilateral decompression with unroofing of the lateral recess by hemilaminectomy. The decompressed nerve root is seen in the left lower corner. For orientation: the upper part of each image is medial, the lower part of each image lateral. Left is cranial, right caudal.

- For hemilaminectomy, the lamina can be directly addressed and resected (**Fig. 16.5**). For foraminotomy, the authors in general recommend starting with an interlaminar fenestration and subsequently enlarging this cranially until the upper area of the neuroforamen is reached. The working channel may have to be repositioned to get a better view onto the surgical field.
- In cases of hypertrophied facet joints, the medial third of the facet has to be resected to allow access to the ipsilateral aspect of the lateral recess and the neuroforamen.
- The extent of decompression can be checked intraoperatively by lateral fluoroscopy with insertion of a nerve hook (**Fig. 16.6**).
- Bilateral decompression is also performed from cranial to caudal and from medial to lateral. The risk of an incidental durotomy can be reduced by pushing the dural sac gently away from the tip of the Kerrison punch with the suction device (**Fig. 16.7**).

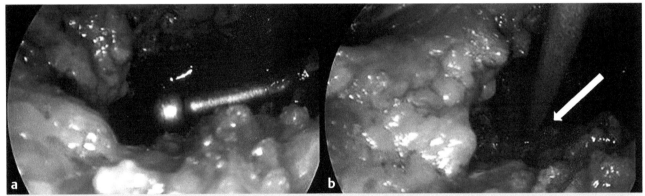

Fig. 16.6 (a) A nerve hook can be used cranial–caudal or (b) it can be brought into the neuroforamen to verify the extent of decompression. For orientation: the upper part of each image is medial, the lower part of each image lateral. Left is cranial, right caudal.

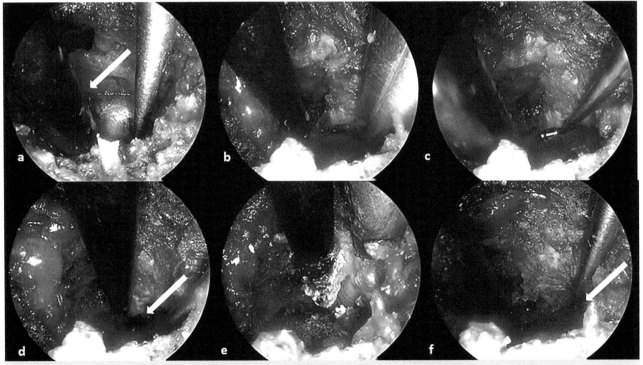

Fig. 16.7 (a,b,c) For contralateral decompression, the work sheath is directed more medially. The decompression is performed from cranial to caudal and from medial to lateral. The risk of an incidental durotomy can be reduced by pushing the dural sac gently away from the tip of the Kerrison punch with the suction device (*arrow*). (d) The extent of decompression can be controlled with a nerve hook (*arrow*). (e,f) Subsequently, remnant osseous or ligamentous structures can be drilled with a diamond bur until sufficient decompression is reached (*arrow* = nerve hook). For orientation: Since it is a contralateral decompression, the upper part of each image is lateral, and the lower part of each image is medial. Left is cranial, right caudal.

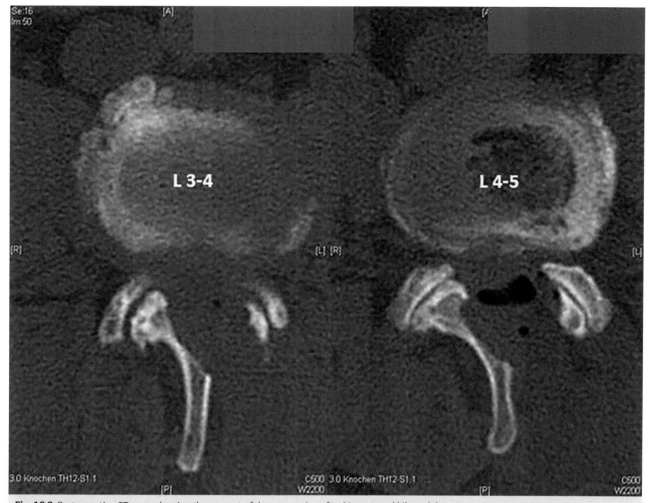

Fig. 16.8 Postoperative CT scans showing the amount of decompression after bisegmental bilateral decompression.

- A nerve hook is used to control the extent of decompression at the contralateral side.
- If necessary, remnant osseous or ligamentous structures can be drilled and/or resected to achieve adequate decompression.
- Postoperatively, CT and/or MRI can be performed to demonstrate the extent of decompression (**Fig. 16.8**).

16.8 Tips

- The trajectory of the approach should be directly to the area of decompression. If the work sheath is tilted, remnant connective and muscle tissue will prolapse into the surgical field.
- For bisegmental decompression, the working trocar should be positioned perpendicular to the lamina between both segments.
- Also, for bilateral decompression, the skin incision should be a little bit more lateral (~ 3 cm) than for a unilateral approach, for better angulation.
- The deeper the surgical field (obese patients) the more difficult it is to angulate the work sheath. Thus, a larger work sheath should be applied in very obese patients to allow as much space for manipulation as possible.

- To avoid dural tear and nerve root injury, decompression should always be performed from cranial to caudal and from medial to lateral, to follow the natural course of the nerve roots and the natural shape of the dural surface. This is particularly important in very severe lumbar canal stenosis.

16.9 Postoperative Management (See Also Chapter 14)

- Postoperative pain medication consists of a nonsteroidal anti-inflammatory drug (NSAID) in combination with a proton pump inhibitor.
- If necessary, low-potency oral narcotics may be used for postoperative management.
- Mobilization on the day of surgery should be the goal in all patients.
- In cases of dural tear, bed rest for 3 to 5 days is prescribed by some surgeons.
- Lifting heavy weights or excessive rotation of the lumbar spine should be avoided for 4 to 6 weeks postoperatively.
- Physical therapy for strengthening of the core muscles is recommended.

References

1 Mixter WJ. Rupture of the lumbar intervertebral disk: an etiologic factor for so-called "sciatic" pain. *Ann Surg* 1937;*106*(4):777–787

2 Caspar W. A new surgical procedure for lumbar disc herniation causing less tissue damage through a microsurgical approach. *Adv Neurosurg.* 1977;*4*:74–80

3 Yasargil MG. Microsurgical operation of herniated lumbar disc. *Adv Neurosurg* 1977;*(4)*:81

4 Khoo LT, Fessler RG. Microendoscopic decompressive laminotomy for the treatment of lumbar stenosis. *Neurosurgery* 2002;*51*(5, Suppl):S146–S154

5 Palmer S, Turner R, Palmer R. Bilateral decompression of lumbar spinal stenosis involving a unilateral approach with microscope and tubular retractor system. *J Neurosurg* 2002;*97*(2, Suppl):213–217

6 Rosen DS, O'Toole JE, Eichholz KM, et al. Minimally invasive lumbar spinal decompression in the elderly: outcomes of 50 patients aged 75 years and older. *Neurosurgery* 2007;*60*(3):503–509

7 O'Toole JE, Eichholz KM, Fessler RG. Surgical site infection rates after minimally invasive spinal surgery. *J Neurosurg Spine* 2009;*11*(4):471–476

8 Kim KT, Lee SH, Suk KS, Bae SC. The quantitative analysis of tissue injury markers after mini-open lumbar fusion. *Spine* 2006;*31*(6):712–716

9 Full Endoscopic Interlaminar Lumbar Disc Surgery: Is it the Gold Standard Yet? Benedikt W. Burkhardt, Mohsin Qadeer, Joachim M. K. Oertel, Salman Sharif World Spinal Column Journal, Volume 5 / No: 2 / 2014

10 Endoscopic Posterior Cervical Foraminotomy as a Treatment for Osseous Foraminal Stenosis. Joachim M. Oertel, Mark Philipps, Benedikt W. Burkhardt World Neurosurg. 2016; Vol 91, p50-57

11 The influence of prior cervical surgery on surgical outcome of endoscopic posterior cervical foraminotomy for osseous foraminal stenosis. Benedikt W. Burkhardt, Simon Müller, Joachim Oertel World Neurosurg. 2016 Jul 29. pii: S1878-8750(16)30619-2. doi: 10.1016/j.wneu.2016.07.075..

12 Endoscopic Surgical Treatment of Lumbar Synovial Cyst. Joachim M. Oertel, Benedikt W. Burkhardt World Neurosurg. 2017 Feb 26. pii: S1878-8750(17)30248-6. doi: 10.1016/j.wneu.2017.02.075.

13 Endoscopic Intralaminar Approach for the Treatment of Lumbar Disc Herniation. Joachim M. Oertel, Benedikt W. Burkhardt World Neurosurg. 2017 Apr 5. pii: S1878-8750(17)30455-2. doi: 10.1016/j.wneu.2017.03.132.

14 The visualization of the surgical field in tubular assisted spine surgery: Is there a difference between HD-endoscopy and microscopy? Benedikt W. Burkhardt, Melanie Wilmes, Salman Sharif, Joachim M. Oertel Clin Neurol Neurosurg. 2017 Apr 11;158:5-11. doi: 10.1016/j.clineuro.2017.04.010.

15 Full Endoscopic Treatment of Dural Tears in Lumbar Spine Surgery Joachim M. Oertel, Benedikt W. Burkhardt Eur Spine J. 2017, May 20 doi: 10.1007/s00586-017-5105-8.

16 Oertel JM, Mondorf Y, Gaab MR. A new endoscopic spine system: the first results with "Easy GO". *Acta Neurochir (Wien)* 2009;*151*(9):1027–1033

17 Philipps M, Oertel J. High-definition imaging in spinal neuroendoscopy. *Minim Invasive Neurosurg* 2010;*53*(3):142–146

17 Ultrasonic Bone Dissectors in Minimally Invasive Spine Surgery

Shrinivas M. Rohidas

17.1 Introduction

In the past two decades, spinal surgery has advanced greatly with the help of operating microscopes, high-speed drills, and endoscopes with high-definition (HD) cameras, and spinal surgery is entering a new era of minimalism with the help of the endoscope and HD camera. The angulation ability of the endoscope makes it easy to access the narrow corridors of the opposite side inside the spinal canal. However, when the endoscopic drill is used adjacent to soft tissues in narrow corridors, such as dura, nerve roots, spinal cord, and vessels, there is always some risk of damaging these important tissues by drilling, even under endoscopic magnified HD camera vision. The risks are high during removal of masses with hard consistency near delicate tissues. In addition, cooling fluid is required to protect soft tissues from heat injury, and endoscopic surgery may have to be interrupted frequently for irrigation and suction to clean the debris off the lens, as well as to clear fogging of the lens. Protection of the surrounding soft tissue using cotton is not recommended because of the risk of cotton tangling with the high-speed drill. The kicking movement is dangerous, particularly in deep corridors with delicate structures.

For several decades, ultrasonic aspirators have been effectively used to debulk large brain tumors and some spinal tumors.[1,2,3] Now ultrasonic bone curets are available for skull base surgery and spinal surgery.[4,5] This chapter discusses the clinical application of ultrasonic bone dissectors in minimally invasive spine surgery using Endospine—Destandau's technique. Its advantages and disadvantages in comparison to drills are included.

17.2 Clinical Material and Methods

The author has used the ultrasonic bone dissector/rasp/cutter, Sonoca 300, in conjunction with the Endospine system in surgery for spinal degenerative disorders. The surgical device is composed of a power supply unit with irrigation and suction, foot switch, handpieces, and various tips. The handpiece is bayonet-shaped, with irrigation and aspiration channels (**Fig. 17.1**).

The dissector handpiece weighs 80 g. It has a working length of 100 mm, the tip width is 4.5 mm, and the height is 3.5 mm. Irrigation is from the outside through a sheath, and aspiration is through the central channel, with a frequency of 35 kHz (**Fig. 17.2**, **Fig. 17.3**, **Fig. 17.4**).

The bone-cutting handpiece/cool knife has a working length of 100 mm, a frequency of 35 kHz, a cutting tip diameter of 3 mm, a cutting tip length of 7 mm, and a cutting width of 0.8 mm. Irrigation is from outside with no aspiration (**Fig. 17.5**, **Fig. 17.6**).

The rasp has a frequency of 35 kHz, with working length of 100 mm, and the rasp area is 4 mm². Irrigation is from the outside and inside with no aspiration. The dissector handpiece is reusable because it can be autoclaved, but the rasp and cutter

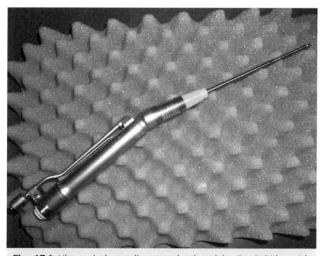

Fig. 17.1 Ultrasonic bone dissector developed by Dr. Rohidas with Soering.

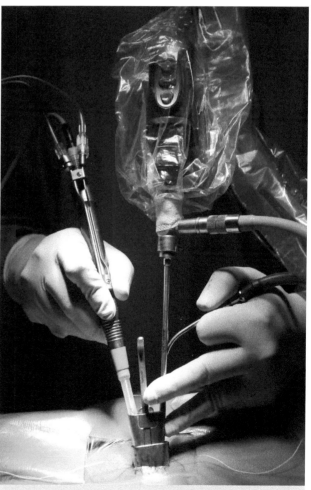

Fig. 17.2 Ultrasonic bone dissector used with Endospine.

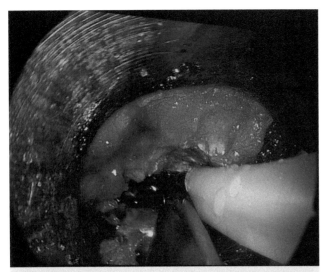

Fig. 17.3 Ultrasonic bone dissector used to undercut opposite lamina in lumbar spine.

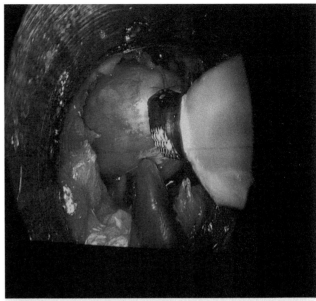

Fig. 17.4 Serrations on the ultrasonic bone dissector tip.

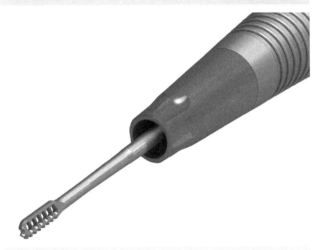

Fig. 17.5 Cool knife/ultrasonic bone cutter/loop.

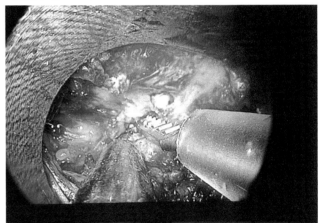

Fig. 17.6 Cool knife used with Endospine.

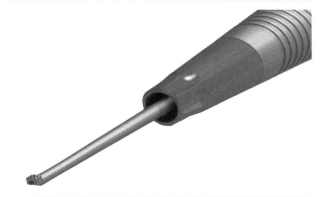

Fig. 17.7 Ultrasonic rasp.

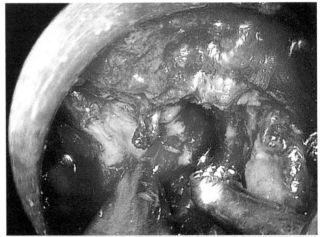

Fig. 17.8 Rasp used with Endospine in the cervical spine.

tips are not reusable, because the tips become blunt after use on bone (**Fig. 17.7**, **Fig. 17.8**).

The ultrasonic bone dissector/rasp/cutter is used to remove bone near dura, nerve root, and blood vessels in endoscopic bilateral decompression using a unilateral approach in the lumbar spine, posterior cervical diskectomy and canal decompression for stenosis, and endoscopic anterior cervical diskectomy.

17.3 Ultrasonic Basics

Ultrasonic movement is measured in Hertz. For example, 25 kHz is 25,000 Hz, equal to 25,000 cycles per second. One cycle is one Hz (**Fig. 17.9**). Less than 20 Hz is infrasound; 20 Hz to 20 kHz is the audible spectrum of sound. Ultrasound is 20 kHz to 20 MHz. Frequencies suitable for ultrasonic dissection are from 20 kHz to 60 kHz (**Fig. 17.10**).

The generator converts the main voltage into electric energy of the desired frequency. Then the converter transforms the electric energy into mechanical energy. The stack of piezoelectric quartzes transforms the electric energy of the generator into longitudinal, deformational, mechanical vibration of the sonotrode tip. The sonotrode is designed so that the entire system—converter, final mass, sonotrode—is in resonance. The stroke at the distal tip is 120 μm. The deformation movement is around 10 μm (**Fig. 17.11**).

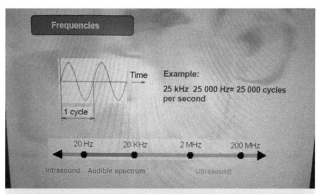

Fig. 17.9 Basic physics of ultrasonic energy.

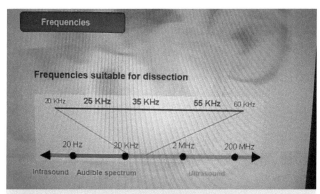

Fig. 17.10 Ultrasonic frequencies used for dissection.

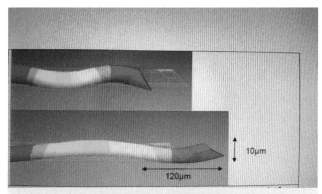

Fig. 17.11 Diagram showing tip to-and-fro and deformation movement.

Three physical effects are used: cavitation, mechanical abrasion, and thermal effect.

17.3.1 Cavitation

Pressure fluctuations are caused by the vibrating sonotrode. Forward movement of the sonotrode tip displaces the surrounding liquid, while backward movement forces the liquid to return. The pressure of the surrounding liquid changes rapidly between high and low values. Due to the high speed and mass inertia of the surrounding medium, the volume cannot be fully compensated by returning liquid. During backward movement, the pressure drops so much that the liquid evaporates and small bubbles are formed. During forward movement, the pressure rises, and the bubbles collapse. The imploding bubbles transmit high-energy pulses into their immediate vicinity. So the cascade of events is as follows:

1. Small gas bubbles are formed.
2. The gas bubbles grow because the surrounding liquid evaporates.
3. The bubbles then reach maximum volume.
4. Then implosion starts by unilateral inversion.
5. The liquid perforates the bubble wall and generates a shock wave.

Abrasion

On a hard, rigid, firm surface, the oscillating movement of the sonotrode acts like a file. Bone tissue incapable of following the vibrating sonotrode is pulverized by friction and abrasion on the edges and tips. On soft tissue, no abrasion occurs because soft tissue is pushed away from the sonotrode tip due to the tissue's elasticity. This is the basic principle of ultrasonic bone dissectors.

17.3.2 Thermal Effect

The vibrating sonotrode generates friction heat in the liquid and directly on the tissue concerned. The benefit of heat is its coagulation effect on soft tissue. For bone, local overheating is prevented by continuous irrigation of the tip.

17.4 Surgical Techniques

17.4.1 Endoscopic Bilateral Lumbar Canal Decompression Using a Unilateral Approach

Endospine is used for endoscopic bilateral canal decompression with a unilateral approach in degenerative lumbar canal stenosis. Angulation of the Endospine is used to approach the contralateral lateral recess. Here the endoscope and the working instrument are inside the spinal canal underneath the base of the spinous process in a narrow lateral recess. In degenerative canal and lateral recess stenosis due to severe medial facet hypertrophy, the lateral recess is compromised by edematous compressed nerve root. Using a drill in this narrow corridor is difficult. Slipping or kick-back of the drill may traumatize the nerve root. We use the ultrasonic bone dissector/rasp/cutter

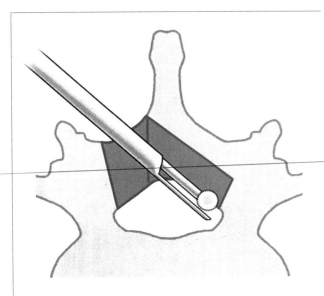

Fig. 17.12 Diagram of use of the drill to undercut the opposite lamina in lumbar canal stenosis.

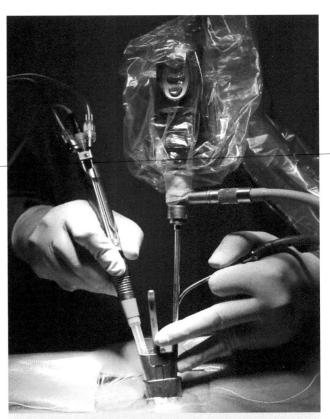

Fig. 17.13 Use of the ultrasonic bone dissector with Endospine.

to undercut the opposite lamina and medial facet. The tip of dissector/rasp/cutter is kept near the bone, and then the foot switch is turned on. Use of a scraping movement of the tip from side to side and to and fro will remove bone. Irrigation is used at approximately 7 to 9 mL/minute, with aspiration for the dissector at 80 Torr. The endoscope lens gets fogged due to irrigation fluid and bone dust. During use, the ultrasonic tip is withdrawn a little bit so that the irrigating fluid cleans the lens, and then dissection can be continued. This maneuver cleans both the lens tip and the operating area. It also helps to decrease the heat generated during use.

Over a nearly six-year period, in 755 lumbar endoscopic cases, the author has used the ultrasonic bone dissector/rasp/cutter for 100 cases. The ultrasonic bone dissector/rasp/cutter is used to shave off thick osteophyte stretching the nerve root, to undercut the opposite lamina, and to undercut the medial facet. Furthermore, in the transforaminal approach, the neural foramen is enlarged at the isthmus to decompress the exiting nerve root. The ultrasonic bone cutter is used to undercut the thick base of the spinous process at a higher lumbar level. In the lumbar region, the interlaminar distance and the interpedicular distance narrow as one proceeds cranially from the lowermost level, L5–S1. Because of this, the base of the spinous process also becomes thicker. We use the cutter to cut the base of the spinous process at a higher lumbar level in order to reach the opposite lateral recess and spinal canal (**Fig. 17.12**, **Fig. 17.13**, **Fig. 17.14**).

17.4.2 Endoscopic Posterior Cervical Diskectomy and Canal Decompression

We use Endospine with a posterior cervical approach to perform foraminotomy and opposite canal decompression with a unilateral approach. The neural foramen is widened with the ultrasonic dissector/rasp to decompress the nerve root.

Cervical canal decompression is achieved with undercutting of the base of the spinous process and opposite lamina. The endoscope and working instrument are inside the spinal canal. In the cervical region, there is very little space and the cervical cord cannot be pushed aside with cotton, unlike in the lumbar region, where the dural tube can be pushed to create some more space. Slipping or kicking of the drill over the slippery lamina in this narrow corridor can have serious complications,

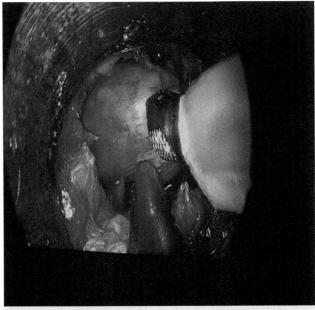

Fig. 17.14 Ultrasonic bone dissector and Endospine.

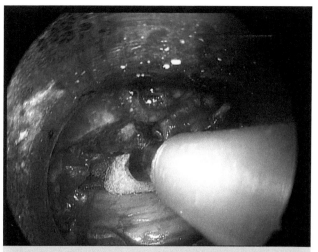

Fig. 17.16 Ultrasonic bone dissector used to undercut the opposite lamina in cervical canal stenosis. Tip is in the opposite spinal canal under the lamina.

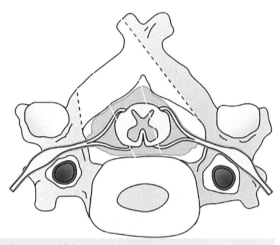

Fig. 17.15 Diagram of the angulation to show the undercutting of the opposite lamina in cervical canal stenosis.

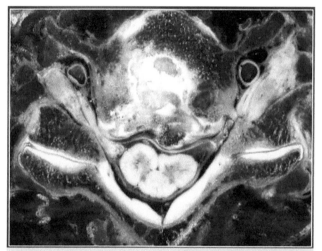

Fig. 17.17 Cervical cord and nerve root compression in degenerative pathology.

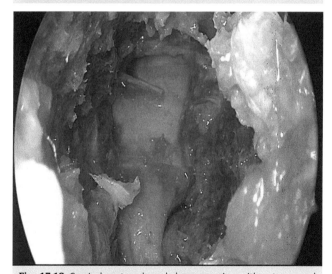

Fig. 17.18 Cervical root and cord decompression with a transuncal approach—cadaver dissection.

such as cord injury leading to quadriplegia. The ultrasonic bone dissector/rasp/cutter is used over cotton wool without pushing the cervical cord. The cotton wool and irrigating fluid help to prevent heat transfer. Out of 31 posterior cervical cases, we have used the ultrasonic dissector/rasp/cutter in 23 cases (**Fig. 17.15**, **Fig. 17.16**).

17.4.3 Endoscopic Anterior Cervical Diskectomy and Canal Decompression

The author uses Endospine to approach disk hernia through a transuncal approach. In this approach, the operating window is around 8 to 10 mm. The nerve root length from the dural sleeve to the medial border of the vertebral artery is around 6 mm. The ultrasonic bone dissector is used to remove bone over the medial border of vertebral artery. This helps to protect the vertebral artery and the venous plexus around it. For canal decompression using this approach and this small window, we have to use suction and a working instrument. While using the working instrument, one cannot put pressure over the cord. Here we use a rasp with an up-cutting edge to undercut the bone of the cranial and caudal vertebral bodies. Using the rasp is safe because the cutting edge is always away from the cord. In 52 cases of anterior cervical endoscopic diskectomy, we have used the ultrasonic dissector/rasp in 44 cases (**Fig. 17.17**, **Fig. 17.18**, **Fig. 17.19**).

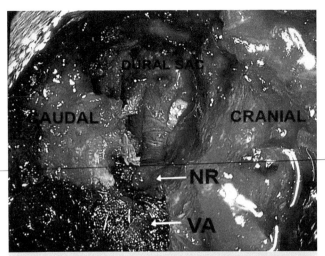

Fig. 17.19 Endoscopic view of decompressed nerve root and cord in cervical pathology.

17.5 Results

There was no major procedure-related intraoperative complication, such as cord injury, nerve root injury, or vertebral artery injury. Postoperative cerebrospinal fluid leakage did not occur. Neither intraoperative dural injury nor wound infection occurred in any case where the ultrasonic bone dissector was used.

17.6 Discussion

Complications related to spinal surgery are reported to occur with a frequency of 8.6% (1,569/18,334).[6] The complications include general complications, neurological and meningeal complications, vascular complications, infections, bone graft failure, and mechanical problems. Among these, complications related to a drilling procedure include spinal cord and nerve root injury, esophageal perforation, vascular injury, and cerebrospinal fluid leak. Thus, iatrogenic complications are relatively rare but are sometimes life-threatening, as in cord injury, vascular injury, and pharyngeal injury in anterior cervical spine surgery. With the minimal incision used in minimally invasive spinal surgery, the operative corridor is narrow. Using an endoscopic drill in such a narrow corridor requires skill and training. Due to the risk of iatrogenic injuries while drilling, training of young endoscopic spine surgeons is a very challenging task. Use of the ultrasonic bone dissector reduces the surgical complication rate.

The ultrasonic aspirator was first developed in 1947 for removal of dental plaque.[3] Flamm et al tested the ultrasonic aspirator in 1978, in studies on animal brains, to assess its efficacy and safety. They applied the ultrasonic aspirator to removal of meningiomas and schwannomas in the same year.[7]

There is always some risk of injury to the dura, neural tissue, and vessels when using high-speed drills in spine surgery, and minimally invasive spine surgery is not immune to it, in spite of the very good vision it allows in narrow corridors due to HD images. To avoid drill-related complications, the surgeon has to use both hands to hold the drill in spine surgery. When using

Endospine, we hold the drill shaft like a pencil and support it over the working channel so that it does not drop inside, and therefore the surgeon can use the drill sideways rather than to and fro. The drill tip is always at an angle of 12° from the suction and endoscope, but it is difficult to maintain the angle of the drill away from cottonoid. It is difficult to use cottonoid in a narrow corridor at depth.

The handpiece is very light (80 g), which helps to reduce operator fatigue while using it for a long period. To prevent direct thermal damage to delicate neural tissues, we use continuous irrigation. For even more safety in avoiding thermal injury, we recommend intermittent drill usage. Also, wherever possible, we use cottonoid over the nerve root and cord to prevent direct mechanical injury due to slippage or kick-back of the handpiece. Unlike with a mechanical drill, the ultrasonic drill has no risk of gripping the cottonoid.

The endoscope lens becomes dirty due to bone dust and irrigating fluid during use. The simple trick of pulling out the ultrasonic handpiece will clean the endoscope lens, rather than taking out the drill to clean it up. This is possible with the rasp and cutting tip, but with the dissector tip, which has the aspiration channel inside, a large bone fragment can block the aspiration channel. In this situation, the surgeon has to take out the handpiece and remove the block. This can be a time-consuming step.

The ultrasonic bone dissector/rasp/cutter cannot replace the routine endoscopic drill. It is very time consuming to remove large amount of bone away from neural structures. Hence it has to be used specifically to remove bone near a nerve, over cord, or near blood vessels so as to reduce operative time.

The ultrasonic bone dissector/rasp/cutter technique used for the procedures described here is the same as for other routine instruments, like the drill and Kerrison punch. In lumbar canal stenosis, to achieve bilateral canal decompression through a unilateral approach, the opposite lateral recess decompression is difficult due to the hypertrophied medial facet compressing the edematous traversing root. The challenges include the depth, narrow space, and lack of control over the tip of the instrument. The ultrasonic bone dissector/rasp cutting edge is always away from the nerve and dura. In addition to the basic safety of ultrasonic equipment, the angle between the hypertrophied facet and the cutting edge of the dissector/rasp helps to minimize trauma to neural structures. The same is true for cervical posterior canal decompression and anterior cervical diskectomy with cord decompression. Here, too, the cutting edge of the ultrasonic instrument is away from neural structures. Using a Kerrison punch in a posterior cervical approach is not possible because there is no space to maneuver the punch over the cord. Using a drill is also difficult because of the slippery edges of the lamina and ligamentum flavum. The ultrasonic dissector/rasp is safer, because even if it accidentally slips over the lamina, it does not have an effect on dura, cord, and nerve root. Also, there is no possibility of tangling the cottonoid in the drill tip.

Use of the ultrasonic bone dissector/rasp/cutter is obviously helpful and safe, and it reduces complications in endoscopic spinal surgery. However, use of this new technology involves a steep learning curve.

References

1   Flamm ES, Ransohoff J, Wuchinich D, Broadwin A. Preliminary experience with ultrasonic aspiration in neurosurgery. *Neurosurgery* 1978;2(3):240–245

2   Inoue T, Ikezaki K, Sato Y. Ultrasonic surgical system (SONOPET) for microsurgical removal of brain tumors. *Neurol Res* 2000;22(5):490–494

3   Sawamura Y, Fukushima T, Terasaka S, Sugai T. Development of a handpiece and probes for a microsurgical ultrasonic aspirator: instrumentation and application. *Neurosurgery* 1999;45(5):1192–1196

4   Hadeishi H, Suzuki A, Yasui N, Satou Y. Anterior clinoidectomy and opening of the internal auditory canal using an ultrasonic bone curette. *Neurosurgery* 2003;52(4):867–870

5   5. Inoue H, Nishi H, Shimizu T, et al. Microsurgical ligamentectomy for patients with central lumbar stenosis: a unilateral approach using an ultrasonic bone scalpel. *Spinal Surgery* 17(2)

6   Yamamoto H. Nationwide survey for spine surgery. Japan Spine Research Society, a committee report. *Spine Surgery* 1999;10(2):332–339

7   Epstein F. The Cavitron ultrasonic aspirator in tumor surgery. *Clin Neurosurg* 1983;31:497–505

18 Minimally Invasive Tubular Decompression for Foraminal Stenosis

Jung-Woo Hur and Jin-Sung Luke Kim

18.1 Introduction

Radiculopathy is most commonly caused by nerve root canal stenosis, which can be the result of various pathologies of the spine, including spondylosis, spondylolisthesis, osteophytes, and disk herniation. Lumbar spinal stenosis can be subdivided based on the location of the stenotic pathology: central stenosis (referring to medial stenosis affecting especially the cauda equina), lateral recess stenosis, and foraminal stenosis (**Fig. 18.1**). Foraminal stenosis can be further categorized into intraforaminal and extraforaminal stenosis. Lumbar foraminal/extraforaminal spinal stenosis (LFSS) is a troublesome disease that can be easily overlooked by surgeons and can result in failed back surgery syndrome (FBSS). Decompression of the whole length of the nerve root from the spinal canal to the extraforaminal zone is often challenging due to the difficulty in identifying the exact site of nerve compression, making preservation of the posterior elements difficult.

18.2 Pathophysiology and Clinical Symptoms

LFSS is defined as compression of a nerve at a site between the medial and lateral borders of the pedicle.[1] Various types of degenerative change can cause LFSS, such as narrowing of the intervertebral disk space, degenerative lumbar scoliosis, bulging of the intervertebral disk, vertebral body osteophyte formation, anterior and posterior spondylolisthesis, and hypertrophy of the ligamentum flavum.

Although LFSS is considered a relatively uncommon disease, Kunogi et al[1] reported that 8% of cases of surgical treatment of lumbar degenerative disease involved LFSS. Furthermore,

Burton et al[2] reported that 60% of cases of failed back syndrome were due to a missed diagnosis of LFSS.

The symptoms of LFSS are similar to those of radiculopathy caused by general lumbar spinal canal stenosis. Patients may present with unilateral foraminal compression and clinical symptoms that are characterized by unilateral radicular pain with or without weakness. Back pain is usually minimal. Surgical intervention is recommended for patients whose symptoms persist despite nonoperative management.[3]

18.3 Treatment Option for LFSS

Current surgical strategies for treating LFSS can be separated into two categories: strategies that require fusion of the lumbar spine, and strategies that do not require fusion. The traditional surgical approach for LFSS has been to perform a wide, bilateral decompressive laminectomy along with resection of the medial portion of the facet joints to decompress the affected neural elements. Although this approach can successfully alleviate nerve compression symptoms, there are drawbacks of the open approach, including amount of soft tissue dissection, blood loss, postoperative pain, and the potential for iatrogenic instability of the spinal segment. These concerns are magnified when treating an elderly, fragile patient. Fusion is usually performed if the removal of spinal tissue presents a risk for spinal instability or in the presence of a significant spinal deformity, such as scoliosis or spondylolisthesis.

Since there is no established imaging technique for the diagnosis of LFSS, it is usually difficult to identify the site of nerve entrapment. Consequently, the entire length of the nerve (nerve root, dorsal root ganglion, and spinal nerve) from the inside of the spinal canal to the outside of the intervertebral foramen (IVF) must be decompressed in most cases. Total

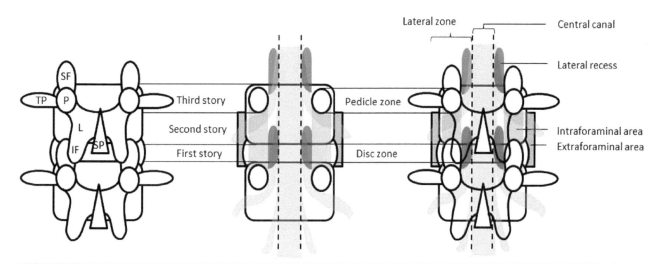

Fig. 18.1 Illustration of lumbar foraminal anatomy. SF, superior facet; IF, inferior facet; L, lamina; P, pedicle; SP, spinous process; TP, transverse process.

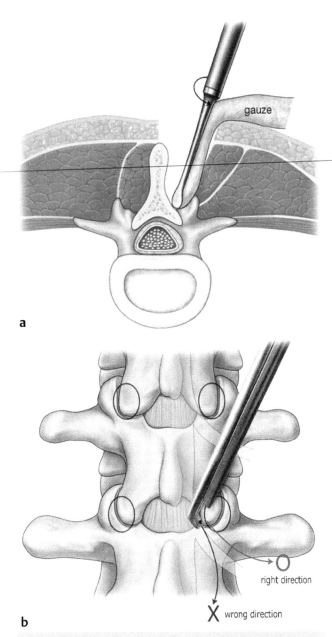

a

b

right direction

X wrong direction

Fig. 18.2 (a,b) Conventional midline open foraminotomy for the treatment of lumbar radiculopathy.

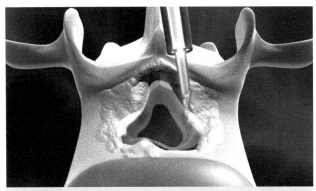

Fig. 18.3 Illustration of full endoscopic interlaminar approach for spinal and foraminal stenosis.

facetectomy combined with spinal fusion using spinal instrumentation, which is unnecessary in many cases, is therefore normally performed. Although it is possible to preserve the posterior elements by combining medial facetectomy and lateral fenestration, the nerves running under the preserved pars interarticularis cannot be decompressed with this method.[1] Additionally, the deep location of intraforaminal lesions makes the surgery technically challenging and more invasive.

Surgical strategies that avoid fusion include conventional open foraminal decompression, full endoscopic percutaneous interlaminar/transforaminal decompression, the relatively novel flexible microblade shaver decompression technique,[4] and less invasive techniques using tubular or similar retractors via a far-lateral intertransverse approach or facet-sparing contralateral approach.

Open decompression has been the gold standard for treatment of radiculopathy since the introduction of foraminotomy by Briggs and Krause in 1945.[5] Contemporary open methods are based on either a midline or a paraspinal approach. Although simple and direct, the midline approach has historically been associated with tissue damage and blood loss (**Fig. 18.2**).

A full endoscopic interlaminar approach was recently introduced for the treatment of central and foraminal stenosis (**Fig. 18.3**). Although the endoscopic approach is theoretically the least invasive, the limited mobility of the instruments, the difficulties in repairing any iatrogenic dural injury, and the demanding learning curve are still problems to overcome.

The newest technique in lumbar foraminal decompression is a flexible blade shaver method to enable inside-out widening of the foramen. The major benefit of the technique is the ability to perform decompression of all four nerve roots at any disk level (two exiting and two traversing nerve roots) with only a single incision and a laminotomy in the intervening interlaminar space. As in the minimally invasive contralateral approach, very little bony tissue is removed for access to the pathology site (**Fig. 18.4**). However, the microblade approach is not suitable for pathologies of the anterior wall of the foramen, nor is it suitable for patients with concomitant central stenosis unless the stenosis is treated first. The inability to directly visualize the exiting nerve root during the procedure is another major limitation. Further studies are required to establish the efficacy and safety of the flexible blade shaver method.

The paraspinal approach was described by Wiltse and Spencer in 1988[4] and is associated with less tissue damage. A far-lateral approach is effective for treating foraminal stenosis but is not suitable for combined central pathologies and foraminal stenosis at L5–S1, due to bony hindrance (**Fig. 18.5**).

With a contralateral approach, the contralateral foramen as well as the bilateral lateral recesses and central canal can all be accessed and decompressed with a single incision and with preservation of mechanical stability. The contralateral approach, therefore, can be applied to many forms of stenotic pathologies of the lumbar foramen, including disk herniations, osteophyte formation, or bony hypertrophy and grade I spondylolisthesis. It is also ideal for treating foraminal stenosis at L5–S1, as the position of the ilium may preclude far-lateral approaches to the foramen.

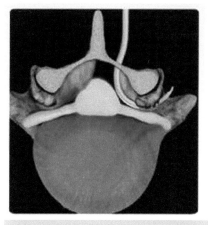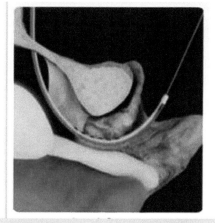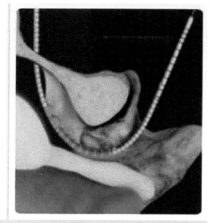

Fig. 18.4 Schematic illustrations of flexible blade shaver method.

18.4 Minimally Invasive Decompression Technique

Microendoscopic diskectomy (MED), developed by Foley and Smith,[6] has been widely used for the treatment of lumbar disk herniation. Recently, as a result of advancements in surgical techniques and instruments, spinal microendoscopy has also come to be applied in various other conditions, such as lumbar spinal canal stenosis and LFSS. Central decompressions and microdiskectomies are now routinely performed at many institutions with the use of minimally invasive techniques.

For foraminal/extraforaminal lumbar lesions, such as far-lateral lumbar disk herniation (FLDH), and far-out syndrome in particular, spinal microendoscopy, which can reach deeper into the back muscles less invasively, is surpassing conventional methods and becoming the standard procedure. While previously there was no possibility of avoiding spinal fusion for decompression in many cases of LFSS, with the help of MED, spinal fusion can be avoided. Benefits of a minimally invasive approach include less tissue dissection, the avoidance of fusion, decreased blood loss, decreased postoperative pain, shortened hospital stay, and earlier mobilization.

18.5 Tubular/Transmuscular Approach

Recently, novel minimally invasive techniques have become available for lumbar decompression, utilizing a tubular retractor system to limit paraspinal muscle trauma.[6] With the use of a tubular retractor system, a surgeon can reach deep into the body and provide relatively free angles, making the existing MED method even lesser invasive. As experience has grown with this surgical approach, surgeons are routinely treating patients with lumbar stenosis using a combination of a tubular retractor system and an operative microscope.

The METRx system (Medtronic Sofamor Danek, Memphis, TN) was the first commercially available tubular retractor system (**Fig. 18.6**). Before this system was introduced, a speculum or a polyethylene tube had been used as a kind of tubular dilator system. The biggest advantage of using this system is the application of endoscopic techniques to conventional surgery. The system enables both endoscopic images and direct surgical

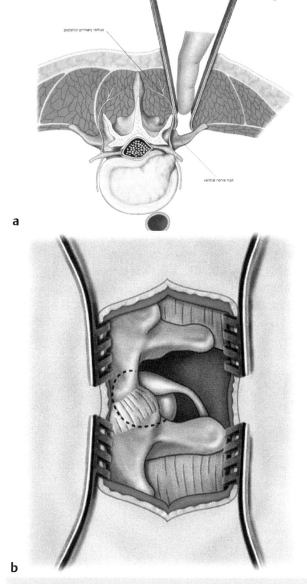

Fig. 18.5 (a,b) Illustrations of paraspinal muscle-splitting approach for the treatment of lumbar foraminal stenosis.

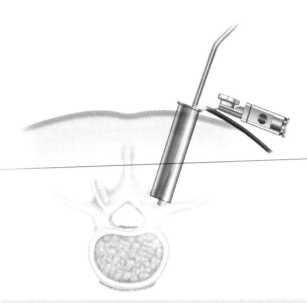

Fig. 18.6 METRx tubular retractor system.

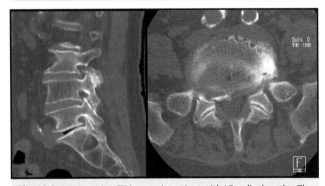

Fig. 18.8 Preoperative CT images in patient with L5 radiculopathy. The L5 nerve root is pinched in the lateral part of the intraforaminal zone.

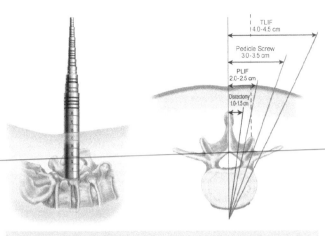

Fig. 18.7 Insight tubular retractor system.

can occur immediately if a small hematoma is generated in the space. Surgery under a microscope can provide direct surgical images, as in conventional surgeries, but the images may be obstructed or disturbed by the use of tools in a narrow space with limited light. To solve these problems, the use of a high-performance microscope with excellent collimation capabilities and good lighting is recommended. Another solution is to attach a fiberoptic light source to one end of the tube for enhanced viewing, but this requires considerable additional cost, because the device is expensive and its uses are limited. There is another problem not to be overlooked. The original purpose of being "less invasive" is impaired with overuse of a monopolar coagulator. Also, increased damage to the attached ligaments and muscles can occur when cleaning the operating field.

18.6 Patient Selection: Inclusion and Exclusion Criteria

The inclusion criteria are: the presence of unilateral radicular symptoms correlated with foraminal/extraforaminal disk herniation or stenosis; evidence of foraminal stenosis on preoperative imaging, such as CT images after radiculography revealing entrapment of the nerve root in the intraforaminal zone (**Fig. 18.8**) and parasagittal MRI depicting obliteration of fat tissue surrounding the nerve root in the intraforaminal zone (**Fig. 18.9**); and failure of nonoperative management for a minimum of 6 weeks. In certain ambiguous cases, selective nerve root block is performed to achieve temporary pain relief.

Patients are included if they have had symptoms that were notably more severe on the unilateral side with foraminal and/or extraforaminal compression.

Exclusion criteria are: bilateral radiculopathy; instability, which is defined as a translation of 4 mm or 10° of angular motion; concomitant intracanal disk herniation/stenosis at the same level; and previous history of spine surgery. Patients are also excluded if they have presented with significant mechanical back pain. Similarly, among patients without slippage, cases are excluded if they are mainly presenting with back pain rather than unilateral radiculopathy. They are also excluded if the etiology of their symptoms was facet joint cyst, tumor, or trauma.

images to be viewed under a microscope. The images can then be used according to the surgeon's goals. Moreover, because the METRx system splits the muscle instead of cutting it, it is possible to minimize postoperative back pain by reducing muscle damage.

When a tubular retractor system is used for lumbar decompression, a paramedian incision is localized fluoroscopically. Serial dilation of the paraspinal muscles (rather than muscle stripping) is used to create a working portal down to the spinal lamina, which allows insertion of the tubular retractor (**Fig. 18.6**, **Fig. 18.7**). The surgeon may then use either an endoscope or a microscope for magnification and lighting, thus providing visualization of the spinal anatomy. Use of a tubular retractor system theoretically limits paraspinal muscle trauma, decreases operative blood loss, and improves early recovery.

Despite the benefits, there are some drawbacks to overcome before effective results can be achieved. First, appropriate surgical tools and manual skills are required, since the surgeon must work in a narrow space. Further, there may be confusion regarding anatomical structures in such a limited space. Another problem is the limitations of effective decompression. The surgeon must be aware that even though the surgery was completed effectively in the narrow space, symptoms

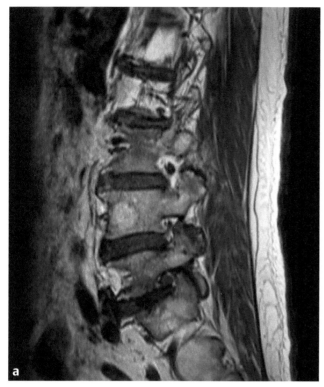

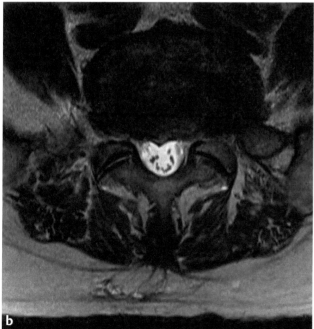

Fig. 18.9 (a,b) Preoperative MRI shows obliteration of fat tissue surrounding the L5 nerve in the intraforaminal zone.

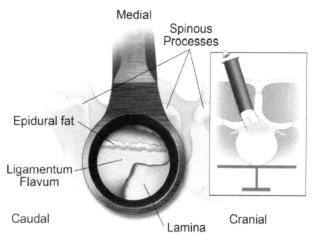

Fig. 18.10 Illustration of far-lateral intertransverse approach decompression procedure. The arrow indicates the area of unroofing at the foramen. Additional decompression is performed depending on the stenotic condition: partial pediculectomy, diskectomy, and extraforaminal decompression.

18.7 Surgical Techniques and Strategies

The procedure is typically performed under general anesthesia, although epidural or spinal anesthesia can be used according to surgeon preference. Prophylactic antibiotics are usually provided at the initiation of the procedure. The patient is positioned prone on a radiolucent spinal frame, which allows decompression of the abdomen and access for fluoroscopic imaging. After a sterile prep and drape, the operative levels are confirmed using an X-ray image intensifier and are marked on the skin with ink.

18.7.1 Far-Lateral Intertransverse Approaches

See **Video 18.1** and **Video 18.2**. A longitudinal skin incision of ~ 16 to 22 mm is made ~ 2.5 to 3.5 cm lateral to the midline. (A 16- to 22-mm skin incision is usually sufficient for decompression at as many as three levels using an octagonal maneuver. An additional skin incision is made if the skin does not move sufficiently in the craniocaudal direction to allow decompression at three levels.) Various tubular retractor systems can be used for the surgery. After incision of the lumbosacral fascia, the multifidus and longissimus muscles are identified and are dissected away using the fingertips. A guidewire is not generally used. Dilators with increasing diameters are inserted sequentially, and a tubular retractor with a diameter of 16 to 22 mm is finally put in place.

The first step is to fully expose the caudal half of the base of the transverse process (TP) of the upper vertebra and the lateral edge of the isthmus using electrocautery. Since the surgery involves a precise approach and it is difficult to visualize the entire area, complete exposure of this region as a landmark is essential to avoid disorientation of the surgeon in the narrow operating view.

Using a diamond drill, approximately one-third of the pedicle is excavated caudally from the base of the TP toward the spinal canal, from the inner side, preserving the medial and caudal cortex. The medial and caudal cortex of the pedicle is thinned from the inner side, little by little, using the drill. The nerve root becomes visible after the cortex of the pedicle has been resected. Compression factors around the nerve are excised from the spinal canal to the extraforaminal zone to decompress the nerve root, dorsal root ganglion, and spinal nerve (**Fig. 18.10**). Up–down stenosis can be eliminated by removing the caudal aspect of the pedicle, and front–back stenosis can be eliminated by removing the ligamentum flavum or the cranial part of the superior articular process (SAP) of the lower vertebra. The decompression can reach the lateral border of the spinal canal without damaging posterior elements, such as the facet joints and pars interarticularis, since the tubular retractor is placed in an inward-tilting fashion.

In patients in whom L5–S1 is affected, the iliac crest may become an obstacle, limiting lateral approaches to the lesion. In such cases, the tubular retractor is inserted from the cranial side, avoiding the iliac crest. CT or MRI should be used to make presurgical decisions regarding the direction of insertion of the tubular retractor and the point of skin incision. Surgical landmarks in the L5–S1 level are the L5 transverse process, pars interarticularis, and sacral ala. Under microscopic view, the lower margin of the L5 transverse process, the lateral part of the pars interarticularis, the lateral margin of the superior facet, and the sacral ala can be removed by high-speed drill. After removal of the lumbosacral ligament, the ganglion of the L5 nerve root is exposed.

In this operative procedure, the caudal part of the pedicle can be partially excavated first, and the nerve root is identified within the foraminal zone. As an alternative, Yoshimoto et al[7] proposed a method whereby the spinal nerve in the extraforaminal zone is identified first and then decompression is begun toward the foraminal zone. However, it is relatively difficult to identify the spinal nerve in the extraforaminal zone in some cases because of bleeding from the dorsal branch of the radicular artery coming through the intertransverse ligaments to the dorsal side.[8] Moreover, adhesion or compression occasionally makes it difficult to identify the involved spinal nerve. Excavation of the caudal part of the pedicle first can minimize the risk of bleeding, can make identification of the nerve root in the foraminal zone easier, and is thus safer.

18.7.2 Facet-Sparing Contralateral Approach

With the patient under general anesthesia and in a prone position, a small skin incision is made overlying the target level ~ 1.5 to 2.0 cm lateral to the midline, more in obese patients. An 18- or 19-mm tubular retractor is placed over a series of tubular dilators for retraction, and under the microscope, the inferior edge of the lamina and the inferior edge and base of the spinous process are exposed. The decompression is performed step by step, starting with an ipsilateral laminotomy using a pneumatic drill and 2- and 3-mm Kerrison punches. To achieve appropriate visualization of contralateral sublaminar structures, the operating table is tilted away from the surgeon and the tubular retractor is angled medially. Next, the base of the spinous process and the contralateral lamina are undercut using the drill and rongeurs. The ligamentum flavum is exposed bilaterally and cranially up to its insertion under the lamina. During the drilling, the ligamentum flavum is preserved to protect the dura. Next, a nerve hook is inserted in the midline where the two leaves of the ligamentum flavum meet, an area that is typically identified by the presence of epidural fat, and the ligamentum flavum is removed using Kerrison rongeurs. Dural exposure and decompression are achieved after complete removal of the ligamentum flavum. This technique minimizes the risk of injury to the dura.

The contralateral lateral recess and the traversing contralateral nerve root are completely decompressed (**Fig. 18.11**).

At this point, a small ball-tip probe is inserted into the foramen, and the correct level and positioning are confirmed with lateral fluoroscopy. It is usually necessary to tilt the table away from the surgeon to allow medial angling of the retractor and to achieve a better trajectory into the contralateral foramen. The contralateral facet is then undercut with the drill while protecting the dura with the narrow tip suction. The superior pedicle is palpated, and the exiting nerve root is visualized. A complete decompression of the exiting nerve root is then performed using Kerrison rongeurs. Sufficient lateral extension of the decompression is confirmed with a nerve hook and anteroposterior fluoroscopy. As the next and final step, the table and retractor are brought back into the initial position, and an ipsilateral decompression is completed, if clinically indicated. In patients with bilateral lower extremity symptoms, the ipsilateral side is decompressed by angling the tubular retractor more vertically, and in some cases even toward the surgeon's side (hence, ipsilateral); on occasion, the table also is tilted toward the surgeon's side. This allows excellent visualization of the ipsilateral aspect of the thecal sac, the traversing ipsilateral nerve root, and decompression of the ipsilateral lateral recess.

18.8 Postoperative Care

The fascia, subcutaneous tissues, and skin are closed in a routine fashion. A skin sealant is placed along the skin edges to allow early showering. The subcutaneous tissues are injected with a long-acting local anesthetic to reduce incisional pain, followed by placement of a small dressing. Patients are encouraged to walk on the first postsurgical day with a soft brace. The drain is usually pulled out 2 days after the operation. Most patients are discharged from the hospital within several days of the surgery. Early return to ambulation and normal activities of daily living is encouraged. Pain management is generally provided by

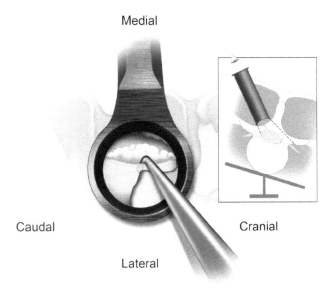

Fig. 18.11 Illustration showing the tubular retractor in the vertical position and in a medially angulated position to access the contralateral side.

either a mild oral narcotic or an NSAID analgesic, depending on the preferences of the patient. Rehabilitation with core muscle stabilization and aerobic activities is encouraged in the early postoperative period, and it is usually started the day after the operation.

18.9 Complications

Although the list of potential complications with tubular decompression is no different from that with traditional open surgery, the rate of certain complications is significantly reduced. For instance, the rates of blood loss, wound infection, iatrogenic instability, and medical deterioration after lumbar decompression using a tubular retractor system are lower than with open laminectomy.[9]

The most frequent complications related to this surgery are incomplete decompression and dural tear. Special care must be taken not to tear the dura mater, because most patients with foraminal stenosis are old and the dura mater is thin. Dural laceration (incidental durotomy) may be managed with either suture repair or dural sealants, depending on the location, size, and severity of the durotomy. Because exposure with the tubular retractor system produces minimal "dead space," the risk of postoperative dura-cutaneous fistula is reduced in comparison to traditional laminectomy. Small, stable tears may be successfully managed with a small pledget of a hemostatic agent followed by a dural sealant (e.g., fibrin glue). Larger tears or tears with exposed nerve root should be treated with direct suture repair. Although technically demanding, this can be achieved using a small needle and a micropituitary instrument as the needle driver and an arthroscopic knot pusher to assist with knot tying. In most cases, prolonged bed rest is not required for patients after a satisfactory dural repair.

Absolute control of bleeding is crucial. Even minimal hematoma may cause serious nerve compression and may require reoperation, because the operated part is narrow and deep.

Infection rates following tubular access surgery are very low. In the rare event of a wound infection, treatment should be instituted with debridement and antibiotic therapy. Due to the avoidance of prolonged anesthesia, heavy blood loss, and prolonged bed rest, medical complications after tubular access decompression are uncommon even in the elderly population.

18.10 Advantages

The largest advantage of use of tubular technique is that it can reach deep into the body with relatively free angles, less invasively. It is unnecessary to stick to the paraspinal posterior approach reported by Wiltse et al,[10] and the tubular retractor can be inserted from an extreme lateral position at a strongly tilted angle. Moreover, an oblique viewing endoscope makes the visual field wider. This technique facilitates decompression of the entire length of the nerve from the spinal canal to the extraforaminal zone, without damaging posterior elements, such as the facet joints and pars interarticularis. Also, use of the tubular retractor minimizes invasion of muscles. In the study by Yoshimoto et al,[7] postoperative C-reactive protein and visual analog scores indicating surgical-site pain were equal to those in patients who underwent MED.

The conventional ipsilateral midline approach, which is used for a repertoire of proven interventions, such as foraminotomy, laminectomy, and laminotomy, has traditionally been, and continues to be, the most common approach for treating all forms of spinal stenosis. Major limitations of conventional approaches include obligatory partial or full removal of the facet joint to access the foramen (which can cause instability), difficulties in visualization of the intraforaminal content, and increased surgical blood loss.

18.11 Disadvantages

The disadvantages of tubular surgeries include the steep learning curve for surgeons, who must establish hand–eye coordination and are unable to rely on three-dimensional vision. Moreover, surgeons are obliged to view the foraminal zone significantly obliquely from lateral to medial in this method. This is not something experienced during general, direct-view surgery. Therefore, it is important to understand the oblique configuration in advance to avoid disorientation during surgery. Use of a fluoroscope is recommended until surgeons become familiar with the method.

18.12 Conclusion

Minimally invasive tubular decompression for foraminal and extraforaminal stenosis can provide good clinical results and avoid complications of lumbar fusion.

References

1. Kunogi J, Hasue M. Diagnosis and operative treatment of intraforaminal and extraforaminal nerve root compression. *Spine* 1991;*16*(11):1312–1320
2. Burton CV, Kirkaldy-Willis WH, Yong-Hing K, Heithoff KB. Causes of failure of surgery on the lumbar spine. *Clin Orthop Relat Res* 1981; (157):191–199
3. Weinstein JN, Tosteson TD, Lurie JD, et al; SPORT Investigators. Surgical versus nonsurgical therapy for lumbar spinal stenosis. *N Engl J Med* 2008;*358*(8):794–810
4. Lauryssen C. Technical advances in minimally invasive surgery: direct decompression for lumbar spinal stenosis. *Spine* 2010;*35*(26, Suppl):S287–S293
5. Briggs H, Krause J. The intervertebral foraminotomy for relief of sciatic pain. *J Bone Joint Surg Am* 1945;*27*:475–478
6. Foley KT, Smith MM. Microendoscopic discectomy. Techniques in neurosurgery 3. Philadelphia: Lippincott-Raven; 1997:301–307
7. Yoshimoto M, Takebayashi T, Kawaguchi S, et al. Minimally invasive technique for decompression of lumbar foraminal stenosis using a spinal microendoscope: technical note. *Minim Invasive Neurosurg* 2011;*54*(3):142–146
8. Yoshimoto M, Terashima Y, Kawaguchi S, et al. Microendoscopic discectomy for extraforaminal lumbar disc herniations. *Jpn J Spine Research Society* 2008;*19*:305
9. Khoo LT, Fessler RG. Microendoscopic decompressive laminotomy for the treatment of lumbar stenosis. *Neurosurgery* 2002;*51*(5, Suppl):S146–S154
10. Wiltse LL, Spencer CW. New uses and refinements of the paraspinal approach to the lumbar spine. *Spine* 1988;*13*(6):696–706

19 Destandau's Technique: Interlaminar Approach (Lumbar Diskectomy with Canal Decompression)

Shrinivas M. Rohidas

19.1 Introduction

Lumbar intervertebral disk prolapse is a common occurrence. The standard surgical treatment is diskectomy with a posterior approach. With the Endospine operating tube, the same approach and surgical technique can be used while reducing the size of the skin incision and approach-related tissue trauma, especially in obese patients. Endospine helps in any deeply located pathology in the lumbar spine, such as disk herniation, stenosis, and foraminal disk herniation. With Endospine, the surgeon's eye is focused right inside the body close to the pathology that is to be treated. In addition to the cosmetic benefit of the reduced length of the incision, the short access route and reduced length of the incision help to decrease postoperative incision discomfort and aid in rapid resumption of routine activities.

19.2 Indications

The technique is indicated for lumbar disk herniation—central, paracentral, extruded, and migrated with neural compression and associated canal stenosis—not relieved by adequate conservative treatment. All levels from L5–S1 to L1–L2 can be approached with the technique. Central and far-lateral lumbar disk extrusions, as well as foraminal and extraforaminal disk extrusions, can be treated with Endospine. Canal stenosis in the lumbar region can be treated with a unilateral approach while achieving bilateral lateral recess and central decompression. The versatility of Endospine lies in its ability to treat various lumbar pathologies, including disk herniations of any kind, along with canal stenosis.[1,2]

19.3 Contraindications

Severe lumbar instability with radiculopathy.

19.4 Patient Positioning

Various patient positions can be used for lumbar diskectomy, such as the prone position, lateral position, and knee-chest position. The prone and knee-chest positions are the natural positions for use of Endospine. With the lateral position, it is difficult to support the Endospine system. The author uses the knee-chest position on a flat operating table with flexion at the patient's knees and hips. In this position, the abdomen is completely lax in between the two thighs at the same time that there is adequate interspinous distraction, which is necessary in cases of canal stenosis. With a pillow under the patient's chest, the head is lower than the caudal end, allowing natural gravitational venous flow toward the heart, which helps in minimizing venous bleeding (**Fig. 19.1**).[3]

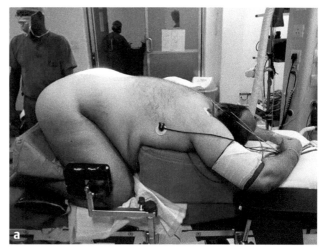

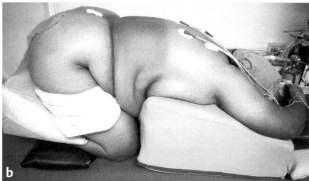

Fig. 19.1 (a) Knee-chest position. **(b)** Knee-chest position showing completely lax abdomen between the two thighs.

19.5 Localization of Disk Space

When the surgeon limits the size of the incision, it is necessary to exactly localize the target disk space. Exact localization of disk space is performed with help of a localizing pin available in the Endospine set. The localizing pin is used in lateral fluoroscopy with the patient placed in the knee-chest position. The localizing pin moves in all three spatial planes, and only lateral fluoroscopy is necessary to confirm the direction to the disk space. The entry point is obtained while determining the direction to the disk space. Hence there is no need for separate anteroposterior and lateral localization (**Fig. 19.2**, **Fig. 19.3**).[4]

19.6 Surgical Technique

Skin Incision

While marking the disk space level in lateral fluoroscopy, the surgeon also determines the entry point in the coronal plane. The incision is ~ 10 to 15 mm from the midline spinous process. The length of the incision is ~ 15 to 20 mm. The fascia is cut in the same direction, and then the paraspinal muscles are separated

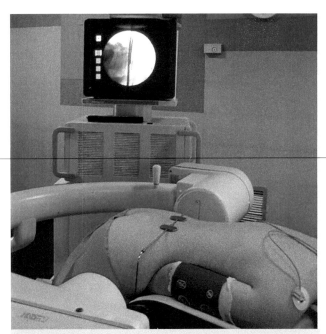

Fig. 19.2 Localizing pin with C-arm fluoroscopy in lateral view to localize the disk space.

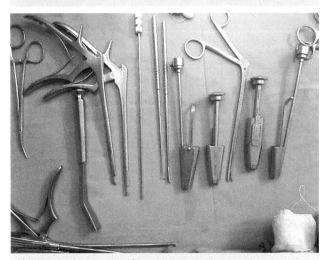

Fig. 19.4 Endospine set with routine spine instruments.

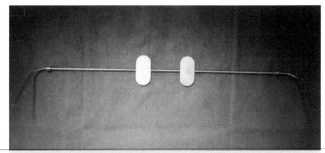

Fig. 19.3 Lumbar localizing pin in Endospine set.

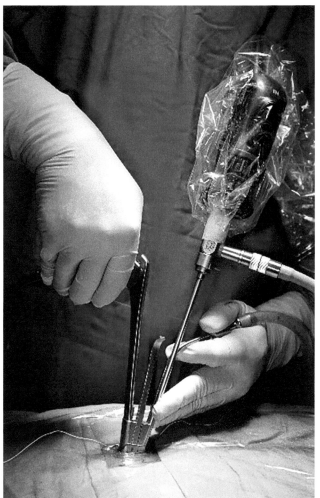

Fig. 19.5 Hand movements with Endospine.

off the midline from the spinous process and interspinous ligament with a 12-mm osteotome. Bleeding from retracted muscles is controlled with bipolar coagulation.

The author uses two gauze pieces with thread to retract separated muscles laterally. One gauze piece is pushed cranially over the lamina and another is used caudally in a similar fashion. Then the outer tube of the Endospine is placed between the spinous process medially and the separated muscles laterally. The outer tube should fit snugly between the spinous process and muscle. With the outer tube in place, the surgeon should see the exposed lamina in the cranial half of the outer tube and the ligamentum flavum in the caudal half. Then the surgeon is assured of the exact localization of the concerned disk space.

Preparation of the Endospine Assembly

The Endospine outer tube and inner tube/working insert with routine instruments are arranged on an instrument trolley. Next, the inner tube/working insert of Endospine is placed in the outer tube and is fixed in the proximal position with the built-in lock. This has to be in the proximal position so that an artificial space is created between the outer tube and the inner tube/working insert. If the inner tube is placed more distally, then the endoscope will touch the underlying tissue and the surgeon will not have space for movement of the instruments. (This is one of the mistakes the surgeon faces during the learning curve.) Then the endoscope is placed in the endoscope channel and is fixed. Suction is used with

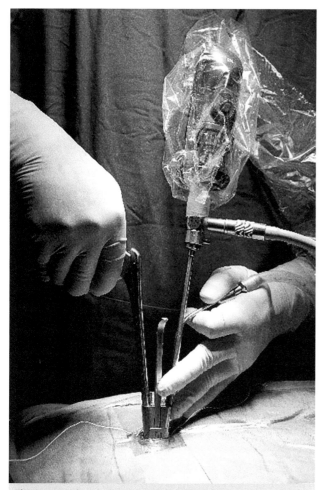

Fig. 19.6 Hand movements with Endospine.

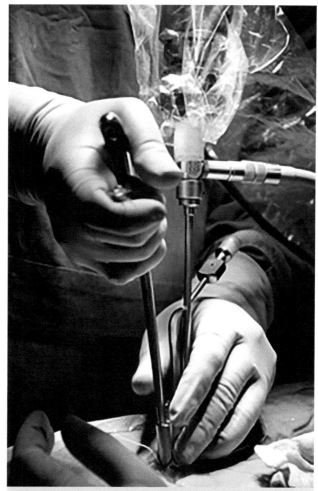

Fig. 19.7 Hand movements with Endospine.

the left hand through a 4-mm channel that is parallel to the 4-mm channel for the endoscope. The channel for working instruments is the widest channel in the Endospine system: 12 mm. The two 4-mm channels for the endoscope and suction are parallel to each other, but the channel for working instruments is at an angle of 12° to the two 4-mm channels. The 12° angle between suction/endoscope and working instruments avoids intermingling of the instruments, while at the same time allowing the surgeon to use a 0° endoscope as an angled scope (**Fig. 19.4**).

Basic Philosophy of Mobility and Stability of Endospine

When the endoscope and suction are attached to the camera and suction tube, respectively, the whole system should remain relatively stable without any pull over the cables. The suction in the left hand is used to move the whole system with the left hand. The working instrument in the right hand is used to move the system with the right hand. With both hands, the surgeon can move the whole system—i.e., endoscope and instruments—in all four directions, cranial, caudal, medial, and lateral. This means that, while using the Endospine system, the surgeon has to balance the forces of both hands so that the whole assembly can be moved in any direction. Thus, when the surgeon moves the Endospine system with suction in the left hand, the system is

stabilized by the working instrument in the right hand (**Fig. 19.5, Fig. 19.6, Fig. 19.7**). Similarly, when the Endospine system is moved to use working instruments in the right hand, the system is stabilized by the suction in the left hand (**Fig. 19.8, Fig. 19.9**).

The surgeon has to look at the monitor while balancing Endospine with suction in the left hand and working instrument in the right hand. The surgeon has to learn the basic movements to balance and at the same time to stabilize the system (**Fig. 19.10**). These are the basics of mobility of Endospine.[4,5]

Excision of Lamina

The excision of lamina is usually started at the spinolaminar junction at the base of the spinous process. A 45° Kerrison punch is used to excise lamina. Excision of lamina is continued laterally and cranially so as to detach the anteroinferior attachment of the ligamentum flavum from the lamina (**Fig. 19.11, Fig. 19.12**). Once the learning curve is mastered, the surgeon can change the approach according to the interlaminar and interpedicular window size.

For example, at the L5–S1 level, where the interlaminar window is wider, the surgeon can detach the ligamentum flavum first and then, if necessary, part of lamina is excised to decompress the traversing nerve root. Part of the cranial lamina and the articular process is excised to expose the lateral edge of the dural sac and the shoulder of the traversing nerve root.

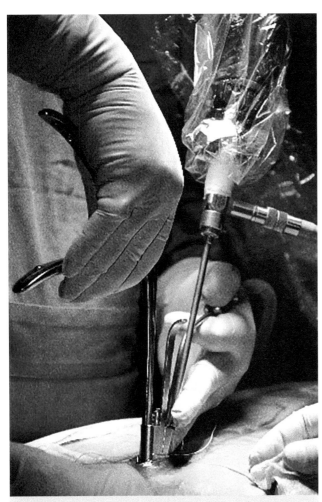

Fig. 19.8 Right hand movement with the Kerrison punch.

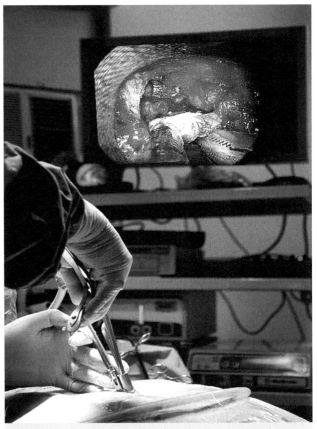

Fig. 19.10 Hand–eye coordination with Endospine held with two hands.

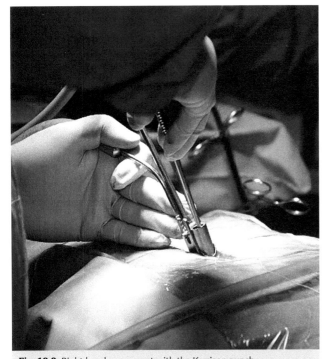

Fig. 19.9 Right hand movement with the Kerrison punch.

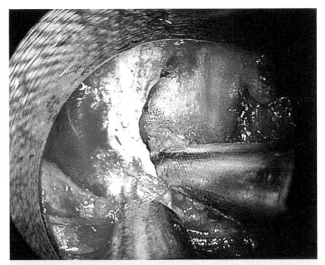

Fig. 19.11 Detachment of ligamentum flavum from lamina.

Excision of Flavum

Next, a cottonoid is used to push the dura anteriorly so that accidental dural injury is avoided during excision of the ligamentum flavum. A 90° Kerrison punch is usually used to excise the ligamentum flavum. Attachment of the ligamentum flavum to the caudal lamina and the medial facet is excised to decompress the traversing nerve root.

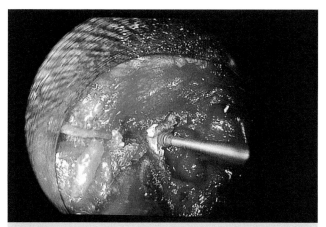

Fig. 19.12 Use of drill to remove lamina.

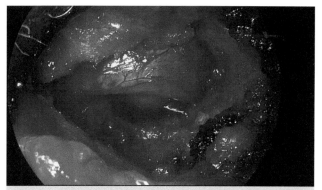

Fig. 19.13 Decompressed left-sided traversing nerve root stretched over huge disk bulge.

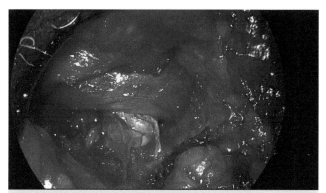

Fig. 19.14 Extruded disk lateral to traversing nerve root.

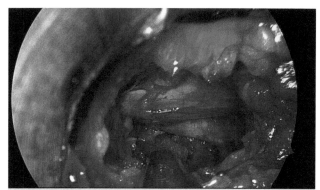

Fig. 19.15 Adequately decompressed traversing nerve root after diskectomy.

Decompression of Traversing Nerve Root

Once the lateral edge of the dural sac is identified, the shoulder of the traversing nerve root is identified. If necessary, the medial facet can be undercut to adequately decompress the traversing nerve root. A cottonoid is pushed cranially and laterally to decompress the shoulder of the nerve root. If the nerve root is not adequately decompressed, the surgeon will not be able to pass the cottonoid easily. Then it is advisable to undercut the medial facet to create some more space lateral to the nerve root. The cottonoid will retract the shoulder of the nerve root medially. Then, with the help of a 45° Kerrison punch, the medial facet formed by the superior articular process is undercut so that the nerve root is adequately decompressed up to the exit into the neural foramen. Another cottonoid is then passed caudally, lateral to the decompressed nerve root, so that the nerve root is retracted medially. This exposes the disk space.

The author uses two cottonoids to retract the nerve root after it is adequately decompressed because, although there is a built-in nerve retractor in the working insert/inner tube, it is better not to use the nerve root retractor in the initial learning phase. Endospine is a mobile system, and when the nerve root retractor is used, the surgeon is using three instruments at a time—i.e., suction, the working instrument (Kerrison punch or disk forceps), and the nerve root retractor. While using the three instruments, the surgeon has to keep the system stable, because if the system doesn't remain stable, the retracted nerve root may be traumatized during movement. Thus, the author uses two cottonoids to judge the adequacy of nerve root decompression.

If the two cottonoids can be passed easily lateral to the nerve root over the shoulder and caudally over the nerve root, then the nerve root is adequately decompressed (**Fig. 19.13**).

After retraction of nerve root, epidural veins over the exposed disk space can be cauterized with endoscopic bipolar cautery. After retraction of the nerve root, extruded disk fragment can be seen and sequestrectomy is performed. If the annulus is lax and still intact, an annulotome is used to open the annulus. A 15-mm blade can also be used to open the annulus, with the cutting edge of the blade facing away from the nerve root. Adequate diskectomy is advised, rather than aggressive diskectomy (**Fig. 19.14**).

The disk space is irrigated with saline to remove any loose disk fragments. The endoscope is passed through the working channel into the disk space in order to inspect the space created after diskectomy. This is the endpoint of diskectomy (**Fig. 19.15**).

Closure

The Endospine is withdrawn as a single unit under endoscopic vision. Endoscopic bipolar cautery is used to achieve hemostasis in the muscles. Fascia is closed with 3–0 Vicryl and the skin is reapproximated with 3–0 Vicryl. A drain is not required.

Postoperative Care

The patient is moved to the recovery room after extubation. Because most patients are not catheterized, when the patient wants to urinate, he is mobilized and then moved to a room. Oral analgesics are started after 6 hours, and the patient is discharged

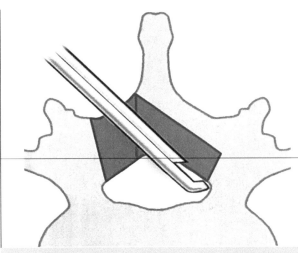

Fig. 19.16 Diagram of undercutting of the opposite lamina with the Kerrison punch in lumbar canal stenosis.

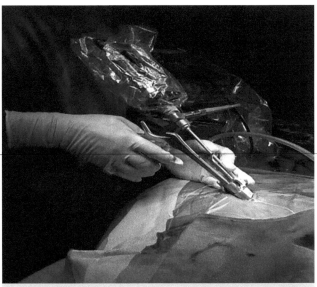

Fig. 19.17 Angulation of Endospine with Kerrison punch to undercut opposite lamina.

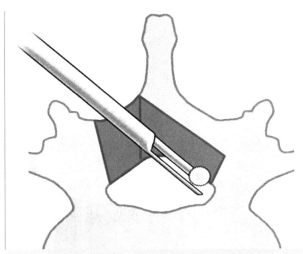

Fig. 19.18 Schematic diagram of endoscopic drill used to undercut opposite lamina.

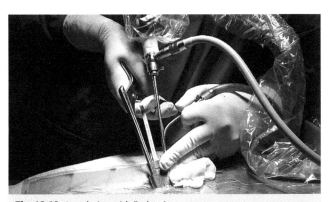

Fig. 19.19 Angulation with Endospine.

after 24 hours. Medically compromised patients are discharged only after they are medically stable.

19.7 Surgical Technique for Lumbar Canal Stenosis

A unilateral approach is used with Endospine to achieve bilateral canal decompression. The same incision as for diskectomy is used for canal decompression (**Fig. 19.16**).[4] The ipsilateral decompression of the traversing nerve root is performed the same way as in diskectomy with a unilateral approach. Then the whole Endospine assembly is angulated to the opposite side. First the base of the spinous process is undercut using a 45° Kerrison punch, so that a wide opening is created to accommodate the outer tube. The Endospine system is angulated for an angle of ~ 30° (**Fig. 19.17**).

After undercutting of the base of the spinous process with 30° angulation, the opposite lamina is tangentially in the same plane as the working instruments. A 45° Kerrison punch is used to undercut the opposite lamina. During undercutting of the opposite lamina, the ligamentum flavum is kept intact,

to protect the dura. Cranially opposite lamina is undercut to detach the ligamentum flavum. Then the ligamentum flavum is detached caudally from the caudal lamina. This detachment proceeds from the midline to the opposite lateral edge. Then the medial facet of the opposite side is undercut with the help of the 45° Kerrison punch. After the flavum is detached from all of its attachments, it is removed with the 90° Kerrison punch. A cottonoid is used under the ligamentum flavum to protect the dura. Once the flavum is resected, a cottonoid is passed over the shoulder of the opposite traversing nerve root, which will retract the nerve root medially. Then a 45° Kerrison punch is used to decompress the lateral edge of the dura and nerve root. The cutting edge of the Kerrison punch is always away from the nerve root and dura while undercutting the opposite lamina, facet, and flavum. The endoscopic drill can be used to undercut the opposite lamina and facet (**Fig. 19.18**, **Fig. 19.19**, **Fig. 19.20**).

The author uses an endoscopic drill with a protection sheath that protects the dura; in addition, a cottonoid is used to protect the dura. Since 2009, the author has used an ultrasonic bone dissector to undercut the opposite lamina and facet in severe canal stenosis. The ultrasonic bone dissector, knife, or rasp emulsifies bone, but at the same time it does not injure soft tissue (**Fig. 19.21**).

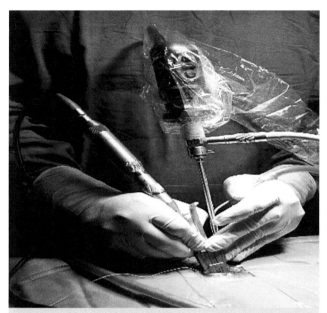

Fig. 19.20 Undercutting of the opposite lamina with the endoscopic drill.

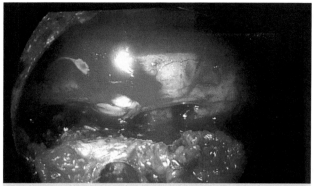

Fig. 19.21 Two-level endoscopic canal decompression with a single incision.

19.8 Results

At Prakruti clinic, the author's center for minimally invasive spinal surgery and neurosurgery, between 2002 and 2014, the Endospine system was used in 1,000 cases of lumbar spine diskectomy, diskectomy with canal decompression, and canal decompression without diskectomy at one level and, if necessary, two or multiple levels. All 1,000 surgeries were done by one surgeon. (Since September 2002, the surgeries performed per year were: 2002, 8; 2003, 38; 2004, 47; 2005, 48; 2006, 80; 2007, 83; 2008, 86; 2009, 104; 2010, 129; 2011, 140; 2012, 111; 2013, 105; and before March 2014, 27 cases.) The pathologies treated were due to degenerative changes in the lumbar spine, but, adhering to the basic principle of adequate nerve decompression with preservation of stability to maintain the motion segment meant that some patients needed only diskectomy, some needed adequate diskectomy with canal decompression, and some needed only canal decompression. Endospine allowed bilateral canal and bilateral nerve root decompression with a unilateral approach.[4,6,7]

Out of 1,000 patients, 642 were male and 358 were female, with a minimum age of 14 years and a maximum of 82 years. MRI was used in 997 cases, with myelography in the initial three cases. In 990 cases, general anesthesia was used, with spinal anesthesia in two cases and local anesthesia in eight. The common levels endoscopically treated were L4–L5, L5–S1, and L4–L5 with L5–S1, because degenerative changes are more common at these levels. Out of 452 cases at the L4–L5 level, diskectomy was performed in 129, diskectomy with canal decompression was performed in 286 cases, and canal decompression alone without diskectomy was performed in 37 cases. At L5–S1, out of 239 cases, diskectomy was performed in 146 cases, diskectomy with canal decompression in 92 cases, and canal decompression alone without diskectomy was done in one case. In the cases involving both L4–L5 and L5–S1, the two levels were approached endoscopically in 89 cases. Out of 89 cases, 50 were approached through a single incision, by angulating Endospine caudally. In eight cases diskectomy was performed, in 77 cases diskectomy with canal decompression was performed, and in four cases only canal decompression was performed. In

surgery at L4–L5 and L5–S1 for canal decompression through a single incision, most often L5 hemilaminectomy was performed for adequate canal decompression. The L3–L4 level was endoscopically treated in 55 patients. Of these 55 patients, 33 had only diskectomy, 18 needed diskectomy with canal decompression, and for four patients only canal decompression was sufficient. In the remaining 165 patients with more than one level of endoscopic surgery, 85 cases were at the L3–L4 and L4–L5 levels, and 13 cases were at the L2–L3 and L4–L5 levels. To approach these levels, two separate incisions were used. In comparison to the incidence of foraminal disk herniations in the Western literature, which is ~ 8%, we have used the transforaminal approach for far-lateral disk herniation in only five cases out of 1,000. Of these five cases, one case was a recurrent disk herniation at L3–L4 after open laminectomy and diskectomy at L4–L5 in 1989. Three cases had a synovial cyst of the facet compressing the nerve root—two at L4–L5 and one at L5–S1. The L5–S1 synovial cyst was on the contralateral side of endoscopic diskectomy performed a year earlier, causing compressive recurrent radiculopathy. A summary of findings is shown in **Box 19.1**.

Box 19.1. Summary of Endospine surgery results

Conjoint root was found in two cases (0.2%).
T12–L1: (CD + D) = 2.
L1–L2: 5(D), 1 (CD + D) = 6.
L2–L3: 7(D), 5 (CD + D) = 12.
L3–L4: 33(D), 18(CD + D), 4(CD) = 55.
L4–L5: 129(D), 286(CD + D), 37(CD) = 452.
L5–S1: 146(D), 92(CD + D), 1(CD) = 239.
L4–L5 & L5–S1: 8(D), 77(CD + D), 4(CD) = 89.
• More than one level lumbar disk surgery:
T12–L1 & L4–L5 = 1.
L1–L2 & L4–L5 = 1.
L1–L2 & L2–L3: 2(CD + D) = 2.
L1–L2 & L3–L4: 2(CD + D) = 2.
L1–L2, L4–L5, & L5–S1: 1(CD) = 1.
L1–L2 & L5–S1: 1(CD + D) = 1.
L2–L3 & L4–L5: 2(D), 11(CD + D) = 13.
L3–L4 & L4–L5: 4(D), 66(CD + D), 15(CD) = 85.
L2–L3 & L3–L4: 1(D), 6(CD + D), 1(CD) = 8.
L3–L4 & L5–S1: 1(D), 7(CD + D), 1(CD) = 9.
L3–L4, L4–L5, & L5–S1: 7(CD + D) = 7.
L2–L3, L3–L4 & L4–L5: 4(CD + D), 6(CD) = 10.
L2–L3, L3–L4 & L5–S1: 1(CD + D) = 1.
L2–L3, L3–L4, L4–L5, & L5–S1: 1(CD) = 1.
L1–L2, L2–L3, L3–L4, & L4–L5: 1(CD) = 1.
L1–L2, L2–L3, L4–L5, & L5–S1: 1(CD + D) = 1.
S1–S2: 1(CD + D) = 1.
Abbreviations: D = diskectomy only; CD + D = diskectomy and canal decompression; CD = canal decompression only (no diskectomy).

In his series, the author has had 29 dural punctures related to the endoscopic procedure. Initially, in two cases where the dural rent was significant, the approach was converted to an open procedure and the dural rent was closed. Incidentally, in these two cases, open laminectomy had been done in the past for diskectomy and there was recurrence of disk herniation. In the rest of the cases, packing with small Gelfoam pieces was sufficient. Pieces of muscle can be used to plug into the tear, as well as fibrin glue to seal the tear. We had four procedure-related nerve injuries that led to weakness. Of the four nerve injuries, two were in cases of listhesis with canal stenosis. Six cases had spondylodiscitis after endoscopic treatment; four received antibiotics and rest, and two underwent decompressive laminectomy with debridement, antibiotics, and complete bed rest. Nine cases had wound infections that required local debridement and increased antibiotics. Of the nine cases, four were cases where a piece of gauze was forgotten underneath the fascia in the muscle, which led to the wound infection. Of the 1,000 cases operated endoscopically, 12 had recurrence of disk herniation. One disk herniation was on the opposite side, and in another case a synovial cyst on the opposite side caused recurrent symptoms. The remaining ten cases had recurrent disk herniation on the same side as the endoscopic approach in the past. Of these ten cases, eight underwent endoscopic diskectomy at our center and two underwent open laminectomy at another center. We had # of spinous process at base in 11 cases while angulating the Endospine to approach opposite side in canal decompression. If the incision is relatively close to spinous process and bone is osteoporotic in elderly patient. Degenerative angulation of the spinous process toward the side of the endoscopic approach is another factor responsible for this. This is one of the factors causing pain at the approach site postoperatively. In spinal canal stenosis above the L4–L5 level, the interlaminar and interpedicular distances become smaller and smaller. In 45 cases we had to excise the ipsilateral facet to decompress the canal and nerve root. In all these cases, the opposite facet was intact, with undercut lamina and muscle attachment. This maintained the stability of the motion segment.

We had 95% excellent results with endoscopic diskectomy, diskectomy and canal decompression, and bilateral canal decompression with a unilateral approach. We used modified McNab's criteria for evaluation, with a good result in 2%, fair result in 1%, and poor result in 1% of cases.[4]

19.9 Conclusion

Endoscopic spine surgery with Endospine—Destandau's technique—is a safe procedure, although with a very steep learning curve. Once the surgeon has passed through the initial learning curve safely, any lumbar degenerative pathology without instability can be successfully treated. The incision may remain the same in thin average-build patients, but the mobile tubular retractor helps in achieving the same results through a small incision in obese patients and in lumbar canal stenosis.

References

1   Isaacs RE, Podichetty V, Fessler RG. Microendoscopic discectomy for recurrent disc herniations. *Neurosurg Focus* 2003;15(3):E11
2   Maroon JC. Current concepts in minimally invasive discectomy. *Neurosurgery* 2002;51(5, Suppl):S137–S145
3   Park CK. The effect of patient positioning on intraabdominal pressure and blood loss in spinal surgery. *Anesth Analg* 2000;91(3):552–557
4   Destandau J. Endoscopically assisted lumbar microdiscectomy. *J Minim Invasive Spine Surg Tech* 2001;1(1):41–43
5   Nowitzke AM. Assessment of the learning curve for lumbar microendoscopic discectomy. *Neurosurgery* 2005;56(4):755–762
6   Khoo LT, Khoo KM, Isaacs RE, et al. Endoscopic lumbar laminotomy for stenosis. In: Perez-Cruet MJ, Fessler RG, eds. *Outpatient Spinal Surgery*. St. Louis: Quality Medical Publishing; 2002:197–215
7   Yadav YR, Parihar V, Namdeo H, Agrawal M, Bhatele PR. Endoscopic interlaminar management of lumbar disc disease. *J Neurol Surg A Cent Eur Neurosurg* 2013;74(2):77–81

20 Endoscopic Transforaminal Lumbar Interbody Fusion and Instrumentation

Faheem A. Sandhu

20.1 Introduction

In the early 1900s, dorsal lumbar fusion techniques were often unsuccessful. This led Muller to attempt to treat patients who had Potts disease through an anterior approach.[1] In the 1930s, Burns performed a successful transabdominal lumbar interbody fusion for traumatic spondylolisthesis.[1] In the 1940s, interbody fusion techniques were further modified to include placement of an autograft, in the form of the removed spinous process and lamina, into the intervertebral space.[2,3] In 1953, Cloward reintroduced the concept of the posterior approach for lumbar interbody fusion and advocated that this technique replace stand-alone lumbar diskectomy and laminectomies.[4] Through Cloward's posterior lumbar interbody fusion (PLIF), 360° of stabilization was achieved via a single dorsal incision, eliminating the need for additional anterior surgery.[5] However, the risks involved with the approach were not insignificant and included neural injury from significant retraction of the thecal sac and nerve root, as well as CSF leak.

In an attempt to reduce the complications associated with PLIF, Harms and Rolinger introduced an alternative method to achieve circumferential lumbar fusion in 1982.[6] By means of a unilateral facetectomy, a transforaminal window was created for placement of a titanium mesh and bone graft. In comparison to the PLIF, the transforaminal approach for lumbar interbody fusion (TLIF) decreases retraction of the neural elements and is performed from a unilateral approach.[6] TLIF also allows for more anterior placement of a larger interbody graft, thereby achieving greater foraminal decompression and restoration of lumbar lordosis. Furthermore, the TLIF avoids disruption of the contralateral facet and pars and is also associated with significantly less blood loss.[7,8,9]

The most recent advancement in lumbar interbody fusions is the development of minimally invasive (MI)/endoscopic techniques.[10,11,12] The open TLIF approach causes disruption of the musculoligamentous complex and requires significant lateral retraction of the musculature for adequate exposure of the surgical anatomy. This has been negatively correlated with long-term lumbar fusion outcomes.[13,14] The development of tubular retractor systems has allowed the achievement of lumbar arthrodesis while minimizing soft tissue damage.[15,16,17] This chapter reviews the appropriate candidates for the procedure, the surgical technique, and details on how to avoid the complications and pitfalls of the MI/endoscopic TLIF.

20.2 Choice of Patient

Indications

The indications for the procedure include:

- Grade I/II spondylolisthesis with dynamic instability
- Pseudoarthrosis
- Postlaminectomy lumbar kyphosis
- Degenerative disk disease and mechanical back pain with reproducible symptoms on provocative testing
- Recurrent disk herniation with mechanical back pain
- Interspace collapse with radiculopathy after diskectomy
- Three or more recurrent disk herniations with radiculopathy
- Instability secondary to trauma
- Lumbar deformity with coronal/sagittal imbalance

Contraindications

Contraindications to the procedure are:

- Multilevel degenerative disk disease without deformity
- Single-level disk disease without mechanical back pain or instability
- Severe osteoporosis

20.3 Technique

Surgical Equipment

- The open Jackson table is preferred, because it promotes lumbar lordosis and decreases intra-abdominal pressure and epidural vein congestion.
- C-arm fluoroscopy
- Expandable tubular retractor
- Endoscope, loupe with headlight, or microscope
- High-speed drill
- Standard laminectomy/fusion surgical set
- Distractors (7–14 mm), rotating cutters, end plate scrapers
- Interbody graft material (polyether ether ketone [PEEK] cage or titanium cage)
- Bone graft material
- K-wire
- Cannulated pedicle screws

Operating Room Setup

- Operating table is placed in the center of the room.
- Anesthesia is positioned at the head of the table.
- C-arm fluoroscopy base is placed on the side opposite the surgical approach.
- Equipment tables should be situated behind the primary surgeon, with the Mayo stand over the patient's feet.

Anesthesia/EMG

- Anesthesia should be asked to avoid paralytics, nitrous oxide, and muscle relaxants, to prevent any interference with EMG recordings.
- Intubation

- Placement of the Foley catheter, EMG leads on the lower extremities, and sequential compression devices should be completed prior to placing the patient in the prone position.
- Preoperative antibiotic should be administered. (We prefer cefazolin or vancomycin if the patient has a penicillin allergy.)

Positioning and Localization

- The patient is placed in the prone position on an open Jackson table.
- The C-arm is used to localize and mark the level(s) of pathology (**Fig. 20.1**) (**Video 20.1**).

Exposure

- A 2.5-cm longitudinal incision is made 4 cm from the midline on the symptomatic side.
- The incision should be carried down to the dorsal lumbar fascia (**Fig. 20.2**).
- A Steinmann pin is inserted at 35° to 45° to rest on the facet complex, and this is confirmed with fluoroscopy (**Fig. 20.3**).
- Sequential soft tissue dilators and tubular retractors are used to split muscle (**Fig. 20.4**).
- The tubular retractor is secured to the table with a flexible arm clamp and the correct level is confirmed with C-arm fluoroscopy (**Fig. 20.5**).

- Soft tissue overlying the lamina and facet complex is then removed using monopolar cautery (**Fig. 20.6**).

Laminectomy/Facetectomy

- The working channel is then angled medially for performance of the laminectomy and facetectomy.
- Using a straight curet, the inferior edge of the lamina is defined.
- Using angled curets, a plane is developed between the undersurface of the lamina and the ligamentum flavum.
- The lamina is thinned with a high-speed drill (**Fig. 20.7**) and then is removed using angled Kerrison rongeurs. This decompression should extend from pedicle to pedicle at the levels above and below the interspace.
- Alternatively, an osteotome can be used to remove the facet by making cuts along the medial aspect of the facet and one perpendicular to this at the base of the pars (**Fig. 20.8**). The remainder of the lamina is then removed with Kerrison rongeurs.
- A total facetectomy is also performed in preparation for placement of the interbody cage.
- The bone removed in the laminectomy and facetectomy is saved for use as part of the interbody and lateral fusion mass.

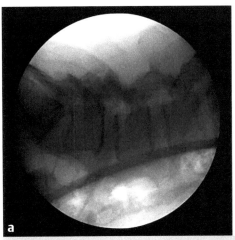
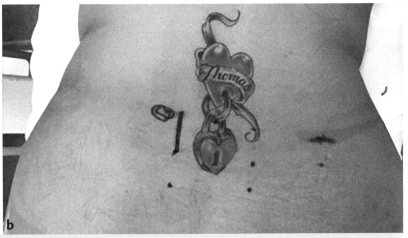

Fig. 20.1 (a,b) Patient in the prone position, level of pathology localized with C-arm fluoroscopy, and 2.5- cm incision marked on the patient's symptomatic left side.

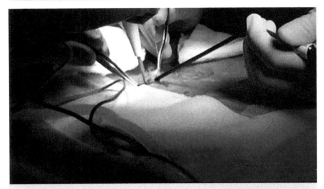

Fig. 20.2 After the incision has been made, the exposure is carried down through the lumbar dorsal fascia with monopolar electrocautery.

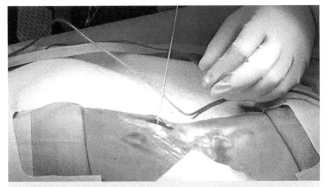

Fig. 20.3 Steinmann pin is inserted to rest on the facet complex, and correct operative level is confirmed with fluoroscopy.

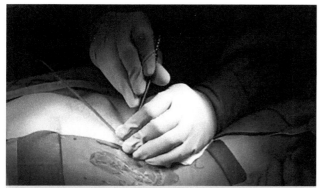

Fig. 20.4 Sequential muscle-splitting dilators are placed; the tubular retractor is placed over the dilators and is secured to the table with a clamp.

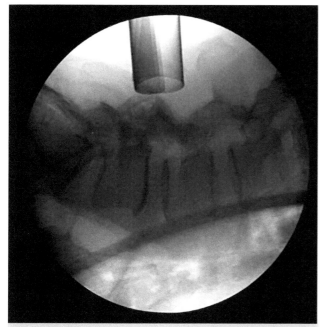

Fig. 20.5 Tubular retractor has been placed over the lamina and facet complex, and the correct level is reconfirmed with C-arm fluoroscopy.

- To complete the decompression, the ligamentum flavum is also removed with the use of Kerrison rongeurs (**Fig. 20.9**, **Fig. 20.10**).
- At this point, the lateral thecal sac, traversing nerve root, and disk space should be visualized. We do not attempt to fully expose the exiting nerve root since there is usually adequate exposure of the disk space without visualizing it, and this helps to protect the dorsal root ganglia from injury during cage placement.

Interbody Fusion

- The epidural veins are coagulated using a bipolar cautery (**Fig. 20.11**).
- A No. 15 blade scalpel is used to incise the annulus.
- Ipsilateral and contralateral disk material is removed using straight and angled pituitary rongeurs (**Fig. 20.12**).
- A variety of end plate scrapers and rotating cutters are used to clean the cartilaginous end plates (**Fig. 20.13**).

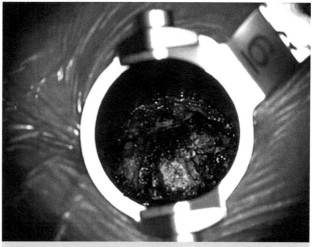

Fig. 20.6 Soft tissue overlying the lamina and facet complex has been removed with monopolar electrocautery.

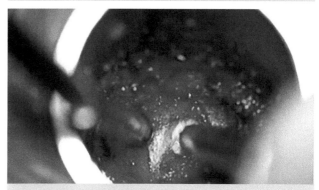

Fig. 20.7 Lamina is thinned with a high-speed drill.

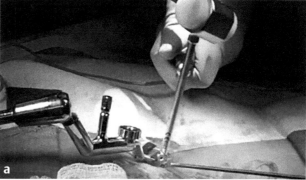

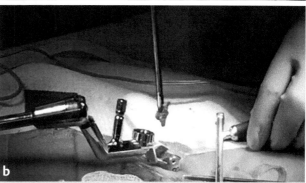

Fig. 20.8 (a,b) Alternatively, the lamina and facet complex may be removed using an osteotome by making a cut at the medial aspect of the facet and a perpendicular cut at the base of the pars.

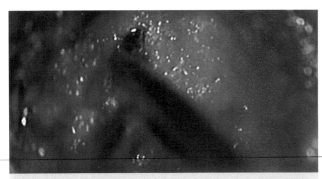

Fig. 20.9 An angled curet is used to develop a plane between the ligamentum flavum and thecal sac.

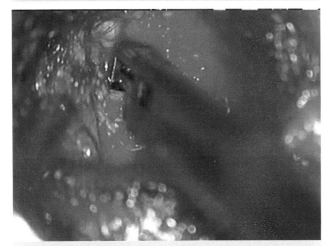

Fig. 20.10 Kerrison rongeurs are used to remove the ligamentum flavum and to complete the decompression of the thecal sac.

- Debris is removed with pituitary rongeurs, and the operative site is irrigated copiously with antibiotic saline.
- We rely heavily on up- and down-angled curets to ensure that end plates are appropriately prepared for arthrodesis (**Fig. 20.14**).
- Using sequential disk space dilators, the interspace is dilated to a height similar to that of the adjacent levels.
- A crescent-shaped cage is packed with bone graft material (**Fig. 20.15**).
- The crescent-shaped cage is then placed in the interspace, and correct placement is confirmed with fluoroscopy (**Fig. 20.16**).
- Hemostasis is then obtained with a flowable hemostatic agent.
- Tubular retractors are then angled laterally and the transverse processes are exposed, as well as the mammillary process.
- A high-speed bur is used to create an entry point into the pedicle, and this is extended into the vertebral body with a probe. Lateral fluoroscopy is helpful when placing screws.
- Screws, rod, and caps are then placed under direct visualization. Alternatively, the retractor can be removed and percutaneous pedicle screws can be placed.
- The transverse processes are decorticated using a high-speed drill, and autograft bone is packed in between.
- Cancellous bone chips can be used to supplement the autograft (**Fig. 20.17**).

Instrumentation (Illustrated in Chapter 14)

- Another C-arm is brought in to visualize the level of interest in both the AP and lateral planes. A Jamshidi needle is placed

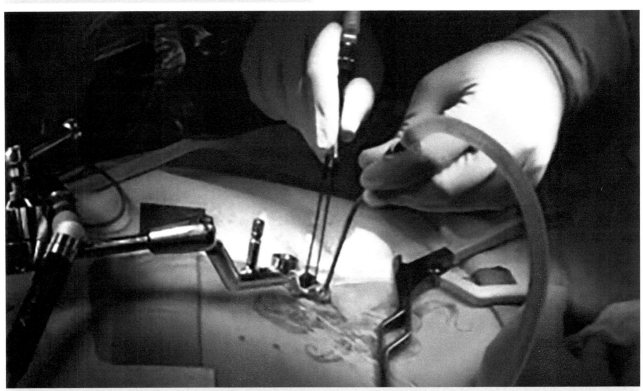

Fig. 20.11 Epidural veins are coagulated using bipolar electrocautery

on the lateral wall of the pedicle (at 3 and 9 o'clock positions on AP images) and is carefully advanced through the pedicle using serial imaging until it enters the vertebral body.

- The stylet is removed, and a K-wire is pushed ~ 1 cm into the vertebral body.
- The Jamshidi needle is now removed, with the surgeon taking care not to dislodge the K-wire, and a fluoroscopic image is taken to confirm good position of the K-wire.
- The soft tissue in the path of the K-wire is dilated using sequential dilators.
- The pedicles are tapped, and then cannulated pedicle screws are placed.
- K-wires are removed once the cannulated screw traverses the pedicle.
- Rod size is determined using calipers.
- The rod is attached to a delivery system specific to the instrumentation system and is pushed through soft tissue and screw heads.
- A final AP fluoroscopy film is taken to confirm good placement of the rods if they cannot be directly visualized in the screw heads.
- Set caps are applied, the pedicle screws are compressed, and final tightening is performed using a torque-limiting wrench.
- Screw extenders are removed.
- Wounds are adequately irrigated with antibiotic saline and are closed in layers using absorbable sutures.
- Dressings are applied per surgeon preference. We dress the wound with Steri-Strips, Telfa non-adherent dressing, and clear Tegaderm.

20.4 Complication Avoidance

As with any surgical procedure, there are several complications that may occur during MI/endoscopic TLIF. Dural tears and nerve injury can occur if the Steinmann pin or dilators slip into the interlaminar space. This can be avoided by removing the pin after the initial dilator is passed and is confirmed by fluoroscopy to be docked on bone. The same complications can be avoided during decompression by using straight and angled curets to develop a well-defined plane. Good illumination and visualization should be present throughout the course of the surgery. Anterior displacement of the interbody cage can be avoided by taking care to preserve the anterior longitudinal ligament during disk preparation.

Bone can be breached during placement of pedicle screws. Taking adequate fluoroscopic images to ensure that K-wires are well centered through the axis of the pedicle and are parallel to the vertebral body superior end plate can minimize risk of this complication. Intraoperative EMG monitoring also provides continuous feedback about nerve function throughout placement of the interbody and instrumentation. Pseudarthrosis, although not an immediate complication, can be minimized by meticulous preparation of the end plates. For this reason, disk preparation is often the lengthiest portion of the procedure. In experienced hands, complications can be avoided with great care and attention to detail.

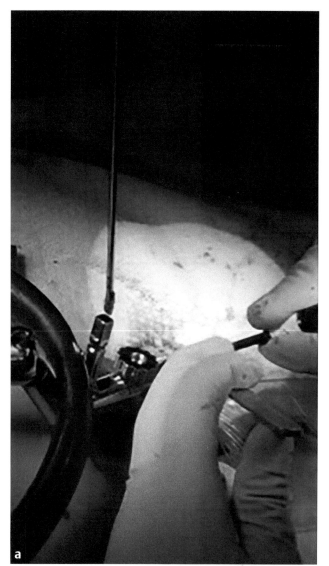

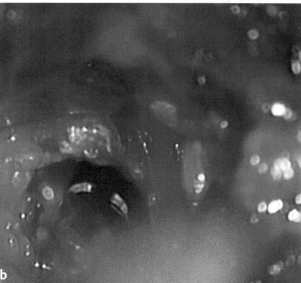

Fig. 20.12 (a,b) After the annulus has been incised with a No. 15 blade, a combination of straight and angled pituitary rongeurs are used to remove disk material.

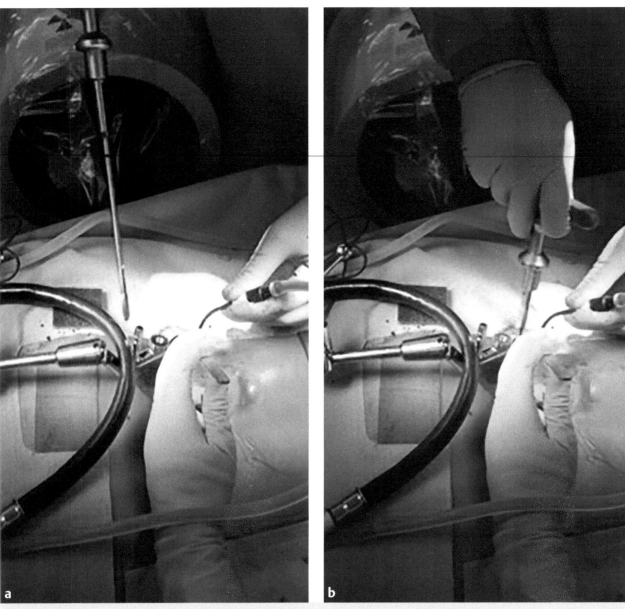

Fig. 20.13 (a,b) The cartilaginous end plate of adjacent vertebral bodies is cleaned with a variety of scrapers and cutters.

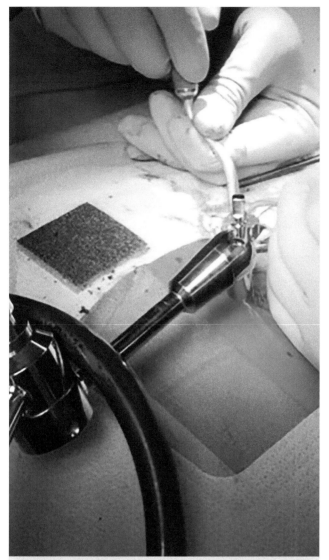

Fig. 20.14 Up- and down-angled curets are used to confirm that the end plates are well prepared for arthrodesis.

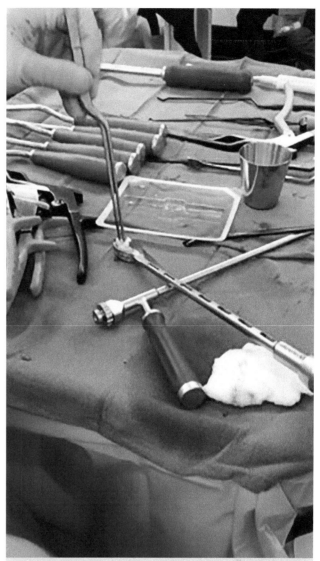

Fig. 20.15 A crescent-shaped interbody cage is prepared with bone graft material.

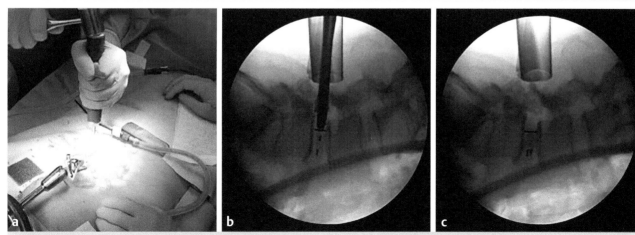

Fig. 20.16 (a,b,c) The interbody cage is placed in the interspace. Correct placement is confirmed using C-arm fluoroscopy.

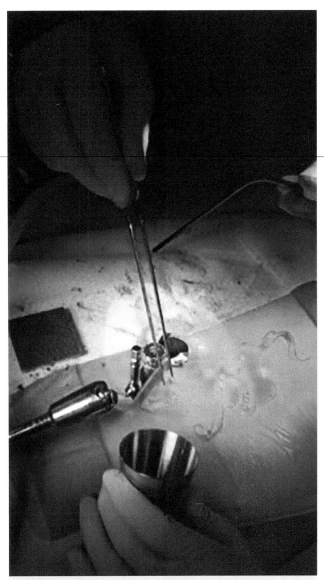

Fig. 20.17 Cancellous bone chips are placed to supplement the bone graft material.

References

1. Mummaneni PV, Lin FJ, Haid RW, et al. Current indications and techniques for anterior approaches to the lumbar spine. *Contemp Neurosurg* 2002;*24*(10):1–8
2. Briggs H, Milligan P. Chip fusion of the low back following exploration of the spinal canal. *J Bone Joint Surg.* 1944;*26*:125–130
3. Jaslow IA. Intercorporal bone graft in spinal fusion after disc removal. *Surg Gynecol Obstet* 1946;*82*:215–218
4. Cloward RB. The treatment of ruptured lumbar intervertebral discs by vertebral body fusion. I. Indications, operative technique, after care. *J Neurosurg* 1953;*10*(2):154–168
5. Cloward RB. Posterior lumbar interbody fusion updated. *Clin Orthop Relat Res* 1985;(193):16–19
6. Harms J, Rolinger H. [A one-stage procedure in operative treatment of spondylolisthesis: dorsal traction-reposition and anterior fusion (author's transl)]. *Z Orthop Ihre Grenzgeb* 1982;*120*(3):343–347
7. Whitecloud TS III, Roesch WW, Ricciardi JE. Transforaminal interbody fusion versus anterior-posterior interbody fusion of the lumbar spine: a financial analysis. *J Spinal Disord* 2001;*14*(2):100–103
8. Humphreys SC, Hodges SD, Patwardhan AG, Eck JC, Murphy RB, Covington LA. Comparison of posterior and transforaminal approaches to lumbar interbody fusion. *Spine* 2001;*26*(5):567–571
9. Hee HT, Castro FP Jr, Majd ME, Holt RT, Myers L. Anterior/posterior lumbar fusion versus transforaminal lumbar interbody fusion: analysis of complications and predictive factors. *J Spinal Disord* 2001;*14*(6):533–540
10. Mummaneni PV, Haid RW, Rodts GE. Lumbar interbody fusion: state-of-the-art technical advances. *J Neurosurg Spine* 2004;*1*:24–30
11. Isaacs RE, Podichetty VK, Santiago P, et al. Minimally invasive microendoscopy-assisted transforaminal lumbar interbody fusion with instrumentation. *J Neurosurg Spine* 2005;*3*(2):98–105
12. Foley KT, Holly LT, Schwender JD. Minimally invasive lumbar fusion. *Spine* 2003;*28*(15, Suppl):S26–S35
13. Kawaguchi Y, Yabuki S, Styf J, et al. Back muscle injury after posterior lumbar spine surgery. Topographic evaluation of intramuscular pressure and blood flow in the porcine back muscle during surgery. *Spine* 1996;*21*(22):2683–2688
14. Wetzel FT, LaRocca H. The failed posterior lumbar interbody fusion. *Spine* 1991;*16*(7):839–845
15. Cloward RB. Spondylolisthesis: treatment by laminectomy and posterior interbody fusion. *Clin Orthop Relat Res* 1981;(154):74–82
16. Hutter CG. Spinal stenosis and posterior lumbar interbody fusion. *Clin Orthop Relat Res* 1985;(193):103–114
17. Branch CL Jr. The case for posterior lumbar interbody fusion. *Clin Neurosurg* 1996;*43*:252–267

21 Endoscopic/Percutaneous Lumbar Pedicle Screw Fixation Technique

Faheem A. Sandhu, Josh Ryan, and R. Tushar Jha

21.1 Introduction

The desire to minimize the surgical morbidity caused by excessive muscle dissection and retraction, which is typical of traditional open procedures, has been a major impetus in the development of minimally invasive spine procedures. The first description of a paraspinal muscle-splitting approach between the multifidus and longissimus muscles for insertion of pedicle screws was done by Wiltse and Spencer in 1988.[1] This procedure served as a gateway through which surgeons have continued to advance minimally invasive lumbar spine techniques. Percutaneous pedicle screw insertion was first described in 1982 by Magerl, but it was intended to be used as part of an external fixation construct.[2] In 2001, Foley et al described the insertion of a longitudinal connector rod between the percutaneous pedicle screws via a minimally invasive approach, which heralded the use of percutaneous pedicle screws for internal fixation.[3] Other systems for percutaneous pedicle screw fixation (PPSF) have since emerged, and the endoscope can be employed with these systems in various ways. The traditional percutaneous method and the endoscopic method of pedicle screw insertion are both be described here.

21.2 Choice of Patient

21.2.1 Indications

Indications for lumbar pedicle screw fixation include:

- Symptomatic grade I or II spondylolisthesis, including postlaminectomy spondylolisthesis and spondylolisthesis caused by spondylolysis
- Augmentation of anterior element fusion procedures, such as anterior lumbar interbody fusion (ALIF), lateral lumbar interbody fusion (LLIF), minimally invasive transforaminal lumbar interbody fusion (MI-TLIF), or minimally invasive posterior lumbar interbody fusion (MI-PLIF)
- Recurrent lumbar disk herniation leading to radiculopathy that is not responsive to conservative management
- Fractures of the lumbar vertebral body, pedicle,[4] or facet causing instability in a neurologically intact patient. Pedicle screw fixation has also been described as an option for lumbar Chance fractures to avoid long periods of external casting and to facilitate early mobilization of the patient.[5]
- Degenerative scoliosis
- Stabilization of osteotomies

21.2.2 Relative Contraindications

Relative contraindications are:

- Morbid obesity, as retractor tubes may not be long enough and radiographic anatomy may be obscured
- Patients with osteoporosis, as K-wires can advance easily through the bone

- Patients with prior posterior surgery at the same level in whom an open procedure may be safer because of the risk of encountering abnormal anatomy
- Patients with multiplanar deformity
- Active systemic or spinal infection
- Allergy to metals

21.3 Percutaneous Technique

21.3.1 Position and Anesthesia

- General anesthesia is used and the patient is placed in the prone position, with the hips and knees in flexion and the abdomen supported, on a Jackson table (**Fig. 21.1**).
- If PPSF is being used as an augmentation to ALIF or LLIF, the patient may need to be repositioned to prone after the prior procedure before the procedures can be staged.
- Percutaneous transfacet screw insertion has been described with the patient in the lateral decubitus position after LLIF, and this position could also be used for percutaneous pedicle screw insertion, but description of this technique is outside the scope of this chapter.[6]
- Either intraoperative 3D imaging or C-arm fluoroscopy may be used. Two C-arm machines may be utilized simultaneously in the AP and lateral planes to avoid moving a single C-arm between planes (**Fig. 21.1**).
- If the C-arm is used, true AP and lateral views must be obtained. A true AP view is indicated by a flat superior end plate with spinous processes centered between pedicles. A true lateral view is indicated by a flat superior end plate with pedicles superimposed.
- Prep and drape the patient in the same fashion as for an open procedure.

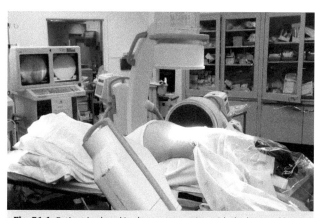

Fig. 21.1 Patient is placed in the prone position with the hips and knees flexed. Two C-arms are used in the AP and lateral positions to expedite the procedure.

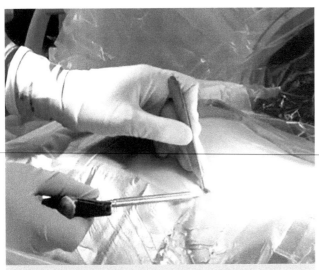

Fig. 21.2 A vertical incision is made with a scalpel and is extended through the lumbodorsal fascia.

21.3.2 Marking and Skin Incision

- Two vertical incisions are made for each level of interest, each 1.5 cm in length and ~ 4 cm from the midline on either side, centered at the level of the pedicles (**Fig. 21.2**).
- Patients with larger or smaller body habitus may require incisions farther from or closer to the midline, respectively, to account for the amount of soft tissue traversed.
- Extend the incision through the lumbodorsal fascia using either sharp dissection or monopolar electrocautery.

21.3.3 Needle Insertion and Dilation

- Use the index finger to extend through the fascial incision and palpate the base of the transverse process.
- Alternatively, just insert a Jamshidi needle through the skin and fascial incisions down to the junction of the base of the transverse process and the facet (**Fig. 21.3**).

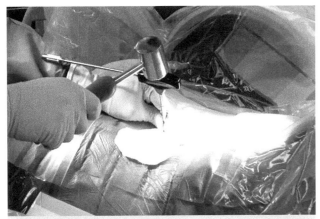

Fig. 21.4 Mallet is used to advance the Jamshidi needle through the pedicle to the junction of the pedicle and vertebral body. The distance is ~ 20 mm deep from the docking point.

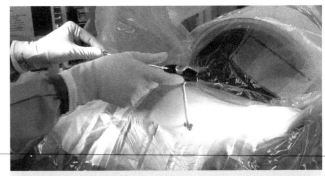

Fig. 21.3 Jamshidi needle is placed through the skin and fascial incision down to the base of the transverse process and facet junction.

- The Jamshidi needle should be docked on the lateral border of the pedicle in the AP fluoroscopic views.
- Tap the Jamshidi needle gently with a mallet (**Fig. 21.4**) until it has advanced through the pedicle and to the border of the pedicle and vertebral body. Intermittently check both AP and lateral fluoroscopic views as the needle is advanced. The Jamshidi should be ~ 20 mm deep from the docking point as it passes from the pedicle into the vertebral body. The final AP view should show that the tip of the Jamshidi needle has not advanced past the medial border of the pedicle.

21.3.4 Screw Insertion

- With the Jamshidi needle in place, remove the inner cannula (**Fig. 21.5**) and then pass the K-wire through the Jamshidi needle (**Fig. 21.6**). With gentle pressure, advance the K-wire into the vertebral body.
- Remove the Jamshidi needle over the K-wire, ensuring not to inadvertently pull the K-wire out (**Fig. 21.7**).
- All previous steps up to this point are repeated for each pedicle until K-wires have been placed in all pedicles of interest. Fluoroscopic AP and lateral confirmation of adequate position of all K-wires is now obtained (**Fig. 21.8**).

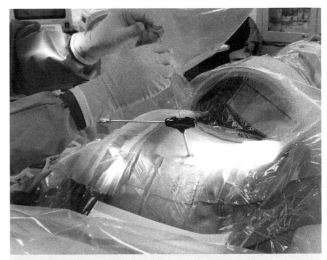

Fig. 21.5 Inner cannula of Jamshidi needle is removed.

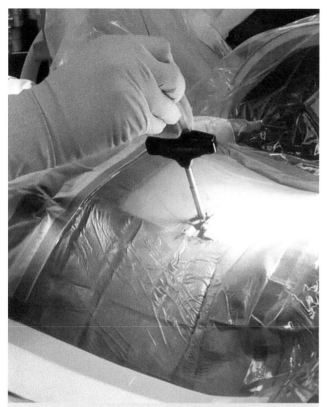

Fig. 21.6 K-wire is inserted and gently advanced to the vertebral body.

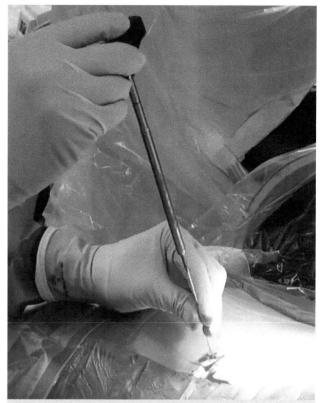

Fig. 21.7 Jamshidi needle is removed over the K-wire.

- Advance a cannulated tap (if desired) over the K-wire and tap the pedicle down to its base. Electromyography (EMG) stimulation of the tap can be used to detect medial or inferior wall breaches.
- Remove the tap over the K-wire. Advance the pedicle screw over the K-wire, through the pedicle, and into the vertebral body (**Fig. 21.9a**). The K-wire is removed as the screw enters

the vertebral body (**Fig. 21.9b**). Align the screw heads in the rostral-caudal direction to facilitate passage of the rod. Each screw has removable extenders attached to the head to create a small working channel through which the screw head can be visualized and a rod may be passed.

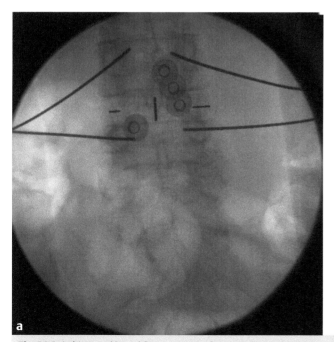

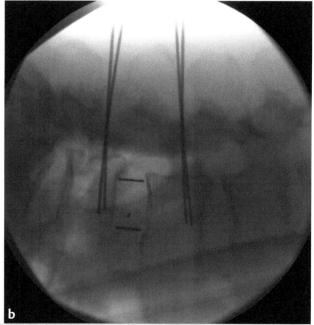

Fig. 21.8 (a,b) AP and lateral fluoroscopy confirming appropriate placement of all K-wires.

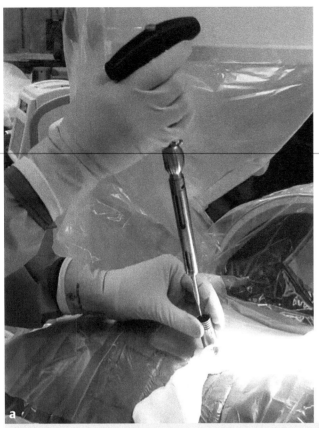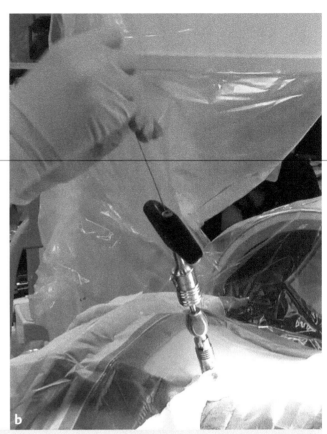

Fig. 21.9 (a,b) Pedicle screw is passed over the K-wire and the K-wire is removed once the pedicle screw has entered the vertebral body on fluoroscopy. Screw is advanced to its final position.

21.3.5 Rod Insertion

- The appropriate length of rod is determined by placing a caliper in the heads of the rostral- and caudal-most screws (**Fig. 21.10**). The rod is rigidly attached to a rod holder, which grips the rod at one end. Advance the free end of the rod longitudinally into either the superior-most or inferior-most incision (**Fig. 21.11a**) and down to the head of the closest screw (**Fig. 21.11b**).

- With an arc-like movement, advance the free end of the rod toward the next screw head while gradually moving the rod from a vertical to a horizontal position as it is advanced (**Fig. 21.12**). For long rod constructs, a new remote incision may be required to complete the arc movement.

- Continue until the rod is seated appropriately in the head of each screw. If a lordotic rod is used, a marking pen can be used to mark longitudinally on the rod prior to insertion so that the lordotic side of the screw can be visualized in situ.

- An endoscope can be introduced into the working channel of each screw to better visualize correct passage of the rod through the screw heads.

- With the rod in the appropriate position, place the guide over the first screw head and hand-tighten a cap onto the screw head. If performing a two-level operation, place the middle screw cap first. Most systems have reduction tools to help manipulate spinal alignment if desired. Continue until all screw caps have been hand-tightened.

- Use a torque wrench for final tightening of each screw cap in place, using the guide to apply counter-torque. Final imaging shows good positioning of the screws and rods (**Fig. 21.13**).

21.4 Endoscopic Technique

This technique can be used for up to two-level operations and allows the surgeon to incorporate a posterolateral fusion along with the pedicle screw instrumentation. This is due to the expanded working channel through which decortication of the posterolateral elements can be achieved. The technique also allows the surgeon to perform a simultaneous minimally invasive decompression or interbody fusion through the same incision (**Video 21.1**).

21.4.1 Position and Anesthesia

General anesthesia is used, and the patient is positioned, prepped, and draped in the same fashion as for percutaneous pedicle screw insertion.

21.4.2 Marking and Skin Incision

- Two vertical incisions are made, each ~ 2.5 cm long and ~ 4 cm from the midline on either side, centered at the level of the pedicles. The technique requires only two incisions total, rather than two incisions at each level.

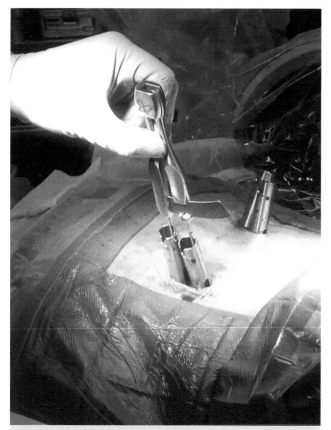

Fig. 21.10 Caliper is inserted onto the most rostral and caudal screw heads to determine the appropriate rod length.

- Patients with larger or smaller body habitus may require incisions farther from or closer to the midline, respectively, to account for the amount of soft tissue traversed.
- Extend the incision through the lumbodorsal fascia using either sharp dissection or monopolar electrocautery.

21.4.3 Needle Insertion and Dilation

- Use the index finger to extend through the fascial incision and palpate the base of the transverse process.
- Alternatively, just insert a Jamshidi needle through the skin and fascial incisions down to the junction of the base of the transverse process and the facet.
- The Jamshidi needle should be docked on the lateral border of the pedicle in the AP fluoroscopic views.
- Tap the Jamshidi needle gently with a mallet until it has advanced through the pedicle and to the border of the pedicle and vertebral body, intermittently checking both AP and lateral fluoroscopic views as it is advanced. The Jamshidi should be ~ 20 mm deep from the docking point as it passes from the pedicle into the vertebral body. The final AP view here should show that the tip of the Jamshidi needle has not advanced past the medial border of the pedicle.

21.4.4 Screw Insertion

- With the Jamshidi needle in place, remove the inner cannula and then insert the fiducial pin through the needle. Tap the

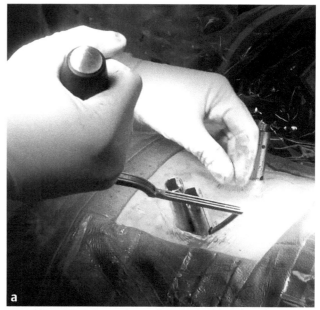

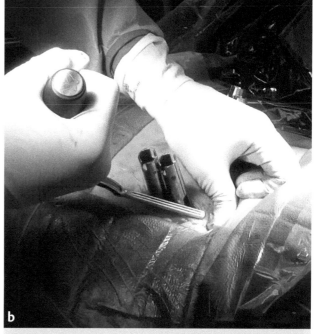

Fig. 21.11 (**a,b**) The rod is rigidly attached to a rod holder and the free end is longitudinally advanced down to the screw head located in the superior-most incision.

pin lightly with a mallet and advance the pin until 1 to 2 cm of the pin is still visible above the posterior bony margin on lateral fluoroscopy.[7]

- Remove the Jamshidi needle over the fiducial pin, taking care not to inadvertently pull the pin out.
- Repeat the prior steps through the same two incisions until fiducial pins have been placed in all pedicles of interest. Obtain AP and lateral fluoroscopic confirmation of adequate position of all pins.
- Serial soft tissue dilators can now be advanced over an inserted guidewire to create a channel through the fascia. An expandable, minimally invasive tubular retractor, such as the

FlexPosure device, can be used for a two-level operation to adequately visualize all levels of interest.

- The tubular retractor can be used to perform a decompression or interbody fusion procedure at this time, or it can be centered over the fiducial pins to move forward with pedicle screw insertion.

- Introduce the endoscope through the working channel and clear soft tissue from around the pedicle screw entry sites with monopolar electrocautery. Again, the endoscope can also be used to assist in decompression or interbody fusion at this time, if desired.

- The high-speed drill may be used at this time or after screw insertion to decorticate the posterior bony elements for posterolateral fusion.

- With the fiducial pins adequately in view, advance a tap over each pin and tap the pedicle down to its base. Electromyography stimulation of the tap can be used to detect medial or inferior wall breaches.

- Remove the tap and fiducial pin. Then advance the pedicle screw into the prepared entry hole, through the pedicle, and into the vertebral body. Align the screw heads in the rostral-caudal direction to facilitate passage of the rod.

21.4.5 Rod Insertion

- The rod is inserted through each screw head in the same fashion used for percutaneous pedicle screw insertion.

- The endoscope is used through the working channel to visualize adequate insertion of the rod into each screw head.

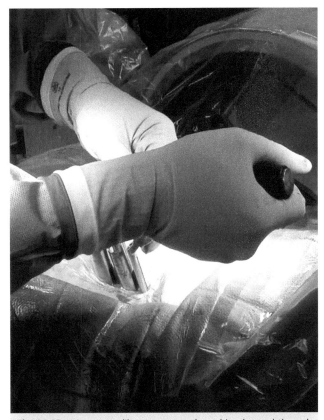

Fig. 21.12 Using an arc-like movement, the rod is advanced through soft tissue and is appropriately seated on the inferior screw's head.

21.5 Complications and Avoidance

Several potential complications with endoscopic/percutaneous pedicle screw insertion have been reported in the literature. A complication that is frequently discussed in the recent literature is violation of the superior articular facet during screw insertion. The concern with facet violation (FV) is that it could possibly contribute to adjacent-segment disease, although more investigation is needed to evaluate if this is the case. A cadaveric study by Patel et al in 2011 evaluated the incidence of superior-level FV during the insertion of 48 lumbar percutaneous pedicle screws by four blinded orthopedic surgeons on four specimens.[8] They found that 28 screws (58%) had FV and that 8 screws (16.7%) were intraarticular. A comparative study was done by Babu et al in 2012 to evaluate the incidence of superior-level FV between open (N = 126 operations) and percutaneous (N = 153 operations) lumbar pedicle screw placement.[9] This retrospective analysis used postoperative CT scans to evaluate for the presence of FV. The investigators found that the incidence of grade 3 (intra-articular) FV was significantly higher in the percutaneous group than the open group (8.5% vs 2.0%, p = 0.0059). They found no significant difference between the two groups in grade 1 (extraarticular, 25.0% vs 26.8%, p = 0.70) or grade 2 ($\leq$ 1 mm articular penetration, 7.1% vs 4.9%, p = 0.34) FV. A similar retrospective analysis by Jones-Quaidoo in 2013 showed that 36 of 264 (13.6%) percutaneous lumbar pedicle screws versus 16 of 263 (6.1%) open pedicle screws were intraarticular (p = 0.005).[10]

However, a 2013 retrospective analysis by Yson et al was done to compare FV rates between open and percutaneous lumbar pedicle screw insertion while using intraoperative 3D CT (O-arm) navigation (the previously reported studies had used C-arm fluoroscopy).[11] Yson and colleagues found that the FV rate was significantly higher in the open group than in the percutaneous group (26.5% vs 4%, p < 0.0001) when using 3D intraoperative guidance. Avoidance of superior-level FV hinges on adequate intraoperative imaging. If biplanar fluoroscopy is used, it is crucial to achieve true AP and true lateral views to avoid malposition of the screw. As suggested by the previous study, 3D intraoperative guidance may lead to lower rates of FV for percutaneous cases. Also, the endoscopic technique provides the surgeon with direct visualization of the surrounding anatomy and pedicle screw insertion site in addition to intraoperative imaging.

Breach of the pedicle during screw insertion is another potential complication encountered during endoscopic/percutaneous pedicle screw insertion. In 2012, Raley and Mobbs performed a retrospective analysis of 424 percutaneously inserted thoracic and lumbar pedicle screws using postoperative CT evaluation.[12] In total, 41 of 424 (9.7%) were misplaced, although only two of the breaches were grade 3 (both caused pedicle fractures) and only one patient had an associated neurologic deficit (L4 radiculopathy). A similar study was done by Heintel et al in 2013 to evaluate thoracic and lumbar percutaneous pedicle screw placement for patients with traumatic fractures.[13] The authors reported eight malpositioned screws total, and only three medial breaches (all thoracic) in 502 inserted screws. One of the patients required reoperation due to a postoperative neurologic deficit. Oh et al retrospectively compared open and percutaneous lumbar pedicle screw accuracy in 2013.[14] They found no significant difference between the two groups in incidence of

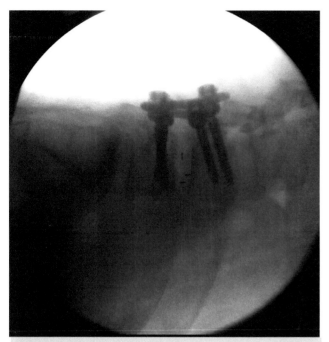

Fig. 21.13 Fluoroscopic image showing pedicle screws and rods in adequate position at the end of the procedure.

pedicle wall penetration (13.4% for open vs 14.3% for percutaneous, p = 0.695). As with superior-level FV, avoidance of pedicle breach during endoscopic/percutaneous pedicle screw insertion is largely dependent upon achieving and utilizing adequate radiographic navigation.

In addition to ensuring true AP and lateral fluoroscopic views (or using 3D navigation), it is critical to intermittently monitor the AP plane during advancement of the Jamshidi needle. The needle tip should initially be docked on the lateral-most aspect of the pedicle on AP view and should not exceed three-quarters the distance from the lateral to medial pedicle border once the needle enters the vertebral body.[15] If the Jamshidi needle does not pass easily, it may be in cortical bone of the pedicle or facet and intraoperative imaging should be used to redirect the needle if necessary. In addition, stimulus-evoked EMG stimulation of the tap once it has traversed the pedicle is another tool the surgeon can use to attempt to detect a pedicle wall breach, particularly if the breach is medial or inferior. Wang et al prospectively evaluated 93 patients who underwent percutaneous placement of 409 lumbar pedicle screws using intraoperative EMG stimulation of the tap with an insulating sleeve and a threshold of < 12 mA indicating a breach.[16] Patients were evaluated with either intraoperative or postoperative CT scans and a total of five breaches were found, none of which was indicated by intraoperative EMG (false-negative rate of 1.2%). Three of the breaches were medial and two resulted in postoperative neurologic symptoms. Thirty-five screws stimulated below the 12 mA threshold and were found to be in the correct position, indicating a false-positive rate of 8.6%. In two instances, the screw trajectory was revised intraoperatively due to stimulation below threshold, with subsequent correct position confirmed. EMG tap stimulation is thus a tool in the surgeon's armamentarium to avoid pedicle breaches, but due to its unreliable nature, radiographic guidance remains a critical tool for avoidance of this complication. Last, careful preoperative radiographic review

of the bony anatomy and measurements of the pedicle allow the surgeon to choose an appropriately sized pedicle screw, thereby avoiding inducing a pedicle breach by a screw too large for its intended pedicle.

A rare but potentially devastating complication is perforation of the structures anterior to the vertebral body (aorta, iliac vessels, bowel, etc.) by either the K-wire or the pedicle screw itself. Raley et al reported four anterior radiographically detected breaches of the vertebral body with the K-wire in 424 inserted percutaneous pedicle screws (0.94%).[12] Only one of the patients experienced a complication, which was a retroperitoneal hemorrhage and ileus that resolved with conservative measures. The single most important factor in preventing this complication is firmly stabilizing the K-wire as multiple instruments are passed and advanced over it. The K-wire can be inadvertently pushed deeper into the soft cancellous bone, especially as the tap is advanced over it, and particularly in osteoporotic patients. If there is any question of advancement of the K-wire during passage or advancement of other instruments over it, lateral fluoroscopic imaging should be done to confirm that the K-wire has not advanced past the anterior border of the vertebral body. Again, a true lateral view is critical to discern actual position of the wire tip.

Alternatively, a "K-wireless" system has been developed, which consists of a Jamshidi needle with an attached tap and dilator system. This system allows placement of percutaneous pedicle screws without the use of a K-wire, and thus it eliminates complications associated with the wire.[17] Finally, like the K-wire, the pedicle screw itself may cause injury to structures anterior to the vertebral body, which can be avoided with careful insertion and intermittent radiographic confirmation as the screw is advanced.

References

1. Wiltse LL, Spencer CW. New uses and refinements of the paraspinal approach to the lumbar spine. *Spine* 1988;13(6):696–706
2. Magerl F. External skeletal fixation of the lower thoracic and the lumbar spine. In: Uhthoff HK, ed. *Current Concepts of External Fixation of Fractures.* Berlin: Springer-Verlag; 1982:353–366
3. Foley KT, Gupta SK, Justis JR, Sherman MC. Percutaneous pedicle screw fixation of the lumbar spine. *Neurosurg Focus* 2001;10(4):E10
4. Johnson JN, Wang MY. Stress fracture of the lumbar pedicle bilaterally: surgical repair using a percutaneous minimally invasive technique. *J Neurosurg Spine* 2009;11(6):724–728
5. Schizas C, Kosmopoulos V. Percutaneous surgical treatment of chance fractures using cannulated pedicle screws. Report of two cases. *J Neurosurg Spine* 2007;7(1):71–74
6. Voyadzis JM, Anaizi AN. Minimally invasive lumbar transfacet screw fixation in the lateral decubitus position after extreme lateral interbody fusion: a technique and feasibility study. *J Spinal Disord Tech* 2013;26(2):98–106
7. Kwon JW, Jahng TA, Chung CK, Kim HJ, Kim DH. Endoscope-assisted pedicle screw fixation using the pedicle guidance system. *Korean J Spine* 2008;5(3):190–195
8. Patel RD, Graziano GP, Vanderhave KL, Patel AA, Gerling MC. Facet violation with the placement of percutaneous pedicle screws. *Spine* 2011;36(26):E1749–E1752
9. Babu R, Park JG, Mehta AI, et al. Comparison of superior-level facet joint violations during open and percutaneous pedicle screw placement. *Neurosurgery* 2012;71(5):962–970
10. Jones-Quaidoo SM, Djurasovic M, Owens RK II, Carreon LY. Superior articulating facet violation: percutaneous versus open techniques. *J Neurosurg Spine* 2013;18(6):593–597
11. Yson SC, Sembrano JN, Sanders PC, Santos ER, Ledonio CG, Polly DW Jr. Comparison of cranial facet joint violation rates between open and percutaneous pedicle screw placement using intraoperative 3-D CT (O-arm) computer navigation. *Spine* 2013;38(4):E251–E258
12. Raley DA, Mobbs RJ. Retrospective computed tomography scan analysis of percutaneously inserted pedicle screws for posterior transpedicular stabilization of the thoracic and lumbar spine: accuracy and complication rates. *Spine* 2012;37(12):1092–1100

13 Heintel TM, Berglehner A, Meffert R. Accuracy of percutaneous pedicle screws for thoracic and lumbar spine fractures: a prospective trial. *Eur Spine J* 2013;*22*(3):495–502

14 Oh HS, Kim JS, Lee SH, Liu WC, Hong SW. Comparison between the accuracy of percutaneous and open pedicle screw fixations in lumbosacral fusion. *Spine J* 2013;*13*(12):1751–1757

15 Harris EB, Massey P, Lawrence J, Rihn J, Vaccaro A, Anderson DG. Percutaneous techniques for minimally invasive posterior lumbar fusion. *Neurosurg Focus* 2008;*25*(2):E12

16 Wang MY, Pineiro G, Mummaneni PV. Stimulus-evoked electromyography testing of percutaneous pedicle screws for the detection of pedicle breaches: a clinical study of 409 screws in 93 patients. *J Neurosurg Spine* 2010;*13*(5):600–605

17 Spitz SM, Sandhu FA, Voyadzis JM. Percutaneous "K-wireless" pedicle screw fixation technique: an evaluation of the initial experience of 100 screws with assessment of accuracy, radiation exposure, and procedure time. *J Neurosurg Spine* 2015;*22*(4):422–431

22 360° Endoscopically Assisted Minimally Invasive Transforaminal Lumbar Interbody Fusion

Alvaro Dowling, Sebastián Casanueva Eliceiry, Gabriela C. Chica Heredia, and Jonathan S. Schuldt

22.1 Introduction

In recent years it has become a common trend in most spinal surgery units to seek minimally invasive and effective solutions. Initially, due to the learning curve, the results of minimally invasive surgery (MIS) were similar to those of conventional surgery, presenting some complications.[1,2] Subsequently, after investment in the development of MIS surgery, it has become common and with significant casuistry. Nowadays the results of both types of interventions are similar, but it is important to mention that MIS presents lower complication rates.[3,4] Minimally invasive transforaminal lumbar interbody fusion (MIS-TLIF) has no significant disadvantages when compared with open TLIF or other standard lumbar fusion techniques.[5] Recent studies have shown that the risks of blood loss, narcotic administration, pseudarthrosis, and infection all decreased when MIS-TLIF was used.[6] Various postoperative recovery and pain rating scales often showed consistent improvement.[5]

The combination of MIS with the endoscope allows direct visualization of important anatomical structures and release of nerve roots from compression or adhesions. Also, it is possible to create enough space for cage placement in the intervertebral space by performing a foraminoplasty, which is especially relevant for the L5–S1 level.

We add biological therapy to increase the patient's intervertebral fusion, combining three essential pillars for the procedure: BMC (stem cells), PRP (platelet-rich plasma and its growth factors), and bone allograft (**Fig. 22.1**). This approach obtains an increased percentage of somatic fusion.[7,8]

With MIS endoscopically assisted TLIF, generally one to three levels can be fused, and occasionally four, depending on the anatomy of the patient.[9,10]

22.2 Preoperative Planning

For preoperative imaging, the authors prefer to use MRI and sitting-standing dynamic X-rays (**Fig. 22.2**, **Fig. 22.3**). When

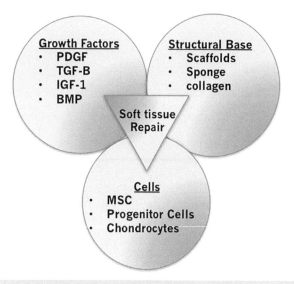

Fig. 22.1 Biologic pillars. A structural base, cells, and growth factors are needed for optimal soft tissue repair and intervertebral fusion.

feasible, we use CT, since it is more accurate for assessing the size of bony structures. Neutral X-ray (**Fig. 22.4**) provides information about alterations of physiological curvatures of the spine. Anatomical structures to consider include:

1. Vertebral pedicle: Pedicles are measured in their diameter, length, and orientation. Axial and sagittal views are necessary for accurate measurement (**Fig. 22.5**). This is relevant for planning screw placement.
2. Facet joint: The orientation of the facet joint is important when transfacet screws are being utilized (**Fig. 22.6**).
3. Spinal stenosis: Stenosis can be anatomically classified as central and lateral. Lateral stenosis is subdivided into lateral recess, medial, and foraminal (**Fig. 22.7**).[11,12] The decompression is planned according to the type of stenosis.

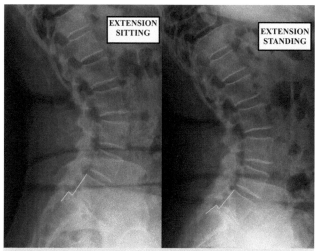

Fig. 22.2 Extension dynamic X-ray, showing significant instability.

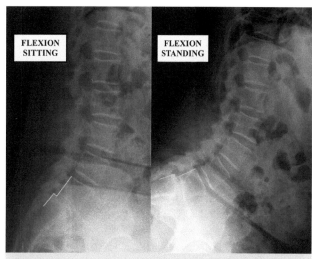

Fig. 22.3 Flexion dynamic X-ray, showing significant instability.

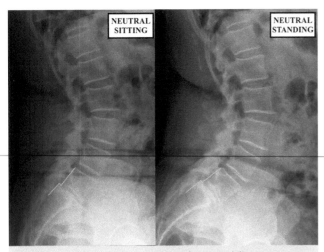

Fig. 22.4 Neutral X-ray, showing no significant instability.

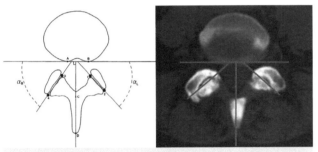

Fig. 22.6 Facet angle. A greater α angle makes transfacet screw placement more difficult.

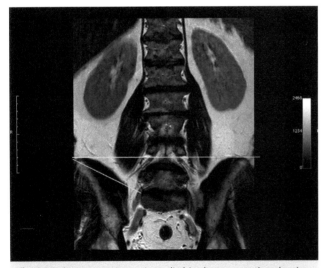

Fig. 22.8 Iliac crest anatomy is studied in the preoperative planning. If a high iliac crest is combined with a large facet joint and a horizontal L5–S1 disk, the transforaminal approach has to be reconsidered.

Considerations for the L5–S1 level include:

1. Iliac crest: A high iliac crest can obstruct trocar passage to the L5–S1 disk. Occasionally, a wide ilium opening angle (evaluated preoperatively) allows access to this level (**Fig. 22.8**).

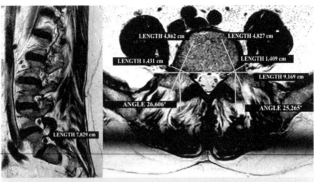

Fig. 22.5 Axial and sagittal MRI. Pedicle length, diameter, and orientation are analyzed during preoperative planning.

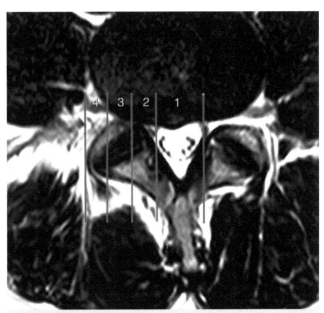

Fig. 22.7 Canal stenosis classification: 1, central stenosis, 2, lateral recess stenosis, 3, foraminal stenosis, and 4, extra foraminal stenosis.

2. Disk obliquity: A horizontal disk will present more difficulty in placement of an intersomatic cage. A sagittal imaging view is employed to assess obliquity (**Fig. 22.9**).

3. Facet size: Larger facets may require a manual foraminoplasty with a trephine if the trocar is unable to reach the intervertebral disk. Manual drills may also be utilized. Once the endoscope can access the neuroforamen, a bur drill can expand the area, releasing the exiting nerve root from compression and allowing the surgeon to reach the intervertebral space.

In our experience, when preoperative planning is performed thoroughly, complications and surgical times are significantly improved.[13] With a sterilized marker and with the help of the C-arm, the midline is traced following the spinous processes, 8 to 12 cm from which are marked laterally on the skin (**Fig. 22.10**). Intervertebral spaces are marked on a lateral and posteroanterior (PA) view. In a PA view, we mark the affected level after lordosis has been corrected by tilting the C-arm. Vertebral pedicles are also marked. In a lateral view, we mark the obliquity of the disks.

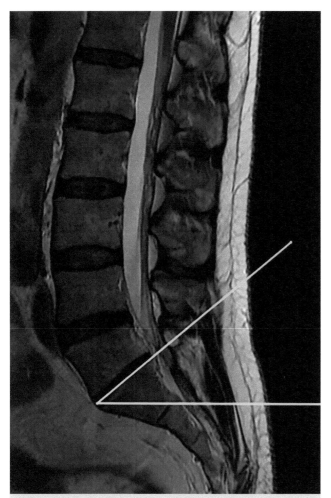

Fig. 22.9 Disk obliquity is especially relevant when a high iliac crest is present.

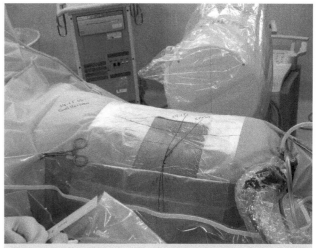

Fig. 22.10 Preoperative landmarks. L4–L5 and L5–S1 are marked on PA and lateral views.

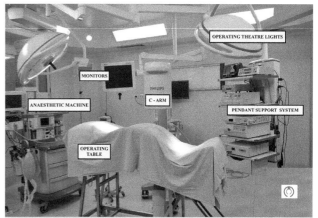

Fig. 22.11 Operating table and different components of the operating room.

22.3 Position and Anesthesia

The evolution of spinal surgery technology has helped improve other fields of medicine. New techniques in anesthesia have been developed to aid with monitoring and better outcomes for the patients. It is the authors' and the anesthesiologist team's preference to use a continuous infusion of dexmedetomidine and propofol, to obtain conscious sedation under monitored anesthesia care (MAC).[14] When the correct sedation state is achieved, the surgeon can perform procedures using local anesthesia and, indeed, achieve adequate anxiolysis and analgesia for the patient.[15,16,17,18] Two-percent lidocaine is used to provide local anesthesia in the skin, while 1% lidocaine is used in the entire intramuscular working tract.

Surgeons cannot get a more accurate response (physically and verbally) than from the awake patient.

Because of the continuous neuromonitoring, complications can be diminished and success rates improved. Although the patient can speak up if there's a problem, the anesthesiologist is always checking for changes in vital signs. Several studies have supported the alliance between MIS and this anesthetic method.[18]

The patient is placed in the prone position with slight flexion of the spine. A specially designed operating table is used to improve surgical performance, allowing the C-arm to freely move under and above the table. Also, there is an empty space designed to receive the patient's abdomen. This reduces intra-abdominal pressure and therefore decreases bleeding, due to proper drainage of the Batson plexus.[19] C-arm fluoroscopy is placed contralateral to the operation site (**Fig. 22.11, Video 22.1**).

22.4 Posterior Decompression

In cases with central spinal stenosis, the surgery starts with central decompression, with placement of progressive dilators and tubular retractors up to 13 mm directly onto the pedicle (**Fig. 22.12**). Decompression begins with a proximal hemilaminectomy, then a complete facetectomy followed by a distal hemilaminectomy. Dissection of the ligamentum flavum is performed to achieve complete decompression of neural structures.

Due to the inverted cone effect (**Fig. 22.13**), where through a small incision we rotate and change our approach angle, we can use a single incision and obtain contralateral nerve root decompression by tilting the tubular retractors medially. Because of this advantage, we prefer not to fix the tubular retractors and to perform a free-hand technique (**Fig. 22.14**).[9] In cases where

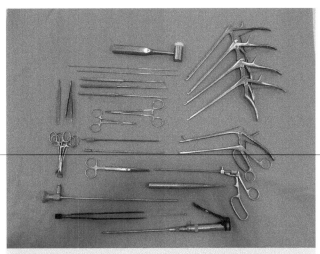

Fig. 22.12 Surgical equipment for posterior decompression.

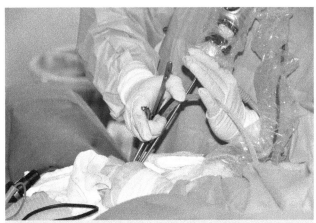

Fig. 22.14 Free-hand technique. This allows the surgeon to use both hands to freely move surgical instrumentation.

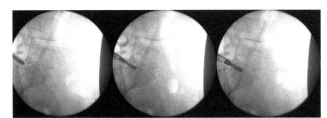

Fig. 22.16 Manual foraminoplasty using drill bits.

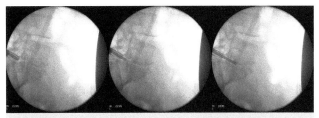

Fig. 22.17 Manual foraminoplasty using a trephine.

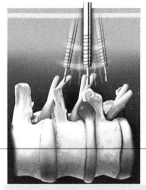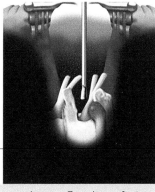

Fig. 22.13 Inverted cone. Left: Inverted cone effect, less soft tissue disruption and wide surgical area through a small incision. Right: Open approach, soft tissue damage by retraction, and smaller surgical area.

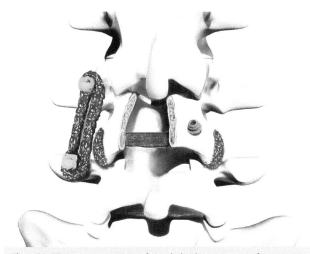

Fig. 22.15 Posterior view of a hybrid system. Left posterior decompression. Two pedicle screws on the left with bone allograft in the interpedicular area. One transfacet screw on the right.

the spine after a left laminectomy has been performed is shown in **Fig. 22.15**.

22.5 Instrument Placement for the Posterolateral Approach

A standard dilation system is used to place a 7-mm working cannula for a 20° high-definition (HD) endoscope. The endoscope accesses the area at a 45° angle, and, depending on the patient's size and fat tissue, the incision is made 8 to 12 cm from the midline.

22.6 Foraminoplasty: Disk and End Plate Preparation

Foraminoplasty is performed to achieve proper decompression and release of both exiting and traversing nerve roots, with two principal goals: to decrease compressive symptoms and to enable cage and allograft entry into the intervertebral space. The patient is under conscious sedation, so any nerve root irritation due to the procedure will be noticed. Foraminoplasty is performed using the outside–in technique (**Fig. 22.16**, **Fig. 22.17**). Decompression begins on the facet joint toward the

symptoms are clearly bilateral, a contralateral approach with tubular retractors can be performed, although it is fairly rare.

Decompression is finalized when we are able to move the traversing nerve root with no associated pain. A posterior view of

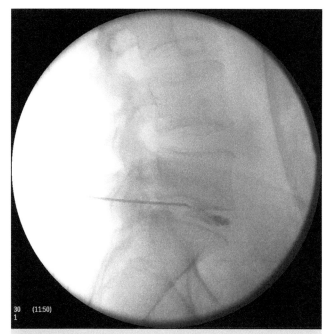

Fig. 22.18 L5–S1 diskography. Dallas IV.

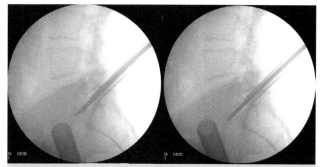

Fig. 22.19 Intervertebral disk extraction using a grasper punch.

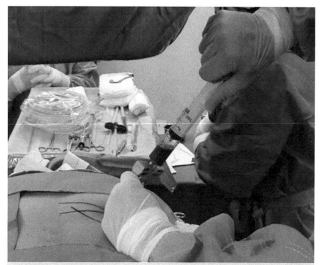

Fig. 22.21 Extraction of bone marrow cells from iliac crest.

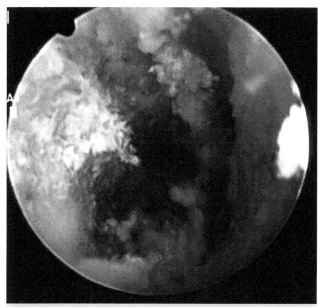

Fig. 22.20 Intervertebral end plates eburnated using trephines and drill bits.

pars articularis, releasing the exiting nerve root, and concluding on the caudal pedicle, releasing the traversing nerve root. The endoscopic decompression allows a wide foraminoplasty and greatly improves access to the now exposed intervertebral disk. The endoscope and interbody fusion instruments are widely movable in both the axial and the sagittal plane. Nerve roots must be visualized with a pulsatile dura and proper coloration.

It is the authors' preference to routinely perform diskography to visualize and confirm the affected level (**Fig. 22.18**). Quantitative diskometry may be performed on the compromised surgical lumbar level by documenting opening pressures and filling volumes.

A grasper punch is used to extract protruded or extruded disk fragments (**Fig. 22.19**). This is of particular help since cage placement could press against any remaining disk fragments, resulting in a continuation of compressive symptoms.

In some situations, especially when accessing the L5–S1 level, if a high iliac crest is encountered and the articular process interferes with trocar passage, a trephine decompression must be performed to create an adequate work area for direct root visualization (**Fig. 22.16**, **Fig. 22.17**).

Vertebral end plates are prepared using 4-mm round drill bits, reamers, and trephines for end plate eburnation, rupturing segments of the haversian system, thus producing punctate bleeding spots. This blood supplies nutrients necessary for bone formation (**Fig. 22.20**).[20] Bipolar radiofrequency (RF) and physiological saline are used.

22.7 Biological Factors

Two syringes are used to extract 30 cc of bone marrow tissue from the patient's iliac crest (**Fig. 22.21**). (Bone marrow aspirate seems to contain a greater percentage of hematopoietic cells, endothelial cells, and mesenchymal stem cells [MSCs] than peripheral blood. The ability of multipotent MSCs to form osteoblasts for bone regeneration makes transplanted bone marrow aspirate a promising tool for enhancing bone regeneration.[21] Studies designed to quantify the MSC population in bone marrow samples obtained for cell therapy used flow cytometry and revealed

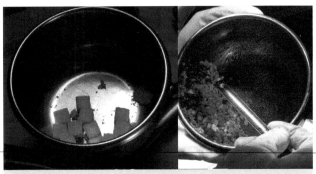

Fig. 22.22 Bone allograft. Left: Bone allograft before mixture. Right: Bone allograft + BMC + PRP.

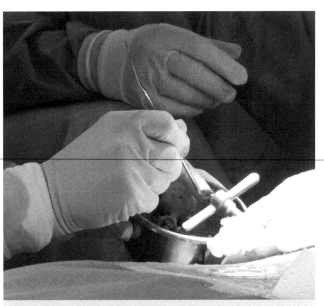

Fig. 22.23 Bone allograft placement in the intervertebral space.

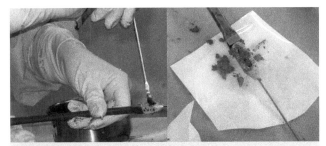

Fig. 22.24 Intersomatic cage with allograft bone.

a low percentage as well as high variability among patients, ranging from 0.0017 to 0.0201%. All cultured MSC adhered to plastic dishes and showed a capacity to differentiate into adipogenic and osteogenic lineages.[22]) The bone marrow tissue is processed and then is brought back to the OR to be mixed with allograft scaffold and platelet-rich plasma (PRP; **Fig. 22.22**).

PRP is defined as a portion of the plasma fraction of autologous blood having platelet concentrations above baseline. Normal platelet counts in blood range between 150,000/μL and 350,000/μL, with an average of ~ 200,000/μL. When activated, the platelets release growth factors that play an essential role in bone healing, such as platelet-derived growth factor, transforming growth factor-β, vascular endothelial growth factor, and others.[23]

Growth factors have a crucial role in this process because they influence chemotaxis, differentiation, proliferation, and synthetic activity of bone cells, thereby regulating physiological remodeling and bone healing.

Recent research on animal models has demonstrated that PRP, when used in combination with a proper scaffold, is a potent growth factor that promotes bone formation in vivo. Allograft with bone marrow concentrate and activated PRP can achieve the same fusion rates as autograft (**Fig. 22.1**).[24]

22.8 Cage Measurement, Bone Allograft, and Cage Placement

A cage meter is positioned in the intervertebral space to measure the intersomatic cage size that will be employed. Depending on the patient's anatomy, ~ 10 cc of bone allograft mixed with bone marrow concentrate (BMC) and growth factors (**Fig. 22.23**) is impacted on the anterior and lateral areas of the intervertebral space, forming an anchor shape and leaving enough space for

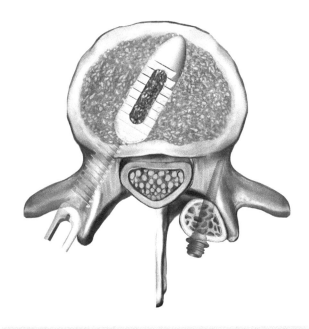

Fig. 22.25 Axial view of a hybrid system. Pedicle screw on the left and transfacet screw on the right. Intersomatic cage placed at approximately 45°.

placement of the cage, which has been previously been filled with bone allograft (**Fig. 22.24**). This increases the contact surface for the cage. PA and lateral X-ray views are used to check the position of the cage, which should be in the midline.

After placement of the interbody fusion cage, meticulous cleaning of the neural foramen is performed under direct visualization of the cage to make certain there are no bone graft residues left in the area and to recheck the cage position.

An oblique cage position must be aimed in an approximate 45° angle relative to the posterior annulus across the interspace to achieve better stability (**Fig. 22.25**). The interspace is filled with the same graft material. In the authors' clinical experience,

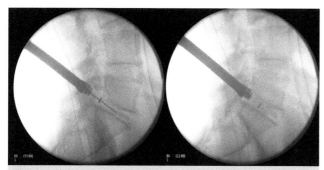

Fig. 22.26 X-ray guide for cage placement. Lateral view of cage placement sequence.

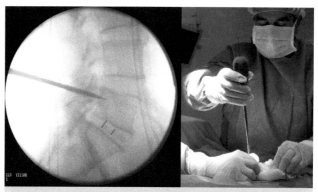

Fig. 22.27 Cannulated tap allows creation of a path on which the screw will be placed.

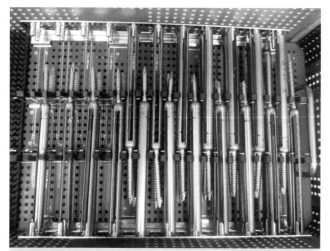

Fig. 22.28 Pedicle screws. Different lengths and diameters are used depending on the preoperative plan.

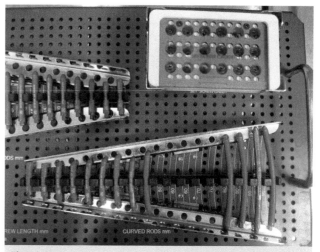

Fig. 22.29 Rods are placed between two pedicle screws to fix them.

this surgical technique improves the biomechanical stability of the reconstructed motion segment and decreases the incidence of cage subsidence.

PA and lateral X-rays are used to check correct cage placement through the visualization of two X-ray markers (**Fig. 22.26**). Once the interbody fusion cage is satisfactorily placed between the two vertebral bodies, intervertebral height is increased. Expandable devices and other systems can be used, reaching up to 9 to 13 mm in height.

22.9 Screw Placement Preparation

A facet tip introduction needle of 12.7 cm is used to reach the pedicle. A metallic guide is placed on the pedicle. A dilator is used to stretch the muscle path. A cannulated tap using a palm ratcheting handle will follow the guide and create the space needed for the screw (**Fig. 22.27**).

22.10 Pedicle and Facet-Pedicle Screws

Pedicle screw placement is planned using preoperative axial MRI or CT images through the surgical level. Cannulated pedicle screws are available in different sizes, from 5.5 to 7.5 mm in diameter and 30 to 65 mm in length (**Fig. 22.28**). Lateral-to-medial and rostral-to-caudal screw trajectories are determined

to avoid injury to nerve roots or dural sac. Once the bone tunnel is achieved and fluoroscopically controlled, the definitive screw is placed. X-ray control can be used while the screw is advanced to maintain the correct direction.

When pain radiates, screw placement is checked and the orientation is modified if needed.

After screw placement, the scissor caliper is inserted to obtain the length of the rod that will be used. The selected rod is then bent according to the surgeon's preference. Insertion of the rod (**Fig. 22.29**) is achieved with an angled rod inserter. Fluoroscopy control can be used at this point.

To lock the fusion system, a set screw is placed on top of the rod, locking it to the head of the pedicle screw. Break-away towers can be detached from the system (**Fig. 22.30**). Eburnation of the transverse process and interpedicular bone surface is performed with drill bits and curets. Part of the bone allograft, BMC, and PRP mixture is placed bilaterally on top of the previously prepared bone surface to increase fusion (**Fig. 22.31**).

An alternative to pedicle screw fixation, but with the same rate of success, is transfacet fixation.[25,26,27,28] It is the authors' preference to use 360° transpedicular fusion when possible or, according to the clinical case or the anatomy of the patient, 270° fusion. A hybrid of the two fusion techniques can be developed,[29,30] placing pedicle screws on one side and a transfacet screw contralaterally (**Fig. 22.25**).

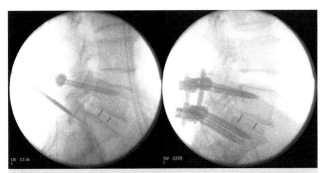

Fig. 22.30 Radiological check. Left: Pedicle screw being placed on the right S1 pedicle. Right: Four pedicle screws and two rods fixing them. Correct cage placement.

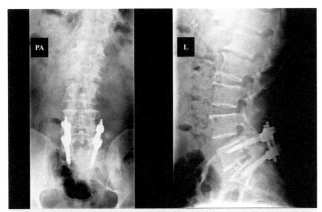

Fig. 22.32 Radiological check after surgery: 360° L5–S1 lumbar interbody fusion.

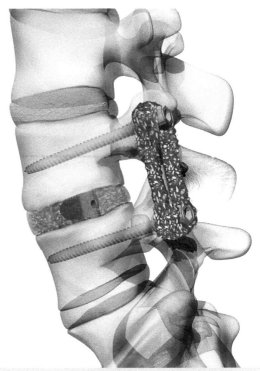

Fig. 22.31 Illustration of a hybrid system in a sagittal view. Two pedicle screws have been placed on the left and one transfacet screw on the right. Interpedicular allograft is positioned. Intersomatic cage with bone allograft surrounding it.

Facet screw systems are available in different sizes, from 4.3 to 5.0 mm in diameter and 20 to 40 mm in length, with drill markers for depth relation. The screws are placed medial-to-lateral and rostral-to-caudal, securing the facet joint toward the pedicle.

It is important to mention that transfacet screw fixation has its own indications and contraindications according to the pathology or the anatomy of the patient. It can be considered a helpful alternative when small or fractured pedicles are found, but it is not a viable choice when the facet has to be removed or there is a spondylolysis.[31] Postoperative radiology is performed to check the screw and cage placement. PA and lateral views are needed (**Fig. 22.32**).

22.11 Clinical Experience

22.11.1 Materials and Methods

Our study included 65 patients who underwent transforaminal lumbar interbody fusion (TLIF) in our clinic between 2010 and 2013. Preoperatively, each patient's functioning was assessed using the Oswestry Disability Index (ODI; two) and the lumbar visual analog scale (VAS) score specific to gluteal, leg, and foot pain. Postoperatively, patients were evaluated at 1 month, 3 months, 1 year, and 2 years. Data collection was performed by a staff member in our outpatient clinic not involved in the clinical

care of the patient. A certified statistician then analyzed the data.

22.11.2 Patients and Outcome Analysis

Sixty-five patients were included in the study; 62 out of 65 reached 2-year follow-up postoperatively. In all 62 patients, an endoscope was used during TLIF. All patients signed an informed consent form prior to being included in the study. Four patients were eventually excluded from the study because of missing intermittent follow-up visits. Clinical outcomes of the remaining 58 TLIF patients were analyzed. Hence, 89.2% of patients were finally included with complete 2-years of follow-up. There were 35 males and 23 females, with a median age of 53 years.

The variables measured on the ODI questionnaire were pain intensity, daily living activities, lifting of objects, walking, sitting down, standing up, sleeping, sexual activity, social activities, and traveling. They were all measured on a 0 to 5 scale, 0 being having no pain or disability and 5 being having severe pain and disability. In this longitudinal cohort study, there were no replicates and no control group.

22.11.3 Results

Significant ODI differences between preoperative and 1-year postoperative assessments were noted. Patients improved 94.25% of the time. Evaluating the lumbar VAS and gluteal VAS score results, we found postoperative improvements of 86.36%. Average improvement of the leg VAS score was 95.65%. Our results with endoscopically assisted MIS-TLIF showed ODI scores of 50.9, 25.7, 16.3, 13.2, and 9.1 at the preoperative, 1 month postoperative, 3 months postoperative, 1 year postoperative, and 2 years postoperative, respectively. Fusion reached 92% in our patients. CT scans were employed to assess fusion status at 3 and 6 months.

22.12 Complications

One patient suffered neurologic complications, with L5 neuropraxia and foot drop. Function returned 3 months postoperatively with excellent results. In another patient, facet-pedicular screws had to be converted to a nonsegmental pedicle screw construct due to loosening. An additional patient had an asymptomatic medially placed pedicle screw revealed on a postoperative CT scan. The patient underwent revision surgery within 12 hours to reposition the pedicle screw. A dural tear was encountered in one patient and was treated with a collagen patch (Duragen). The patient was discharged after 24 hours and was advised to observe an additional 5 days of bed rest at home. This patient had an otherwise uncomplicated recovery without headaches or development of a CSF fistula. Another patient presented with deep vein thrombosis and was treated with a standard anticoagulant therapy.

One case had important postoperative axial lumbar pain. MRI showed inflammation of the disk, while all blood tests were between normal parameters. Aseptic diskitis was diagnosed and was treated with analgesics and a lumbar belt. The patient was brought back to the OR, where a sample was taken for microbiological culture and the intervertebral disk was irrigated with saline and antibiotic solution. All tests came back negative. The patient's symptoms subsided in less than 5 days. Each one of these complications represented 1.53% of all patients.

In patients with complications requiring revision surgery, it became clear that revision of MIS pedicle screw instrumentation is suitable for percutaneous reattachment of pedicle screws to extension tabs and tubular retractors. However, reattachment of extension tabs and delivery tools onto the pedicle screw construct may present some degree of difficulty and may require some practice.

During the pedicle screw repositioning maneuver, we use progressive dilation tubes to access the area with an endoscope. Reattachment of the delivery instrumentation to the pedicle screw can be monitored under direct visualization on the video screen. Repositioning of the pedicle screw rod construct may considerably increase surgical time, even in the hands of an experienced surgeon.

22.13 Discussion

The MIS-TLIF technique has been shown to reduce the trauma to the paraspinal musculature, postoperative recovery, length of hospital stay, and risk of infection. It creates small surgical wounds, resulting in minor bleeding.[32,33] Using the MIS-TLIF technique, we discharge our patients in less than 24 hours. In comparison, one study reported that the average discharge after conventional open TLIF was at 9.3 ± 2.6 days.[34]

General anesthesia with total intravenous anesthesia or in combination with minimal use of anesthetic gases may have some advantages over MAC. These include reduced postoperative nausea and faster wake-up. However, MAC under local anesthesia and sedation offers the advantage of being able to communicate with the patient during surgery. Prevention of neural injury is obviously of concern and the ability to perform a quick wake-up test during surgery, rather than relying on intraoperative neuromonitoring with EMG or sensory or motor evoked potentials, may prove useful, particularly to the novice surgeon. It is clearly the authors' preference; we consider performing endoscopically assisted MIS-TLIF risky under general anesthesia. However, each surgeon should discuss the appropriate choice of anesthesia with the patient and anesthesia team in the context of the local community standard.

In the authors' experience, one of the most relevant aspects of endoscopically assisted surgery is the ability to access the L5–S1 level. In an attempt to reduce tissue damage and improve the release of the compromised nerve root under direct endoscopic visualization, the posterior decompression is performed through a tubular retractor, which is placed via progressive dilation tubes.

After our experience with more than 100 cases to date in which we used an endoscope during MIS-TLIF, we recommend its use for direct visualization at the L4–L5 and L5–S1 levels to achieve a proper release and decompression of the symptomatic nerve roots.

Accessing the intervertebral disk via Kambin's triangle to perform the diskectomy and end plate preparation for placement of an interbody fusion cage allows direct and facile access to the interspace while producing minimal scarring around the neural elements, and the lateral recess in particular.

In the authors' opinion, direct root visualization (DRV) of the L5 nerve root during foraminoplasty and its mobilization by release of adhesions due to foraminal ligaments and the intraforaminal venous complex is integral to accessing the interbody space to facilitate cage placement. The combination of nerve root exposure and mobilization during foraminoplasty lowers the risk of nerve root injury at this otherwise difficult-to-access level. Endoscopically assisted TLIF allows direct visualization of both the neural elements and the vertebral end plates during diskectomy, as well as end plate preparation: this is a clear advantage in comparison to traditional TLIF or the nonvisualized version of the procedure.

At the L5–S1 level, a foraminoplasty is practically mandatory in almost every case, given the narrow entry point into Kambin's triangle that can be obliterated by a hypertrophic facet joint complex, the transverse process, and sacral wing. Transitional anatomy may pose an additional hindrance to accessing the foramen via the outside-in technique. The foraminoplasty may greatly reduce the risk of postoperative neuropraxia, nerve damage, and pain, which is frequently caused by irritation of the dorsal root ganglion.

Foraminoplasty may facilitate better preparation of the end plates to achieve a most complete interbody fusion. In addition to the interbody fusion cage, the authors advocate the use of bone graft, such as allograft, placed anterior to the cage and laterally on the sides so that the graft surrounds the cage. Posterior unilateral facet-pedicular screw fixation may reduce surgical time and postoperative pain.

Assessing the configuration of the iliac crest is of importance for both the L5–S1 and the L4–L5 level. The latter may be problematic as well when there is a high-riding iliac crest. The surgeon should be wary of the feasibility of the transforaminal approach when the iliac wing projects above the L4–L5 disk level on the lateral X-ray projection or if there is posterior pelvic tilt with a horizontal L5–S1 intervertebral disk. A conventional TLIF approach may be more appropriate for these patients. A significant learning curve may also be associated with endoscopically assisted MIS-TLIF and should be taken into consideration when selecting patients for the procedure.

The authors' technique capitalizes on traditional transforaminal lumbar interbody fusion. The combination of smaller incisions, reduced postoperative pain, less blood loss, and MAC allows patients to be discharged within 24 hours.

22.14 Conclusion

On the basis of our experience, the authors recommend the use of an endoscope to assist during MIS-TLIF in combination with percutaneous pedicular screws as an alternative to open TLIF. Our favorable clinical findings have been corroborated by others, who also reported shorter hospital stays, fewer complications, reduced postoperative drug use, and lower cost with MIS-TLIF.[35,36]

The interbody fusion cage and the transpedicular screw fixation system employed in our patients have been extensively described in the literature.[17] Endoscopically assisted TLIF via the posterolateral transforaminal approach occurs through the existing neuroforamen, with minimal disruption of the supporting dynamic paraspinal muscles and minimal removal of bone. In contrast, during a classic TLIF, the inferior portion of the lamina and the superior and inferior articular processes, or some variation thereof, are typically resected with the ligamentum flavum.

Hence, the endoscopically assisted TLIF approach seems to be an advanced, less invasive surgical technique, which in most cases requires only partial removal of the lumbar facet joint—namely, its anterior portion directly facing the lumbar intervertebral disk. The overall strain on the patient is significantly reduced, making this procedure more suitable for the elderly. Overall, endoscopically assisted TLIF may be possible in higher-risk patients who would not consider open surgery in spite of chronic pain syndromes.

References

1   Goldstein CL, Macwan K, Sundararajan K, Rampersaud YR. Perioperative outcomes and adverse events of minimally invasive versus open posterior lumbar fusion: meta-analysis and systematic review. *J Neurosurg Spine* 2015:1–12
2   Li YB, Wang XD, Yan HW, Hao DJ, Liu ZH. The long-term clinical effect of minimal-invasive TLIF technique in 1-segment lumbar disease. *J Spinal Disord Tech* 2015
3   Sidhu GS, Henkelman E, Vaccaro AR, et al. Minimally invasive versus open posterior lumbar interbody fusion: a systematic review. *Clin Orthop Relat Res* 2014;472(6):1792–1799
4   Khan NR, Clark AJ, Lee SL, Venable GT, Rossi NB, Foley KT. Surgical outcomes for minimally invasive vs open transforaminal lumbar interbody fusion: an updated systematic review and meta-analysis. *Neurosurgery* 2015;77(6):847–874
5   Wong AP, Smith ZA, Stadler JA III, et al. Minimally invasive transforaminal lumbar interbody fusion (MI-TLIF): surgical technique, long-term 4-year prospective outcomes, and complications compared with an open TLIF cohort. *Neurosurg Clin N Am* 2014;25(2):279–304
6   Phan K, Mobbs RJ. Minimally invasive versus open laminectomy for lumbar stenosis—a systematic review and meta-analysis. *Spine* 2015
7   Gupta A, Kukkar N, Sharif K, Main BJ, Albers CE, El-Amin III SF. Bone graft substitutes for spine fusion: a brief review. *World J Orthop* 2015;6(6):449–456
8   Landi A, Tarantino R, Marotta N, et al. The use of platelet gel in postero-lateral fusion: preliminary results in a series of 14 cases. *Eur Spine J* 2011;20(Suppl 1):S61–S67
9   Lee WC, Park JY, Kim KH, et al. Minimally invasive transforaminal lumbar interbody fusion in multilevel: comparison with conventional transforaminal interbody fusion. *World Neurosurg* 2015
10 Min SH, Yoo JS. The clinical and radiological outcomes of multilevel minimally invasive transforaminal lumbar interbody fusion. *Eur Spine J* 2013;22(5):1164–1172
11 Azimi P, Mohammadi HR, Benzel EC, Shahzadi S, Azhari S. Lumbar spinal canal stenosis classification criteria: a new tool. *Asian Spine J* 2015;9(3):399–406
12 Weber C, Rao V, Gulati S, Kvistad KA, Nygaard ØP, Lønne G. Inter- and intraobserver agreement of morphological grading for central lumbar spinal stenosis on magnetic resonance imaging. *Global Spine J* 2015;5(5):406–410
13 Harasymczuk P, Kotwicki T, Koch A, Szulc A. The use of computer tomography for preoperative planning and outcome assessment in surgical treatment of idiopathic scoliosis with pedicle screw based constructs—case presentation. *Ortop Traumatol Rehabil* 2009;11(6):577–585
14 Das S, Ghosh S. Monitored anesthesia care: an overview. *J Anaesthesiol Clin Pharmacol* 2015;31(1):27–29
15 Avitsian R, Manlapaz M, Doyle J. Dexmedetomidine as a sedative for awake fiberoptic intubation. *Trauma Care J* 2007;17:19–24
16 Chen HT, Tsai CH, Chao SC, et al. Endoscopic discectomy of L5–S1 disc herniation via an interlaminar approach: prospective controlled study under local and general anesthesia. *Surg Neurol Int* 2011;2:93
17 Gertler R, Brown HC, Mitchell DH, Silvius EN. Dexmedetomidine: a novel sedative-analgesic agent. *Proc Bayl Univ Med Cent* 2001;14(1):13–21
18 Tobias J. Dexmedetomidine in trauma anesthesiology and critical care. *Trauma Care J* 2007;17:6–18
19 Shriver MF, Zeer V, Alentado VJ, Mroz TE, Benzel EC, Steinmetz MP. Lumbar spine surgery positioning complications: a systematic review. *Neurosurg Focus* 2015;39(4):E16
20 Johnson RG. Bone marrow concentrate with allograft equivalent to autograft in lumbar fusions. *Spine* 2014;39(9):695–700
21 Smiler D, Soltan M, Albitar M. Toward the identification of mesenchymal stem cells in bone marrow and peripheral blood for bone regeneration. *Implant Dent* 2008;17(3):236–247
22 Alvarez-Viejo M, Menendez-Menendez Y, Blanco-Gelaz MA, et al. Quantifying mesenchymal stem cells in the mononuclear cell fraction of bone marrow samples obtained for cell therapy. *Transplant Proc* 2013;45(1):434–439
23 Rodriguez IA, Growney Kalaf EA, Bowlin GL, Sell SA. Platelet-rich plasma in bone regeneration: engineering the delivery for improved clinical efficacy. *BioMed Res Int* 2014;2014:392398
24 Mayer HM. *Minimally Invasive Spine Surgery: A Surgical Manual.* Springer Science & Business Media; 2005
25 Chin KR, Newcomb AG, Reis MT, et al. Biomechanics of posterior instrumentation in L1–L3 lateral interbody fusion: pedicle screw rod construct vs transfacet pedicle screws. *Clin Biomech (Bristol, Avon)* 2015
26 Kretzer RM, Molina C, Hu N, et al. A comparative biomechanical analysis of stand alone versus facet screw and pedicle screw augmented lateral interbody arthrodesis: an in vitro human cadaveric model. *J Spinal Disord Tech* 2013;1:40–7
27 Agarwala A, Bucklen B, Muzumdar A, Moldavsky M, Khalil S. Do facet screws provide the required stability in lumbar fixation? A biomechanical comparison of the Boucher technique and pedicular fixation in primary and circumferential fusions. *Clin Biomech (Bristol, Avon)* 2012;27(1):64–70
28 Beaubien BP, Mehbod AA, Kallemeier PM, et al. Posterior augmentation of an anterior lumbar interbody fusion: minimally invasive fixation versus pedicle screws in vitro. *Spine* 2004;29(19):E406–E412
29 Zeng ZY, Wu P, Mao KY, et al. [Unilateral pedicle screw fixation versus its combination with contralateral translaminar facet screw fixation for the treatment of single segmental lower lumbar vertebra diseases]. *Zhongguo Gu Shang* 2015;28(4):306–312
30 Awad BI, Lubelski D, Shin JH, et al. Bilateral pedicle screw fixation versus unilateral pedicle and contralateral facet screws for minimally invasive transforaminal lumbar interbody fusion: clinical outcomes and cost analysis. *Global Spine J* 2013;3(4):225–230
31 Hsiang J, Yu K, He Y. Minimally invasive one-level lumbar decompression and fusion surgery with posterior instrumentation using a combination of pedicle screw fixation and transpedicular facet screw construct. *Surg Neurol Int* 2013;4:125
32 Sulaiman WAR, Singh M. Minimally invasive versus open transforaminal lumbar interbody fusion for degenerative spondylolisthesis grades 1-2: patient-reported clinical outcomes and cost-utility analysis. *Ochsner J* 2014;14(1):32–37
33 Peng CW, Yue WM, Poh SY, Yeo W, Tan SB. Clinical and radiological outcomes of minimally invasive versus open transforaminal lumbar interbody fusion. *Spine* 2009;34(13):1385–1389
34 Dhall SS, Wang MY, Mummaneni PV. Clinical and radiographic comparison of mini-open transforaminal lumbar interbody fusion with open transforaminal lumbar interbody fusion in 42 patients with long-term follow-up. *J Neurosurg Spine* 2008;9(6):560–565
35 Shunwu F, Xing Z, Fengdong Z, Xiangqian F. Minimally invasive transforaminal lumbar interbody fusion for the treatment of degenerative lumbar diseases. *Spine* 2010;35(17):1615–1620
36 Morgenstern R, Morgenstern C. *Endoscopically Assisted Transforaminal Percutaneous Lumbar Interbody Fusion. Endoscopic Spinal Surgery.* London: JP Medical Ltd; 2013:138–145

23 Percutaneous Translaminar and Ipsilateral Facet Fixation Technique

Ricardo B. V. Fontes and Richard G. Fessler

23.1 Introduction

The pioneering description of the ipsilateral facet fixation technique was made by King in 1948. As a stand-alone construct, the technique was associated with significant failure rates and a necessity for bed rest that were virtually the same as for noninstrumented (Hibbs) fusion: particularly in multilevel cases, fusion rates declined to ~ 50%.[1,2] In 1984, Magerl described a translaminar modification of the trajectory, but with the advent of pedicle-based instrumentation and its more favorable biomechanical properties, facet fixation fell into disuse. Facet fixation has regained popularity in the 21st century due to increased numbers of interbody fusions and its ease of percutaneous placement. It is a particularly attractive form of posterior supplementation to lateral lumbar interbody fusion because it maintains the minimally invasive philosophy of the latter operation (**Video 23.1**).[3]

23.2 Patient Selection

Indications for the procedure are:

- Posterior supplementation for interbody fusion, particularly anterior lumbar interbody fusion (ALIF) and lateral lumbar interbody fusion (LLIF), from L1 to S1

Contraindications are:

- Extensive laminectomy or facetectomy
- Nonreduced degenerative spondylolisthesis after insertion of the interbody graft
- Isthmic spondylolisthesis or spondylolysis
- More than two levels of fixation

23.3 Technique

23.3.1 Preoperative Planning

MRI or CT myelography (preferred) of the lumbar spine is obtained, as well as flexion/extension lumbar spine radiographs.

23.3.2 Anesthesia and Positioning

General anesthesia (without neuromuscular blockade) and neurophysiological monitoring (SSEP and EMG) are used. The patient is positioned prone on a Jackson open-frame table to maximize lumbar lordosis (**Fig. 23.1**). Checks are made for ocular pressure or contact points.

23.3.3 Localization

Fluoroscopic localization of the levels to be operated in the lumbar spine is used. Anteroposterior (AP) fluoroscopy is preferred for marking the incision; lateral fluoroscopy is utilized during most of the case.

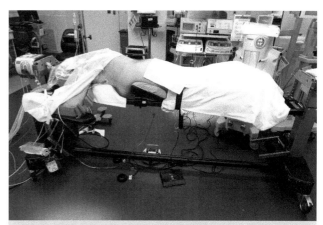

Fig. 23.1 Patient positioned prone on a Jackson open-frame table to maximize lordosis.

23.3.4 Entry Point

Under AP fluoroscopy, the midline over the caudal margin of the spinous process of the level cranial to be operated is marked longitudinally (e.g., the caudal margin of the spinous process of L3 is marked for L4–5 fixation) (**Fig. 23.2**).

Skin and soft tissue analgesia is obtained using lidocaine 2% with 1:100,000 epinephrine. A longitudinal 1-cm skin incision is made.

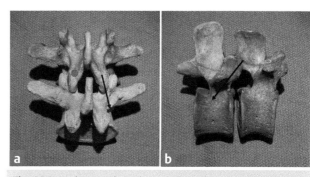

Fig. 23.2 Lumbar vertebrae demonstrating the entry point for facet fixation (*red circle*). The arrow demonstrates the planned trajectory of fixation across the zygapophysial joint. (**a**) Posterior view. (**b**) Lateral view.

23.3.5 Guidewire Insertion

The Jamshidi needle is inserted aiming caudally and laterally until it is docked in the medial margin of the inferior articular process of the cranial level to be fused (**Fig. 23.3**). The Jamshidi needle orientation is then confirmed on lateral fluoroscopy to ensure it aims at the pedicle of the caudal level. Under fluoroscopy, a K-wire is inserted and sequentially traverses the superficial cortex of the inferior articular process and the zygapophysial joint, and proceeds into the pedicle (**Fig. 23.4**). Do not advance the guidewire beyond 15 mm past the posterior wall of the vertebral body.

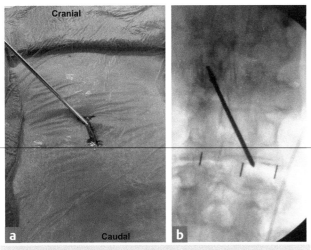

Fig. 23.3 Midline incision over the spinous processes and Jamshidi trocar angled caudally and laterally to contact the inferior articular process of the cranial level to be fused. The midline incision is typically located one level cranial to allow for the caudal trajectory of the trocar.

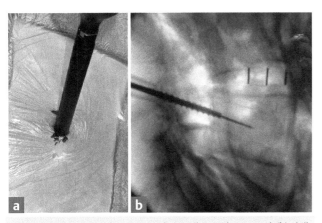

Fig. 23.5 (a) Dilator shown passed over the guidewire and (b) drill advanced over guidewire.

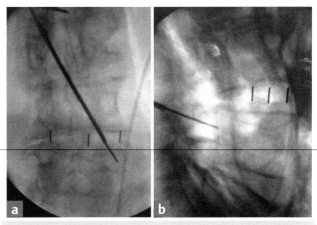

Fig. 23.4 Guidewire being advanced through the joint and into the pedicle. (a) Anteroposterior fluoroscopic view. (b) Lateral view. Great care is taken not to advance the guidewire past 15 mm from the posterior wall of the vertebral body.

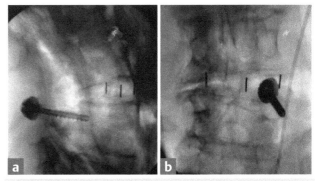

Fig. 23.6 The screw and its polyaxial ring are passed over the guidewire, which is then removed. (a) AP view. (b) Lateral view.

23.3.6 Dilation, Drilling, and Tapping

The tubular working channel is advanced over the guidewire until docked at the articular process. A cannulated drill is advanced over the guidewire and is drilled through the joint and into the pedicle. Do not advance more than 15 mm beyond the posterior wall of vertebral body (**Fig. 23.5**).

Use of a cannulated tap is optional but useful in patients with a sclerotic zygapophysial joint, poor bone quality, or use of a larger-diameter (6-mm) screw.

23.3.7 Screw Assembly and Insertion

Facet fixation is a form of lag fixation. A partially threaded screw is utilized so the articular processes can be locked together. Screws of 5- or 6-mm diameter can be utilized; the authors normally employ a screw length between 30 and 40 mm.

A polyaxial ring serves as a base for the screw head, so it can turn smoothly and accomplish lag fixation. The polyaxial ring is assembled over the screw before insertion.

The screw is inserted over the guidewire under lateral fluoroscopy. Once the screw is in the pedicle, the guidewire can be

safely removed. Once the screw is firmly seated on its polyaxial base, the working channel is removed (**Fig. 23.6**).

Unilateral fixation is possible, because this is a supplementation to interbody fusion, but bilateral screws are preferred.

23.3.8 Complication Avoidance and Treatment

Never advance the guidewire more than 15 mm beyond the posterior wall of the vertebral body.

Make sure the guidewire is firmly seated on the inferior articular process before advancing it. We recommend attempting the first few procedures in patients with an intact lamina to avoid inadvertent placement of the guidewire through the dura.

Avoid off-axis pressures when handling the guidewire to avoid bending it.

Avoid over-tightening the screw, because it may strip the zygapophysial joint and result in loss of fixation. If this occurs, insert the guidewire again and switch the screw for a larger-diameter screw or revert to pedicle-based fixation.

23.3.9 Closure

If the fascia is visible, it can be approximated with a Vicryl 0 suture. Otherwise, the subcutaneous plane is approximated with interrupted 3–0 Vicryl and the skin with a running 5–0 Monocryl dermal suture.

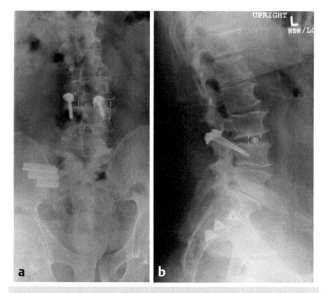

Fig. 23.7 Final radiographs demonstrating bilateral facet fixation supplementing a transpsoas interbody fusion. **(a)** AP view. **(b)** Lateral view. On AP view, screw trajectory is slightly divergent.

23.4 Postoperative Care

Patients may ambulate immediately after surgery. Discharge is more dependent on the type of interbody fusion and recovery from the bigger part of the operation (anterior or transpsoas approach). Patients may be discharged home as soon as they are able to ambulate and urinate without problems. Usually, they require a one- to three-night hospital stay.

Muscle spasm may be a problem because the nerve supply to the paraspinal muscles is kept intact. Spasm may be controlled with the anti-spasm medication of the surgeons' choice (e.g., methocarbamol 500 mg PO four times a day or baclofen 10 mg PO three times a day; **Fig. 23.7**).

References

1   Boucher HH. A method of spinal fusion. *J Bone Joint Surg Br* 1959;*41-B*(2):248–259
2   King D. Internal fixation for lumbosacral fusion. *J Bone Joint Surg Am* 1948;*30A*(3):560–565
3   Su BW, Cha TD, Kim PD, et al. An anatomic and radiographic study of lumbar facets relevant to percutaneous transfacet fixation. *Spine* 2009;*34*(11):E384–E390

24 Direct Lateral Endoscopic Lumbar Interbody Fusion and Instrumentation

Jin-Sung Luke Kim and Choon Keun Park

24.1 Introduction

Lumbar interbody fusion (LIF) methods, such as posterior lumbar interbody fusion (PLIF),[1,2,3] transforaminal lumbar interbody fusion (TLIF),[4,5,6] anterior lumbar interbody fusion (ALIF),[7,8] and axial lumbar interbody fusion (axial LIF),[9] have been effective surgical treatment for degenerative lumbar spondylosis with instability and persistent chronic pain. Since Pimenta first introduced the retroperitoneal transpsoas minimally invasive lateral LIF in 2006,[10] cases of lateral lumbar interbody fusion (LLIF) have been increasing for spine surgeons. LLIF has strong advantages, such as cortex-to-cortex wide interbody graft, less tissue damage, preservation of posterior ligaments and muscles, minimal blood loss, short operation time, and early return to work. For these reasons, many surgeons prefer LLIF, especially in elderly and debilitated patients.

24.2 Choice of Patient

Indications for the procedure are:

- Degenerative disk disease with instability
- Recurrent disk herniation
- Postlaminectomy syndrome
- Adjacent segment pathology requiring additional surgery (problems at a level adjacent to a previous fusion surgery)
- Degenerative/isthmic spondylolisthesis
- Degenerative scoliosis (right/left curvature of the spine)
- Posterior pseudarthrosis (previous fusion surgery that did not fuse)

  Contraindications to LLIF are:
- Symptomatic level at L5–S1
- Symptomatic level at L4–L5 with high iliac crest
- Lumbar deformities with more than 30° of rotation
- Degenerative spondylolisthesis greater than Grade 2
- Retroperitoneal scarring on both left and right sides (e.g., due to abscess or prior surgery)
- Need for direct decompression through the same approach.

24.3 Surgical Technique

The procedure is performed with the patient under general anesthesia and in the lateral decubitus position (**Fig. 24.1**). The intervertebral disk and margins of vertebrae are marked under C-arm fluoroscopic guidance. The surgeon can be positioned in front or in back of the patient. A skin incision of about 2 to 2.5 cm is made, and serial dissection of the external oblique, internal oblique, and transversalis abdominis muscles is performed using the muscle-splitting technique (**Video 24.1**). Then, the retroperitoneal space is exposed. The surgeon identifies the psoas muscle using the index finger, and a guide pin is inserted at the disk space under fluoroscopic guidance with neuromonitoring. Serial

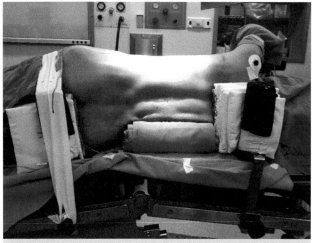

Fig. 24.1 Position for direct lateral interbody fusion (DLIF).

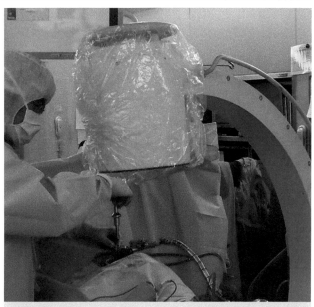

Fig. 24.2 Tubular retractor and flexible arm mounted on operating table.

dilators are sequentially applied and a 22-mm diameter tubular retractor is attached to the table using a flexible arm (**Fig. 24.2**).

The intervertebral disk is removed and the end plate is prepared using curets, a shaver, and long pituitary forceps by the usual methods under C-arm fluoroscopic guidance. Finally, a large lordotic cage (6 or 12°) is carefully placed through the direct lateral interbody fusion (DLIF) corridor at the affected level as an interbody device containing allograft bone chips mixed with demineralized bone matrix (DBM; **Video 24.2**). In the case of moderate to severe osteoporosis, cancellous bone can be harvested from the iliac bone. The wound is closed layer by layer after removal of the retractor systems. After changing the patient to the prone position, additional posterior fixation is performed using percutaneous pedicle screws (**Fig. 24.3**).

The patient is allowed to recover from anesthesia and may be discharged in as little as two to three days. The patient is supplied with an opioid analgesic, nonsteroidal anti-inflammatory drug, and muscle relaxant.

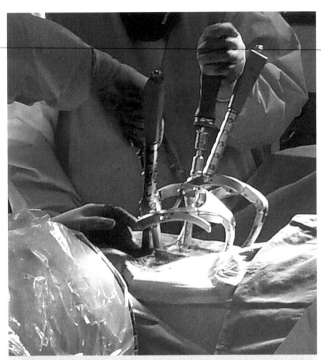

Fig. 24.3 After changing the patient to the prone position, only percutaneous pedicle screws are used for fixation.

24.4 Case Illustration

A 67-year-old female presented with right leg pain along the L3 and L4 dermatome, chronic low back pain, and neurogenic intermittent claudication. Physical examination revealed no positive straight leg raising sign on either side and there was weakness of the ankle dorsiflexion, graded 4. Preoperative X-rays and MRI showed right-sided foraminal stenosis at the L3–L4 and L4–L5 levels, degenerative spondylolisthesis, and degenerative scoliosis (**Fig. 24.4**, **Fig. 24.5**).

Foraminal stenosis at L3–L4 and L4–I5 was successfully decompressed (**Fig. 24.6**). Restoration of the disk heights and correction of the anterolisthesis were confirmed on postoperative MRI and radiography (**Fig. 24.6**, **Fig. 24.7**, **Fig. 24.8**). Preoperative symptoms, including leg pain on the right side and intermittent claudication, subsided completely.

24.5 Complications

There is still some debate about approach-related morbidities with LLIF, including the high possibility of psoas plexus injury in the procedure, abdominal wall paresis, the impossibility of direct decompression of lumbar stenosis, and subsidence of the cage in osteoporotic patients (**Fig. 24.9**, **Fig. 24.10**).[11,12,13,14,15,16] The most important issue for spine surgeons who oppose LLIF is lumbar plexus injury during the procedure. Although many investigators have reported that approach-related psoas plexus injuries are temporary,[11,12,13] most patients do not have these symptoms before surgery.

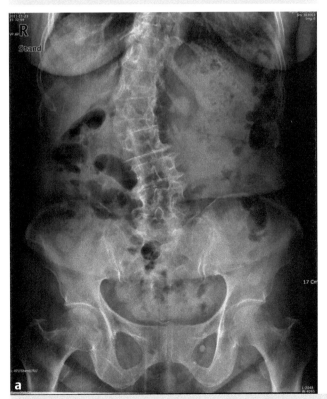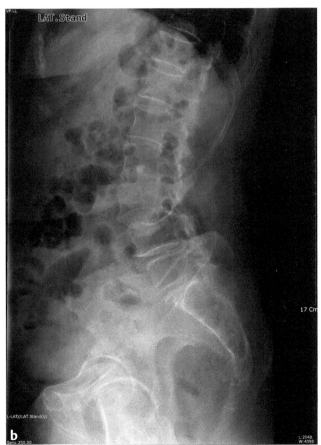

Fig. 24.4 (a,b) Preoperative X-rays show degenerative spondylolisthesis at L3–L4 and L4–L5 levels, with scoliosis.

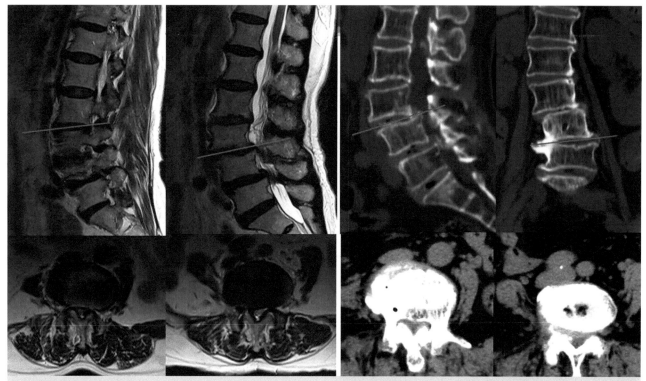

Fig. 24.5 Preoperative MRIs show right foraminal and central stenosis at L3–L4 and L4–L5. CT shows calcified traction spurs at L4–L5, right, and foraminal to central stenosis.

24.6 Discussion

Lumbar interbody fusion (LIF) has been the gold standard for the surgical treatment of unstable spinal segments in adults with chronic and debilitating clinical symptoms. Owing to recent advancements in minimally invasive spinal instruments, LIF is being done more frequently than ever before and minimally invasive spinal surgery (MISS) has gained popularity, especially in LIF.[6,7] However, there still remains significant variation in, and debates about, surgical strategies, and there is limited evidence to guide decision-making about which kind of LIF is better. The preferred surgical techniques for LIF have been posterior lumbar interbody fusion (PLIF), transforaminal lumbar interbody fusion (TLIF), anterior lumbar interbody fusion (ALIF), and direct or extreme lateral interbody fusion (DLIF or XLIF). Recent advances in minimally invasive techniques have generated much interest in DLIF and XLIF as technical variants of ALIF, and spine surgeons have come to consider DLIF and XLIF as being less invasive.[10] The direct lateral approach to the lumbar spine has been considered effective for access to the intervertebral lumbar spine. The two direct lateral transpsoas approaches (XLIF, Nuvasive; DLIF, Medtronic, Inc.) were developed from techniques reported by Mayer and McAfee separately in 1997 and 1998.[17,18] The transpsoas approach relies on entering the retroperitoneal space from the lateral retroperitoneal space and splitting the psoas muscle. This also allows the anterolateral lumbar spine to be approached through a small incision, in minimally invasive fashion, with preservation of the paraspinal musculature.

The XLIF approach to the spine has evolved due to work done by many spine surgeons and companies, and it has many advantages, such as wide interbody graft, preservation of the posterior back muscles, minimal blood loss, and rapid return to daily

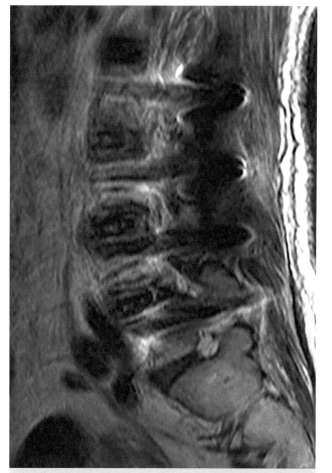

Fig. 24.6 Postoperative MRI shows well-decompressed foraminal canal.

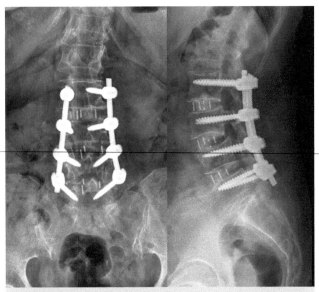

Fig. 24.7 Postoperative X-rays show the correction of scoliotic change and restoration of spondylolisthesis.

activity. Nevertheless, many investigators have reported a high rate of approach-related complications of XLIF: lumbar plexus injury during the transpsoas approach, abdominal wall paresis, subsidence of the cage in osteoporotic patients, and the impossibility of direct decompression of the spinal canal. Although most symptoms related to lumbar plexus injury have been reported to be transient and recovery occurs within several weeks, motor deficit and pain are still present for more than a year in some cases. Moreover, considering the neural anatomy of the lumbar plexus, neural complications related to the lumbar plexus after XLIF are higher at the L4–L5 level than at other lumbar levels.

24.7 Conclusion

Although DLIF and XLIF are relatively new, evidence suggests that they may achieve high rates of fusion while minimizing morbidity and mortality. Moreover, oblique LIF, a variant of D(X) LIF, was recently introduced and decreases lumbar plexus injury through use of the oblique corridor, although its clinical results are still under evaluation.

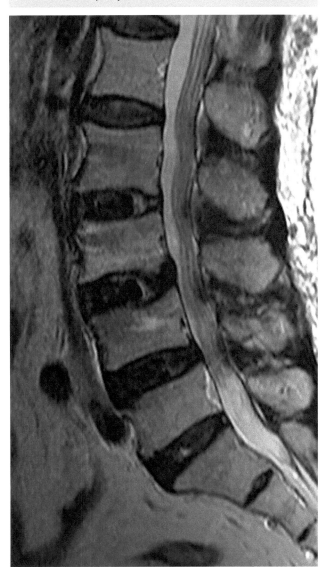

Fig. 24.8 Postoperative MRI shows well-decompressed central canal.

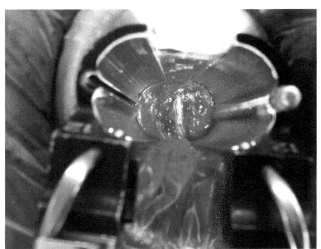

Fig. 24.9 Intraoperative surgical image shows variant of lumbar plexus inside the tubular retractor.

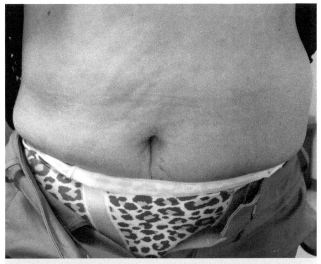

Fig. 24.10 Atony of truncal muscles after direct lateral interbody fusion (DLIF).

References

1 DiPaola CP, Molinari RW. Posterior lumbar interbody fusion. *J Am Acad Orthop Surg* 2008;*16*(3):130–139

2 Sears W. Posterior lumbar interbody fusion for degenerative spondylolisthesis: restoration of sagittal balance using insert-and-rotate interbody spacers. *Spine J* 2005;*5*(2):170–179

3 Ekman P, Möller H, Tullberg T, Neumann P, Hedlund R. Posterior lumbar interbody fusion versus posterolateral fusion in adult isthmic spondylolisthesis. *Spine* 2007;*32*(20):2178–2183

4 Rosenberg WS, Mummaneni PV. Transforaminal lumbar interbody fusion: technique, complications, and early results. *Neurosurgery* 2001;*48*(3):569–574

5 Sclafani JA, Kim CW. Complications associated with the initial learning curve of minimally invasive spine surgery: a systematic review. *Clin Orthop Relat Res* 2014;*472*(6):1711–1717 Review

6 Kim JS, Jung B, Lee SH. Instrumented minimally invasive spinal-transforaminal lumbar interbody fusion (MIS-TLIF); minimum 5-year follow-up with clinical and radiologic outcomes. *J Spinal Disord Tech* 2012;

7 Kim JS, Choi WG, Lee SH. Minimally invasive anterior lumbar interbody fusion followed by percutaneous pedicle screw fixation for isthmic spondylolisthesis: minimum 5-year follow-up. *Spine J* 2010;*10*(5):404–409

8 Ishihara H, Osada R, Kanamori M, et al. Minimum 10-year follow-up study of anterior lumbar interbody fusion for isthmic spondylolisthesis. *J Spinal Disord* 2001;*14*(2):91–99

9 Hofstetter CP, Shin B, Tsiouris AJ, Elowitz E, Härtl R. Radiographic and clinical outcome after 1- and 2-level transsacral axial interbody fusion: clinical article. *J Neurosurg Spine* 2013;*19*(4):454–463

10 Ozgur BM, Aryan HE, Pimenta L, Taylor WR. Extreme lateral interbody fusion (XLIF): a novel surgical technique for anterior lumbar interbody fusion. *Spine J* 2006;*6*(4):435–443

11 Rodgers WB, Gerber EJ, Patterson J. Intraoperative and early postoperative complications in extreme lateral interbody fusion: an analysis of 600 cases. *Spine* 2011;*36*(1):26–32

12 Phillips FM, Isaacs RE, Rodgers WB, et al. Adult degenerative scoliosis treated with XLIF: clinical and radiographical results of a prospective multicenter study with 24-month follow-up. *Spine* 2013;*38*(21):1853–1861

13 Castro C, Oliveira L, Amaral R, Marchi L, Pimenta L. Is the lateral transpsoas approach feasible for the treatment of adult degenerative scoliosis? *Clin Orthop Relat Res* 2014;*472*(6):1776–1783

14 Ahmadian A, Verma S, Mundis GM Jr, Oskouian RJ Jr, Smith DA, Uribe JS. Minimally invasive lateral retroperitoneal transpsoas interbody fusion for L4–5 spondylolisthesis: clinical outcomes. *J Neurosurg Spine* 2013;*19*(3):314–320

15 Graham RB, Wong AP, Liu JC. Minimally invasive lateral transpsoas approach to the lumbar spine: pitfalls and complication avoidance. *Neurosurg Clin N Am* 2014;*25*(2):219–231

16 Ahmadian A, Deukmedjian AR, Abel N, Dakwar E, Uribe JS. Analysis of lumbar plexopathies and nerve injury after lateral retroperitoneal transpsoas approach: diagnostic standardization. *J Neurosurg Spine* 2013;*18*(3):289–297

17 Mayer HM. A new microsurgical technique for minimally invasive anterior lumbar interbody fusion. *Spine* 1997;*22*(6):691–699

18 McAfee PC, Regan JJ, Geis WP, Fedder IL. Minimally invasive anterior retroperitoneal approach to the lumbar spine. Emphasis on the lateral BAK. *Spine* 1998;*23*(13):1476–1484

25 Endoscopic Removal of Intradural Extramedullary Space-Occupying Lesions

Shrinivas M. Rohidas

25.1 Introduction

The last two decades have seen the emergence of minimalism in spine surgery aimed at preventing approach-related trauma to tissue. MISS—minimally invasive spine surgery—is a term that is now used often. In fact, it is a misleading term, because MISS is potentially maximally invasive at the target area. There is no compromise in achieving the precise goal—that is, adequate decompression of compressed neural structures—in MISS, but approach-related trauma to surrounding tissue is minimized.

As MacNab wrote, "It really does not matter what technique you use to decompress the nerve root, if you fail to fully decompress the nerve root or introduce complications to the equation, you have failed to serve the patient." It is advisable to remember this principle in spine surgery. In MISS, every patient's symptoms, clinical signs, and radiology have to be evaluated separately and carefully. If the decompression of the compressed nerve root/cord is inadequate, then the compressive symptoms and signs will persist. If the decompression is aggressive or more than necessary, then there are chances that existing stability will be compromised. Hence there has to be an equilibrium between adequate decompression and not compromising existing stability. This equilibrium will be different for every patient, every level to be operated, the extent of stability/instability, and the pathology to be treated. It is dependent on each spine surgeon, along with the technique used by the surgeon. This is one of the many factors that are responsible for the steep learning curve in MISS and endoscopic spine surgery.

25.2 Destandau's Technique

Jean Destandau, a neurosurgeon from Bordeaux, France, developed a technique for endoscopic spine surgery in 1993.[1,2] His technique is based on the triangulation between an endoscope and suction with working instruments.

For Destandau's technique, the authors use Endospine, a set of outer tube/insert and inner tube/working insert with an endoscope. The endoscope used with Endospine is an 18-cm, rigid, straight, 0° endoscope (that is, a universal endoscope used for cystoscopy, arthroscopy, sinoscopy, etc.). Endospine was initially used for lumbar disk herniation. The target area in the lumbar region is elliptical, between two laminae, medially the spinous process and laterally the medial facet, so the outer tube is elliptical rather than round. The inner tube/working insert fits into the outer tube with a ratchet-type lock. There is an inherent telescoping movement between the tubes (**Fig. 25.1**).

The working insert has four built-in channels. On the left side of the working insert, there are two 4-mm-diameter channels that are parallel to each other. The medial 4-mm channel hosts the endoscope and the endoscope remains fixed with the lock. The second 4-mm channel is for the suction tube. The largest channel, which has a 9-mm diameter, is for the working instrument (**Fig. 25.2**).

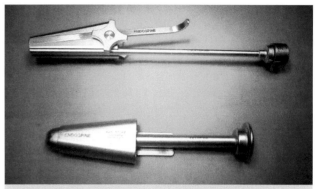

Fig. 25.1 Endospine outer tube and inner tube (working insert).

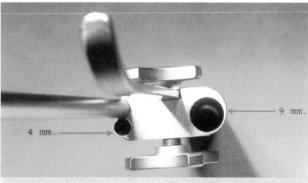

Fig. 25.2 Endospine inner tube with all channels. Working channel of 9-mm and 4-mm channels for suction and endoscope.

The channels for the endoscope and suction are at an angle of 12° to the wide channel of the instrument. Because of this angle, the 0° endoscope can be used as an angled scope. This helps to minimizing fogging of the endoscope tip. When the endoscope and the instrument are working parallel to each other, there is intermingling of the instruments, and the surgeon has to use an angled endoscope when endoscope and instrument work parallel to each other. The fourth channel is for the nerve root retractor, which retracts the nerve root medially to expose the disk space. The outer tube and inner tube are fixed in such a way that there is an artificial space created between the two tubes. This is the working space for the instruments. Once the excision of bone is achieved, then the inner tube can be pushed inside/down. If there is no space maintained between the outer tube and inner tube, then the endoscope will touch the tissue in front and will hamper the surgeon's vision. Also, there will be splashing of fluid over the endoscope lens if adequate space is not maintained between the tubes.

The suction is used with the left hand and the working instrument is in the right hand. With suction in the left hand, the surgeon can move the whole system in medial, lateral, cranial, and caudal directions. The same movements are possible with the instrument in the right hand. The suction in the left hand and

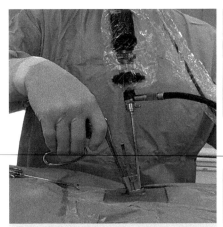
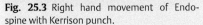

Fig. 25.3 Right hand movement of Endospine with Kerrison punch.

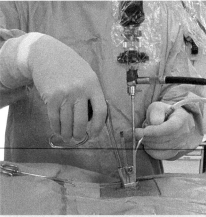

Fig. 25.4 Stable Endospine with Kerrison in right hand and suction tube in left hand.

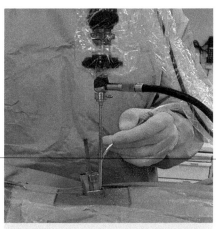

Fig. 25.5 Left hand supporting the Endospine.

instrument in the right hand work to maintain the stability of the system. When the surgeon is using suction to clean the operative area, the instrument in the right hand keeps the system stable, and vice versa—when the surgeon is using the instrument, the suction in the left hand keeps the system stable. Synchronization of movements of both hands is necessary while looking at the image on the screen. The surgeon should learn the synchronization of both hands' movements, along with using both hands while looking at the screen image. These are the basics of Destandau's technique in spine surgery (**Fig. 25.3**, **Fig. 25.4**, **Fig. 25.5**).

Once sufficient experience is gained, Endospine can be used for excision of small intradural extramedullary tumors, mostly posterior or lateral. Anteriorly placed tumors in the thoracic region are difficult. Exact localization of the level is done with the localizing pin and C-arm fluoroscopy. Rather than a paramedian incision, a midline incision is preferred. Subperiosteal dissection of muscles with excision of the spinous process is done. Then the outer tube with two small retractors is fixed in the Endospine system. Under endoscopic vision, laminectomy is performed with a Kerrison punch. Small, thin pieces of Gelfoam are placed over the lateral edge of the dural sac to control epidural oozing, rather than cauterizing the epidural veins. The dura is opened

with a 15-mm knife and the incision is extended with scissors. Two stay sutures are made on the dural edges through the outer tube. Again, the outer tube is placed with stay sutures retracting the dural edges. If the localization is correct, with no shift of the space-occupying lesion (SOL) due to positioning, then mostly the SOL is seen compressing the cord. Dissection of the SOL is done with small curets and endoscopic angulated cautery. Attachment of the nerve root is resected with scissors or cautery. The SOL, carefully held with biopsy forceps, and the whole Endospine system are removed (**Fig. 25.6**, **Fig. 25.7**, **Fig. 25.8**).

Closure of the dura is achieved with 2-mm titanium AnastoClips. These are used in cardiac surgery to close arterial walls. The dural stay suture holds the dural edges together and the shaft of AnastoClips is sufficiently slender to be passed through the working channel of the Endospine system. Muscle and skin are closed with 2–0 Vicryl (**Fig. 25.9**, **Fig. 25.10**, **Fig. 25.11**, **Fig. 25.12**).

From 2004 through 2011, the author treated 14 intradural tumors with Endospine; patients were six males and eight females, with a minimum age of 22 years and a maximum age of 73 years. Eleven tumors were neurofibromas at the lumbar and thoracic levels and three were meningiomas (**Table 25.1**).

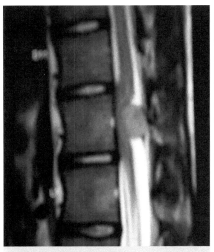

Fig. 25.6 MRI showing thoracic intradural space-occupying neuro-fibroma.

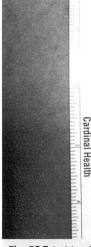

Fig. 25.7 Incision for endoscopic excision of space-occupying lesion.

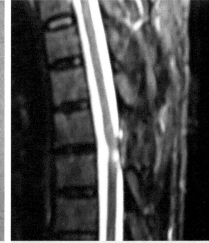

Fig. 25.8 Postoperative MRI.

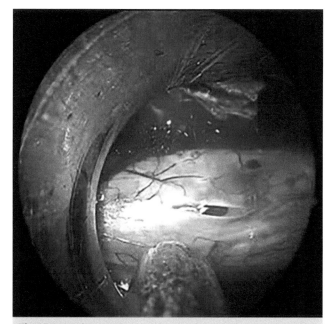

Fig. 25.9 Dural incision.

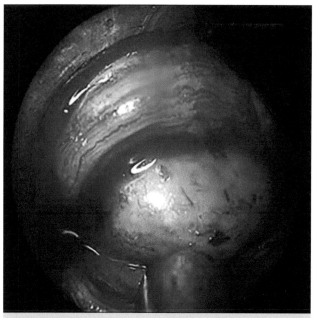

Fig. 25.10 Exposed intradural space-occupying neurofibroma.

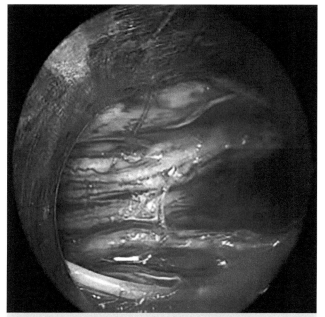

Fig. 25.11 Cord after excision of space-occupying neurofibroma.

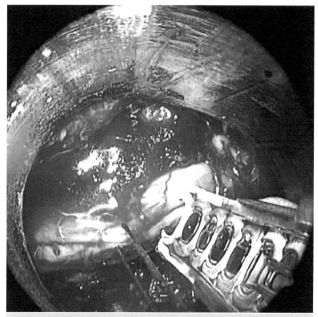

Fig. 25.12 Dural closure with AnastoClips.

Postoperatively, 13 patients recovered completely. One patient had partial recovery of preoperative spastic paraplegia. She is able to walk with minimal support but did not have complete recovery of spasticity in both lower limbs. This patient had a meningioma at dorsal level T9–T10 that was anteriorly placed. No postoperative CSF leak or wound infection was noted.

25.3 Conclusion

Small intradural extramedullary neoplasms can be safely and effectively treated with Endospine—a minimally invasive mobile technique. Small incision, relatively less blood loss, and shorter hospitalization suggest that, in the hands of an experienced surgeon, Endospine may be an alternative to the traditional open technique.

Table 25.1 Demographic data for patients who underwent surgery for space-occupying lesions

Number	Age (years)/Sex	Location	Pathology	Preoperative symptoms	Postoperative 6-week review
1. 747/2004	22/M	T12 intradural	Neurofibroma	Paraparesis	Complete recovery
2. 142/2005	60/F	T8–T9 intradural	Meningioma	Paraparesis, sphincter involvement	Complete recovery
3. 1311/2006	50/M	T4–T5 intradural	Neurofibroma	Spastic paraplegia	Complete recovery
4. 1317/2006	62/M	T12–L1 intradural	Neurofibroma	Paraparesis	Complete recovery
5. 821/2007	84/F	T6–T7 intradural	Neurofibroma	Paraparesis	Partial recovery
6. 1363/2007	69/F	T7–T8 intradural	Meningioma	Paraparesis	Complete recovery
7. 256/2009	60/F	L3–L4 intradural	Neurofibroma	Radiculopathy, weakness	Complete recovery
8. 1061/2009	73/F	T6–T7 intradural	Meningioma	Spastic paraplegia, sphincter involvement	Complete recovery
9. 981/2010	48s/M	L2–L3 extradural in left axilla	Neurofibroma	Radiculopathy, weakness	Complete recovery
10. 516/2011	41/F	L3 dumbbell-shaped intradural + extradural	Neurofibroma	Radiculopathy, weakness	Complete recovery
11. 1479/2011	41/M	L1–L2 intradural	Neurofibroma	Paraparesis	Complete recovery
12. 1592/2012	58/F	L4–L5 intradural	Neurofibroma	Radiculopathy	Complete recovery
13. 735/2013	30/M	Right L5–S1 intraneural	Neurofibroma	Radiculopathy, weakness	Complete recovery
14. 1926/2013	65/F	T9–T10 intradural left & anterior	Neurofibroma	Spastic paraplegia	Partial recovery

References

1   Tredway TL, Santiago P, Hrubes MR, et al. Minimally invasive resection of intra-
    dural extramedullary spinal neoplasms. *Neurosurgery 58*(Operative neurosur-
    gery Suppl. 1): 52–57
2   Destandau J. Endoscopically assisted lumbar microdiscectomy. *J Minimally
    Invasive Spinal Technique* 2001;*1*(1):41–43

26 Laparoscope- and Endoscope-Assisted Oblique Lumbar Interbody Fusion

Ji-Hoon Seong and Jin-Sung Luke Kim

26.1 Laparoscope-Assisted OLIF

26.1.1 Background

Laparoscope-assisted spine surgery via a retroperitoneal approach is not a new surgical technique. Peretti et al[1] presented a technical description of laparoscope-assisted lumbar interbody fusion with a lateral retroperitoneal approach in four patients in 1996. Henry[2] and Regan[3] demonstrated that anterior lumbar fusion via a laparoscope-assisted retroperitoneal approach was safe and effective.

The laparoscope had been used for minimally invasive surgery, but recently the popularity of the laparoscope has decreased, perhaps because of development of surgical devices and instruments for lumbar spinal surgery, especially the tubular retractor system for an anterior or lateral retroperitoneal approach. However, there may be cases requiring a laparoscope, such as when a tubular retractor would be positioned at a dangerous location in the oblique lumbar interbody fusion (OLIF) procedure. If the OLIF corridor is blocked by retroperitoneal vessels or if the ureter or a nerve has an abnormal course, a tubular retractor in the OLIF procedure can injure the anatomic structures. In these cases, a laparoscope-assisted surgical procedure can give a surgical field of vision and decrease approach-related complications.

26.1.2 Clinical Findings

A 72-year-old female presented with long-standing low back pain and right leg radiating pain. Preoperative imaging studies

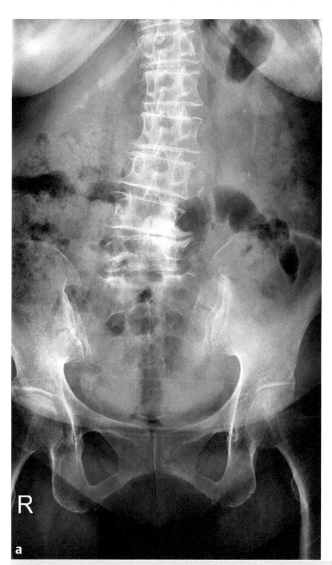 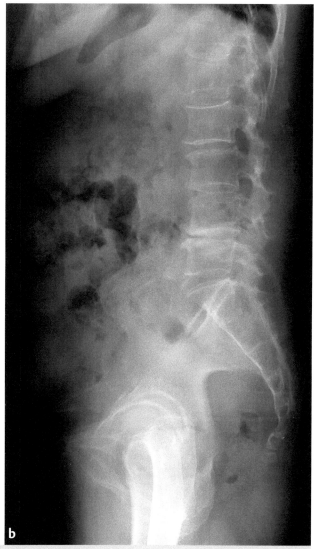

Fig. 26.1 (a,b) Plain radiographs showing lumbar degenerative kyphosis and scoliosis.

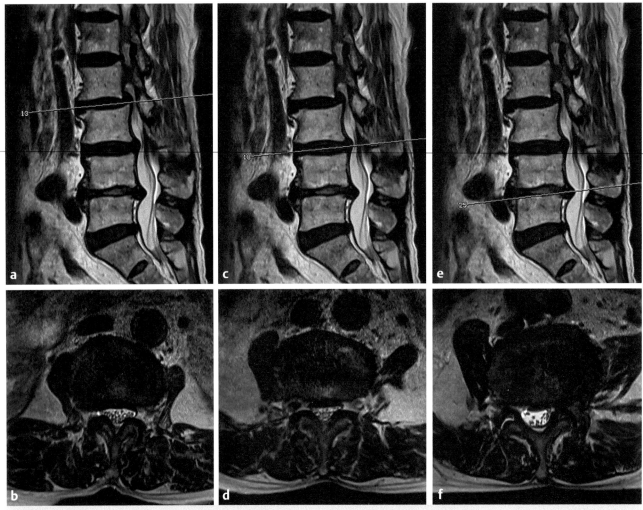

Fig. 26.2 (a–f) Sagittal and axial MRIs showing multilevel degeneration of lumbar spine.

were performed. Plain radiographs showed lumbar degenerative kyphotic and scoliotic change (**Fig. 26.1**). MRI sagittal and axial views showed degenerative lumbar kyphosis, degenerative spondylolisthesis of L2 on L3, and central canal stenosis with foraminal stenosis at the L3–L4 and L4–L5 levels (**Fig. 26.2**).

26.1.3 Preoperative Plan

It was determined that the patient would undergo a laparoscope-assisted OLIF via a retroperitoneal approach. A right-sided approach was selected.

26.1.4 Surgical Procedures

The first skin incision, for the laparoscopic port, was made, and the Veress needle was inserted. Next, that CO_2 gas filled the retroperitoneal space was confirmed through the Veress needle.

The 10-mm diameter trocar was carefully placed, and the laparoscope was introduced through the trocar. The retroperitoneal space was inspected and it was determined that there was no intraperitoneal injury. The second and third trocar sites were incised and two 5-mm trocars were placed.

Under C-arm and laparoscopic guidance, serial dilators and the retractor for OLIF were introduced above the disk space (**Fig. 26.3, Fig. 26.4, Fig. 26.5**).

26.1.5 Results

The procedure resulted in sufficient decompression, and improvement of scoliosis and kyphosis were shown on postoperative radiographs (**Fig. 26.6**).

26.2 Endoscope-Assisted OLIF

26.2.1 Background

The advantages of direct lateral interbody fusion (DLIF) include indirect decompression based on a wide interbody graft, with less tissue damage, preservation of the posterior ligaments and muscles, minimal blood loss, short duration of surgery, and rapid recovery.[4,5]

Therefore, many investigators promoted the use of DLIF in the elderly and debilitated patients. However, many authors do not agree on the effectiveness of transpsoas DLIF due to the disadvantages of a lateral approach: a high risk of lumbar plexus injury during the procedure, abdominal wall paresis, and the impossibility of direct decompression of lumbar stenosis.[6]

OLIF, as a variant of DLIF, was introduced to decrease lumbar plexus injury by using the oblique trajectory, even though its clinical results are still under evaluation.

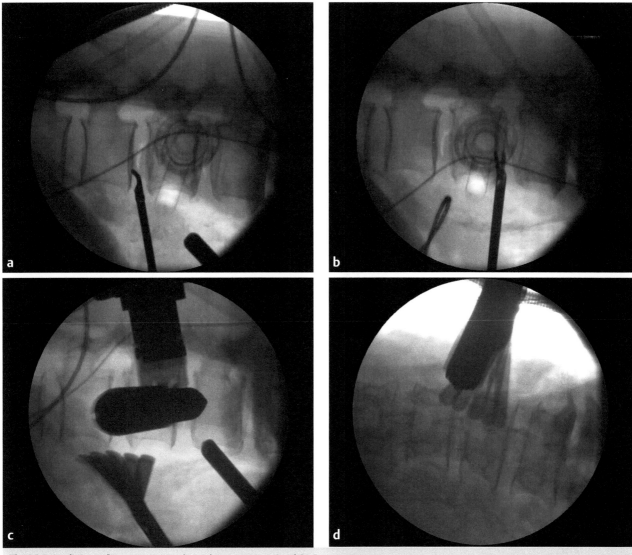

Fig. 26.3 (a–d) C-arm fluoroscopic view during laparoscope-assisted OLIF.

To overcome the drawbacks of DLIF, the authors use spinal endoscopic systems through the OLIF corridor. With the specialized aid of the spinal endoscope, spine surgeons can remove the disk fragments directly under endoscopic visualization. The oblique trajectory of OLIF may help spine surgeons to directly access the target lesion and to decompress intracanal or contralateral foraminal lesions.

26.2.2 Preoperative Plan

OLIF was recommended to the patient for restoration of the disk heights and correction of the anterolisthesis.

Before the insertion of the OLIF cage, endoscopic removal of the ruptured disk was planned. It is impossible to directly remove herniated disk during DLIF or OLIF. The deeply located disk and shallow diameter of the tubular retractor interfere with direct decompression and removal of ruptured disk material.

26.2.3 Surgical Procedures

The procedure is performed with the patient under general anesthesia, in the right true lateral decubitus position. The

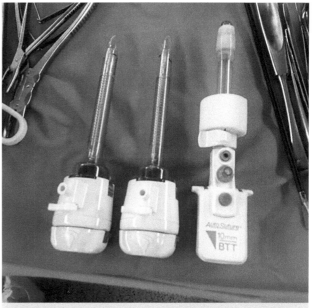

Fig. 26.4 Laparoscopic trocars.

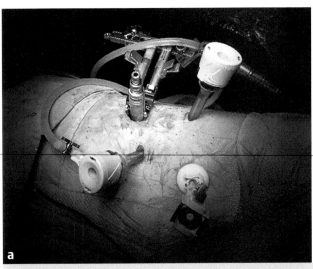
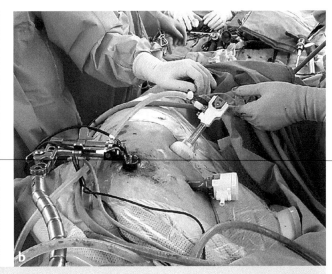

Fig. 26.5 (a,b) Laparoscope-assisted OLIF.

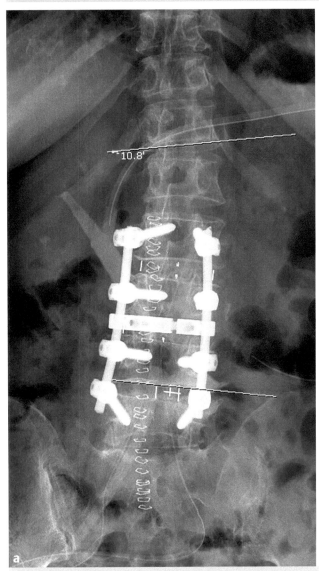
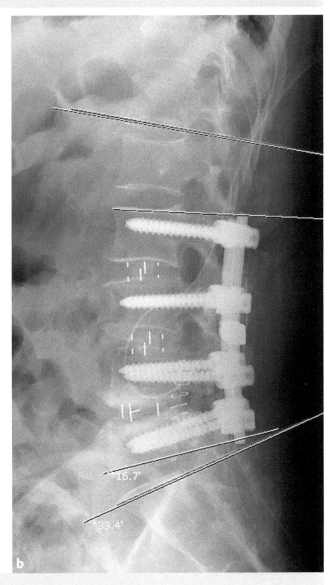

Fig. 26.6 (a,b) Postoperative plain radiographs.

intervertebral disk and anterior margin of the vertebrae are marked using a sterile marking pen using C-arm fluoroscopic guidance. In contrast to DLIF, OLIF procedures are always performed with the surgeon in front of the patient. An oblique skin incision of about 2.0 to 2.5 cm is made for one segmental fusion, and serial muscle dissection is performed parallel to muscle fibers from the external oblique, internal oblique, and transversalis abdominis muscles. The retroperitoneal fat and psoas muscle are identified, and the anterior portion of psoas muscle is palpated and retracted to prevent lumbar plexus injury. A guide pin is inserted into the intervertebral disk space under fluoroscopic guidance, and serial dilators of increasing diameter are sequentially applied. A 22-mm-diameter tubular retractor is attached to the table using a flexible arm.

The disk materials are removed and the end plate is prepared using curets, a shaver, and long pituitary forceps under C-arm fluoroscopic guidance.

Spinal endoscopic systems are used in the diskectomy area for additional disk removal before insertion of the cage. After removal of the intervertebral disk, the obturator and the working channel are advanced in the diskectomy area for additional disk removal before insertion of the cage (**Fig. 26.7**).

The posterior portion of the disk is removed under endoscopic magnetic visualization until identification of the posterior longitudinal ligament (PLL). If the PLL floats well with saline irrigation, the surgeon removes the dorsally located ruptured disk.

The surgeon can explore not only the central part of the spinal canal but also the contralateral side of the neural foramen for removal of ruptured disk particles. The surgeon also can resect the PLL for exploration of the epidural space, as required. Finally, a cage for lateral interbody fusion via the oblique corridor is inserted. The wound is closed layer by layer after removal of the retractor systems. After the patient is place prone, additional posterior fixation is performed using percutaneous pedicle screw systems.

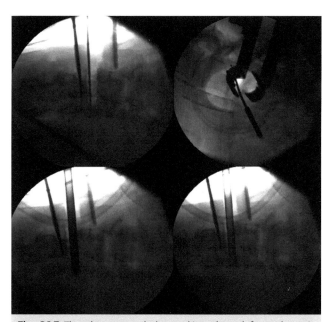

Fig. 26.7 The obturator and the working channel for endoscopic diskectomy are advanced under C-arm fluoroscopic guidance.

26.2.4 Case Presentations

Case 1

A 61-year-old female presented with right leg pain along the L3 and L4 dermatomes, chronic low back pain, and neurogenic intermittent claudication. Physical examination revealed a positive straight leg raising sign at 30° on the right side and there was weakness of the ankle dorsiflexion, graded 4. MRI showed right-sided foraminal disk herniation at L3–L4, and bilateral foraminal stenosis with central disk herniation at L4–L5 (**Fig. 26.8**, **Fig. 26.9**, **Video 26.1**).

● *Case 1 Results*

Foraminal disk fragments were successfully removed at L3–L4. Restoration of the disk heights and correction of the anterolisthesis were confirmed on postoperative MRI and radiography (**Fig. 26.10**, **Fig. 26.11**). Preoperative symptoms, including leg pain on the right side and intermittent claudication, subsided completely.

Case 2

The video of this case is available on YouTube (https://www .youtube.com/watch?v=9YCSx9ttTyw&feature=youtu.be).

A 70-year-old female presented with leg pain in both legs along the posterolateral thigh and calf. Because of severe radiating leg pain and neurogenic intermittent claudication, the patient could not walk more than 10 m.

Physical examination revealed a positive straight leg raising sign at 30° on both sides and there was weakness of the ankle and great toe dorsiflexion of both legs, graded 4. X-ray and MRI showed right-sided paracentral disk herniation at L3–L4 combined with central stenosis and slight instability at L3–L4. Moderate degrees of disk height loss were observed at the L4–L5 and L5–S1 levels, but were not associated with recent-onset symptoms (**Fig. 26.12**, **Fig. 26.13**, **Fig. 26.14**).

● *Case 2 Results*

Restoration of the disk heights and correction of the anterolisthesis were confirmed on postoperative X-rays (**Fig. 26.15**). Central and paracentral disk fragments were successfully removed at L3–L4, which was confirmed on postoperative MRI (**Fig. 26.16**). Preoperative symptoms subsided completely.

Case 3

A 72-year-old female presented with both sciatica and neurogenic intermittent claudication.

Pre- and postoperative X-rays and MRIs showed changes of disk herniation and restoration of coronal imbalance and spondylolisthesis at the L4–L5 level (**Fig. 26.17**, **Fig. 26.18**).

Intraoperative C-arm images show semi-flexible forceps and hooks (upper images) and cage inserted (lower images) (**Fig. 26.19**).

26.2.5 Complications

Complications of the procedure include sympathetic dysfunction (**Fig. 26.20**) and abdominal ileus.

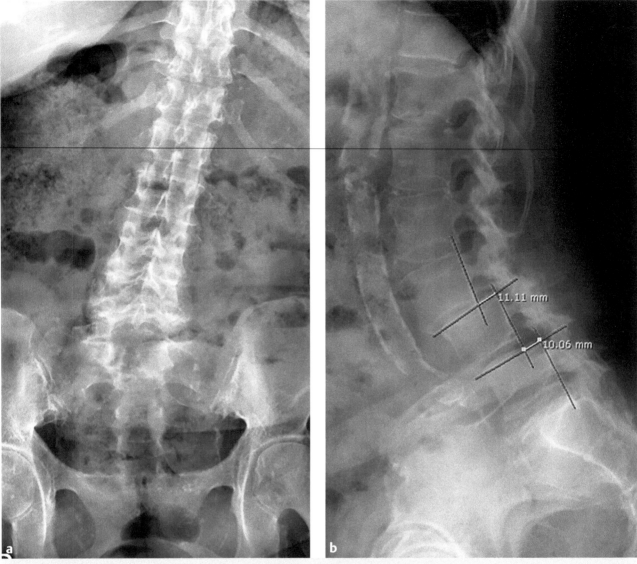

Fig. 26.8 (a,b) Preoperative X-rays show degenerative spondylolisthesis at L3–L4 and L4–L5 and scoliotic change.

26.2.6 Conclusion

With the specialized aid of the spinal endoscope, spine surgeons can remove disk fragments directly under endoscopic visualization in selected cases. Due to the oblique trajectory of OLIF, it can help spine surgeons to directly access the target lesion and decompress the intracanal or contralateral foraminal lesion.

References

1. de Peretti F, Hovorka I, Fabiani P, Argenson C. New possibilities in L2–L5 lumbar arthrodesis using a lateral retroperitoneal approach assisted by laparoscopy: preliminary results. *Eur Spine J* 1996;5(3):210–216
2. Henry LG, Cattey RP, Stoll JE, Robbins S. Laparoscopically assisted spinal surgery. *JSLS* 1997;1(4):341–344
3. Regan JP, Cattey RP, Henry LG, Robbins S. Laparoscopically assisted retroperitoneal spinal surgery. *JSLS* 2006;10(4):493–495
4. Kepler CK, Sharma AK, Huang RC, et al. Indirect foraminal decompression after lateral transpsoas interbody fusion. *J Neurosurg Spine* 2012;16(4):329–333

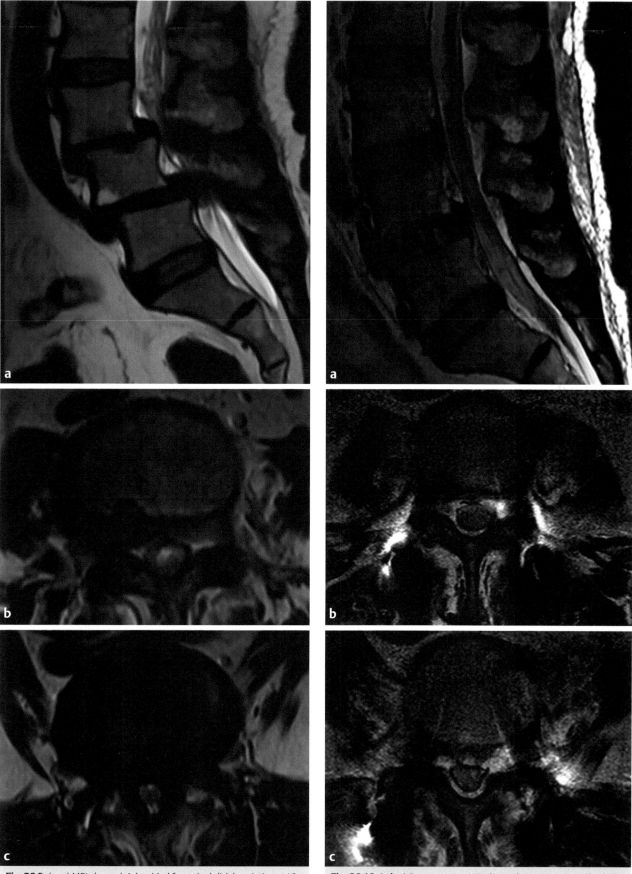

Fig. 26.9 (a–c) MRI showed right-sided foraminal disk herniation at L3–L4 and bilateral foraminal stenosis with central disk herniation at L4–L5.

Fig. 26.10 (a,b,c) Postoperative MRI shows decompression in both the central and the foraminal area.

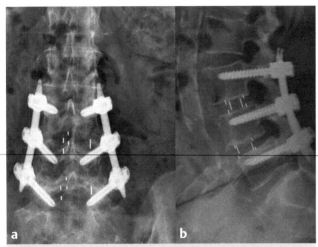

Fig. 26.11 (a,b) Restoration of disk heights and correction of the anterolisthesis and scoliosis were confirmed on postoperative X-ray.

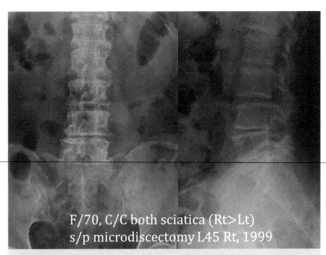

F/70, C/C both sciatica (Rt>Lt)
s/p microdiscectomy L45 Rt, 1999

Fig. 26.12 Preoperative X-ray shows degenerative spondylolisthesis at L3–L4 and loss of disk height at L4–L5 and L5–S1.

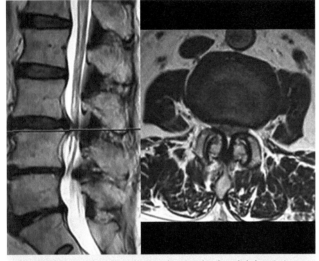

Fig. 26.13 Sagittal and axial MRIs showing lumbar disk herniation at L3–L4.

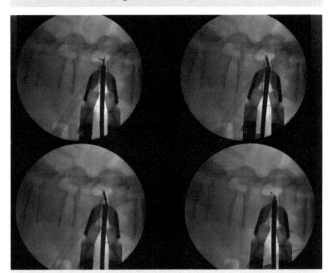

Fig. 26.14 The working channel and spinal endoscope for endoscopic diskectomy are advanced under C-arm guidance. Semiflexible endoscopic forceps and probe are observed in C-arm views.

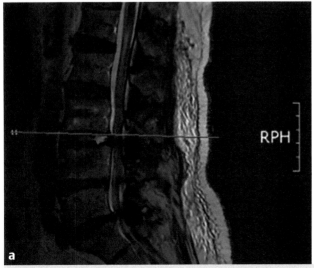

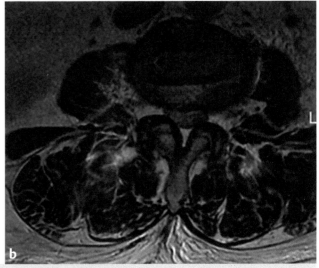

Fig. 26.16 (a–d) Postoperative sagittal and axial MRI reveals decompression of the thecal sac at L3–L4.

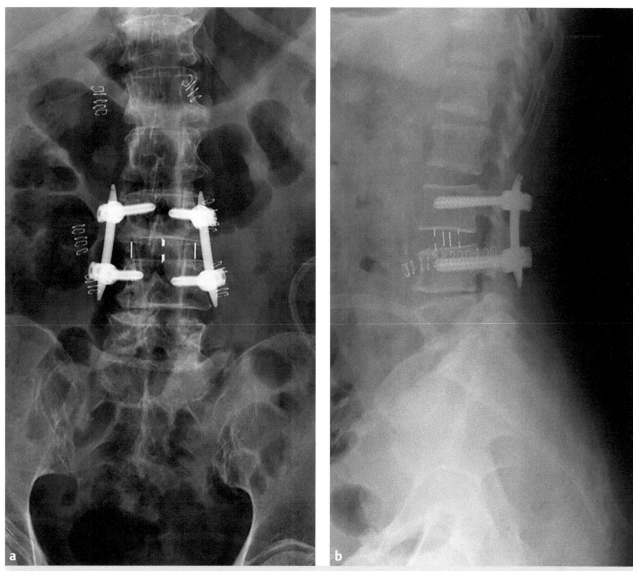

Fig. 26.15 (**a,b**) Postoperative X-ray shows OLIF cage and percutaneous screws.

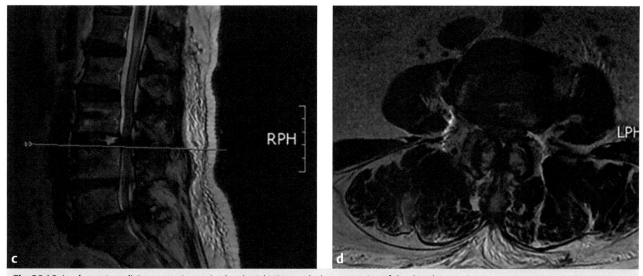

Fig. 26.16 (**a–d, continued**) Postoperative sagittal and axial MRI reveals decompression of the thecal sac at L3–L4.

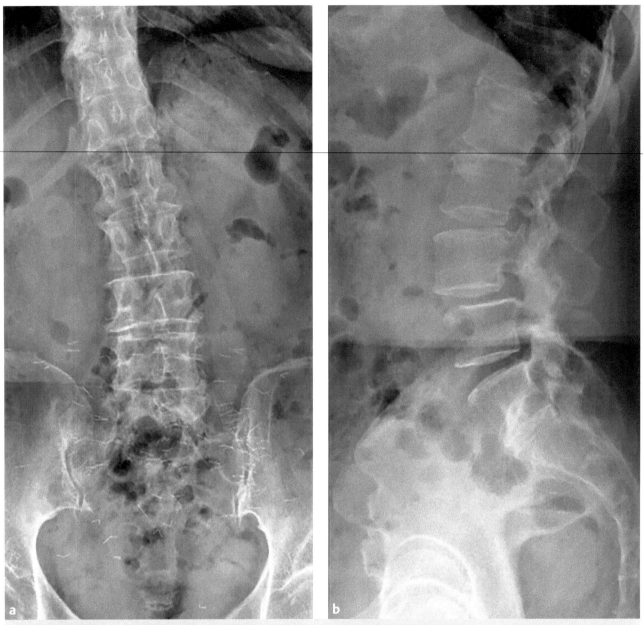

Fig. 26.17 (**a–d**) Pre- and postoperative X-rays show the restoration of coronal and sagittal alignment at L4–L5.

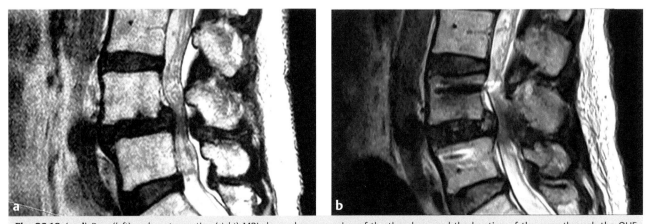

Fig. 26.18 (**a–d**) Pre- (*left*) and postoperative (*right*) MRI shows decompression of the thecal sac and the location of the cage through the OLIF corridor.

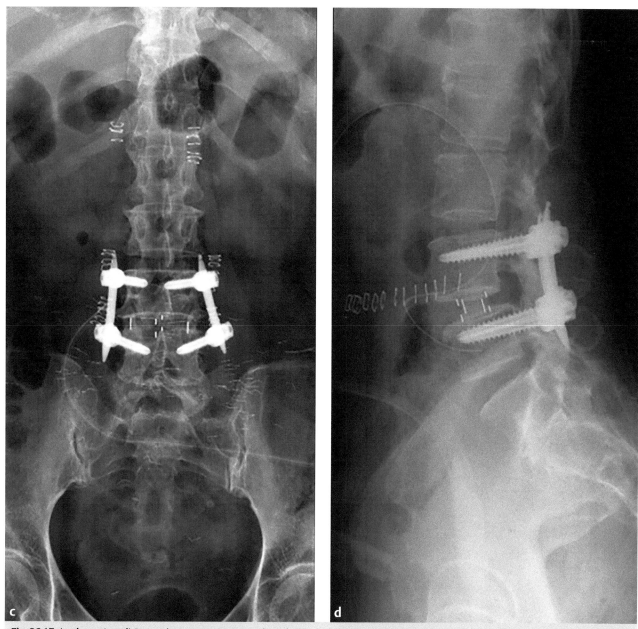

Fig. 26.17 (a–d, continued) Pre- and postoperative X-rays show the restoration of coronal and sagittal alignment at L4–L5.

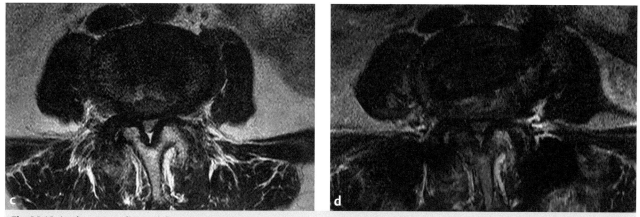

Fig. 26.18 (a–d, continued) Pre- (*left*) and postoperative (*right*) MRI shows decompression of the thecal sac and the location of the cage through the OLIF corridor.

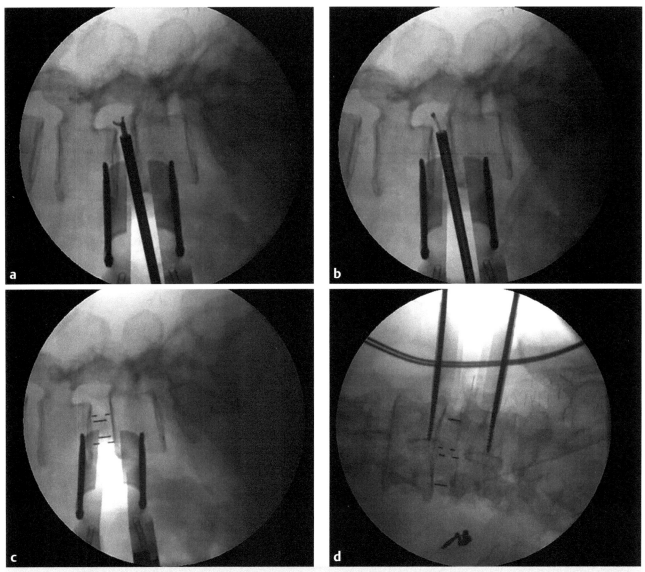

Fig. 26.19 (a–d) Intraoperative C-arm views show semiflexible endoscopic forceps and probe (*upper images*) and the location of the cage (*lower images*).

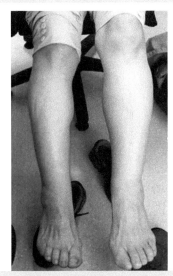

Fig. 26.20 Swelling of the left leg and discomfort are complications due to sympathetic dysfunction associated with direct injury to the sympathetic chain during OLIF. Most complications are transient.

5   Oliveira L, Marchi L, Coutinho E, Pimenta L. A radiographic assessment of the ability of the extreme lateral interbody fusion procedure to indirectly decompress the neural elements. *Spine* 2010;*35*(26, Suppl):S331–S337

6   Houten JK, Alexandre LC, Nasser R, Wollowick AL. Nerve injury during the transpsoas approach for lumbar fusion. *J Neurosurg Spine* 2011;*15*(3):280–284

27 Endoscopic Radiofrequency Denervation for Treatment of Chronic Low Back Pain

Won-Suh Choi and Jin-Sung Luke Kim

27.1 Introduction

The lifetime prevalence of low back pain is estimated to be 60 to 80%.[1,2] Chronic low back pain (CLBP) that persists for 3 months or more is reported to have a lifetime prevalence of 4 to 10%.[3] CLBP can be caused by various sources of pain generation, including intervertebral disk, back musculature, facet joints, and sacroiliac joints. It can also be caused by a combination of these pain generators, and identification of the source of pain is the first step in successful treatment of CLBP.

Low back pain arising from the facet joint, also known as facet joint syndrome (FJS), is a major source of CLBP and is reported to be responsible for 15 to 45% of the total population suffering from CLBP.[4,5] Symptoms can be similar to those of herniated disk, and pain can be exacerbated by back extension after flexion.

The sacroiliac joint (SIJ) complex is also a major, but often overlooked, source of CLBP, accounting for ~ 10 to 33% of CLBP.[1,6,7,8,9,10] The symptoms are nonspecific and can sometimes mimic symptoms of lumbar herniated disk, which makes the diagnosis difficult. SIJ pain can develop as a form of adjacent-segment pathology, especially after fusion surgery.

The current standard treatment for FJS and SIJ pain is steroid injection of the joint itself, the medial branch of the dorsal ramus in the case of FJS[4,11] or lateral sacral nerve branches in the case of SIJ-mediated CLBP.[12,13,14] These procedures can be performed on an outpatient basis, are easy to perform, and have additional diagnostic value. However, patients may experience symptom recurrence due to short duration of effect,[15] and there are always risks of possible local and systemic complications associated with repeated steroid injection.

Fluoroscopy-guided radiofrequency ablation (RFA) of the aforementioned structures provides a longer-lasting effect.[16,17] However, often extensive ablation is required to achieve satisfactory relief of patients' pain. Extensive ablation can also scar adjacent muscular and ligamentous structures, and the scarring itself can become a source of CLBP. With direct visualization under endoscopic guidance, more precise lesioning and effective neural ablation are possible without damaging nearby structures (**Video 27.1**).

27.2 Indications and Contraindications

27.2.1 Medial Branch RFA

- A minimum of 2 months of conservative and medical treatment, including analgesics and physical therapy.
- Two diagnostic medial branch blocks performed on separate occasions, with greater than 50% pain reduction after the procedure on both occasions.
- Any patient with CLBP arising from fracture, infection, or pathologic origin, or with issues of possible secondary gain, is excluded.

27.2.2 Sacroiliac Joint RFA

- A minimum of 2 months of conservative and medical treatment, including analgesics and physical therapy.
- Two diagnostic intraarticular and/or periforaminal SIJ blocks performed on separate occasions, with greater than 50% pain reduction after the procedure on both occasions.
- Any patient with CLBP arising from fracture, infection, or pathologic origin, or with issues of possible secondary gain, is excluded.

27.3 Surgical Technique

The patient is placed in the prone position on chest rolls on a radiolucent table. A small dose of intravenous fentanyl and midazolam is administered for light anesthesia. Before the procedure is started, patients are fully informed of all the details of the procedure. Patients are monitored and maintain communication with the surgeon throughout the procedure.

The patient is prepped and draped in a sterile manner. Fluoroscopic equipment, such as the C-arm, is required for confirmation of landmarks and for checking the position of the endoscope (**Fig. 27.1**).

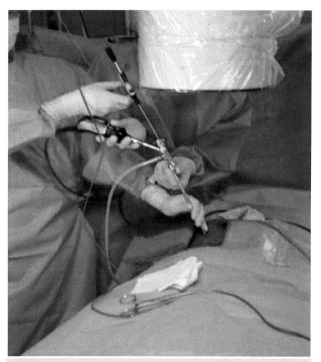

Fig. 27.1 The patient should be prepped and draped in a sterile manner, as in open surgery. A C-arm is set up to confirm the position of the endoscope at various points during the procedure. An assistant can help hold the cannula or the scope, which can decrease the surgeon's fatigue.

27.4 Technique

27.4.1 Medial Branch RFA

The facet joint is innervated by the medial branch of the dorsal ramus at the target vertebral level and one level above it (**Fig. 27.2**).[18,19] Therefore, to successfully treat pain arising from a facet joint, the medial branch one level above the target needs to be ablated as well. The target point for ablation is the junction of the transverse process and the base of the superior articular process (SAP) (**Fig. 27.3**). After verification of the target level with the C-arm, 0.5% lidocaine is injected at the needle entry site via a 22 G spinal needle. Under fluoroscopic guidance, an 18 G needle is docked on the target point. Next, the skin opening is widened slightly with a No. 11 scalpel, and a K-wire, obturator, and beveled working cannula are serially inserted through the opening (**Fig. 27.4**). After the correct position of the cannula is verified with C-arm fluoroscopy, the endoscope is advanced through the cannula, and the bipolar electrocoagulator is advanced through the opening in the endoscope.

Continuous irrigation is maintained throughout the procedure to obtain a clear view of the working field, and also to prevent charring of the bipolar tip. We start by ablating soft tissue at the base of the transverse process. Ablating this area should elicit pain, because the medial branch, and sometimes the lateral branch, course through this region. The medial branch is visible in this location with the endoscope (**Fig. 27.5**), but not in all cases. However, even when the medial branch is not visible, we are able to see the bony landmarks and ablated areas under endoscopic view. Occasionally, the pain elicited during ablation

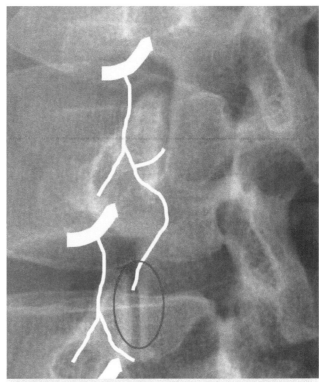

Fig. 27.2 The lumbar zygapophysial joint, or facet joint, has dual innervations. It is innervated by the ascending medial branch at the index level, as well as by the descending medial branch from the level above it.

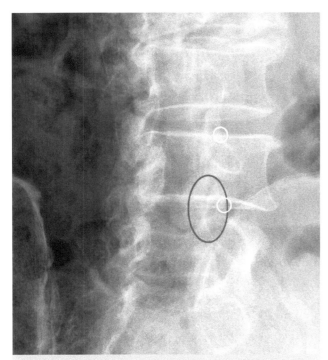

Fig. 27.3 The target for RFA is at the junction of the transverse process and the superior articular facet. This location is best visualized on the oblique image of the C-arm. In treating L4–L5 facet joint arthropathy (*red circle*), the targets for RFA are two locations (*yellow circles*).

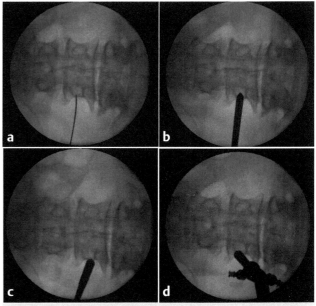

Fig. 27.4 C-arm anteroposterior images during the procedure. (**a**) First, an 18 G needle is docked on the target point, at the junction of the transverse process and superior articular process. (**b,c**) After widening of the opening with a No. 11 blade, the obturator and then the beveled working cannula are inserted through the trajectory made by the 18 G needle. (**d**) Finally, the endoscope is introduced through the working cannula.

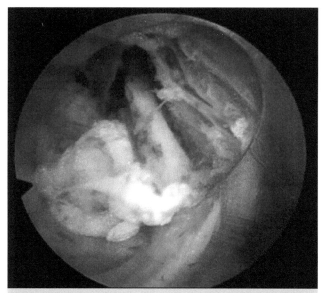

Fig. 27.5 Endoscopic view of the medial branch as it courses caudally over the junction of the superior articular process (SAP) and transverse process (TP). Arrow denotes medial branch.

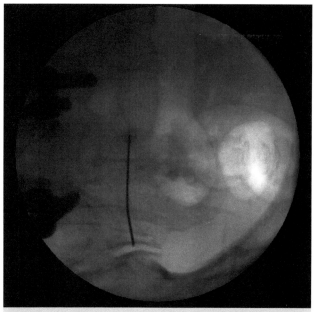

Fig. 27.6 An 18 G needle is docked on the posteroinferior portion of the SIJ capsule.

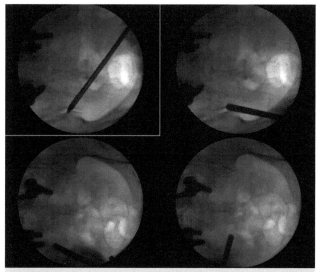

Fig. 27.7 Fluoroscopic view of the endoscopic cannula tip in various positions during the procedure. The cannula tip can be moved in the subcutaneous plane and can be repositioned without causing too much discomfort.

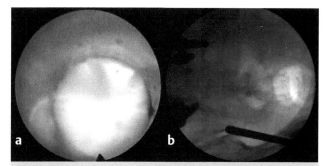

Fig. 27.8 (**a**) Long posterior ligament (*arrowheads*) overlying the posterior capsule of the SIJ. (**b**) Corresponding position of the cannula tip on an anteroposterior fluoroscopic image.

is too much for the patient to bear, and in such cases we inject 0.5 to 1 mL of lidocaine at the target through an 18 G needle prior to ablation. The ablation is done preferably in short bursts of 2 to 3 seconds to prevent excessive charring. The process is continued until stimulation of the previously ablated area does not elicit any significant pain.

27.4.2 Sacroiliac Joint RFA

The C-arm transducer is tilted cephalad ~ 10° to 15° and obliqued 10° to 15° contralaterally to optimally visualize the posterior aspect of the SIJ. The skin entry point is the inferior aspect of the posterior SIJ (**Fig. 27.6**), and 1% lidocaine is injected into the entry point. An 18 G needle is docked on the interosseous ligament overlying the posterior SIJ. Then a guidewire is

advanced through the needle, the needle is removed, and the entry opening is widened with a No. 11 blade. A cannulated obturator is inserted along the guidewire through the skin incision, and a nonbeveled working cannula is advanced along the obturator until it touches the posterior SIJ. After the obturator is removed, the endoscope is introduced through the cannula. The final position of the cannula is confirmed again with fluoroscopy (**Fig. 27.7**).

Under endoscopic view, the posterior sacroiliac ligament and the soft tissue overlying it are ablated using the bipolar electrocoagulator introduced through the working channel in the endoscope. First, we ablate the perforating branches that innervate the posterior capsule of the SIJ (**Fig. 27.8**). After visual confirmation of the long posterior sacroiliac ligament, RFA is carried out along the course of the ligament in the cranial direction up to the level of posterior superior iliac spine. The fluoroscope is then tilted back to an anteroposterior view, and tilted cephalad until S1–S3 sacral foramina are clearly visible. Next, using a wanding maneuver of the cannula, the tip of the cannula is moved along the subcutaneous plane toward the region lateral to the S1–S3 sacral foramina, and a long strip of lesion is made along the line connecting the lateral margins of the S1–S3 sacral foramina.[20]

Position of the cannula tip is occasionally checked with the fluoroscope. When possible, an attempt is made to visually confirm the lateral branches exiting from the sacral foramina and coursing toward the SIJ for accurate lesioning of the nerve. Constant communication with the patient is maintained to see how much pain each stimulus elicits and in which area the stimulus causes the most pain. Continuous saline irrigation is maintained throughout the procedure to minimize thermal injury to the surrounding structures and excessive charring.

After ablation of target points is completed, endoscope and cannula are removed, one nylon point suture is made, and sterile dressing is applied.

27.5 Avoiding Complications

The endoscopic view may sometimes be obscured by blood and debris. In such instances, always touch the bone with the bipolar probe before initiating ablation. If uncertain about the location of the bipolar tip, always check with the C-arm. Do not ablate unless perfectly certain of the location. Ablation of nerve roots and vascular structures can lead to devastating consequences.

Be careful not to enter into the sacral foramina with the bipolar tip when performing periforaminal RFA. If unsure, check with the C-arm.

27.6 Postoperative Considerations

- The patient can be mobilized immediately after the procedure.
- The patient can be discharged on the postoperative day.
- The patient may experience discomfort on the operated levels on the postoperative day but will gradually feel better. Pain medication should be prescribed to alleviate pain in the interim period.

References

1. Boswell MV, Trescot AM, Datta S, et al; American Society of Interventional Pain Physicians. Interventional techniques: evidence-based practice guidelines in the management of chronic spinal pain. *Pain Physician* 2007;*10*(1):7–111
2. Katz JN. Lumbar disc disorders and low-back pain: socioeconomic factors and consequences. *J Bone Joint Surg Am* 2006;*88*(Suppl 2):21–24
3. Freburger JK, Holmes GM, Agans RP, et al. The rising prevalence of chronic low back pain. *Arch Intern Med* 2009;*169*(3):251–258
4. Poetscher AW, Gentil AF, Lenza M, Ferretti M. Radiofrequency denervation for facet joint low back pain: a systematic review. *Spine* 2014;*39*(14):E842–E849
5. Manchikanti L, Pampati V, Fellows B, Bakhit CE. Prevalence of lumbar facet joint pain in chronic low back pain. *Pain Physician* 1999;*2*(3):59–64
6. Schwarzer AC, Aprill CN, Bogduk N. The sacroiliac joint in chronic low back pain. *Spine* 1995;*20*(1):31–37
7. D'Orazio F, Gregori LM, Gallucci M. Spine epidural and sacroiliac joint injections—when and how to perform. *Eur J Radiol* 2015;*84*(5):777–782
8. Maigne JY, Planchon CA. Sacroiliac joint pain after lumbar fusion. A study with anesthetic blocks. *Eur Spine J* 2005;*14*(7):654–658
9. Sembrano JN, Polly DW Jr. How often is low back pain not coming from the back? *Spine* 2009;*34*(1):E27–E32
10. Bowen V, Cassidy JD. Macroscopic and microscopic anatomy of the sacroiliac joint from embryonic life until the eighth decade. *Spine* 1981;*6*(6):620–628
11. Saito T, Steinke H, Miyaki T, et al. Analysis of the posterior ramus of the lumbar spinal nerve: the structure of the posterior ramus of the spinal nerve. *Anesthesiology* 2013;*118*(1):88–94
12. Cohen SP, Abdi S. Lateral branch blocks as a treatment for sacroiliac joint pain: a pilot study. *Reg Anesth Pain Med* 2003;*28*(2):113–119
13. Hansen HC, McKenzie-Brown AM, Cohen SP, Swicegood JR, Colson JD, Manchikanti L. Sacroiliac joint interventions: a systematic review. *Pain Physician* 2007;*10*(1):165–184
14. Kapural L, Nageeb F, Kapural M, Cata JP, Narouze S, Mekhail N. Cooled radiofrequency system for the treatment of chronic pain from sacroiliitis: the first case-series. *Pain Pract* 2008;*8*(5):348–354
15. Cohen SP, Chen Y, Neufeld NJ. Sacroiliac joint pain: a comprehensive review of epidemiology, diagnosis and treatment. *Expert Rev Neurother* 2013;*13*(1):99–116
16. Cox RC, Fortin JD. The anatomy of the lateral branches of the sacral dorsal rami: implications for radiofrequency ablation. *Pain Physician* 2014;*17*(5):459–464
17. Stelzer W, Aiglesberger M, Stelzer D, Stelzer V. Use of cooled radiofrequency lateral branch neurotomy for the treatment of sacroiliac joint-mediated low back pain: a large case series. *Pain Med* 2013;*14*(1):29–35
18. Cavanaugh JM, Lu Y, Chen C, Kallakuri S. Pain generation in lumbar and cervical facet joints. *J Bone Joint Surg Am* 2006;*88*(Suppl 2):63–67
19. Lakemeier S, Lind M, Schultz W, et al. A comparison of intraarticular lumbar facet joint steroid injections and lumbar facet joint radiofrequency denervation in the treatment of low back pain: a randomized, controlled, double-blind trial. *Anesth Analg* 2013;*117*(1):228–235
20. Roberts SL, Burnham RS, Ravichandiran K, Agur AM, Loh EY. Cadaveric study of sacroiliac joint innervation: implications for diagnostic blocks and radiofrequency ablation. *Reg Anesth Pain Med* 2014;*39*(6):456–464

28 Video Telescope Operating Monitor for Spine Surgery

Doniel Drazin and Adam N. Mamelak

28.1 Introduction

A recent advent in operative technology is the "exoscope." This is a rigid rod lens system that looks and functions much like standard endoscopes but has a long focal distance of 25 to 30 cm and is positioned outside the surgical cavity. The exoscope is used with a mechanical or pneumatic scope holder that permits rapid repositioning and refocusing. The device has been termed the *video telescope operating microscope*, or VITOM (Karl Storz Endoscopy, Tuttlingen, Germany; **Fig. 28.1**). Since operative surgical visualization is performed from the monitor, the surgeon is able to sit or stand in a comfortable, arms flexed position, with minimal strain on his neck or arms, thereby reducing surgical fatigue and endpoint tremor. The authors have previously reported their surgical experiences with this system in limited aspects of intracranial surgery (pineal region, posterior fossa) as well as in surgery on the spine.[1,2,3]

28.2 VITOM: Components

The VITOM consists of a rigid lens telescope, camera head, light source, and video display monitor(s).

28.2.1 Exoscope

The exoscope is an 8-mm autoclavable rigid lens telescope (Model E1051–1, Karl Storz Endoscopy, Tuttlingen, Germany) with a 10-mm outer diameter and a shaft length of 14 cm (**Fig. 28.2**).

28.2.2 Light Source

A commercially available 300-W xenon fiberoptic light source (Xenon Nova 300, Karl Storz) is used (**Fig. 28.3**).

28.2.3 Camera Head

The camera head is a 3-chip sterilizable high-definition (HD) digitized camera (HD A3, Karl Storz), with optical zoom and focus features (**Fig. 28.4**).

28.2.4 Video Display and Documentation

A medical-grade 23-inch HD (2 million pixels) video monitor (NDS Surgical Imaging, San Jose, CA) is used (**Fig. 28.5**).

28.2.5 Telescope Holder

The telescope is held in position by a pneumatic endoscope holder (UniArm, Mitaka Kohki Company, Tokyo, Japan) with a wide range of motion. The device allows for push-button rapid repositioning with minimal drift (**Fig. 28.6**).

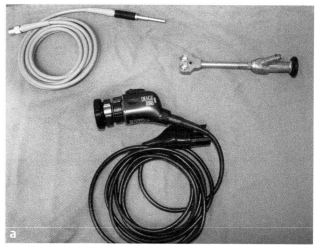
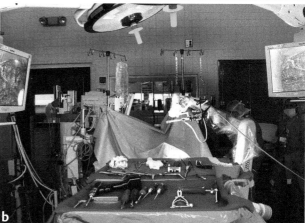
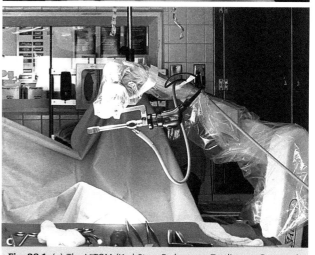

Fig. 28.1 **(a)** The VITOM (Karl Storz Endoscopy, Tuttlingen, Germany). **(b)** The operating room set up with the VITOM exoscope, camera, and light attached to a pneumatic holder, and dual video monitors. **(c)** A close-up view of the VITOM system.

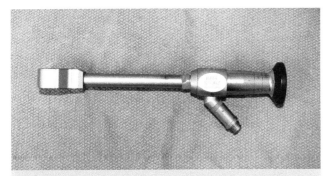

Fig. 28.2 Exoscope.

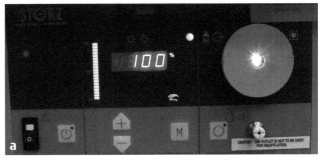

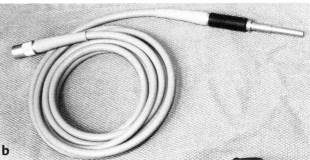

Fig. 28.3 (a) Light source and (b) light cable.

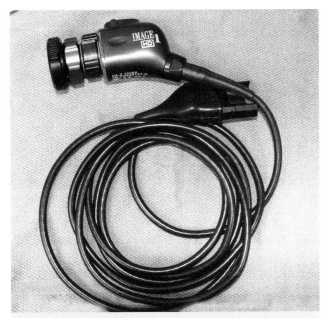

Fig. 28.4 Camera head.

28.3 VITOM: Position and Anesthesia

Positioning the pneumatic telescopic holder is an important part of operative success. Preoperative positioning requires forethought into how the arm should be placed within the operating room and draped into the surgical field. It is important that the arm be a comfortable distance from the surgeon to allow for easy repositioning. Also, the surgeon needs to verify that the rotating universal arm is free to move in all directions prior to draping.

Positioning the HD monitor is a key factor for the surgeon's comfort and for ease of use. The video monitor is most effective when placed 2 to 3 feet from the surgeon, on the opposite side of the operating table, to the right of the assistant, at eye level. This allows the monitor to take up most of the surgeon's field of view (**Fig. 28.5**). A second monitor, placed in a similar position just behind and to the right of the surgeon, allows the assistant an identical field of view (**Fig. 28.7**). VITOM is positioned perpendicular to the skin surface throughout the surgery as the incision is directed toward the spinal cord (**Fig. 28.8**).

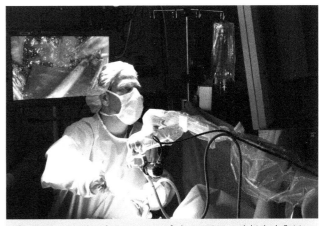

Fig. 28.5 Example of positioning of the VITOM and high-definition (HD) monitor at eye level on the opposite side of the operating table. A second HD monitor is behind the surgeon for the assistant.

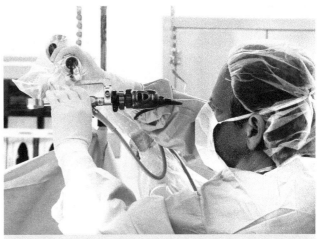

Fig. 28.6 Surgeon adjusting the pneumatic endoscope holder (UniArm, Mitaka Kohki Co., Tokyo, Japan).

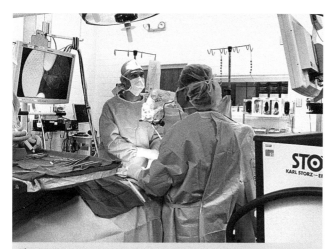

Fig. 28.7 Demonstration of operating room setup for high-definition monitors.

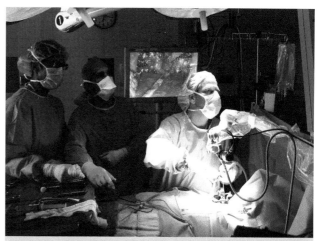

Fig. 28.8 VITOM intraoperative positioning, perpendicular to the skin surface.

28.4 VITOM: Anterior Cervical Diskectomy and Fusion at the C4–C6 Level

28.4.1 Clinical Findings, Illustrative Case (Video 28.1)

A 40-year-old male presented with a history of right upper extremity pain and paresthesia for the preceding 2 years. He had experienced numbness and tingling in the lateral portions of his right arm and forearm as well as in the thumb and fifth finger. He complained of neck pain that occasionally radiated down to the right upper extremity.

The patient had tried acupuncture, chiropractic adjustments, physical therapy, and epidural steroid injections, none of which resolved his symptoms completely. He was taking a significant amount of pain medication to resolve his pain issues.

An MRI showed C4–C5 and C5–C6 disk bulges with significant cervical stenosis and some right-sided C5–C6 foraminal stenosis and degenerative disk disease (**Fig. 28.9**). The patient requested surgical intervention.

A right-sided approach was selected, and the skin entry point was determined at the level of the thyroid cartilage (**Fig. 28.10**). After complete removal of the herniated disk fragment, the decompressed pulsating dura could be seen (**Fig. 28.11**).

It was often possible to leave the VITOM in position over the surgical field while inserting the various spinal tools for instrumentation (**Fig. 28.12**). The procedure resulted in sufficient decompression. The intraoperative X-ray and the postoperative scout and CT films showed excellent position of the C4–C6 anterior cervical diskectomy and fusion (ACDF) (**Fig. 28.13**).

28.5 VITOM: Pearls

The VITOM is similar to an operating microscope in that the VITOM sits outside the body cavity and has a larger focal distance.

For the majority of spine surgeries, the VITOM can be positioned perpendicular to the skin surface throughout the duration of the surgery as the incision is directed toward the spinal cord.

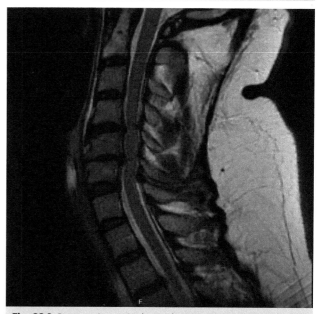

Fig. 28.9 Preoperative sagittal MRI showing C4–C5 and C5–C6 disk herniations with cervical stenosis.

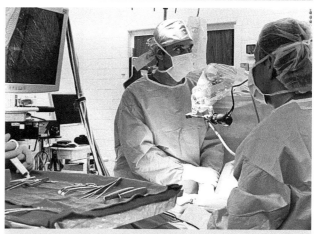

Fig. 28.10 Skin incision planned at the thyroid cartilage for a C4–C6 ACDF.

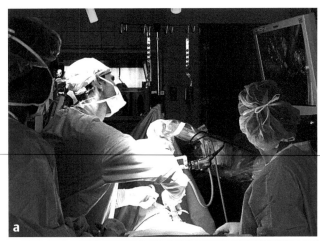

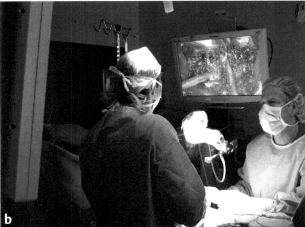

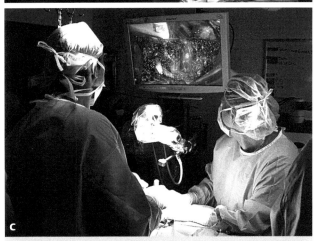

Fig. 28.11 (a) The VITOM view of the Kerrison rongeur removing the disk. (b) Removing the disk fragment. (c) After removal of the disk and ligament, the underlying pulsating dura could be visualized.

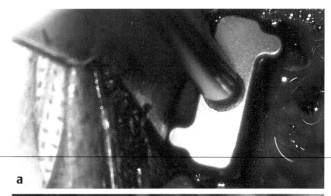

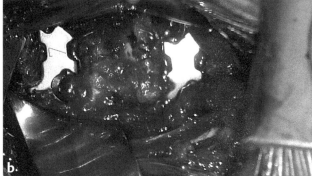

Fig. 28.12 (a) The VITOM view of placement of the implant template without repositioning. (b) The VITOM view of final implants with screws at both levels.

VITOM provides a larger field of view and a long working distance and allows for the placement of traditional spinal instrumentation.

Issues of lateral image inversion are obviated due to the ability of the HD camera head to be rotated 360°, with the VITOM image able to be adjusted to identically match the surgeon's position relative to the anatomy.

Residents and operating room staff enthusiastically endorsed the HD image quality on the monitors that benefited their ability to observe the nuances of microsurgical anatomy in the spine.

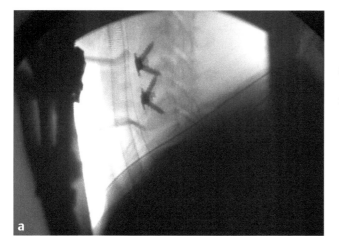

References

1   Birch K, Drazin D, Black KL, Williams J, Berci G, Mamelak AN. Clinical experience with a high definition exoscope system for surgery of pineal region lesions. *J Clin Neurosci* 2014;*21*(7):1245–1249

2   Shirzadi A, Mukherjee D, Drazin DG, et al. Use of the video telescope operating monitor (VITOM) as an alternative to the operating microscope in spine surgery. *Spine* 2012;*37*(24):E1517–E1523

3   Mamelak AN, Drazin D, Shirzadi A, Black KL, Berci G. Infratentorial supracerebellar resection of a pineal tumor using a high definition video exoscope (VITOM). *J Clin Neurosci* 2012;*19*(2):306–309

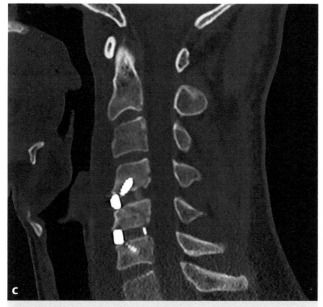

Fig. 28.13 (**a**) Intraoperative X-ray, (**b**) postoperative scout film, and (**c**) CT showing good position of the C4–C6 ACDF.

29 Applied Anatomy and Percutaneous Approaches to the Thoracic Spine

Gun Choi, Alfonso García, Ketan Deshpande, and Akarawit Asawasaksakul

29.1 History

Hans Christian Jacobaeus, a professor of internal medicine in Stockholm, Sweden, is credited with having performed the first thoracoscopic procedure in 1910. The groundbreaking procedure was a technique for lysis of tuberculous pleural adhesions.[1] In 1990, the modern era of thoracoscopy began with the introduction of video imaging to standard endoscopy. Mack and colleagues in 1993 and Rosenthal and colleagues in 1994 first reported the technique of video-assisted thoracoscopic surgery (VATS).[2,3] Thoracic disk herniations were treated first by thoracoscopic spine procedures.

In a further attempt to reduce tissue trauma and enhance postoperative outcome, percutaneous endoscopic thoracic diskectomy (PETD) has been developed to treat thoracic disk herniations from a direct posterior or posterolateral approach. Jho described the technique of endoscopic transpedicular thoracic diskectomy with 0 and 70° 4-mm endoscopes, requiring relatively small 1.5- to 2.0-cm incisions and minimal tissue dissection. The technique avoided the need for separate skin incisions in the chest wall for postoperative chest drainage as were used in thoracoscopic approaches.[4] Also, Chiu et al demonstrated the safety and efficacy of posterolateral endoscopic thoracic diskectomy followed by application of a low-energy nonablative laser for disk thermodiskoplasty using a 4-mm 0° endoscope.[5] Currently, PETD has been described as a safe procedure with outcomes similar to, or better than, those seen with classic procedures for the treatment of thoracic disk herniations.

29.2 Introduction

Thoracic disk herniations present a unique challenge for the spine surgeon in terms of patient selection, surgical technique, and potential complications. Symptomatic thoracic disk herniations are a relatively rare condition, representing less than 1% of all disk herniations.[6,7] The increased rigidity of the thoracic cage, which causes the thoracic spine to have decreased flexion, extension, and rotation compared with the cervical and lumbar spine, is likely the main cause of the low incidence of symptomatic thoracic disk herniations (**Fig. 29.1**, **Fig. 29.2**, **Fig. 29.3**).[7,8,9]

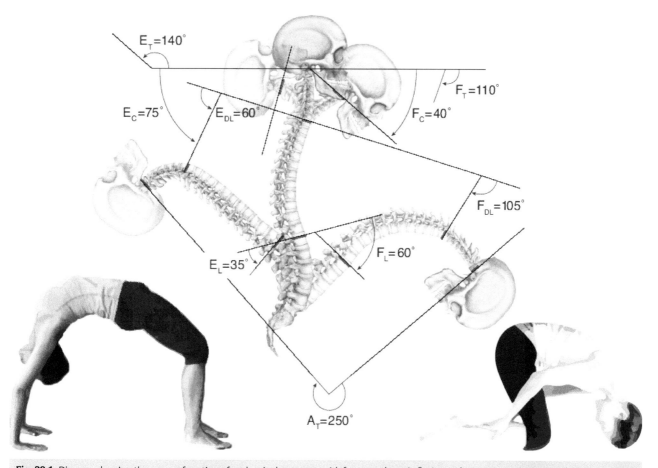

Fig. 29.1 Diagram showing the range of motion of each spinal segment, with focus on thoracic flexion and extension movements. Flexion = F_{DL} 105°, Extension = E_{DL} 60°. (Used with permission from Kapandji AI. *The Physiology of the Joints: The Spinal Column, Pelvic Girdle and Head*, 6th ed., 2011.)

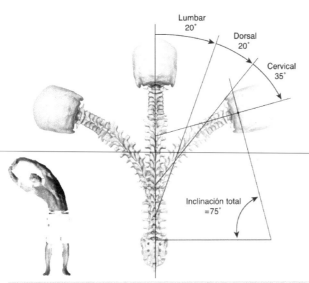

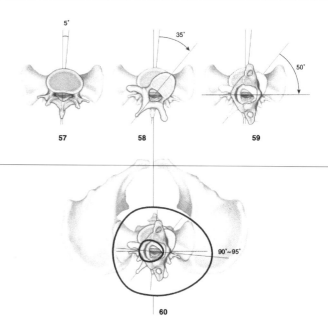

Fig. 29.2 Global lateral flexion of the spine and range of motion experienced in this movement by each segment. The thoracic or dorsal spine has a lateral flexion = dorsal of 20° on each side. (Used with permission from Kapandji AI. *The Physiology of the Joints: The Spinal Column, Pelvic Girdle and Head*, 6th ed, 2011.)

Fig. 29.3 Axial rotation of each spinal segment. For the thoracic spine, the total movement is 35°, as shown. (Used with permission from Kapandji AI. *The Physiology of the Joints: The Spinal Column, Pelvic Girdle and Head*, 6th ed, 2011.)

Thoracic disk herniations are frequently an acute event and manifest clinically with acute paraparesis or even paraplegia. A review of the literature suggests that patient presentation may be extremely variable. Thoracic disk herniations have mimicked systemic, cardiac, renal, and orthopaedic diseases.[10,11] Neurogenic claudication is most commonly attributable to lumbar stenosis, although others have reported this as a presentation of lower thoracic disk herniations.[12,13]

A few patients with thoracic disk herniations may require surgical intervention, and they present with a wide variety of symptoms. In contrast, a large variety of surgical approaches have been developed to treat thoracic disk herniations. These include posterior, posterolateral, and lateral approaches, transthoracic approaches, and thoracoscopic approaches.[14,15,16] The difficulty the spine surgeon encounters when treating these patients is shown clearly by the discrepancy between the small percentage of patients seen with the disease and the large number of surgical techniques developed. Disk herniations in the thoracic region represent a challenging pathology, because although the thoracic spinal canal is the narrowest among all spinal regions, the blood supply to the thoracic cord is precarious, and the approach to the thoracic region is more difficult (**Fig. 29.4**).[17,18] The various approaches to thoracic disk herniations all have advantages and disadvantages.

Anterior and lateral approaches allow the surgeon the greatest access to the intervertebral disk and vertebral body, but these approaches also place the lung, heart, and great vessels at risk. Although posterior approaches are inherently safer, they are correlated with significant blood loss, paraspinal pain, and potential instability.[17,19,20]

PETD is performed as an alternative to classic open diskectomy, with results that are comparable to, and in some cases better than, those of open diskectomy. PETD is usually performed under local anesthesia, postoperative pain is quite minimal, normal paraspinal and thoracic structures are preserved, and

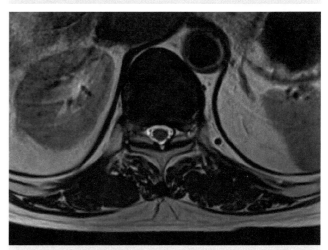

Fig. 29.4 The thoracic region has very little space to accommodate herniated nucleus pulposus, which applies pressure on the thecal sac, while decompression may lead to neural damage.

the risk of postoperative epidural scar formation and instability can be minimized. However, the PETD learning curve is steep, so the surgeon must be familiar with endoscopic lumbar spine surgery before deciding to perform PETD.

Furthermore, despite the low complication rate, minor complications, such as incomplete herniotomy or decompression, and major complications, such as neurovascular injury, lung injury, spinal cord injury, and/or spondylodiscitis, may occur. For these reasons, a new approach to thoracic disk herniations has been developed.

PETD allows the spine surgeon to treat thoracic herniations through a minimally invasive posterior approach, resulting in minimal blood loss, same-day discharge, greatly reduced postoperative pain, and short recovery time.

29.3 Anatomical Considerations

A thorough understanding of spinal anatomy is crucial for a comprehensive evaluation and treatment of the patient with thoracic disk herniation. Several aspects of the thoracic spinal anatomy must be taken into account before deciding to perform an endoscopic diskectomy:

- The size of the thoracic vertebrae increases as one moves down the spinal column.
- The thoracic spine is mechanically stiffer than the rest of the spinal column because of its intimate relationship with the ribs.
- The thoracic spinal canal has less free space for the spinal cord than do the cervical and lumbar regions.
- The foramen is large and oval from cephalad to caudal, similar to that of the upper lumbar spine.
- The intramural component at the thoracic level differs from the lumbar level in that it has many rootlets and less buffer, making it more susceptible to root injury or dural tears from the heat of the laser (**Fig. 29.5**, **Fig. 29.6**, **Fig. 29.7**, **Fig. 29.8**).

29.4 Goals

- Excision of a thoracic herniated disk fragment
- Preservation of the posterior elements of the thoracic spine
- Avoidance of complications associated with a more morbid anterior approach, such as posterior thoracic pain, pleural effusion, pneumothorax, and Horner syndrome
- Minimally invasive surgical option for thoracic disk herniations
- Performing the surgery under local anesthesia, making it an outpatient procedure

29.5 Advantages

- PETD is a minimally invasive procedure performed under local anesthesia with conscious sedation.
- It can avoid complications associated with open surgery.
- It preserves the normal anatomy.
- It has a satisfactory cosmetic result due to the small incision size.

29.6 Patient Selection

- As with any surgical procedure, patient selection is very important.
- A well-performed physical examination with attention to sensory deficits over the anterior and posterior thoracic region may lead to the correct diagnosis.
- A detailed history must be performed, with care to elicit any recent history of trauma, infection, or suggestion of malignancy.
- The clinician must correlate the patient history with the physical examination and radiologic findings.

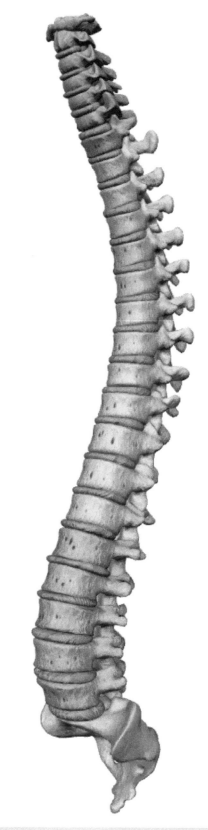

Fig. 29.5 The thoracic spinal segment is shown in green. It is the stiffer part of the spine because of its intimate relationship with the thoracic cage, which provides additional stabilization.

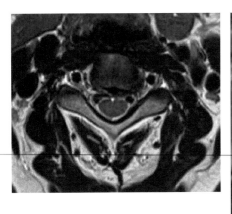
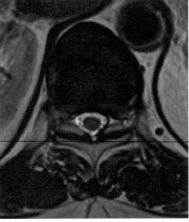
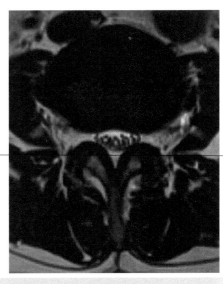

Fig. 29.6 The thoracic canal has less free space than the canal in the cervical and lumbar segments.

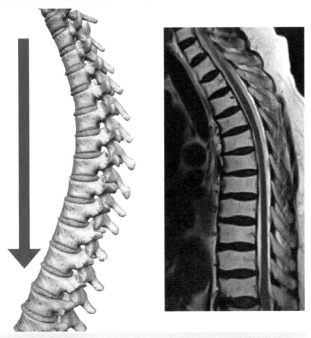

Fig. 29.7 The thoracic vertebrae increase in size as one moves down the spinal column.

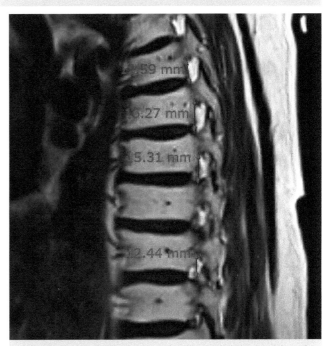

Fig. 29.8 The foramen is large and oval from cephalad to caudal, similar to that of the upper lumbar spine.

29.7 Indications

Indications for PETD include:

- Soft thoracic disk herniation (without calcification) as proven by CT and MRI (**Fig. 29.9**)
- Level confirmed by clinical and radiographic findings and with the help of selective root blocks
- Axial pain and/or radicular pain, including interscapular pain, thoracolumbar pain, anterior radiating chest pain, intercostal pain, or low back pain
- Mild degree of myelopathy due to soft disk herniation without calcification

- Failure of adequate conservative therapy[21]

29.8 Contraindications

Contraindications to PETD include:

- Hard or calcified disk
- Thoracic ossification of the posterior longitudinal ligament
- Evidence of acute progressive degenerative spinal cord disease
- Severe disk space narrowing
- Severe cord compression

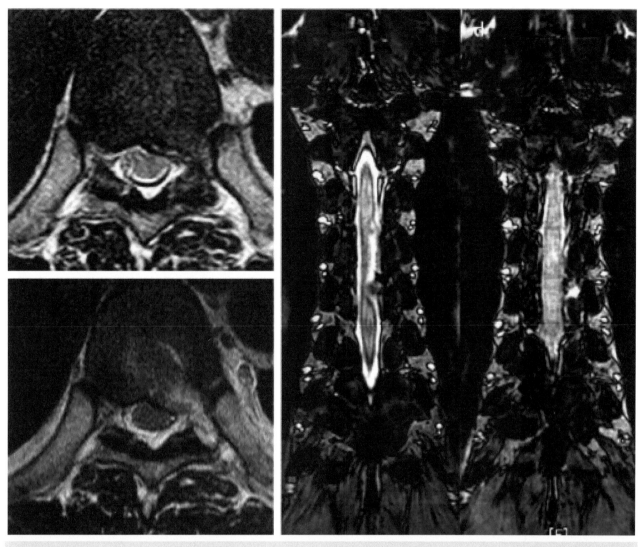

Fig. 29.9 Soft thoracic disk herniation, on preoperative and postoperative MRI. (Used with permission from Choi KY, et al. Percutaneous endoscopic thoracic diskectomy: transforaminal approach. *Minim Invas Neurosurg* 2010;53:25–28.)

References

1   Fessler RG, O'Toole JE, Eichholz KM, Perez-Cruet MJ. The development of mini-mally invasive spine surgery. *Neurosurg Clin N Am* 2006;17(4):401–409

2   Mack MJ, Regan JJ, Bobechko WP, Acuff TE. Application of thoracoscopy for diseases of the spine. *Ann Thorac Surg* 1993;56(3):736–738

3   Rosenthal D, Rosenthal R, de Simone A. Removal of a protruded thoracic disc using microsurgical endoscopy. A new technique. *Spine* 1994;19(9):1087–1091

4   Jho HD. Endoscopic microscopic transpedicular thoracic discectomy. Technical note. *J Neurosurg* 1997;87(1):125–129

5   Chiu JC, Negron F, Clifford T, Greenspan M, Princethal RA. Microdecompressive percutaneous discectomy: spinal discectomy with new laser thermodiskoplasty for non-extruded herniated nucleosus pulposus. *Surg Technol Int* 2000;8:343–351

6   Lee HY, Lee S, Kim D, et al. Percutaneous endoscopic thoracic discectomy: pos-terolateral transforaminal approach. *J Korean Neurosurg Soc* 2006;40(1):58–62

7   Eichholz KM, O'Toole JE, Fessler RG. Thoracic microendoscopic discectomy. *Neurosurg Clin N Am* 2006;17(4):441–446

8   Adams MA, Hutton WC. Prolapsed intervertebral disc. A hyperflexion injury 1981 Volvo Award in Basic Science. *Spine* 1982;7(3):184–191

9   White AA, Panjabi MM. *Clinical Biomechanics of the Spine*. Philadelphia, PA: JB Lippincott; 1990

10 Eleraky MA, Apostolides PJ, Dickman CA, Sonntag VK. Herniated thorac-ic discs mimic cardiac disease: three case reports. *Acta Neurochir (Wien)* 1998;140(7):643–646

11 Georges C, Toledano C, Zagdanski AM, et al. Thoracic disk herniation mimicking renal crisis. *Eur J Intern Med* 2004;15(1):59–61

12 Hufnagel A, Zierski J, Agnoli L, Schütz HJ. [Spinal claudication caused by thoracic intervertebral disk displacement]. [In German.] *Nervenarzt* 1988;59(7):419–421

13 Morgenlander JC, Massey EW. Neurogenic claudication with positionally depen-dent weakness from a thoracic disk herniation. *Neurology* 1989;39(8):1133–1134

14 Isaacs RE, Podichetty VK, Sandhu FA, et al. Thoracic microendoscopic discecto-my: a human cadaver study. *Spine* 2005;30(10):1226–1231

15 Le Roux PD, Haglund MM, Harris AB. Thoracic disc disease: experience with the transpedicular approach in twenty consecutive patients. *Neurosurgery* 1993;33(1):58–66

16 Perez-Cruet MJ, Kim BS, Sandhu F, Samartzis D, Fessler RG. Thoracic microendo-scopic discectomy. *J Neurosurg Spine* 2004;1(1):58–63

17 Fessler RG, Sturgill M. Review: complications of surgery for thoracic disc dis-ease. *Surg Neurol* 1998;49(6):609–618

18 Pait TG, Elias AJ, Tribell R. Thoracic, lumbar, and sacral spine anatomy for endo-scopic surgery. *Neurosurgery* 2002;51(5, Suppl):S67–S78

19 el-Kalliny M, Tew JM Jr, van Loveren H, Dunsker S. Surgical approaches to tho-racic disc herniations. *Acta Neurochir (Wien)* 1991;111(1-2):22–32

20 Lee SH, Lim SR, Lee HY, et al. Thoracoscopic discectomy of the herniated thorac-ic discs. *J Korean Neurosurg Soc* 2000;29(12):1577–1583

21 Choi KY, Eun SS, Lee SH, Lee HY. Percutaneous endoscopic thoracic discectomy; transforaminal approach. *Minim Invasive Neurosurg* 2010;53(1):25–28

30 Surgical Techniques in Percutaneous Endoscopic Thoracic Diskectomy

Gun Choi, Akarawit Asawasaksakul, and Alfonso García

30.1 Introduction

In the era before MRI, symptomatic thoracic disk herniation was a rare condition in spinal surgery, representing only 1% of all disk herniations.[1,2] In the MRI era, thoracic disk herniation can be detected much more easily than in the past, but the treatment is very difficult, since a transthoracic or extrapleural approach may be required.

Recently, with the development of endoscopic spine procedures and instruments, thoracic diskectomy is possible via a percutaneous endoscopic technique,[3] but the procedure is technically demanding. Two methods are now available:

1. Percutaneous endoscopic thoracic diskectomy (PETD)
2. Percutaneous endoscopic thoracic annuloplasty using real-time CT guidance with laser-assisted spinal endoscopy (PETA with LASE)

This chapter focuses on PETD (**Video 30.1**).

30.2 Indications for PETD

- Thoracic paramedian or foraminal soft disk herniation
- In an upper thoracic level, diffuse bulging soft disk herniation
- Pain with no response to conservative treatment

30.3 Contraindications to PETD

- Calcified disk
- Ossification of posterior longitudinal ligament (OPLL)
- Central disk herniation
- Major compression or neurologic deficit
- Abnormal vasculature

30.4 Special Instruments and Preoperative Planning

The operating room setup and instrumentation needed to perform PETD are shown in **Fig. 30.1** and **Fig. 30.2**. CT and MRI are mandatory for preoperative planning, not only to determine if the patient is a candidate for a percutaneous thoracic procedure but also to plan the needle trajectory. Axial MRI or CT is used to calculate the needle's skin entry point (**Fig. 30.3**).

30.5 Position and Anesthesia

- The patient is positioned prone on a radiolucent operating table, with the affected side facing the surgeon. The arms are positioned above the patient.
- Local anesthesia using 1% lidocaine, together with conscious sedation with propofol and fentanyl, allows continuous

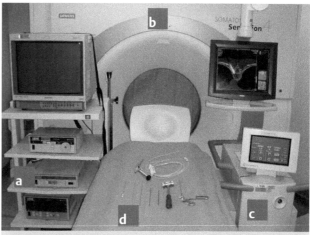

Fig. 30.1 (**a**) Endoscopic set, (**b**) CT scanner, (**c**) Ho-YAG laser, (**d**) endoscope (KESS, Richard Wolf Medical Instruments Corporation, Vernon Hills, IL), dilators, and forceps.

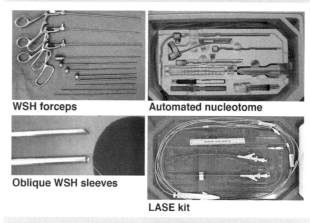

WSH forceps   Automated nucleotome

Oblique WSH sleeves

LASE kit

Fig. 30.2 Instruments needed to perform a percutaneous endoscopic thoracic diskectomy. Need to explain details of each instrument .

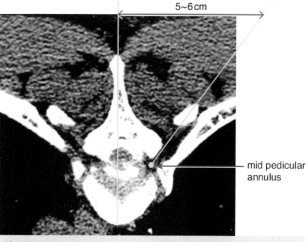

Fig. 30.3 Measurements done on an axial CT scan to determine the skin entry point.

feedback from the patient during the entire procedure to avoid any damage to neural structures.

- Level and landmark marking are done under C-arm imaging. The lateral coordinates of the skin entry point are determined by extrapolating a line from the midpedicular annulus to the lateral margin of the facet and extending up to the skin's surface.

30.6 Needle Insertion Technique

- The appropriate operative level must be precisely located using lateral and anteroposterior (AP) fluoroscopy, counting the level from the sacrum or C1.
- The procedure requires continuous or intermittent CT guidance. CT guidance is more precise but not necessary.
- Because the thoracic disks are more concave than the lumbar disks, lumbar fluoroscopic landmarks cannot be used for thoracic disks. Because of the concavity, thoracic disk herniations can only be approached through the foraminal region.
- The skin entry point is determined based on an imaginary line projected toward the skin from the target area (between the rib and facet). Usually 5 to 6 cm lateral to midline is the point calculated on axial CT scan or MRI.
- Direction of the needle should be parallel to the end plate at the corresponding level.
- The safest route for passing the needle into the thoracic disk is between the rib head and the thoracic facet (**Fig. 30.4**).

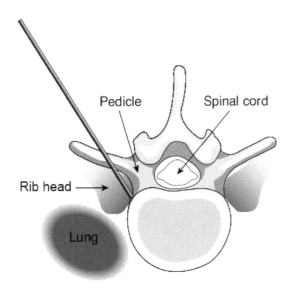

Fig. 30.4 Needle trajectory between the rib head and facet joint.

- A more lateral approach is required for larger patients in order to reduce manipulation of the spinal cord during disk removal.
- Always keep the needle posterior to the rib head, because the pleura is located anterior to the ribs (**Fig. 30.5**).
- The needle tip is advanced into the foramen until it touches the outer annular surface. At this point, periannular infiltration of

1 to 1.5 mL of 1% lidocaine is injected to lessen annular pain due to needle penetration, then the needle is advanced (**Fig. 30.6**).

- Diskography is performed at this stage as a provocative test and to stain the herniated fragments.

30.7 Diskography

- The stylet is withdrawn, and diskography is performed by injecting 2 to 3 mL of a mixture of radiopaque dye, indigo carmine, and normal saline mixed in a 2:1:2 ratio (**Fig. 30.7**).
- The injected mixture usually leaks and tends to follow the track of the sequestrated herniation through the tear in the annulus.
- Indigo carmine, being a base, selectively stains the degenerated acidic nucleus pulposus and aids identification of the herniated disk during endoscopic visualization.
- The spinal needle is now advanced to the center of the disk space.

30.8 Obturator and Working Channel Positioning

- A 0.8-mm blunt-tipped guidewire is passed through the already inserted needle and the needle is withdrawn.
- A skin incision ~ 5 mm in length is made.
- The subcutaneous tract is developed by passing serial dilators of increasing size from 1 to 5 mm. A gentle twisting motion is preferable.
- After withdrawal of the dilators, a blunt, tapered obturator is passed over the guidewire using a gentle twisting motion under an image intensifier and is controlled up to the posterolateral margin of the facet (**Fig. 30.8**).
- The route is further dilated to accommodate the working cannula until the beveled opening is facing medially and inferiorly and the tip of the cannula compresses the annulus

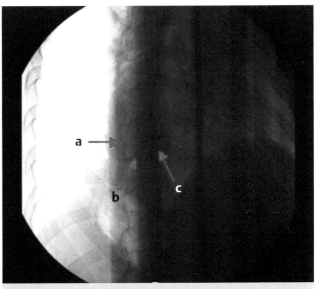

Fig. 30.5 C-arm oblique view. Note the needle (**a**) within the desired disk space, (**b**) between the pedicles, and (**c**) posterior to the rib head.

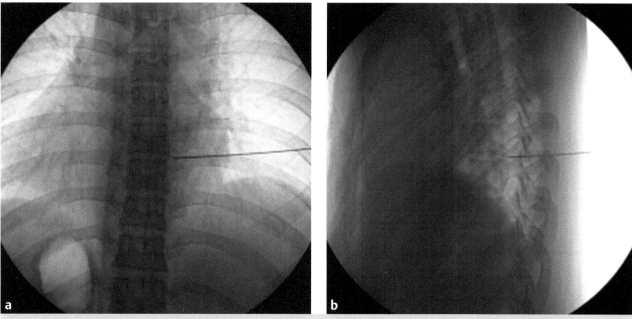

Fig. 30.6 (**a**) C-arm AP view showing the needle tip positioned at the outer annulus, and (**b**) lateral view showing the needle tip in the posterior vertebral line.

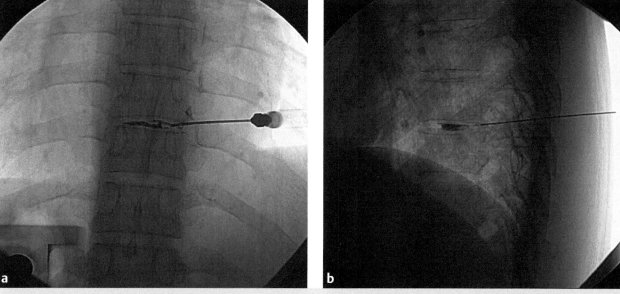

Fig. 30.7 Diskography: (**a**) AP view and (**b**) lateral view.

just lateral to the midpedicular line, after which the working channel endoscope is passed (**Fig. 30.9**).

30.9 Endoscopic Procedure

- It is imperative to maintain a proper orientation to avoid inadvertent entry into the spinal canal, with potential damage to the spinal cord or exiting nerve root.
- Once the endoscope is placed, muscle and soft tissue overlying the field are removed with a radiofrequency bipolar probe or laser.

- The exposure should include the proximal transverse process and lateral facet. It is essential to reduce the lateral manipulation of the spinal cord; therefore, needle insertion and dilator placement are essential.
- Foraminoplasty might be required for insertion of the cannula at the upper thoracic levels.
- The lateral aspect of the superior facet is removed by using an endoscopic drill.
- Once the disk space is visualized, annulotomy is performed (**Fig. 30.10**).
- Initially, a space is created in the posterior subannular region with holmium:yttrium-aluminum-garnet (Ho-YAG) laser

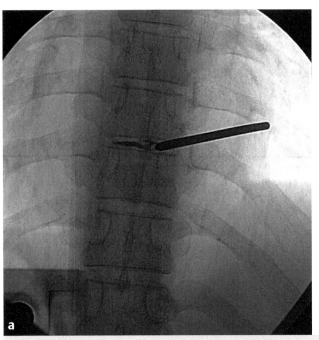
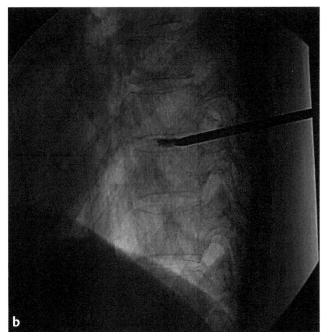

Fig. 30.8 (**a,b**) Passage of a blunt-tapered dilator into the desired disk space under fluoroscopic guidance.

ablation of disk tissue (laser settings: repetition rate 15–25 PPS, 15–25 W, and 2000–5000 J).

- After the initial decompression, the cannula is drawn back slightly or tilted posteriorly to expose the foraminal epidural space (**Fig. 30.11**).
- The remaining extruded portion of the thoracic disk herniation can be removed either by laser ablation, with endoscopic forceps through the working channel endoscope, or by automated nucleotome.

- With a slight twisting motion of the working cannula, the remaining herniated fragment is brought into view and is released from its surrounding adhesions by a side-firing laser probe using a Ho-YAG laser.
- The fragment can also be delivered into the field of vision with the help of a blunt probe.
- The fragment can usually be removed by grasping the tail with the endoscopic grasping forceps and gentle pulling.

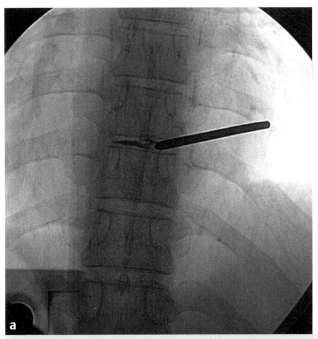
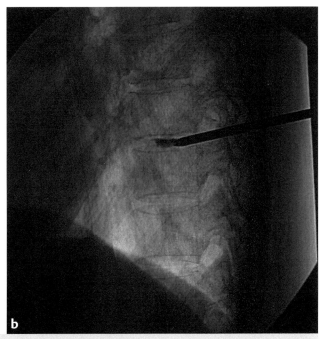

Fig. 30.9 Final working cannula positioning: (**a**) on the AP view, the cannula is lateral to the midpedicular line, and (**b**) on the lateral view, it is the posterior vertebral line.

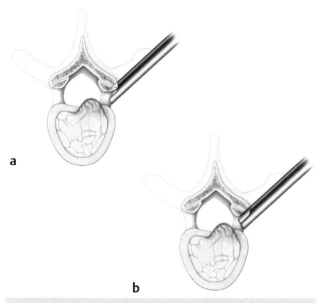

Fig. 30.10 (**a,b**) Adequate beveled cannula positioning for foraminotomy.

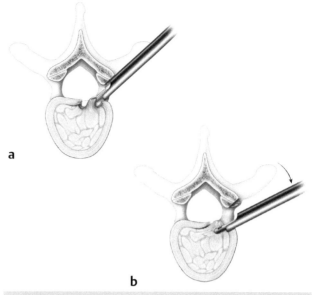

Fig. 30.11 Half–half technique (half intradiskal, half epidural). Initially, after intradiskal sublunar decompression, the cannula is either slightly withdrawn (**a**) or tilted posteriorly (**b**) to expose the epidural portion of the ruptured disk fragment.

- The adequacy of decompression of the exiting nerve root can be checked by visual inspection of the dural sac and by absence of any more fragments lying in its vicinity.
- After the herniated disk is removed, the operative field is copiously irrigated and meticulous hemostasis is obtained.
- Finally, a gentle, circular, twisting motion is used to gradually withdraw the cannula.
- The skin incision is closed with a single nylon suture, and sterile dressing is applied.

30.10 Expert Suggestions

- Only spine surgeons who are well trained in open thoracic surgery and who are familiar with percutaneous spinal endoscopic procedures should perform PETD.
- Proper surgical planning and detailing of the diagnosis can prevent complications.
- Before opting for PETD, it is advisable to be familiar with the lumbar percutaneous endoscopic diskectomy procedure.

30.11 Complication Avoidance

- The surgical treatment of thoracic disk herniations has potentially devastating complications.
- The thoracic spinal cord, especially in the upper thoracic region, is in the watershed region of the spinal vascular supply, leaving it prone to ischemic complications. Although root injury in the thoracic cord does not have the morbidity and neurological deficit that root injury has in the cervical or lumbar region, damage to the thoracic cord, with its tenuous blood supply, can render a patient paraplegic.
- Disk and foramen shape are different in the thoracic region (more concave than in the lumbar spine); therefore, there is a risk of injury to the thoracic tissue if the anatomical differences are not kept in mind.

- The needle tip should be kept between the rib-head shadow and the pedicle shadow on the anteroposterior and oblique views throughout needle insertion.
- Decompression should be done first, with intradiskal decompression followed by intracanal herniectomy after levering of the cannula.
- It is essential to carefully monitor the patient's response to detect any potential neural injury.
- Pain associated with the procedure should be addressed with 1% lidocaine while preserving the neural response.
- A CT-guided approach is safer than using fluoroscopy only.
- Only symptomatic soft disk herniation confirmed by selective root block should be subjected to this procedure.

30.12 Postoperative Considerations

- The patient can be mobilized as soon as the procedure is completed.
- The patient can be discharged on the same day.
- A routine physiotherapy protocol is advised, along with three days of oral antibiotic treatment.

References

1   Adams MA, Hutton WC. Prolapsed intervertebral disc. A hyperflexion injury. 1981 Volvo Award in Basic Science. *Spine* 1982;7(3):184–191
2   Arce CA, Dohrmann GJ. Thoracic disc herniation. Improved diagnosis with computed tomographic scanning and a review of the literature. *Surg Neurol* 1985;23(4):356–361
3   Lee HY, Lee SH, Kim DY, Kong BJ, Ahn Y, Shin SW. Percutaneous endoscopic thoracic discectomy: Posterolateral transforaminal approach. *J Korean Neurosurg Soc* 2006;40:58–61

31 Posterolateral Endoscopic Thoracic Diskectomy

John C. Chiu

31.1 Introduction

An effective alternative procedure for treating symptomatic herniated thoracic disks through an endoscope is posterolateral endoscopic thoracic diskectomy (PETD), which achieves less tissue trauma than is caused by current conventional thoracic disk surgery and thoracoscopic procedures. This chapter discusses the rationale, indications, instrumentation, surgical technique, safety, and efficacy of the PETD procedure, as well as lower-energy nonablative laser applied for shrinkage and tightening of the disk (laser thermodiskoplasty). This minimally invasive spinal surgery has numerous advantages, but it requires thorough knowledge of the PETD procedure, the surgical anatomy, specific surgical training, and hands-on experience in a laboratory and working closely with an experienced endoscopic surgeon through its steep surgical learning curve.

Historically, spinal surgeons have long sought a procedure for treating thoracic disk herniations.[1,2,3,4,5,6,7,8,9,10,11,12] The threat of spinal cord, neural, vascular, and pulmonary injury has stimulated many approaches, including posterior laminectomy (seldom performed, as it is too likely to result in neurologic injury), costotransversectomy, and transthoracic, transpleural, posterolateral, transfacet pedicle-sparing, transpedicular, and, more recently, transthoracic endoscopic and posterolateral endoscopic procedures.[1,2,3,4,5,6,11,12,13]

As a result, many clever minimally invasive endoscopic thoracic procedures have been developed, including video-assisted thoracic surgery (VATS),[1] thoracic sympathectomy, and others attempting to reduce operative trauma. Usually, in the past, surgery was not contemplated unless considerable cord compression and neurologic deficit were present,[5,6,11,12] yet a significant number of patients complain of thoracic spinal and paraspinal pain, intercostal or chest wall pain, upper abdominal pain, and occasionally low back pain due to thoracic disk protrusions without severe neurologic deficit or dramatic radiological abnormalities. With improved diagnostic methods like MRI[8] (the method of choice), CT myelography, and CT, the diagnosis of thoracic disk protrusions is now far more common. Such patients usually receive some period if not cured, are expected to live with their discomfort because potential severe postoperative complications are feared if usual surgical treatment is attempted.

With the advent of laser thermodiskoplasty,[11,12,13] PETD has evolved from a minimally invasive technique used in the lumbar and cervical areas,[10,11,12,13,14,15,16] and from the basic approach for performing thoracic diskography.[9] The author has utilized pre- or intraoperative diskograms and pain provocation tests in almost all cases to confirm the diagnosis and the appropriate levels to treat. This chapter describes the technique, safety, and efficacy of the method for treating thoracic disk protrusions by outpatient PETD.

31.2 Indications

The surgical indications for PETD are:[12]

- Pain in the thoracic spine, often radiating to the chest wall, with possible numbness and paresthesia in an intercostal distribution due to thoracic disk herniation
- No improvement of symptoms after a minimum of 12 weeks of conservative management
- MRI or CT scan positive for disk herniation, consistent with the level of clinical symptoms
- Confirmatory pre- or intraoperative diskogram and pain provocation test
- Multiple thoracic disks may be treated in one procedure.[17,18,19,20,21]

31.3 Contraindications

The PETD approach is contraindicated in the following clinical situations:

- Severe cord compression or total block on radiographic studies
- Advanced spondylosis with severe disk space narrowing or osteophytes blocking entry into the disk space

31.4 Instruments and Preparation

The equipment and surgical instruments[11,12,13] necessary to perform PETD (similar to anterior endoscopic cervical microdiskectomy) are:

- Digital fluoroscopy equipment (C-arm) and monitor
- Full radiolucent C-arm/fluoroscopic carbon-fiber surgical table
- Endoscopic tower equipped with digital video monitor, digital imaging documentation/recording device, light source, photo printer, and high-definition (HD) digital camera system (**Fig. 31.1**)
- Thoracic endoscopic diskectomy set (Karl Storz, Tuttlingen, Germany), including 4-mm 0° endoscope (**Fig. 31.1**)
- Thoracic 3.5-mm 6° operating endoscope, and 2.5-mm 0° and 30° diagnostic endoscopes (**Fig. 31.1**)
- Thoracic diskectomy sets (2.5- and 3.5-mm) (Blackstone Medical, Inc., Springfield, MA) with short and long diskectomes (**Fig. 31.1**)
- Endoscopic grasping and cutting forceps and scissors (**Fig. 31.1**)
- Endoscopic probe, knife, rasp, and bur (**Fig. 31.1**)
- More aggressively toothed trephines used for spurs and spondylitic ridges at the anterior and posterior disk space (**Fig. 31.1**)
- Holmium:YAG laser generator (Trimedyne, Irvine, CA) and 550 μm holmium bare fiber with flat-tip right-angle (side-firing) probe (**Fig. 31.2**)

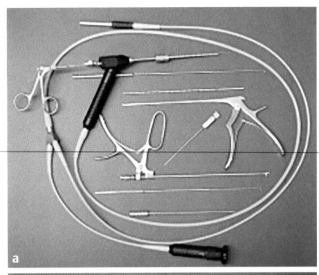
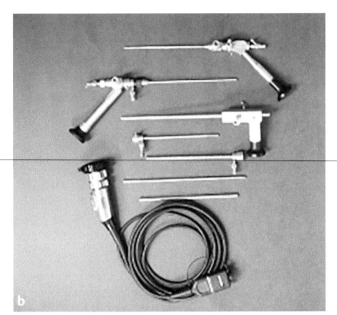
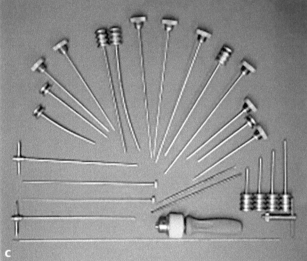
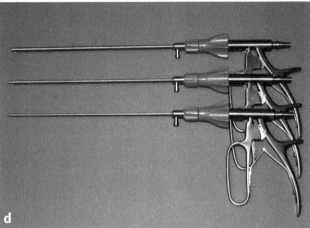

Fig. 31.1 Video digital endoscopic tower and posterolateral endoscopic thoracic diskectomy instruments. (**a**) Video digital endoscopic tower. (**b**) Thoracic endoscopes (0°, 6°, and 30°) and HD digital camera system. (**c**) Endoscopic working cannula systems, trephines, rasp, and burs. (**d**) Long and short diskectomes, various types of forceps and rongeurs.

31.5 Anesthesia

The patient is treated in a digital operating room (DOR) equipped with a digital technology convergence and control system (e.g., SurgMatix), under monitored conscious sedation and local anesthesia. The anesthesiologist maintains mild sedation, but the patient is able to respond. Two grams of Ancef and 8.0 mg of dexamethasone are given intravenously at the start of anesthesia. Surface EEG (SNAP; Nicolet Biomedical, Madison, WI) which can provide an optimal level of anesthesia.

31.6 Patient Positioning

The patient is positioned prone on the table with a radiolucent 20° angled sponge under the symptomatic side of the chest, angling it into an obliquely up position (**Fig. 31.3a**). The arms are supported on arm boards over the head. Because only local anesthesia and mild sedation are used, the extremities, buttocks, and shoulders are restrained from sudden motion with adhesive tape.

31.7 Localization

Levels are identified by counting under C-arm fluoroscopy from the twelfth rib up, and from C7 of the cervical spine down for upper-level thoracic diskectomies. Radiopaque markers are placed on the skin at appropriate sites.[11,12,13] The midline, the levels, and the point of entry (operating portal) for surgery are marked on the skin with a marking pen (**Fig. 31.3b**). Using sterile technique, the level of the disk can be accurately identified by inserting an 18 G needle into a disk under fluoroscopic guidance (**Fig. 31.3c, Fig. 31.4, Fig. 31.5**).

The portal of entry is marked 4 to 5 cm away from the midline at the midthoracic area (T5–T8 inclusive) at the respective thoracic disk level, and 6 to 7 cm from the midline at the lower thoracic area (T9–T12 inclusive) and at the upper thoracic area (T1–T4 inclusive). Positioning of the instruments is checked throughout the procedure by C-arm fluoroscopy in two planes as needed. After the involved levels are identified, sterile needle electrodes are placed in the intercostal muscles innervated from

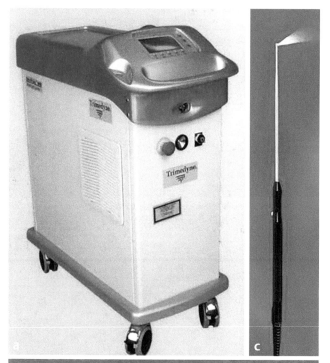

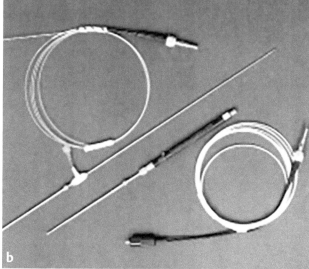

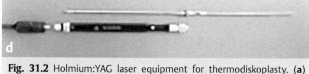

Fig. 31.2 Holmium:YAG laser equipment for thermodiskoplasty. (**a**) An 85 W double-pulse holmium:YAG laser generator. (**b**) A 550-μm holmium bare fiber with flap tip, and right-angle (side-firing) probe. (**c**) Single-use side-firing probes. (**d**) Reusable short side-firing probes.

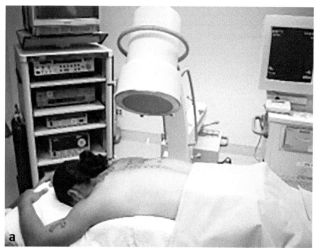

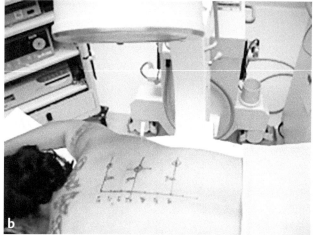

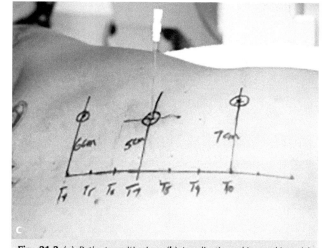

Fig. 31.3 (**a**) Patient positioning. (**b**) Localization—skin marking. (**c**) Placement of needle (portal).

those levels for continuous neurophysiologic EMG monitoring,[22] with ground electrodes having been previously placed.

31.8 Surgical Technique

Under local anesthesia, a beveled, 20 G, 3.5-inch spinal needle is inserted into the portal of entry, as described under localization and fluoroscopic guidance (**Fig. 31.5**). The needle is incrementally advanced under C-arm fluoroscopic guidance at a 35° to 45° angle from the sagittal plane, targeting toward the center of the disk, into the "safety zone," between the interpedicular line medially and the rib head at the costovertebral articulation laterally,[11,12] and medial to the costotransverse junction (**Fig. 31.5**). During needle insertion, the needle tip must be kept immediately along the medial aspect of the rib head to avoid entering the spinal canal medially, and medial to

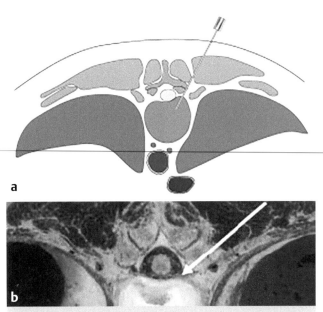

Fig. 31.4 Surgical approach for posterolateral endoscopic thoracic diskectomy for needle and stylet placement into the disk. (**a**) Axial view for needle placement. (**b**) Cadaveric cross-section cryomicrotome: posterolateral surgical approach.

the costovertebral junction to avoid pleural puncture. After the annulus is punctured, the needle is incrementally advanced to the center of the disk. The stylet of the spinal needle is removed. Isovue contrast (Bracco Diagnostics, Inc., Princeton, NJ) is injected, with the surgeon observing the ease and volume of injection, the fluoroscopic appearance in AP and lateral projections, and the patient's description of the location, concordance, and intensity of any pain produced. Surgery is performed if the diskogram and pain provocation tests are confirmatory.

A narrow 12-inch plain guidewire is passed into the center of the disk through the spinal needle placed for the diskogram. The needle is then removed. A 3- to 4-mm skin incision is made at the site. The diskectomy cannula containing its dilator is passed over the guidewire and is advanced to the annulus. A trephine replaces the dilator and incises the annulus. The cannula then advances a short distance into the disk space. The disk is decompressed using curets, trephine, microforceps, diskectome, and the laser (**Fig. 31.6**, **Fig. 31.7**, **Fig. 31.8**, **Fig. 31.9**).

Disk removal is aided by a rocking excursion of the cannula in a 25° arc, a "fan sweep" motion from side to side, that creates an oval cone-shaped area of removed disk totaling up to 50° (**Fig. 31.7**). During the procedure, the endoscope is utilized for visualization, and under magnification additional disk material and osteophytes are removed with microcurets, rasps, forceps,

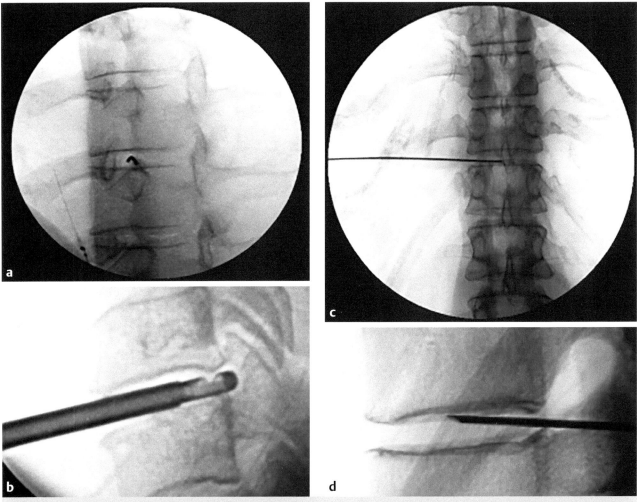

Fig. 31.5 Fluoroscopic views for placement of needle/stylet. (**a,b**) Needle placement into "safety zone" at the neuroforamen between the interpedicular line and the rib head. (**c,d**) Incremental advance of stylet placement into center of the disk.

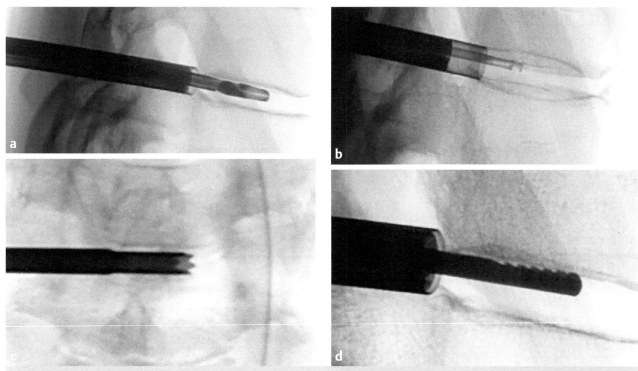

Fig. 31.6 Fluoroscopic view of posterolateral endoscopic thoracic diskectomy (PETD) instruments. (**a**) Micrograsper forceps. (**b**) Trephine. (**c**) Side-firing laser probe. (**d**) Endoscopic rasp.

and diskectome (**Fig. 31.8**, **Fig. 31.9**). Large spurs or a rib head obstructing entry to the disk space can be removed or can be perforated by a set of more aggressively toothed trephines (**Fig. 31.6**). A holmium:YAG laser (**Fig. 31.2**) is used to ablate additional disk (500 J at 10 W, 10 Hz, 5 sec on and 5 sec off), then at a lower power setting (300 J at 5 W; **Table 31.1**) to shrink and contract the disk, further reducing the profile of the protrusion and hardening the disk tissue—laser thermodiskoplasty (**Fig. 31.7**).[9] This may also cause sinovertebral neurolysis or denervation. The diskectome is again used briefly to remove charred debris. The disk space can be directly visualized by endoscopy for confirmation of disk decompression (**Fig. 31.9**). The probe and cannula are removed. Marcaine (0.25%) is infiltrated subcutaneously around the wound. A bandage is applied over the tiny wound.

Table 31.1 Laser setting for thoracic laser thermodiskoplasty*

Stage	Watts	Joules
First	10	500
Second	5	300

*Nonablative levels of laser energy, at 10 Hz, 5 seconds on and 5 seconds off.

31.9 Postoperative Care

The patient is checked neurologically prior to leaving the operating room. An upright portable chest X-ray done in the recovery room rules out a pneumothorax. Ambulation begins immediately after recovery, and the patient is usually discharged 1 hour after surgery. The patient may shower the following day. An ice pack is helpful. Mild analgesics and muscle relaxants are required at times. A progressive exercise program begins the second postoperative day. Patients are usually allowed to return

to work in 1 to 2 weeks, as long as heavy labor and prolonged sitting are not involved. Most patients found the procedure extremely beneficial.

31.10 Outcome

Ninety-six percent of 150 consecutive patients with a total of 197 herniated thoracic disks demonstrated good to excellent relief of symptoms. Six patients (4%) had persistent thoracic pain, although overall their pain improved. The patients postoperatively resumed usual activity in a few days, and fully active lives in 3 to 7 weeks.[13]

31.11 Discussion

PETD is a minimally invasive surgical procedure for treating symptomatic herniated thoracic disks through an operating endoscope with much less tissue trauma and zero mortality. It has numerous advantages, but it requires thorough knowledge of the surgical anatomy, the PETD procedure, specific surgical training, and hands-on experience in a laboratory and working closely with an experienced endoscopic surgeon through its steep surgical learning curve in order for a surgeon to become competent and to avoid possible complications.

31.12 Complications and Avoidance

A thorough knowledge of the procedure and surgical anatomy of the thorax and thoracic spine, careful selection of patients, and preoperative surgical planning with appropriate diagnostic

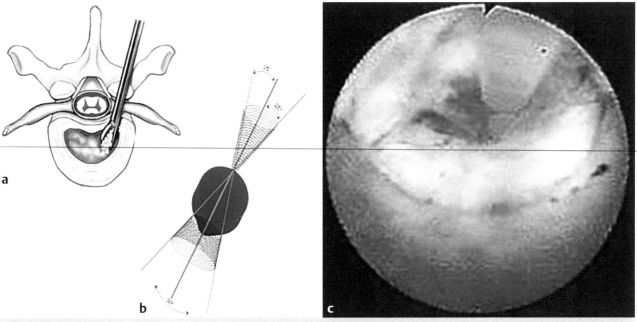

Fig. 31.7 Surgical technique of thoracic diskectomy "fan sweep" maneuver and endoscopic view of laser thermodiskoplasty. (**a**) Thoracic diskectomy (**b**) "Fan sweep" maneuver. (**c**) Holmium bare laser flat-tip fiber in action.

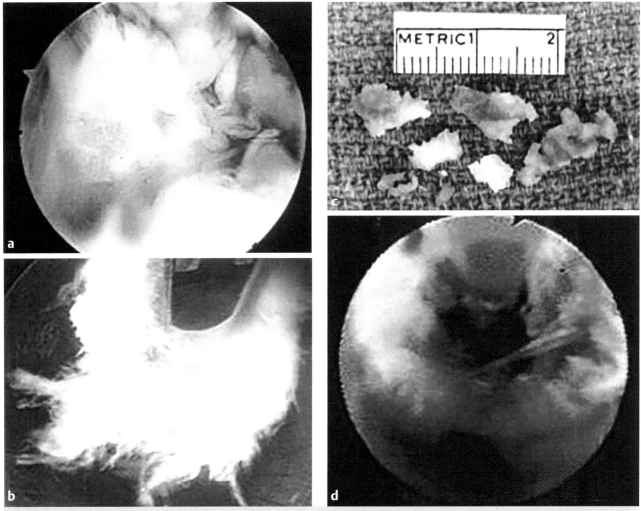

Fig. 31.8 Endoscopic view of thoracic diskectomy. (**a**) Intradiskal endoscopic view. (**b**) Endoscopic disk removal with cutter forceps. (**c**) Disk fragments removed. (**d**) Laser application for disk decompression.

evaluations facilitate PETD and prevent potential complications.[2,3,11,13] All potential complications of open approaches for thoracic disk surgery are possible but are rare or much less frequent[3,7,10,11,21,23] in PETD, with no rib resection or deliberate collapse of the lung required.

- **Pneumothorax, pulmonary injury, and postoperative atelectasis**: Pneumothorax is a potential complication in all approaches to thoracic disks, including PETD. The spinal needle should be introduced into the "safety zone" of the disk, with the interpedicular line medially and rib head laterally at the neuroforamen, to protect it from penetrating the pleura. Direct endoscopic visualization helps to avoid pulmonary injury. Atelectasis is not a problem. Chest X-ray is obtained immediately after the operation is completed to rule out pneumothorax and to initiate treatment if present.

- **Infection** is avoided by careful sterile technique, using prophylactic antibiotics IV intraoperatively, and the much smaller incisional area compared with open posterolateral and transthoracic approaches, as well as the multiport thoracoscopic approaches.

- **Aseptic diskitis** may be prevented by aiming the laser beam in a "bow tie" fashion to avoid damaging the end plates (at 6 and 12 o'clock).

- **Hematoma (subcutaneous and deep)** may occur with PETD but is minimized by careful technique, the small incision (3 mm), allowing the patient no use of aspirin or NSAIDs within 1 week prior to surgery, and application of digital pressure or an IV bag over the operative site for the first 5 minutes after surgery, as well as application of an ice pack thereafter.

- **Vascular injuries:** The thoracic aorta and its segmental branches, the intercostal artery and vein and the azygos, hemiazygos, and accessory hemiazygos veins, are at risk in open procedures and lateral, anterior, and posterolateral approaches to thoracic disks. Strict adherence to the technique and knowledge of the applicable surgical anatomy should avoid such injuries. No vascular injury has been reported with PETD.

- **Neural injury** is extremely rare with PETD; no spinal cord injuries have been reported. Nerve root injury (intercostal nerve) causing intercostal neuralgia, or chest pain, although possible, can be avoided with intraoperative neurophysiologic monitoring (EMG/NCV)[22] of intercostal muscles at and immediately below the operated levels. By using direct endoscopic visualization (**Fig. 31.9**), intercostal injury related to open chest surgery and thoracoscopic surgery can be avoided. No nerve injuries were noted in 300-plus cases at our center. The initial spinal needle placement can be onto the posterior, superior surface of the rib into the "safety zone" at the neuroforamen, avoiding the intercostal nerve lying on the inferior surface of the rib, in the costal groove. This maneuver, as well as observing the strict boundaries of the interpedicular lines, protect the spinal cord.

- **Sympathetic chain and rami communicantes:** Prone position for surgery avoids pressure on the brachial plexus, which can cause compression plexoplasty. Complications are only a remote possibility; observing the surgical anatomy of the parathoracic area and keeping needle placement within the "safety zone" should sufficiently guard against them.

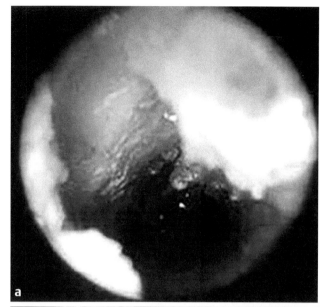
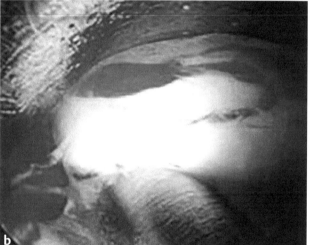
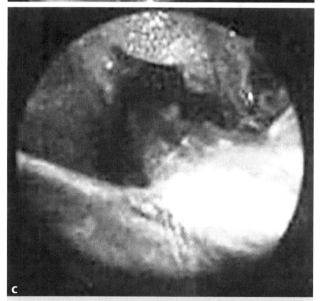

Fig. 31.9 Endoscopic view after PETD. (**a**) After PETD, hollow disk defect and end plates are seen. (**b**) Grasper forceps for disk removal below the intercostal nerve. (**c**) Intercostal nerve after microdiskectomy.

- **Excessive sedation** is avoided by surface EEG monitoring, providing more precise estimation of the depth of sedation and reducing the amount of anesthetics, as well as preventing excessive or insufficient sedation. Patients are able to respond throughout the procedure, and this provides a further means of evaluating their sedation level.
- **Improper localization:** A major complication of all disk surgeries is operating at the wrong level. Proper utilization of C-arm fluoroscopy for anatomical localization avoids complications caused by poor placement of instruments or operating at the wrong disk level. Routine pain provocation test and diskogram give additional verification of the proper level.
- **Dural tears** are common in all other approaches to the thoracic disk, but they have not been reported in PETD.
- **Soft tissue injuries** due to prolonged forceful retraction, as occurs in many disk operations, are not at issue with PETD.
- **Inadequate decompression of disk material** is minimized by using multiple modalities, by using instruments like forceps, trephines, diskectome, bur, and rasp, and by application of laser to both vaporize tissue and to perform thermodiskoplasty.

31.13 Advantages

The advantages[7,10,11,12,14,21] of PETD are numerous. They include:

- No general anesthesia required
- Commonly done under local anesthesia
- Small incision and less scarring without multiple or large incisions
- Minimal blood loss
- Zero mortality
- No need of lung collapse or opening of the pleural cavity
- No postoperative pleural effusion, intercostal neuralgia, and pneumothorax
- No significant infection
- Avoiding injury to blood vessels
- No resection of rib
- No spinal fusion or fixation needed
- No dissection of muscle, bone, ligaments, or manipulation of the dural sac, spinal cord, or nerve roots

- Little or no epidural bleeding
- Minimal use of analgesics postoperatively
- Same-day outpatient procedure
- Less traumatic, both physically and psychologically
- Does not promote further instability of spinal segments
- Early return to usual activities, including work
- Costs less than conventional diskectomy
- Multiple-level diskectomy feasible and well tolerated[17,18,19,20,21]
- Least challenging to medically high-risk patients, such as those with cardiopulmonary problems, the aged, and the morbidly obese
- Exercise programs can begin the same day as surgery
- Direct endoscopic visualization and confirmation of the efficacy of surgery, which contribute to a safe and effective outcome

31.14 Disadvantages

The technique is not appropriate for patients with severe thoracic disk extrusions causing cord compression with severe neurologic deficit (paraparesis) and patients with severe congenital or acquired stenosis of the spinal canal. In patients with severe spondylosis and foraminal stenosis, the technique may not be suitable, because insertion of the endoscope may not be feasible.

31.15 Case Illustration

A 24-year-old man had complained for two months of intractable midback pain and muscle spasm. Past history was noncontributory. Parathoracic muscle spasm was palpable adjacent to the painful level. Neurologic examination showed hypalgesia in T10 and T12 dermatomes. MRI demonstrated two protruded thoracic disks (at the T10 and T12 levels). Physical therapy, analgesics, and epidural steroid injections did not alleviate the patient's discomfort. Chest X-ray demonstrated 13 thoracic vertebrae with 13 ribs, with 7 cervical and 5 lumbar vertebrae. The patient was treated by PETD at T10–T11 and T12–L1. He had excellent relief of his symptoms postoperatively. Comparative preoperative and postoperative MRI scans showed the disappearance of the protruded disks (**Fig. 31.10**).

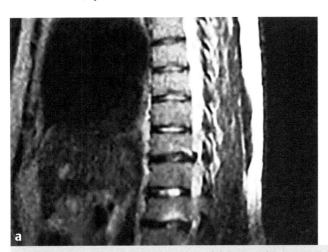
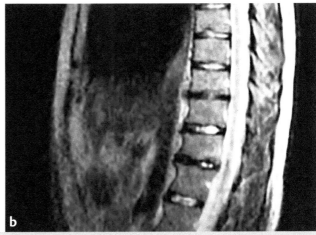

Fig. 31.10 (a,b) Large herniated T10 and T12 disks, pre- and postoperative MRI scans.

31.16 Conclusion

Posterior lateral endoscopic thoracic diskectomy performed for symptomatic herniated thoracic disk with added laser "tightening" of the disk (thermodiskoplasty) is a safe, relatively easy, and efficacious procedure. A minimally invasive, less traumatic outpatient procedure, it results in less morbidity, more rapid recovery, and significant economic savings. The mortality rate was zero in a multicenter study[23] of percutaneous endoscopic spinal diskectomy (26,860 cases), and the morbidity rate was less than 1%, with patient satisfaction of more than 92% for thoracic disks. There were no reported spinal cord injuries, intercostal neuralgia, or dural tears, and no significant infection, vascular injury, or pulmonary complications. PETD requires a knowledgeable and competent surgeon with a thorough appreciation of the surgical anatomy of the thorax and thoracic spine, intercostal nerves and vessels, rib heads, pedicles, disk spaces, and spinal cord. To perform the procedure, the spine surgeon must have specific surgical training with hands-on experience in the laboratory, and, most important, must spend time working through the steep surgical learning curve with an endoscopic spinal surgeon expert in the procedure.

References

1. Kim D, Choi G, Lee S, eds. *History of Endoscopic Spine Surgery. Endoscopic Spine Procedures.* New York: Thieme; 2011:1:1–7
2. Jaikumar S, Kim DH, Kam AC. History of minimally invasive spine surgery. *Neurosurgery* 2002;51(5, Suppl):S1–S14
3. Perez-Cruet MJ, Fessler RG, Perin NI. Review: complications of minimally invasive spinal surgery. *Neurosurgery* 2002;51(5, Suppl):S26–S36
4. Fessler R, Khoo L. Minimally invasive cervical microendoscopic foraminotomy: an initial clinical experience. *Neurosurgery* 2002;51(5):S37–S45
5. Chiu J. Endoscopy-assisted thoracic microdiscectomy. In: Kim DK, Kim KH, Kim YC, eds. Minimally Invasive Percutaneous Spinal Technique, Philadelphia: Elsevier-Saunders 2011;24:320–327
6. Chiu J, Clifford T, Princenthal R. The new frontier of minimally invasive spine surgery through computer assisted technology. In: Lemke HU, Vannier MN, Invamura RD, eds. *Computer Assisted Radiology and Surgery.* New York: Spring-Verlag; 2002:233–237
7. Simpson JM, Silveri CP, Simeone FA, Balderston RA, An HS. Thoracic disc herniation. Re-evaluation of the posterior approach using a modified costotransversectomy. *Spine* 1993;18(13):1872–1877
8. Schellhas KP, Pollei SR, Dorwart RH. Thoracic discography. A safe and reliable technique. *Spine* 1994;19(18):2103–2109
9. Chiu JC, Clifford TJ, Greenspan M, Richley RC, Lohman G, Sison RB. Percutaneous microdecompressive endoscopic cervical discectomy with laser thermodiskoplasty. *Mt Sinai J Med* 2000;67(4):278–282
10. Chiu JC, Clifford TJ, Sison R. Percutaneous microdecompressive endoscopic thoracic discectomy for herniated thoracic discs. *Surg Technol Int* 2002;10:266–269
11. Chiu J, Clifford T. Percutaneous endoscopic thoracic discectomy. In: Savitz MH, Chiu JC, Yeung AD, eds. *The Practice of Minimally Invasive Spinal Technique.* Richmond, VA: AAMISMS Education; 2000:211–216
12. Chiu J, Clifford T. Posterolateral approach for percutaneous thoracic endoscopic discectomy. *J Min Inv Spinal Tech* 2001;1:26–30
13. Chiu JC, Negron F, Clifford T, Greenspan M, Princethal RA. Microdecompressive percutaneous endoscopy: spinal discectomy with new laser thermodiskoplasty for non-extruded herniated nucleosus pulposus. *Surg Technol Int* 1999;8:343–351
14. Savitz MH. Same-day microsurgical arthroscopic lateral-approach laser-assisted (SMALL) fluoroscopic discectomy. *J Neurosurg* 1994;80(6):1039–1045
15. Yeung AT, Chow PM. Posterior lateral endoscopic excision for lumbar disc herniation: surgical technique, outcome, and complications. *Spine* 2002;27:722–731
16. Boriani S, Biagini R, De Iure F, et al. Two-level thoracic disc herniation. *Spine* 1994;19(21):2461–2466
17. Coleman RJ, Hamlyn PJ, Butler P. Anterior spinal surgery for multiple thoracic disc herniations. *Br J Neurosurg* 1990;4(6):541–543
18. Dickman CA, Mican CA. Multilevel anterior thoracic discectomies and anterior interbody fusion using a microsurgical thoracoscopic approach. Case report. *J Neurosurg* 1996;84(1):104–109
19. Shikata J, Yamamuro T, Iida H, Kashiwagi N. Multiple thoracic disc herniations: case report. *Neurosurgery* 1988;22(6 Pt 1):1068–1070
20. Chiu J, Clifford T. Multiple herniated discs at single and multiple spinal segments treated with endoscopic microdecompressive surgery. *J Min Inv Spinal Tech* 2001;1:15–19
21. Clifford T, Chiu J, Rogers G. Neurophysiological monitoring of peripheral nerve function during endoscopic laser discectomy. *J Min Inv Spinal Tech.* 2001;1:54–57
22. Chiu J, Clifford T, Savitz M, et al. Multicenter study of percutaneous endoscopic discectomy (lumbar, cervical and thoracic). *J Min Inv Spinal Tech* 2001;1:33–37
23. Chiu J, et al. Use of laser in minimally invasive spinal surgery and pain management. In: Kambin P, ed. *Arthroscopic and Endoscopic Spine Surgery Text and Atlas.* 2nd ed. Totowa, NJ: Humana Press; 2005;13:259–269

32 Tubular Endoscopic Transpedicular Diskectomy

Ricardo B. V. Fontes, Manish Kasliwal, John O'Toole, and Richard G. Fessler

32.1 Introduction

Symptomatic thoracic disk herniation (TDH) is a relatively uncommon pathology that may present a significant technical challenge to treat because of the anatomical constraints of the narrow thoracic spinal canal, the necessity to minimize cord manipulation, and the frequently calcified nature of TDH. Laminectomy alone was historically associated with poor outcomes, so a variety of anterior and posterolateral approaches were developed to treat TDH, including the transfacet-transpedicular approach first described by Patterson and Arbit in 1978. This technique is especially amenable to minimally invasive concepts and can be very successfully performed through a tubular endoscopic approach.[1,2,3,4,5]

32.2 Patient Selection

Midline TDH causing thoracic myelopathy (**Fig. 32.1**) is the main indication for tubular endoscopic transpedicular diskectomy.

Absolute contraindication is purely paramedian TDH (a transpedicular approach is not necessary), and relative contraindications are broad-based TDH causing bilateral compression (it may require a bilateral approach) and intradural TDH.

32.3 Technique

32.3.1 Preoperative Planning

Preoperative planning includes MRI or CT myelogram of the thoracic spine. If MRI is done, then noncontrast CT of the thoracic and lumbar spines is performed to assess TDH calcification and localization (ribs, transitional lumbar levels).

Cardiac clearance is necessary to maintain blood pressure during the procedure.

Preoperative chest X-ray is obtained to count ribs, and lumbar spine X-ray is taken to confirm the number of lumbar vertebrae.

32.3.2 Anesthesia and Positioning

General anesthesia without neuromuscular blockade (**Fig. 32.2**) is used. Intraoperative neurophysiological monitoring is done with SSEP and EMG. The patient is positioned prone on a Wilson frame, with checks for ocular pressure or contact points.

Mean arterial pressure is kept above 80 mm Hg at all times.

Rail attachment for the retractor arm is caudal and opposite the surgeon.

32.3.3 Localization

Preoperative marking is done with radiopaque material or fluoroscopic localization is accomplished with multiple views (anteroposterior for counting, lateral for lower thoracic levels and ribs). Image guidance may be used with intraoperative acquisition (O-arm), especially if the TDH is calcified. Fluoroscopy or navigation is utilized throughout the procedure.

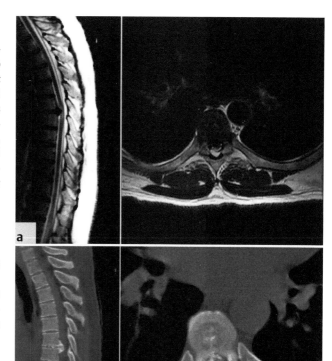

Fig. 32.1 Case example, a 45-year-old male with progressive spastic paraparesis. (**a**) MRI and (**b**) CT demonstrate a large, predominantly midline T7–T8 disk herniation. This is a good example of an ideal patient for an endoscopic transpedicular diskectomy. The herniation is slightly larger on the right.

32.3.4 Entry Point

The entry point is 2 to 3 cm off midline, on the side of the larger TDH component or worse symptoms. Cranial-caudal position at the level of the affected interspace is confirmed with fluoroscopy.

32.3.5 Skin and Soft Tissues

Local anesthesia uses lidocaine 2% with 1:100,000 epinephrine. Skin incision is made and the K-wire is inserted perpendicular to the skin (**Fig. 32.3**).

The initial contact point is the zygapophysial joint, then exploration proceeds medially and the guidewire is docked at the spinous process–lamina junction.

The initial tubular dilator is inserted and the K-wire is removed, followed by sequential dilation.

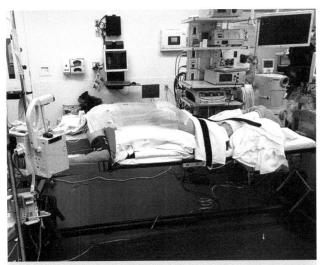

Fig. 32.2 Patient positioned prone on a Jackson table and Wilson frame. The rail attachment is positioned opposite the surgeon at the level of the hips. The tubular retractors are secured to the rail for the duration of the case.

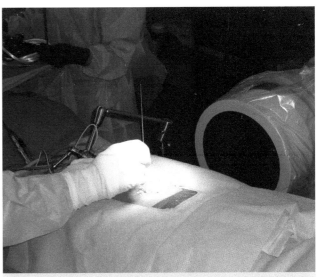

Fig. 32.3 Right T10–T11 diskectomy. Incision is marked 2 to 3 cm off midline and a K-wire is inserted initially, contacting the zygapophysial joint.

After placement of the final working channel, the dilators are removed and connection is made to the retractor arm (**Fig. 32.4**). The 30° endoscope and light source are attached (**Fig. 32.5**).

Residual muscle is resected with cautery.

32.3.6 Transpedicular Approach (Video 32.1)

The correct level is confirmed. Decompression is started with ipsilateral partial laminectomies; a combination of Kerrison rongeurs and high-speed drill may be used. The medial half of the zygapophysial joint is resected (**Fig. 32.6**). Enhanced medial visualization is afforded by selective resection of the pedicle of the caudal vertebra. The medial and cranial two-thirds of the pedicle may be safely removed.

32.3.7 Diskectomy and Decompression

- Do not attempt to remove a large calcified fragment at this point.

- Space can be created to mobilize the TDH fragment *away* from the surgeon.
- Epidural veins are coagulated with bipolar cautery.
- Lateral/paramedian annulus may be incised and soft disk removed to create space.
- Five to 10% of the cranial and caudal vertebral bodies can be resected with a high-speed drill.
- A plane can be created between fragment and dura, then an attempt can be made to mobilize the fragment away from the dura and into the space created. Minimize cord manipulation.
- If intradural, at this point there may be a CSF leak. Once the fragment is released from the dura and is dislodged into the vertebral body cavity, it is safe to remove it.
- Ensure decompression is adequate by sliding an angled instrument anterior to the dura. The instrument should slide cranially and caudally without problems. An angled mirror of the type occasionally used for pituitary surgery or a 70° endoscope can also be used for visual inspection, but we have found it to be of limited value.[3] Image guidance may be useful

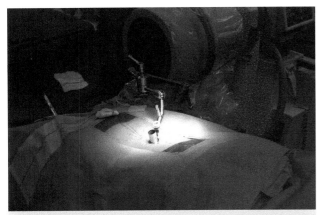

Fig. 32.4 Final tubular retractor secured by the retractor arm and in place. Note slightly medial angulation for the initial part of the laminectomy. The tube is then aimed exactly perpendicular to the floor for the transpedicular approach.

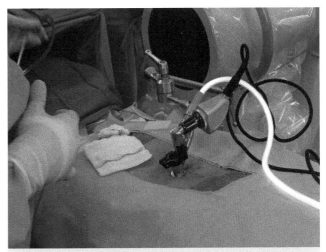

Fig. 32.5 Endoscope and light source secured to the tubular retractor.

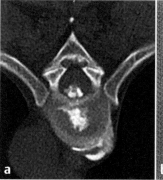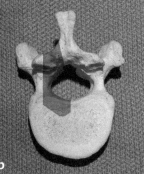

Fig. 32.6 (a) CT example in the prone position and **(b)** anatomical specimen demonstrating the extent of osseous resection for a transpedicular approach. The shadowed area demonstrates the typical transpedicular approach with resection of the medial half of the zygapophysial joint and pedicle. An additional 5 to 10% of the vertebral body may be resected to displace the calcified fragments to enable their removal without retracting the cord.

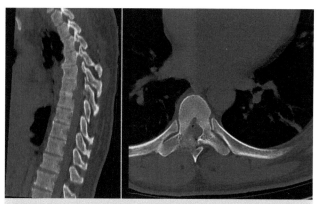

Fig. 32.7 Postoperative CT of the case demonstrated in Fig. 32.1. Adequate surgical result with removal of the disk herniation and cord decompression.

to assess decompression, especially contralaterally, but cannot be relied upon exclusively.

32.3.8 Complication Avoidance and Treatment

- Avoid cord manipulation at all costs.
- Root section is usually not necessary, because it courses caudal to the pedicle and thus is not in close proximity to midline TDHs.
- Anterior cord syndrome may ensue due to anterior spinal artery compression by the fragment; therefore it is important to maintain mean arterial pressure above 80 mm Hg at all times.
- Ensure that the patient is not pharmacologically paralyzed and that the monitoring technician is alert at the start of decompression.
- Unintended posterior or posterolateral durotomies can be managed with direct repair utilizing specially designed instruments, as described elsewhere.[6]
- Direct repair of unintended durotomies or large dural defects due to calcified TDH should not be attempted. Careful packing with muscle or absorbable gelatin sponge (Gelfoam) and the lack of dead space due to the minimally invasive approach are the best measures to address these defects. Onlay dural substitutes and sealants may or may not be used based on the surgeon's preference. Lumbar CSF diversion may also be used for large anterior dural defects.
- Hemostasis is achieved with injectable hemostatic matrix, bone wax, and fine bipolar coagulation of larger epidural

veins. If a more extensive corpectomy was performed, a multiperforated epidural drain may be left in place.

32.3.9 Closure

The retractor/endoscope apparatus is removed as a single unit. Larger bleeding points can be coagulated during the removal process. Fascial and subcutaneous planes are approximated with interrupted 0 and 3–0 absorbable sutures. Skin is closed with a running dermal 5–0 suture and/or surgical adhesive.

32.4 Postoperative Course

The patient may ambulate immediately after surgery and may be discharged home as soon as he or she is able to ambulate and urinate without problems. Alternatively, a single overnight hospital stay may be necessary, especially for older males with urinary retention due to anesthetic side effects.

Overnight bedrest is prescribed if a durotomy occurred and may be extended for 3 to 5 days if CSF diversion is utilized.

Postoperative noncontrast CT is obtained to assess the degree of decompression; reoperation may be considered if decompression is not satisfactory (**Fig. 32.7**).

References

1. Eichholz KM, O'Toole JE, Fessler RG. Thoracic microendoscopic discectomy. *Neurosurg Clin N Am* 2006;17(4):441–446
2. Jho HD. Endoscopic microscopic transpedicular thoracic discectomy. Technical note. *J Neurosurg* 1997;87(1):125–129
3. Jho HD. Endoscopic transpedicular thoracic discectomy. *J Neurosurg* 1999;91(2, Suppl):151–156
4. Patterson RH Jr, Arbit E. A surgical approach through the pedicle to protruded thoracic discs. *J Neurosurg* 1978;48(5):768–772
5. Tan LA, Lopes DK, Fontes RBV. Ultrasound-guided posterolateral approach for midline calcified thoracic disc herniation. *J Korean Neurosurg Soc* 2014;55(6):383–386
6. Fontes RB, Tan LA, O'Toole JE. Minimally invasive treatment of spinal dural arteriovenous fistula with the use of intraoperative indocyanine green angiography. *Neurosurg Focus* 2013;35(2, Suppl):Video 5

33 Thoracoscopic Diskectomy

Victor Lo, Alissa Redko, Ashley E. Brown, Daniel H. Kim, and J. Patrick Johnson

33.1 Introduction

Video-assisted thoracoscopic surgery (VATS) emerged to treat spinal disorders in 1993.[1,2,3] Current uses of thoracoscopy in spinal procedures include spinal canal decompression (e.g., diskectomy, corpectomy), spinal biopsy, deformity correction, and sympathectomy. The thoracoscopic technique parallels an open thoracotomy procedure in that a ventrolateral approach is taken through the chest cavity, providing a full and direct vertebrolateral view of the vertebra and thecal sac. The benefits of the thoracoscopic procedure include minimal tissue retraction, reduced postoperative pain, and decreased hospital length of stay.[4,5,6] The thoracoscopic approach can also be adapted for instrumentation and fusion if required.[7] In addition, innovation in intraoperative navigation technology has led to the incorporation of image-guided VATS.[8,9] This chapter describes the indications and procedure for thoracoscopic diskectomy.

33.2 Indications for Thoracic Diskectomy

The incidence of clinically significant thoracic disk herniation is reported to be as low as 1 per million or 0.25 to 0.75% of all ruptured disks.[10,11] Radiculopathy due to thoracic disk herniation typically causes both axial back pain and radicular pain that manifests as paraspinal muscular spasms and bandlike radiating chest wall pain.

Nonsurgical management of these lesions with nonsteroidal anti-inflammatories, epidural steroid injections, and physical therapy has been successful in treating many patients with solely radicular symptoms. Nonsurgical treatment of tolerable thoracic radiculopathy for 3 to 6 months is reasonable given that a large proportion of cases will improve without surgical intervention.

Although there is no consensus regarding thoracic disk removal, surgery is generally reserved for patients who failed conservative treatment of primarily radicular symptoms or who have myelopathy, especially if it is progressive or severe.

Approaches for thoracic diskectomy are dorsolateral (e.g., transpedicular), lateral (e.g., costotransversectomy, lateral extracavitary, parascapular), ventrolateral (e.g., transthoracic/thoracoscopic, retropleural), and ventral (e.g., transsternal). Approach selection depends on the anatomical location of the disk herniation. All soft herniated disks, calcified lateral disks, and mildly calcified centrolateral disks can usually be treated with posterolateral approaches (**Fig. 33.1**). Centrolateral disks that are densely calcified or certain mildly calcified disks that require any retraction of the spinal cord for diskectomy should be considered for treatment primarily with a ventrolateral or lateral approach (**Fig. 33.2**). When a transthoracic approach is indicated, one may consider a thoracoscopic approach as well.

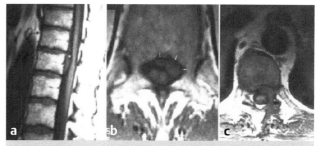

Fig. 33.1 (a) Sagittal T1 MRI of the thoracic spine demonstrating a herniated thoracic disk. **(b)** Axial T1 MRI of the thoracic spine demonstrating a herniated thoracic disk in the ventrolateral aspect of the spinal canal. **(c)** Axial T2 MRI of the thoracic spine demonstrating a herniated thoracic disk in the ventrolateral aspect of the spinal canal.

33.3 Contraindications to Thoracoscopic Diskectomy

Contraindications include:

- Respiratory insufficiency (i.e., inability to tolerate single-lung ventilation)
- Pleural symphysis
- Failed prior open ventral surgery
- Thoracic empyema
- Previous thoracotomy
- Previous tube thoracostomy
- Bullous lung pathology with reduced lung function

33.4 Imaging for Thoracic Disk Disease

MRI is the optimal modality for assessing the thoracic vertebra, intervertebral disk, and neural elements. MRI can characterize the herniated disk's location with respect to the spinal canal (i.e., central, paracentral, lateral; **Fig. 33.2**).

CT defines the bony anatomy and can determine whether the herniated disk is calcified (**Fig. 33.3**) or the posterior longitudinal ligament is calcified (**Fig. 33.4**). CT myelography is useful when the patient is unable to tolerate, or has a contraindication to, MRI (**Fig. 33.5**).

Plain film studies of the thoracic and lumbar spine can be used as an intraoperative reference for localizing the herniated disk.

33.5 Surgical Instruments

The endoscopic equipment needed for a thoracoscopic diskectomy procedure is available in hospital operating rooms where general surgical and gynecological laparoscopy and/or general thoracic endoscopy is performed.[12] The equipment includes:

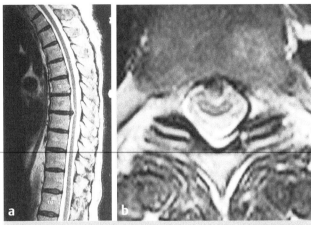

Fig. 33.2 **(a)** Sagittal T2 MRI of the thoracic spine demonstrating a thoracic herniated disk. **(b)** Axial T2 MRI of the thoracic spine demonstrating the herniated thoracic disk in the ventral spinal canal. The anatomical location of this herniated disk suggests it would benefit from the thoracoscopic approach.

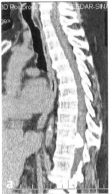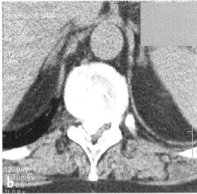

Fig. 33.3 **(a)** Sagittal CT of the thoracic spine demonstrating a large calcified thoracic herniated disk. **(b)** Axial CT of the thoracic spine showing the large calcified thoracic disk causing canal compression.

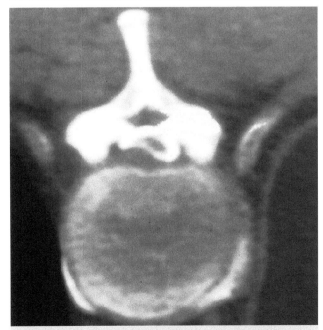

Fig. 33.5 Axial CT myelogram of the thoracic spine demonstrating disk herniation resulting in spinal cord compression.

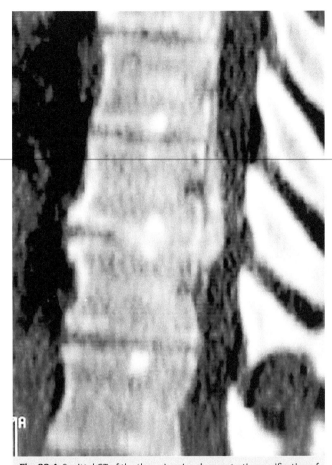

Fig. 33.4 Sagittal CT of the thoracic spine demonstrating ossification of the posterior longitudinal ligament.

- Radiolucent surgical table
- Fluoroscopy equipment (C-arm)
- Endoscope
  - 5-mm or 10-mm diameter optical working channel
  - 0°, 30°, and 45° angled cameras (**Fig. 33.6**)
- Surgical drill
  - Extended drill attachments
  - Pistol grip provides some rotational and angular stabilization (**Fig. 33.7a**)
  - Coarse diamond drill bit and round cutting bit (**Fig. 33.7b**)
- Extended long-handled spine instruments (**Fig. 33.8**)
  - Kerrison rongeurs
  - Straight and angled curets
  - Pituitary grasper
  - Nerve hook
  - Penfield dissectors
  - Dental dissector
- Suction-irrigator
  - Available from the standard endoscopic equipment set
  - Extended Frazier suction tip can also be used
- Endoscopic instruments
  - Endo shears
  - Bipolar endoscopic cautery

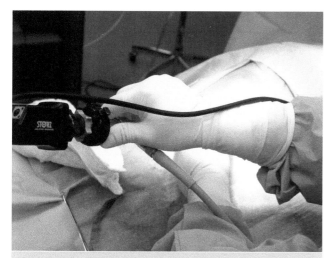

Fig. 33.6 Surgical endoscope used for thoracoscopy.

- ○ Harmonic scalpel
- ○ Endovascular clip and loop ligatures
- • Various cotton-tip applicators for use as soft tissue dissectors or to apply bone wax

33.6 Technique for Thoracoscopic Diskectomy

33.6.1 Anesthetic Considerations

The procedure requires the induction of general anesthesia. Insertion of a double-lumen endotracheal tube for selective ventilation of the contralateral lung from the side of the approach allows for maximal exposure.

33.6.2 Positioning

The patient is secured in a lateral decubitus position with the operative side up. A right-sided approach is generally preferred for access from T11 to L2 and a left-sided approach for access from T3 to T10. The legs are slightly flexed, and an axillary roll is placed under the axilla. The top arm is held in a Krause arm support to expose the chest wall for a thoracotomy (**Fig. 33.9**).

C-arm fluoroscopy is used to ensure the patient and spine are perpendicular to the operating table. Spinal cord somatosensory and motor evoked potential monitoring is utilized during the procedure.

33.6.3 Thoracoscopic Access

The spinal levels are localized with lateral C-arm fluoroscopy. The involved vertebral bodies, disks, anterior spinal line, and posterior spinal line are marked on the lateral chest wall.

Three portals are marked on the chest wall in a triangular pattern, with the port for the endoscope perpendicular and centered over the level of the lesion. The working portal and suction/irrigation portal are placed in the anterior axillary line.

The entire lateral chest wall is prepped in event a conversion to thoracotomy is needed.

After single-lung ventilation has been initiated, the first portal for the endoscope is placed. A minithoracotomy technique, using

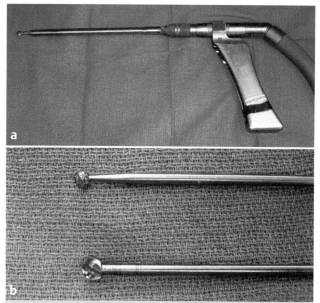

Fig. 33.7 (**a**) Pneumatic drill with extended shaft (8–10 inches) and pistol grip attachment. (**b**) Diamond cutting burs (5 mm in diameter) used for bone removal.

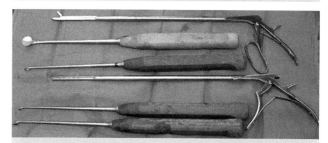

Fig. 33.8 Extended long-shaft and handled thoracoscopic instruments used for diskectomy.

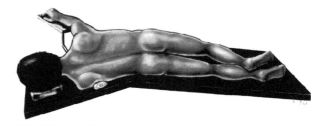

Fig. 33.9 Lateral patient position for thoracoscopy.

blunt dissection through the subcutaneous tissues and intercostal muscles, is used until the parietal pleura is exposed and entered. Proper lung deflation is confirmed under direct visualization.

The 5- or 10-mm (depending on the size of the instrument to be introduced) soft trocars are used, to reduce the incidence of intercostal nerve injury (**Fig. 33.10**). After insertion of the trocar, the 30° endoscope is introduced. The thoracic cavity is inspected and the subsequent trocars are inserted under direct endoscopic visualization.

The endoscopic image is oriented so that the spine is parallel to the lower edge of the monitor.

Once the portals are placed, the lung is retracted anteriorly. Additional retraction of the lung can be accomplished by rotation of the operating table to allow the lung to fall away from the vertebral column.

Localization of the spinal level is done with placement of a Steinmann pin into the presumptive disk space and is confirmed with C-arm fluoroscopy.

33.6.4 Exposure

The segmental vessels lie transversely across the midportion of the vertebral body, and therefore division is usually unnecessary (**Fig. 33.11**). However, if needed, the segmental vessels can be mobilized, ligated, and divided.

The parietal pleura is opened widely over the rib head and over the disk space (**Fig. 33.12**). The proximal end of the rib and the disk space are colinear and help to orient the surgeon during the procedure.

The proximal 2 cm of the rib is removed using a high-speed drill to expose the lateral surface of the pedicle and neural foramen (**Fig. 33.13a**). After drilling of the proximal rib head, the pedicle is visualized (**Fig. 33.13b**). The neural foramen contains

epidural fat and is relatively small, with the segmental nerve and vessels traversing.

33.6.5 Diskectomy

The pedicle is then drilled until the lateral spinal canal is exposed and the dura is visualized (**Fig. 33.14**). Decompression requires adequate bony removal of the posterior end plates, which can be extended to the contralateral pedicle if needed (**Fig. 33.15**).

Bleeding from the cancellous bone can obscure visualization, thus hemostasis during every stage of the procedure is essential. Bone wax applied with an endoscopic cotton tip applicator can effectively control bone bleeding.

A disk fragment that has migrated either cephalad or caudally requires further drilling to undermine the spinal canal adequately for complete decompression.

The posterior longitudinal ligament is identified and is opened with a blunt-tip probe and subsequently resected with curets and Kerrison rongeurs (**Fig. 33.16**). This often requires pulling soft disk material or cracking calcified disk into the defect created by the bony decompression. Prior to closure, bony or disk debris must be irrigated out.

The procedure achieves complete decompression of the dura and spinal cord and spinal canal from a ventrolateral endoscopic exposure (**Fig. 33.17**). Postoperative MRI and CT are shown in **Fig. 33.18**.

33.6.6 Wound Closure and Postoperative Management

A chest tube is placed through the posterior portal with endoscopic guidance and 20 cm H_2O suction is applied while the

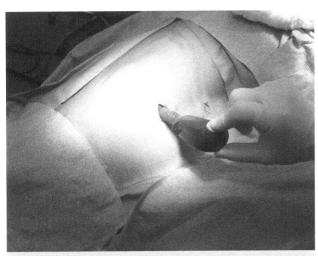

Fig. 33.10 The 5-mm and 10-mm soft trocars are used to reduce the incidence of intercostal nerve injury.

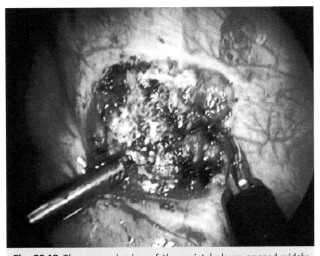

Fig. 33.12 Thoracoscopic view of the parietal pleura opened widely over the rib head and over the disk space.

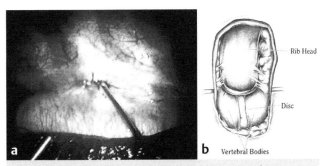

Fig. 33.11 (**a**) Thoracoscopic view of the thoracic spine with Steinmann pin in the disk space for radiographic localization. (**b**) Anatomical relationship between the intervertebral disk and rib head.

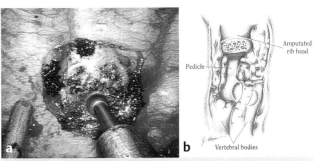

Fig. 33.13 (**a**) The proximal rib head is drilled to reveal the pedicle. (**b**) Anatomical relationship of the pedicle to the disk space after the proximal rib head has been removed.

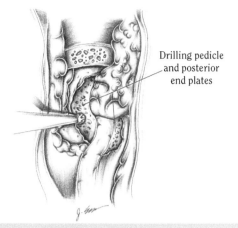

Fig. 33.14 The pedicle and posterior end plates are drilled to allow adequate exposure to the herniated disk.

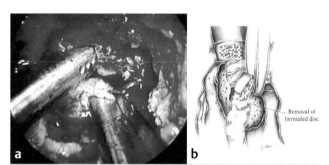

Fig. 33.16 (a) Thoracoscopic view of the diskectomy. (b) Diagram of the diskectomy.

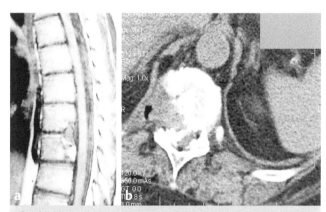

Fig. 33.18 (a) Postoperative sagittal T1 MRI of the thoracic spine demonstrating decompression of the spinal cord and canal. (b) Postoperative axial CT of the thoracic spine illustrating the extent of bony resection for diskectomy.

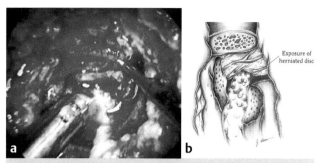

Fig. 33.15 (a) Thoracoscopic view of the herniated disk after pedicle and adjacent end plates have been drilled. (b) Diagrammatic view of the herniated disk after drilling of the pedicle and end plates.

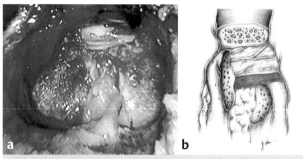

Fig. 33.17 (a) Thoracoscopic view after diskectomy has been completed. (b) Illustration of completed diskectomy.

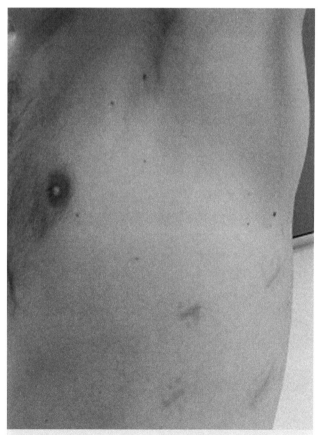

Fig. 33.19 Healed incisions after thoracoscopic diskectomy.

anesthesiologist reinflates the lung. The endoscopic ports are then removed, and the incisions are closed in anatomic layers with absorbable sutures. The patient is extubated at the end of the procedure, and a chest radiograph is obtained in the recovery room to ensure lung inflation. The patient is treated postoperatively with aggressive pulmonary toilet. The chest tube is removed when drainage diminishes to less than 100 mL per day, typically within 24 to 48 hours.

The thoracoscopic approach to diskectomy yields minimal scarring after the wounds are healed (Fig. 33.19).

33.7 Complications

Complications from the thoracoscopic diskectomy procedure have been uncommon, and most were transient and not life-threatening.[13,14] Thoracoscopic complications include intercostal neuralgia, pneumothorax, pleural effusion, atelectasis, hemothorax, chylothorax, and subcutaneous emphysema. Diskectomy complications are retained disk fragment, neurologic deficit, and CSF leak. General complications can be a misidentified level, infection, and blood loss > 2,000 mL.

References

1   Landreneau RJ, Hazelrigg SR, Mack MJ, et al. Postoperative pain-related morbidity: video-assisted thoracic surgery versus thoracotomy. *Ann Thorac Surg* 1993;56(6):1285–1289
2   Mack MJ, Regan JJ, Bobechko WP, Acuff TE. Application of thoracoscopy for diseases of the spine. *Ann Thorac Surg* 1993;56(3):736–738
3   Horowitz MB, Moossy JJ, Julian T, Ferson PF, Huneke K. Thoracic discectomy using video assisted thoracoscopy. *Spine* 1994;19(9):1082–1086
4   Dickman CA, Detweiler PW, Porter RW. Endoscopic spine surgery. *Clin Neurosurg* 2000;46:526–553
5   Johnson JP, Filler AG, Mc Bride DQ. Endoscopic thoracic discectomy. *Neurosurg Focus* 2000;9(4):e11
6   Oskouian RJ Jr, Johnson JP, Regan JJ. Thoracoscopic microdiscectomy. *Neurosurgery* 2002;50(1):103–109
7   Bisson EF, Jost GF, Apfelbaum RI, Schmidt MH. Thoracoscopic discectomy and instrumented fusion using a minimally invasive plate system: surgical technique and early clinical outcome. *Neurosurg Focus* 2011;30(4):E15
8   Johnson JP, Drazin D, King WA, Kim TT. Image-guided navigation and video-assisted thoracoscopic spine surgery: the second generation. *Neurosurg Focus* 2014;36(3):E8
9   Hur JW, Kim JS, Cho DY, Shin JM, Lee JH, Lee SH. Video-assisted thoracoscopic surgery under O-arm navigation system guidance for the treatment of thoracic disk herniations: surgical techniques and early clinical results. *J Neurol Surg A Cent Eur Neurosurg* 2014;75(6):415–421
10 Carson J, Gumpert J, Jefferson A. Diagnosis and treatment of thoracic intervertebral disc protrusions. *J Neurol Neurosurg Psychiatry* 1971;34(1):68–77
11 Arce CA, Dohrman GJ. Thoracic disc herniations. Improved diagnosis with CT scanning and a review of the literature. *Surg Neurol* 1958;23:356–361
12 Regan JJ, McAfee PC, Mack MJ. *Atlas of Endoscopic Spine Surgery*. St. Louis, MO: Quality Medical Publishing; 1995
13 McAfee PC, Regan JR, Zdeblick T, et al. The incidence of complications in endoscopic anterior thoracolumbar spinal reconstructive surgery. A prospective multicenter study comprising the first 100 consecutive cases. *Spine* 1995;20(14):1624–1632
14 Barbagallo GMV, Piccini M, Gasbarrini A, Milone P, Albanese V. Subphrenic hematoma after thoracoscopic discectomy: description of a very rare adverse event and review of the literature on complications: case report. *J Neurosurg Spine* 2013;19(4):436–444

34 Tubular Endoscopic Thoracic Decompressive Laminectomy

Ryan Khanna and Zachary A. Smith

34.1 Introduction

Spinal surgeons are choosing to perform more and more cases using endoscopic instruments due to the advantages offered by minimally invasive approaches. Advances in technology have allowed the incorporation of these techniques in thoracic decompression. While the procedure is still evolving, there are indications for the use of endoscopes in thoracic decompression (**Video 34.1**).

34.2 Choice of Patient

34.2.1 Indications

- Symptomatic compression of the thoracic spinal cord (**Fig. 34.1**)
- Epidural hematoma and infection
- Thoracic epidural tumors
- Degenerative compression: ossified ligamentum flavum, synovial cysts (**Fig. 34.2**)

34.2.2 Contraindications

- Instability of the spinal column
- Any procedure requiring fusion of thoracic vertebrae
- Scoliosis

- Significant postlaminectomy scar (relative)
- Previous instrumentation at operative level

34.3 Technique

34.3.1 Position and Anesthesia

General anesthesia (propofol and remifentanil) is used, along with monitoring of somatosensory and motor evoked potentials. The patient is placed in the prone position, with the head secured in a Mayfield three-point fixation holder.

Surgical levels are identified and marked using lateral fluoroscopy and counting cephalad from the sacrum. Levels are confirmed with anteroposterior fluoroscopy by counting thoracic ribs. The authors commonly employ preoperative fiducial markers (**Fig. 34.3**). It is their experience that a fiducial marker placed at the level of the pedicle aids in minimizing operative time, decreases radiation exposure during the operation, and additionally adds safety in the correct localization of the surgical level. In particular, this is helpful in single-level cases in patients with poorly defined radiographic anatomy.

Skin infiltration is accomplished with a mixture of lidocaine and bupivacaine injected at the incision site.

34.3.2 Skin Entry

The skin entry point is incised 2.0 cm lateral to the midline in a rostral-caudal direction, for 20 to 24 mm.

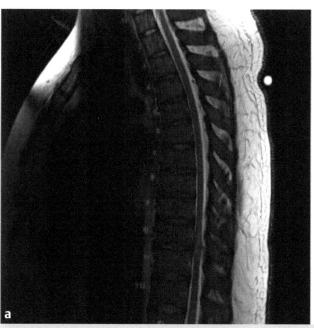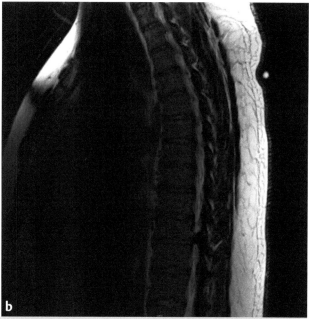

Fig. 34.1 Thoracic MRI demonstrates multilevel degenerative changes of the thoracic spine, superimposed upon prominent dorsal epidural fat. The changes are overall most pronounced at T10–T11, where there is a severe spinal canal stenosis as well as mild to moderate (right greater than left) bilateral neural foraminal stenosis. There is associated cord compression and focal, abnormal, hyperintense T2 signal within the thoracic spinal cord, centered on the T10–T11 level. (**a**) Midline sagittal cut; (**b**) sagittal cut on the right side.

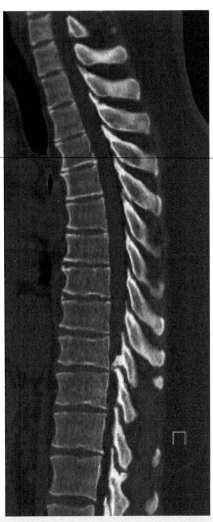

Fig. 34.2 Thoracic CT demonstrates heterotopic bone consistent with the potential ossification of the ligamentum flavum and hypertrophy of the facet. The bone is causing symptomatic compression of the spinal cord.

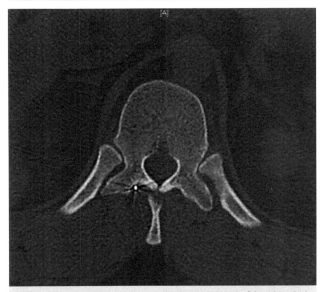

Fig. 34.3 Axial CT shows preoperatively placed fiducial, which facilitated docking and minimally invasive techniques intraoperatively. Interventional radiology placed the fiducial on the day before surgery.

34.3.3 Needle Insertion and Dilation

Either a microscope or an endoscope may be used for the procedure. Here we describe the technique with microscope assist. The same steps can be used with insertion of an endoscope.

The fascia is opened sharply with a No. 15 blade. A spinal needle is not used for docking (as would be done in a lumbar decompression). Instead, the soft tissue is focally spread in a narrow path (5–10 mm wide) down to the thoracic laminar facet junction. The first METRx (Medtronic Inc., Memphis, TN) dilator is then placed down this path with minimal medial angulation of the dilator. Placement is stopped short of the bone, and the location is checked on the lateral C-arm. After the C-arm imaging, we then advance further to bone and begin serial dilations.

Serial dilation is accomplished by insertion of the METRx dilation system into the incision and progressive replacement with successively larger dilators, one around the other, until the Quadrant retractor (Medtronic, Inc.) can be placed through the portal created by the dilators (**Fig. 34.4**). We dilate to a 24-mm diameter in many cases with advanced pathology. (However, in cases with focal, unilateral, or even focal bilateral compression, an 18-mm working channel is quite effective. The smaller working channels are easier to angle and manipulate in the soft tissue and are less likely to get "hung up" on the facet.)

A Quadrant retractor tube is placed and secured to the operating table by a flexible arm. At this juncture, we then angle the tube toward the midline hemilamina. Often, the location of the working channel (18- or 20-mm tubular portal or 24-mm Quadrant) is then confirmed on AP and lateral fluoroscopy.

34.3.4 Decompression

The Quadrant retractor is placed through the portal and expanded in the rostral–caudal direction to expose the lamina of the superior and inferior surgical borders (for example, T3–T5).

To define the laminar edges, curets are used. The soft tissue is removed with Bovie cautery, followed by multilevel hemilaminotomies with Kerrison rongeurs and a high-speed drill. We use the drill to initially remove the ipsilateral hemilamina down to the ligamentum flavum. It is only after ipsilateral removal that we work on the other side. To do so, we often will re-angle the working channel to add 5 to 10° of medial angulation. We then drill the contralateral hemilamina. Here, the surgeon is essentially undercutting the lamina from the inside.

During the removal of bone from the opposite side, the ligamentum flavum is kept intact. This protects the dura from injury during drilling. In the thoracic spine, unlike the lumbar spine, the surgeon cannot compress the dura during contralateral exposure. It is also important to note that during subsequent removal of the ligamentum, there is often a midline opening or fold in the ligamentum that can be used to aid in access to a plane below the ligament. For bilateral decompressions, we often use this to our advantage.

Finally, the same surgical steps are repeated for the lower end of the lesion (for example, T7–T9) on the contralateral side of the posterior tension band.

After decompression, we inspect to confirm a "pedicle-to-pedicle" decompression. However, different pathologies will have unique anatomical requirements. For multilevel cases, we often employ two separate working channels. For example, an epidural infection/bleed extending from T2–T8 may be accessed by two

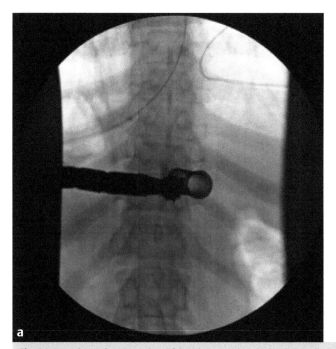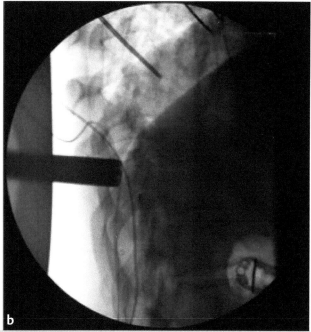

Fig. 34.4 Docking of METRx tube. A fiducial was used to dock a minimally invasive retractor at T10–T11. It was placed at the pedicle and then was used to dock at this site. An 18-mm METRx tube was docked on the hemilamina on this side. (**a**) Coronal and (**b**) sagittal images of the docking apparatus.

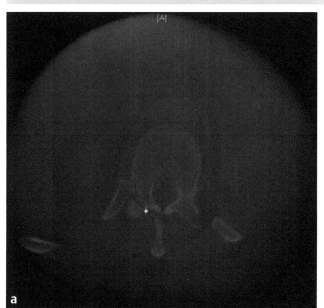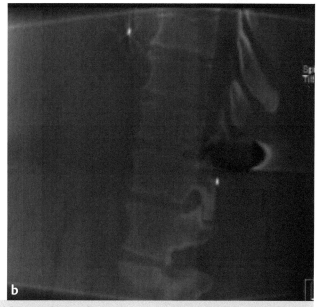

Fig. 34.5 Intraoperative CT is used to confirm correct level: (**a**) axial cut, and (**b**) sagittal cut confirming the location. After surgery, O-arm was used to confirm that all bone was removed.

incisions. The top incision on the left side will allow decompression of T2–T4, while the bottom right incision (also 2 cm off midline), allows T5–T8 access. After decompression of each level, the METRx tube is re-angled and docked at the site of decompression (**Fig. 34.5**).[1]

34.4 Complication Avoidance

Operations in the thoracic spine carry unique risks, whether the approach is open or minimally invasive. For minimally invasive access, the risk of surgery at the wrong level may be magnified. The lack of open anatomical landmarks, obfuscation of anatomy,

radiopaque retractors arms and retractors, and potential for poor radiographic detail in obese and osteoporotic patients can increase the risk of disorientation. In some cases, we have used the placement of preoperative fiducials to prevent issues with anatomical level and site.[2] We believe this is beneficial to both the surgeon who is new to minimally invasive techniques as well as experienced operators. The preoperative fiducial helps minimize fluoroscopy time at the beginning of the case and offers an easy "cross-check" with preoperative planning.

Docking the minimally invasive portal also can pose a significant risk in the thoracic spine. Misadventures with the K-wire or smaller dilators can lead to inadvertent placement in the intralaminar space and potential neurologic injury. Therefore, we do not use K-wires for thoracic decompressions. Focal dilation of an initial working channel is done with curved scissors, and the first dilator is the initial instrument placed on the bone. In addition, we often use a "straight up and down" docking technique. This ensures that the dilators are placed toward the facet or laminar/facet junction. Only after docking do we re-angle the working channel toward the midline.

Bilateral access with minimally invasive techniques can be challenging. To avoid retraction on the theca and contralateral decompression, we suggest frequent angling/repositioning of the Quadrant or METRx access portal. In addition, at times we have utilized either bilateral docking of a METRx tube or sequential left- then right-sided decompression.

Last, hemostasis during closure is critical for these cases. Because there is a small anatomical potential space, even a small hematoma can lead to severe symptoms. Following decompression, all bleeding bone edges are thoroughly waxed, epidural veins are coagulated, and Surgifoam is placed in the lateral gutters. When needed, we have a low threshold for placing a medium Hemovac drain down the working channel. It can be left in place as the channel is removed from the site of decompression.

References

1   Smith ZA, Lawton CD, Wong AP, et al. Minimally invasive thoracic decompression for multi-level thoracic pathologies. *J Clin Neurosci* 2014;21(3):467–472
2   Upadhyaya CD, Wu JC, Chin CT, Balamurali G, Mummaneni PV. Avoidance of wrong-level thoracic spine surgery: intraoperative localization with preoperative percutaneous fiducial screw placement. *J Neurosurg Spine* 2012;16(3):280–284

35 Thoracoscopic Decompression and Fixation for Thoracic and Thoracolumbar Junction Lesions

Ricky Raj S. Kalra, Meic H. Schmidt, and Rudolf Beisse

35.1 Indications

- Anterior reconstruction of unstable fractures of the thoracic spine and thoracolumbar junction[1]
- Posttraumatic and degenerative narrowing of the spinal canal[2]
- Disk–ligament instability
- Posttraumatic deformity of healed fractures with or without instability[3]
- Revision surgery (i.e., implant removal, infection, implant failure and loosening)[4]
- Preparation and release of the anterior column in tumor and metastasis
- Sympathectomy for hyperhidrosis[5]
- Protruded disk removal in degenerative disk disease of the thoracic spine[6]
- Resection of metastatic spinal tumors[7]

35.2 Equipment

35.2.1 Trocars

Reusable, flexible, threaded trocars with a diameter of 11 mm are used. Black trocars eliminate reflection. Air insufflation is not required, and thus valves within the trocars are not necessary.

35.2.2 Image Transmission

A high-intensity xenon light source is required to illuminate the thoracic cavity. A rigid, long, 30° endoscope enables positioning of the camera far away from the working portal, thus facilitating undisturbed working and variable adjustment of the angle of vision. The intraoperative view is transmitted onto two or three flat screens.

35.3 Technique

35.3.1 Preoperative Requirements

Pulmonary function testing and assessment for respiratory therapy should be done preoperatively with single-lung ventilation. Bowel preparation is completed to decrease intraabdominal pressure and tension on the diaphragm.

35.3.2 Anesthesia

General anesthesia is used with double-lumen tube intubation and single-lung ventilation. Bronchoscopy confirms tube positioning.

35.3.3 Patient Positioning

The patient is placed in the lateral position, with the approach side determined by great vessels and location of pathology. The patient is stabilized with four supports and a special U-shaped cushion for the legs (**Fig. 35.1**).

35.3.4 Designing the Entry Portals

Four portals are used: the scope portal, working portal, suction–irrigation portal, and retractor portal. Their location and, in particular, the position of the working portal are crucial for endoscopic surgery.

The lesion is first displayed in the lateral projection (with reference to the patient's body) under precise adjustment of the image intensifier, and a marker is used to draw the injured spinal section on the lateral abdominal and thoracic wall. Careful attention is paid to correct projection of the vertebrae, whose end plates and anterior and posterior margins should be displayed in the central beam, in sharp focus with no double contour. This marking is taken as the sole reference for subsequent placement of the portals.

The working portal is drawn in directly above the lesion. The trocar for the endoscope is marked either caudal or cranial to the working portal, depending on the height of the lesion, and following the axis of the spine. The distance from the working portal is approximately two intercostal spaces.

The entry points for suction and irrigation and for the retractor are then located ventral to these portals (**Fig. 35.1c**).

35.3.5 Localization and Port Entry: Approach to the Thoracolumbar Junction

Anterior Reconstruction Landmarks

Landmarks are set under image intensifier control to serve as orientation points for the surgeon and camera operator during the subsequent course of the operation (**Video 35.1**). For this, the K-wires associated with the implant are used; the K-wires define the later position of the cannulated screws, and they are placed near the end plates between the posterior and central thirds of the vertebra. To achieve this in the thoracolumbar junction region, the psoas muscle must be mobilized in a ventral to dorsal direction, thus avoiding irritation of the fibers of the lumbar plexus.

Positioning of the K-wires near the end plates avoids injury to the segment vessels, and the screws are anchored in a region of higher bone density (**Fig. 35.2**).

Preparation of the Segment Vessels

The pleura is opened along the connecting line between the K-wires, and the segment vessels are exposed with a Cobb periosteal raspatory. The vessels are mobilized subperiosteally from both sides, ligated twice with titanium clips ventrally and dorsally, and raised slightly with a nerve hook.

The vessels are dissected with the endoscopic hook scissors. The lateral aspects of the vertebral body and the disks are exposed with the raspatory (**Video 35.1**).

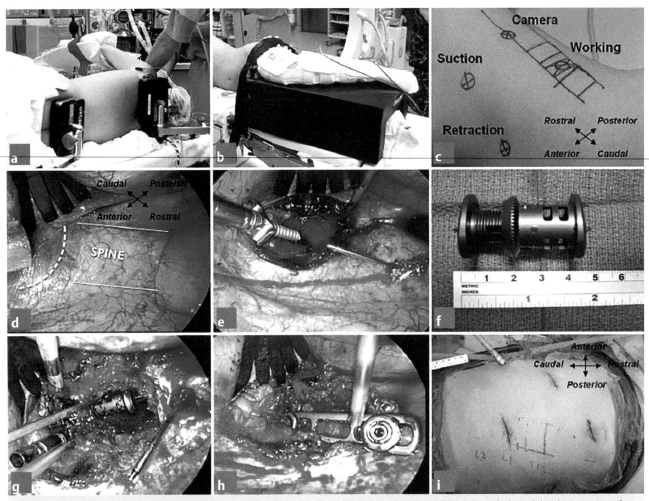

Fig. 35.1 Thoracoscopic decompression and fixation. (**a**) The patient is positioned on a radiolucent table in the right lateral decubitus position for a left-sided thoracoscopic approach to L1. The independent arm is in a Krause frame. Adjustable pads at the pubis, sternum, and lower and upper spine hold the patient in position. (**b**) The independent leg is slightly flexed at the hip to facilitate iliopsoas relaxation, making it easier to dissect this muscle off the lateral aspect of the vertebral bodies at the thoracolumbar junction. (**c**) The level of interest is marked, identifying the vertebral body above and below, and the four chest portals are planned. (**d**) Endoscopic view of the spine (*solid lines*). The diaphragm is swept inferiorly with a fan retractor and a diaphragmatic incision is planned (*dotted lines*). (**e**) A K-wire is placed above the planned corpectomy, and a polyaxial screw-clamp combination is placed below it. (**f**) Lateral view of a fully expanded gear-driven cage. (**g**) The cage is placed and expanded within the central corpectomy. (**h**) Final anterolateral plate construct. (**i**) Closure with chest tube exiting the retraction port. (Used with permission from Ragel BT, Amini A, Schmidt MH. Thoracoscopic vertebral body replacement with an expandable cage after ventral spinal canal decompression. *Neurosurgery* 2007;61(5 Suppl 2):ONS319.)

35.3.6 Instrumentation

Cannulated Screw Insertion

The K-wires are overdrilled with a cannulated broach, and the lateral cortex of the vertebral body is opened (**Video 35.1**).

The working trocar is exchanged for a speculum through a switching stick, and the clamping element is tightened with a screw. The length of the screw has been previously measured against the preoperative CT scan and subsequently defines whether a monocortical or bicortical screw fixation is attempted. The direction of the screw can be altered after removal of the K-wire and checked in both planes under C-arm monitoring.

The connecting line between the screws and the anterior boundary of the clamping elements now defines an area of safety within which the partial removal of the vertebral body and the disks is performed. The ventral and dorsal extent of the partial corpectomy thus defined also then corresponds to the dimensions of the planned vertebral body replacement, which has a transverse diameter between 16 mm (thoracic) and 20 mm (lumbar) (**Fig. 35.3**).

The intervertebral disks are incised laterally with a long-handled knife, and the disk space is opened with a slightly offset osteotome (**Video 35.1**).

The posterior osteotomy is then performed with a straight osteotome from disk space to disk space on the connecting line between the screws. The scale on the osteotome shows the corresponding depth, which in the anterior direction should be about two thirds of the diameter of the vertebra. The line of the anterior osteotomy runs along the anterior boundary of the clamping elements; an osteotome that is slightly angled to the rear is used to be certain of avoiding unintentional perforation of the anterior vertebral wall (and adjacent vessels).

The central section of the vertebral body is removed with a rongeur, and the removed cancellous bone is preserved for later implantation adjacent to the vertebral body replacement (**Video**

35.1). In cases of metastatic disease, the bone is collected and sent for pathological analysis as part of the specimen.

Using a curet and rongeurs, the intervertebral disks are then resected and the end plates are rasped with box cutters. When titanium cages are implanted, any weakening of the load-bearing end plates must be avoided. In monosegmental fusion with a tricortical pelvic crest graft, the subchondral bone lamella on the cranial end plate is removed to assist healing of the bone graft.

Insertion of the Bone Graft

In monosegmental reconstructions and fusion, a tricortical bone graft taken from the iliac crest is used.

After the corpectomy defect has been measured, the iliac crest is prepared and exposed. By using an oscillating saw and chisel, the bone graft is harvested and firmly connected to a graft holder. The graft is inserted into the defect in a centered position; the position has to be checked fluoroscopically in both planes (**Video 35.1**).

For vertebral body replacement in a bisegmental reconstruction, we mostly use the hydraulic Hydrolift (Aesculap, Center Valley, PA) with continuously variable distraction and adaptation of the end plates.

Before the vertebral replacement is implanted, the extent and clean preparation of the implant site in the anterior sagittal direction and in its depth should be verified by palpation with a probe hook under image intensifier control.

Two Langenbeck hooks are inserted into the incision for the working portals, and the incision is widened slightly. The vertebral body replacement is then gradually introduced through the chest wall into the thoracic cavity and positioned over the defect in the vertebral body with a holder. Once again, it is determined that no soft tissue, in particular the ligated segment vessels, has slipped between the corpectomy defect and the vertebral body replacement.

The vertebral body replacement device is then implanted into the planned central position in the vertebral body and distracted. The implant is surrounded with cancellous bone harvested from the partial corpectomy or frozen allograft bone.

Ventral Instrumentation with a Constraint Plate Implant

Because the screws and so-called clamping elements belonging to the implant were placed into position as a first step before the beginning of the partial corpectomy, at this point the plate just has to be fastened and the ventral screws of the four-point fixation inserted (**Video 35.1**). The distance between the screws is defined with a special measuring instrument to select a plate of the correct length.

The plate is introduced lengthwise into the thoracic cavity through the incision for the working portal, laid onto the clamping elements with a holding forceps, and definitively fixed with nuts with a starting torque of 15 Nm. The plate can be brought into direct bone contact with the lateral vertebral body wall by tightening the bone screws. The ventral screws are inserted after temporary fixation of a targeting device and opening of the cortex.

Because of the heart shape of the vertebral body, the ventral screws are usually 5 mm shorter than the dorsal screws. The fixation of the angle-stable implant ends with the insertion of a locking screw that locks the polyaxial mechanism of the dorsal screws (**Fig. 35.4**).

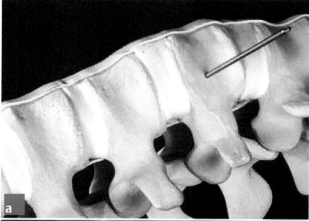

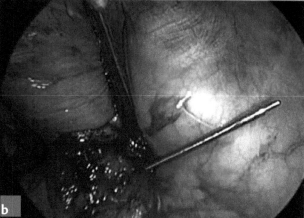

Fig. 35.2 (a) The entry point for the caudal screw is positioned ~ 10 mm ventral to the spinal canal and 10 mm away from the end plate in the upper third of the vertebra. **(b)** A K-wire is driven with a mallet into position away from the midportion of the vertebral body where the segmental blood vessels lie.

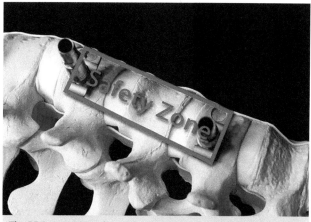

Fig. 35.3 Operative safe zone between cannulated screws for removing anterior lesions, herniated disks, or tumors. The cannulated screws provide a cranial/caudal and anteroposterior safe zone. Courtesy of the Department of Neurosurgery, University of Utah.

Final Stages of the Endoscopic Operation

In every case, radiographs are taken in both planes with the C-arm to check the decompression and position of the implants before the operation is concluded (**Video 35.1**).

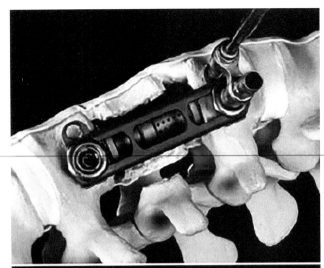

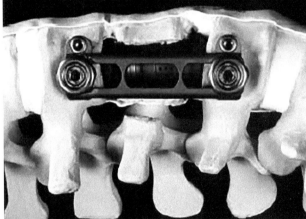

Fig. 35.4 After fixation nuts are secured and the entire assembly is tightened, ventral stabilizing screws are placed through the screw guide sleeve. The construct is completed after securing the locking screws, converting the polyaxial screw-clamp system into a rigid construct.

For operations on the thoracolumbar junction that include incision of the diaphragmatic attachment, an incision longer than 2 cm should be closed with endoscopic suturing. Two or three adapting sutures are sufficient, depending on the extent of the incision. The suture does not need to be watertight.

The entire thoracic cavity is again inspected endoscopically, and the site is irrigated and cleaned of blood residue.

A 20 Charrière thoracic drainage tube is inserted through the suction–irrigation portal. The instruments are removed under endoscopic monitoring.

After consultation with the anesthesiologist, the lung is reinflated and ventilated. The complete reinflation of the lung is checked endoscopically before the endoscope is removed.

In the four incisions for the portals, adapting sutures are applied to the musculature, and the skin is closed by suturing.

The thoracic drainage is connected to a water seal chamber, and suction of 15 cm H_2O is applied.

The patient is usually extubated while still on the operating table. The chest tube is usually kept in place for 24 hours. A postoperative chest X-ray is obtained immediately and again the morning after the procedure. The chest tube is connected to a water seal the next morning and removed on postoperative day 2.

35.4 Conclusion

In the past 10 years, endoscopic procedures on the spine have become an alternative to standardized spine surgery. Through the transdiaphragmatic approach, it has been possible to open up the thoracolumbar junction, including the retroperitoneal segments of the spine, by way of an endoscopic technique. With the extension of the technique to the retroperitoneal sections of the thoracolumbar junction, it became possible to increase the indication spectrum of the endoscopic technique substantially, so that it includes complete fracture treatment with vertebral body replacement and ventral instrumentation as well as anterior decompression of the spinal canal in posttraumatic, metastatic, and degenerative pathologic processes. The complication rate of the endoscopic procedure is on the same scale as that for open procedures, with clear advantages in terms of the reduced access morbidity associated with the minimally invasive technique.

References

1 Beisse R. Video-assisted techniques in the management of thoracolumbar fractures. *Orthop Clin North Am* 2007;*38*(3):419–429, abstract vii
2 Beisse R, Mückley T, Schmidt MH, Hauschild M, Bühren V. Surgical technique and results of endoscopic anterior spinal canal decompression. *J Neurosurg Spine* 2005;*2*(2):128–136
3 Beisse R, Trapp O. Thoracoscopic management of spinal trauma. *Oper Tech Neurosurg* 2005;*8*(4):205–213
4 Beisse R. Endoscopic surgery on the thoracolumbar junction of the spine. *Eur Spine J* 2006;*15*(6):687–704
5 Dickman CA, Rosenthal DJ, Perin NI. *Thoracoscopic Spine Surgery*. New York: Thieme; 1999
6 Rosenthal D, Rosenthal R, Simone A. Removal of a protruded disc using micro-surgery endoscopy. *Spine* 1994;*19*:1087–1091
7 Schmidt M. Minimally invasive thoracoscopic approach for anterior decompression and stabilization of metastatic spine disease. *Neurosurg Focus* 2008;*25*(2):E8

36 Endoscopic Approaches to Thoracic Tumors, Trauma, and Infection

Christopher C. Gillis and John O'Toole

36.1 Introduction

A variety of surgical approaches have been proposed and implemented in the treatment of thoracic spine pathology, with the latest advancements geared toward minimally invasive options.[1,2,3,4,5,6] The direct open posterior approach can be used in cases of purely dorsal disease but otherwise is unfavorable in the thoracic region due to the requirement for retraction of the thoracic cord instead of cauda equina nerve roots.[4,5,6,7] The thoracic cord is especially sensitive to minimal retraction, and this has been postulated to be the cause of the relatively poor outcomes that had traditionally been seen with posterior approaches to more central and ventral pathology.[1,4] This has led surgeons away from direct posterior approaches to postero-lateral approaches, including both costotransversectomy and transpedicular trajectories, which used more extensive bone removal to minimize manipulation of neurologic structures and have thus been shown to be much safer than a direct posterior approach. These posterolateral approaches, however, result in removal of supportive bone structures that often necessitates fusion for prevention of postoperative instability and can also lead to increased postoperative pain and morbidity. Open anterior and lateral approaches have also been used, and are associated with complications related to the approach through the thoracic cavity, such as risk of injury to vital thoracic structures and vessels, pulmonary contusion, hemothorax, chylothorax, intraoperative and postoperative difficulty with ventilation, shoulder girdle dysfunction, and difficulty with wound healing.[4]

36.2 Minimally Invasive Approaches

Minimally invasive options include endoscopic lateral retropleural decompression, minimally invasive transpedicular decompression, and thoracic microendoscopic decompression (TMED).[4] TMED is a modification of the lumbar microendoscopic technique. Benefits of this approach include sparing of the majority pedicle, which must be removed in the transpedicular approach, and the avoidance of rib resection, required in the lateral retropleural approach.[4,5,6] Use of the endoscope is not required for visualization during this approach, and a similar approach using tubular muscle retractors can be used for a variety of thoracic pathologies, with the use of loupe, microscope, or endoscopic visualization.[5,6] Once a laminectomy is performed through either a direct posterior approach or a more lateral transpedicular approach, depending on the angle of pathology presenting, both ventral and dorsal decompression can be achieved, as well as durotomy and resection of intradural lesions. Tredway et al[8] successfully adapted a minimally invasive unilateral laminotomy approach for resection of intradural extramedullary lesions in both the cervical and thoracic spine. The lateral retropleural approach allows easier access for vertebral body decompression and can be performed in a fashion very similar to lateral lumbar interbody fusion (LLIF),

using the same retractor system with long retraction blades. For cases of trauma or instability related to tumor or approach, instrumentation can be achieved through the use of percutaneous screw placement with fluoroscopic or navigation guidance.

36.3 Choice of Patient

36.3.1 Indications

The choice of minimally invasive approach depends on the area to be decompressed, the presence or absence of instability, and the primary location of the pathology. As an example, ventral decompression can be achieved through both the transpedicular and direct lateral retropleural approach, with the lateral retropleural ideal for more central ventral pathology than can be reached through a transpedicular approach. Direct dorsal decompression or paramedian dorsal decompression can be achieved through a more direct posterior approach. Once decompression is achieved, for tumor, trauma, or infection, the next step is determination of the presence of instability, which would require supplemental instrumentation with percutaneous pedicle screw and rod placement.

In the direct lateral approach, as in LLIF, vertebrectomy and cage placement can be used in cases of severe burst fracture or significant bony infiltration of tumor.[9,10] In cases of metastases, however, the need for complete tumor resection has been minimized through the concept of separation surgery,[11,12] which requires decompression of the neural elements with adjuvant (often stereotactic) radiotherapy for treatment. A minimally invasive corpectomy can also be performed through a posterolateral approach by taking a more lateral trajectory (average of 6 cm off midline) and approaching through a corridor similar to that used for an open costotransversectomy.

36.3.2 Contraindications

As in most minimally invasive procedures, the approach is limited by the retractor size and thus is left mostly to lesions spanning one to two spinal levels. Some surgeons have successfully performed staggered contralateral skip laminectomies for larger lesions. Primary bony tumors requiring complete vertebrectomy in the thoracic area are likely best approached through a combination of anterior and posterior approaches, which may involve a combination of minimally invasive and open techniques.[13]

36.4 Procedure

36.4.1 Level Identification

One of the most important steps, irrespective of the technique used, is appropriate identification of the surgical level. Identification of the surgical level in the thoracic spine is more difficult than in the cervical or lumbar spine, where counting of levels facilitates knowledge of the appropriate level. This is due to the distance of the thoracic spine from the skull or sacrum, individual variance in regional anatomy and the number of ribs that can be used for counting, and poor fluoroscopic penetration in upper thoracic levels—especially in patients with increased subcutaneous fat. We have found that careful preoperative examination of ribs and levels combined with careful fluoroscopic intraoperative counting has allowed identification of the appropriate level. Other described adjuncts for level identification include percutaneous placement of radiographic skin markers, percutaneous placement of a radiopaque marker at the periosteum of the pedicle of interest, percutaneous injection of methylene blue dye, and even preoperative vertebroplasty; however, none of these adjuncts has gained widespread use.[14] Depending on the procedure being performed, intraoperative neuronavigation can help with the identification of level, but it requires an intraoperative CT scan and is not usually of benefit in cases without instrumentation placement. At our center, we rely on anatomical landmarks and level counting with both lateral and anteroposterior fluoroscopic views.

36.4.2 Decompression

The lateral transpedicular or direct dorsal decompressive procedure is done with the patient in the prone position and under general anesthetic, in a fashion similar to minimally invasive laminectomy elsewhere in the spine. A radiolucent Jackson table with appropriate chest and hip pads facilitates use of fluoroscopy during the case. Arms can be tucked with sheets for upper thoracic cases, and positioned on arm boards for lower thoracic cases, with care to appropriately pad the elbows, and especially the ulnar nerve, as well avoiding extension of the arms greater than 90°. It is the practice of many surgeons to obtain continuous somatosensory evoked potentials throughout the procedure. Some advocate for motor evoked potentials (MEP) as well.

Once the appropriate level has been identified and marked as described above, an incision is made between 3 and 4 cm lateral to the midline. In cases where thoracic corpectomy is to be performed, an even more lateral trajectory is desired, which averages 6 cm from midline. In obese patients or patients with an increased amount of subcutaneous tissue, it is useful to take a more lateral trajectory. The goal of entering laterally is to minimize manipulation of the thecal sac and spinal cord during the procedure. Through the incision, a K-wire is inserted at the rostral side of the caudal transverse process of the level of interest. Serial tubular muscle dilators are then placed over the K-wire under fluoroscopic guidance. Care is taken to ensure the K-wire remains

on bone throughout the dilation, to prevent migration. After dilation is complete, the tubular retractor is placed over the dilators and fixed to the rigid retractor arm, attached to the operating table. Through the tubular retractor, a microscope, loupes, and a headlight or an endoscope with a 30° lens can be used for visualization. When using the endoscope, it is useful to orient the scope so that medial is located at the top of the monitor and lateral at the bottom, bringing the rostral-caudal axis along the horizontal.

Remnant muscle and soft tissue at the bottom of the tubular retractor is then dissected away using monopolar cautery and can be removed from the field with a pituitary rongeur. With this small amount of soft tissue removal, the proximal transverse process and the lateral facet are exposed. The tubular retractor can be adjusted to bring the facet–transverse process junction into the middle of the field of view for optimal working exposure. The high-speed drill is then used to remove the rostral aspect of the inferior transverse process and the lateral facet until the pedicle of the caudal vertebral body is exposed. The pedicle is then followed ventrally to identify the disk space; drilling a portion of the rostral aspect of this pedicle allows a better working corridor into the disk space if this is required, such as in a case of diskitis. Due to the lateral trajectory, minimal to no manipulation of the thecal sac is required. Laterally placed tumor, bone fragment, or abscess is readily identified and more medial pathology can be dissected away from the thecal sac, underneath the annulus, with downpushing curets into the disk space or resection cavity, where they are then safely retrieved.

In thoracic corpectomy through the posterior approach, greater bony removal involves resection of a longer segment of the rib from medial to lateral. This provides a greater space for expansion and angling of a retractor for visualization. From a unilateral approach, the disk above, the vertebral body, and the disk below can all be resected through a combination of curets and drilling. After bone removal, an expandable intervertebral cage can be placed, supported by the remaining cortical bone from the contralateral side. If contralateral decompression is desired, a bilateral approach can be used. An illustration of the approach angle and bone removal is seen in **Fig. 36.1a,** and postoperative CT from a thoracic minimally invasive corpectomy is seen in **Fig. 36.1b**.

After decompression, the field is irrigated and meticulous hemostasis is achieved, especially in the muscle edges, which are carefully inspected as the tubular retractor is removed. Absorbable Vicryl sutures are used in the fascia and then in the subcutaneous tissue. For the skin, skin glue, a continuous subcuticular monofilament suture, or skin tape can be used to augment the subcutaneous stitch.

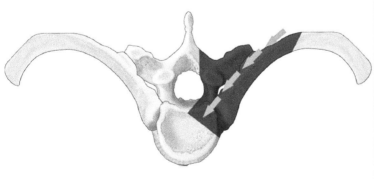
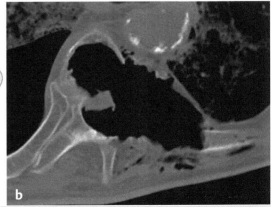

Fig. 36.1 (a) Illustration of the trajectory (*arrows*) and bone removal (*coloration*) in minimally invasive posterior approach for thoracic corpectomy. (b) CT scan of cadaveric model illustrating postoperative results of a left-sided minimally invasive posterior approach for thoracic corpectomy.

36.4.3 Lateral Retropleural Approach

For the lateral retropleural approach, the patient is placed in the lateral decubitus position with either the left or right side up, depending upon the side of the pathology and the great vessels. All pressure points are padded adequately and, as mentioned, neuromonitoring is performed. The fluoroscopic C-arm is positioned and draped to allow acquisition of lateral and anteroposterior X-ray images of the operative area. The incision is marked with fluoroscopy so as to be directly above the posterior vertebral body border of the index level and spinal canal. Following appropriate localization, a 2-cm incision is made and is carried down to the rib using monopolar cautery. The space between the ribs can be limited, and removal of part of the rib using a Kerrison rongeur can widen the interspace for retractor placement. Blunt dissection between the pleura and the rib is carried down as far as possible, down to the head of the rib. Though the exposure can be completely extrapleural, the pleural cavity is often entered, and this is not usually an issue as long as the visceral pleura is not violated. The rib head usually lies over the pedicle disk space and the spinal canal. The initial dilator is then introduced into the thoracic cavity and is passed posteriorly along the ribs down the intersection of the rib head and spine.

After insertion of further dilators, the final working portal is introduced and centered over the identified area of pathology—e.g., the disk space or the vertebral body. The retractors are then secured to the table in the standard fashion and can be expanded if needed to enhance the exposure. The operative microscope is then brought into the field. The heads of the ribs are identified. After removal of the head of the rib with a pneumatic drill, the pedicle is exposed. Partial drilling of the pedicle exposes the dura and the disk space. Decompression can be achieved using a combination of a Kerrison punch, curets, and pituitary rongeurs to adequately decompress the dura. After decompression and, when needed, reconstruction, a red rubber catheter is then inserted in the thoracic cavity. The wound is then closed in layers, with several interrupted 2–0 Vicryl sutures used for the musculature; the red rubber catheter is pulled out at the closure of the subcutaneous tissue under Valsalva maneuver, allowing evacuation of air and blood products from the pleural cavity. Subcutaneous tissue is closed with absorbable sutures followed by application of Dermabond over the skin. Placement of a chest tube is not routinely required.

36.5 Complications Avoidance

Routine postoperative chest X-ray is indicated to monitor for postoperative pneumothorax. If present, the pneumothorax usually resolves with 100% oxygen by face mask or nasal prongs. During anesthesia for patients with cord compression, it is prudent to maintain a mean arterial pressure of at least 80 mm Hg or above to maintain adequate spinal perfusion pressure, which is especially important in the watershed area of the thoracic spine. As already mentioned, identification of the appropriate level is critical in the thoracic spine, where landmarks and counting can be extremely difficult, depending on the morphology of the patient.

36.6 Case Examples

36.6.1 Case 1

A 27-year-old firefighter presented with acute thoracic back pain after lifting a heavy object. He had no known history of infection or intravenous drug use or any risk factors for immunodeficiency. MRI showed a T7–T8 dorsal epidural enhancing fluid collection (**Fig. 36.2**). Blood cultures were negative and the patient's pain was uncontrollable with patient-controlled analgesia. Options, including empiric medical therapy and surgery, were discussed with the patient and he elected to proceed with a minimally invasive decompression, which would also provide samples for culture. A right-sided posterior thoracic laminectomy was performed through an 18-mm fixed tubular retractor and the operative microscope. Intraoperative cultures were obtained.

Postoperatively (**Fig. 36.3**), the patient's pain improved within 24 hours and the intraoperative culture demonstrated methicillin-sensitive *Staphylococcus aureus*. The patient was placed on home IV therapy and had clinical and radiographic improvement by the sixth postoperative week. Per the recommendation of the infectious disease service, he was maintained on IV antibiotics for a total of 8 weeks.

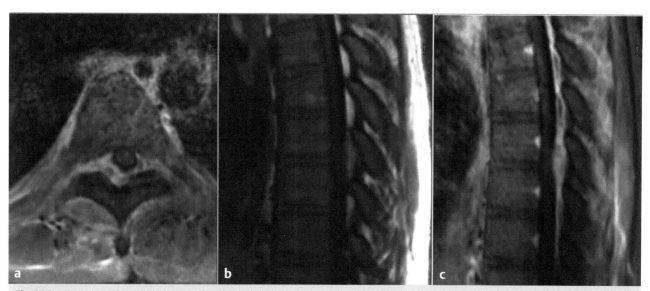

Fig. 36.2 Preoperative MRI. (**a**) Axial T1-weighted image with gadolinium contrast showing small right-sided dorsal enhancing epidural fluid collection at the level of the T7–T8 facets. (**b**) Sagittal T1-weighted MRI without gadolinium contrast and (**c**) sagittal T1-weighted image with gadolinium contrast showing the small dorsal epidural fluid collection enhancing at the T7–T8 level.

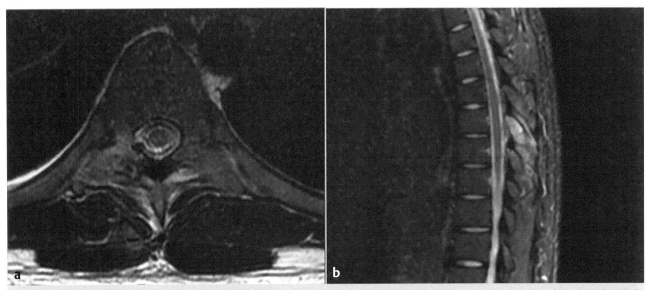

Fig. 36.3 (a) Axial and (b) sagittal images from postoperative T2-weighted MRI showing the limited extent of tissue disruption from the right-sided minimally invasive approach and the improvement in focal compression of the thecal sac.

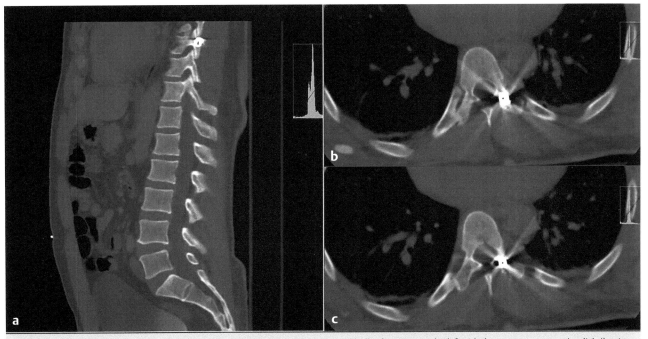

Fig. 36.4 Preoperative (a) sagittal and (b,c) axial CT scan views showing a retained bullet fragment in the left-sided transverse process/pedicle/laminar junction at the level of T9.

36.6.2 Case 2

A 48-year-old male presented with neck, midthoracic, and low back pain radiating into the buttocks bilaterally. He had a history of a T9 gunshot wound 3 months before presentation, with no previous surgery and a retained bullet. He did not have any neurologic symptoms. CT demonstrated a bullet at T9 lodged in the transverse process/pedicle/laminar junction without any canal compromise (**Fig. 36.4**). MRI was not performed due to the retained metal from the bullet.

Nonoperative management and the option of minimally invasive surgery to remove the bullet fragment, with the possibility of its improving his midthoracic pain, were both discussed with the patient. He elected operative management. A minimally invasive T9 laminectomy on the left was performed using a 20-mm retraction tube (**Fig. 36.5**). The bone around the bullet was drilled and then a combination of curets was used to remove the fragment.

36.6.3 Case 3

A 19-year-old female presented with a two-year history of midthoracic back pain with intercostal radiation along the right lateral thorax. She originally treated the pain with ibuprofen, but when the pain did not resolve, she underwent imaging. The patient was neurologically intact. Both

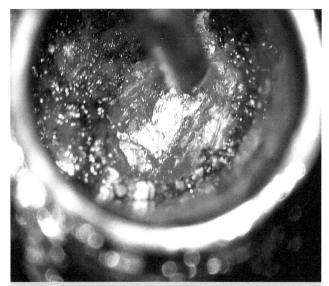

Fig. 36.5 Intraoperative view through 20-mm retractor showing bullet fragment within T9.

MRI and CT were performed, showing T2 hyperintense, contrast-enhancing lesion within the right posteroinferior portion of the T7 vertebral body; the lesion was noted to have a sclerotic nidus (**Fig. 36.6**). The results of a CT-guided biopsy were osteoid osteoma.

A right-sided direct lateral retropleural approach for lesion resection and partial thoracic corpectomy was performed. With the patient in the lateral decubitus position, a 3-cm incision was made and a direct lateral lumbar fusion retractor system was used. The proximal rib was resected to make space for the retractor and the retropleural dissection was bluntly performed; the retractor blades held the lung and pleural contents out of the field. After removal of the hypertrophic soft tissue adjacent to the spine and lesion, an osteotome was used to remove an en bloc portion of the vertebral body in the area of the lesion for pathology. Additional curetting was performed through the resulting defect until the extradural space was reached.

Postoperatively, the patient did very well, with resolution of her pain and pathology confirmation of osteoid osteoma. Postoperative images are shown in **Fig. 36.7**.

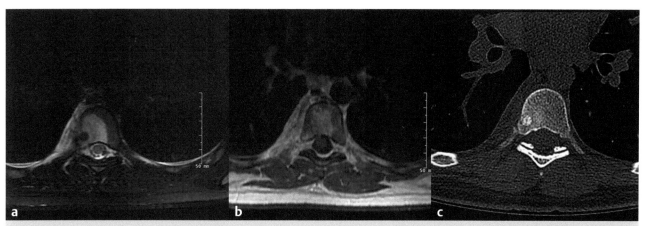

Fig. 36.6 Series of axial MRI images. (**a**) T2-weighted image illustrates edema within the T7 vertebral body with hypertrophic and edematous soft tissue along the right side of the spinal column; the lesion itself is hypointense. (**b**) T1-weighted post-gadolinium image showing that the lesion is contrast enhancing. (**c**) Axial CT image showing the sclerotic nature of the lesion, consistent with osteoid osteoma.

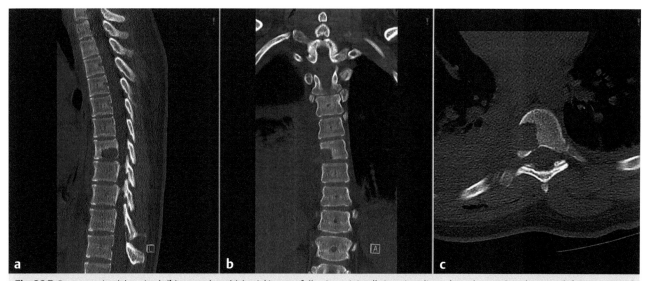

Fig. 36.7 Postoperative (**a**) sagittal, (**b**) coronal, and (**c**) axial images following minimally invasive, direct, lateral, retropleural approach for resection of osteoid osteoma within the right posteroinferior vertebral body of T7.

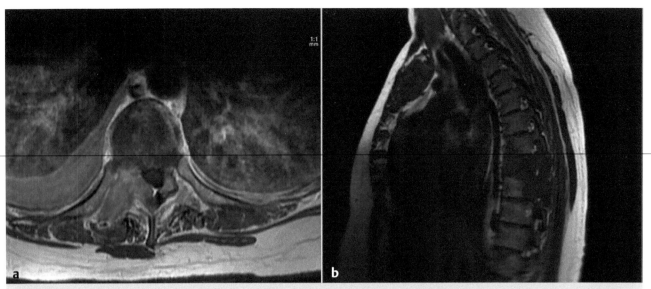

Fig. 36.8 (a) Axial post-gadolinium T1-weighted MRI at T9 showing contrast-enhancing lesion within the lamina, transverse process, and pedicle on the right side causing stenosis of the thoracic spinal canal and compression of the thoracic cord. (b) Sagittal T2-weighted image showing hypointense lesion within the vertebral body and posterior elements of T8 and the posterior elements of T9 on the left.

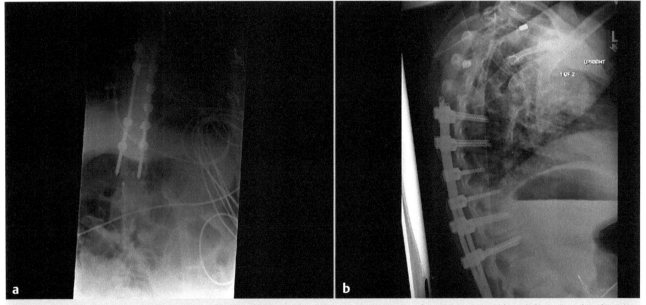

Fig. 36.9 Postoperative (a) anteroposterior and (b) lateral radiographs showing instrumentation from T6 to T11, with pedicle screws placed on the right at levels where left transpedicular decompression was performed.

36.6.4 Case 4

A 56-year-old woman presented with a persistent cough for 6 months; initially she was treated for pneumonia, but she was found on subsequent imaging to have lung and liver nodules. Imaging of the neuraxis showed multiple brain and spine lesions, with a large lesion at T8–T9. She did not have any neurologic symptoms.

MRI (**Fig. 36.8**) showed a contrast-enhancing lesion at T8–T9 on the right, involving mostly the posterior elements and the pedicle. At the T9 level, the mass of the lesion was causing canal stenosis, but the compression and stenosis were minimal at T8.

The patient underwent mini-open right-sided T8–T9 laminectomies and transpedicular decompression followed by T6–T11

percutaneous image-guided placement of pedicle screw and rod instrumentation. One single midline incision was made, with the fascia opened only over T8 and T9. The skin was retracted laterally for placement of the percutaneous screws through separate fascial incisions. To achieve decompression, the T8 nerve root was sacrificed on the right. Postoperative images are shown in **Fig. 36.9**.

References

1. Stillerman CB, Chen TC, Couldwell WT, Zhang W, Weiss MH. Experience in the surgical management of 82 symptomatic herniated thoracic discs and review of the literature. *J Neurosurg* 1998;88(4):623–633
2. Perez-Cruet MJ, Kim BS, Sandhu F, Samartzis D, Fessler RG. Thoracic microendoscopic discectomy. *J Neurosurg Spine* 2004;1(1):58–63

3   Dalbayrak S, Yaman O, Oztürk K, Yılmaz M, Gökdağ M, Ayten M. Transforaminal approach in thoracal disc pathologies: transforaminal microdiscectomy technique. *Minim Invasive Surg* 2014;*2014*:301945

4   Smith JS, Eichholz KM, Shafizadeh S, Ogden AT, O'Toole JE, Fessler RG. Minimally invasive thoracic microendoscopic diskectomy: surgical technique and case series. *World Neurosurg* 2013;*80*(3-4):421–427

5   Snyder LA, Smith ZA, Dahdaleh NS, Fessler RG. Minimally invasive treatment of thoracic disc herniations. *Neurosurg Clin N Am* 2014;*25*(2):271–277

6   Smith ZA, Lawton CD, Wong AP, et al. Minimally invasive thoracic decompression for multi-level thoracic pathologies. *J Clin Neurosci* 2014;*21*(3):467–472

7   Awwad EE, Martin DS, Smith KR Jr, Baker BK. Asymptomatic versus symptomatic herniated thoracic discs: their frequency and characteristics as detected by computed tomography after myelography. *Neurosurgery* 1991;*28*(2):180–186

8   Tredway TL, Santiago P, Hrubes MR, Song JK, Christie SD, Fessler RG. Minimally invasive resection of intradural-extramedullary spinal neoplasms. *Neurosurgery* 2006

9   Karikari IO, Nimjee SM, Hardin CA, et al. Extreme lateral interbody fusion approach for isolated thoracic and thoracolumbar spine diseases: initial clinical experience and early outcomes. *J Spinal Disord Tech* 2011;*24*(6):368–375

10 Park MS, Deukmedjian AR, Uribe JS. Minimally invasive anterolateral corpectomy for spinal tumors. *Neurosurg Clin N Am* 2014;*25*(2):317–325

11 Bilsky MH, Laufer I, Burch S. Shifting paradigms in the treatment of metastatic spine disease. *Spine* 2009;*34*(22, Suppl):S101–S107

12 Amankulor NM, Xu R, Iorgulescu JB, et al. The incidence and patterns of hardware failure after separation surgery in patients with spinal metastatic tumors. *Spine J* 2014;*14*(9):1850–1859

13 Fang T, Dong J, Zhou X, McGuire RA Jr, Li X. Comparison of mini-open anterior corpectomy and posterior total en bloc spondylectomy for solitary metastases of the thoracolumbar spine. *J Neurosurg Spine* 2012;*17*(4):271–279

14 Yoshihara H. Surgical treatment for thoracic disc herniation: an update. *Spine* 2014;*39*(6):E406–E412

37 Thoracoscopic Approaches to Deformity Correction [1]

Leok-Lim Lau and Hee-Kit Wong

37.1 Introduction

The thoracoscopic approach represents a physiological approach to adolescent idiopathic scoliosis with a single, structural, main thoracic curve and classical thoracic hypokyphosis. The approach utilizes the natural body cavity via strategically placed portals to assess the vertebrae, with the potential to save levels needed for instrumentation, to improve thoracic kyphosis, and to preserve the posterior spinal muscle complex. While the learning curve is steep, the following guide facilitates familiarity with the process.

37.2 Preoperative Planning

Thoracoscopic deformity correction can be considered when the scoliotic curves have the following characteristics:

- Single and right-sided structural thoracic curves. In patients with adolescent idiopathic scoliosis, they are classified as Lenke 1 curves.
- The thoracic curve is flexible and bends down to less than 45°.
- The end vertebrae (the most tilted vertebrae on X-rays) situate within T4 to L1 inclusively.
- Thoracic kyphosis is less than 40°.

The contraindications to the procedure include:

- Patients unable to tolerate or to achieve satisfactory single-lung ventilation, especially patients with pre-existing restrictive lung diseases or right heart failure
- Previous thoracotomy or pleural adhesion

Full-length posteroanterior (PA) lateral erect and PA bending spine X-rays, and/or bolster films, are essential for evaluation and surgical planning.

37.3 Position and Anesthesia

With patient in a supine position, single-lung ventilation is achieved with a double-lumen endotracheal tube. The ideal position of the tube is shown (**Fig. 37.1**). Malposition may result in hypoxemia and hypercarbia. The tube position is verified with bronchoscopy both before and after completion of the positioning. There is a tendency for the endotracheal tube to migrate further into the left bronchus on turning the patient from the supine to left lateral position.

The patient is turned to lie on the left lateral side on a standard radiolucent operating table, such as the Amsco table (Steris Corporation, Mentor, OH), with an axillary roll (**Fig. 37.2**). The table is bent at the midsection to open up the interval between the rib cage and the pelvis, and to facilitate clearance between the rigid telescope and camera from the pelvis during surgery.

The neck is supported and maintained in a neutral position. The right shoulder and elbow are flexed at 90° and are supported on an arm rest. Adequate access to the third rib on the

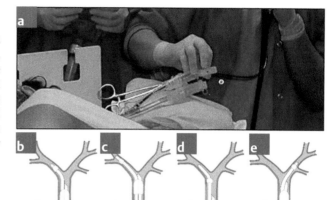

Fig. 37.1 Successful selective left lung intubation is imperative to achieve adequate ventilation in the presence of a completely empty right lung. **(a)** Endotracheal tube position is confirmed with the bronchoscope. **(b)** The intended position and **(c, d, e)** unintended positions are shown.

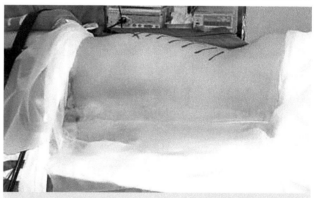

Fig. 37.2 The patient is in the left lateral position. The ribs are marked, starting from the most caudal floating rib.

right lateral chest wall should be checked by palpation of the rib. The left upper limb is flexed and supported. The left hip and left knee are flexed, while the right lower limb is kept straight, with a pillow in between the lower limbs. Additional straps can be used to stabilize the patient's position and to prevent excessive rolling movement.

Pressure areas, such as elbows, knees, and ankles, are padded.

37.4 Portals of Entry

The ribs are identified by palpation of the last floating rib, and are marked accordingly. Useful surface anatomy is that the angle of the scapula overlies the fifth rib.

Four portals are required. The portals are chosen with the aid of preoperative radiographs. Typically, the portals are situated along the third, fifth, seventh, and ninth ribs or, instead, along the fourth, sixth, eighth, and tenth ribs. The portals cover the

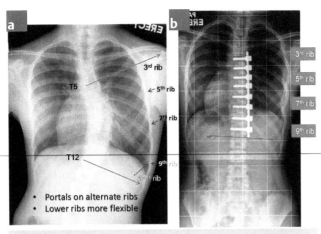

Fig. 37.3 Planning so that the thoracoscopic portals span the end vertebrae of the scoliotic curve. (**a**) In this case, the curve spans the third to tenth ribs. (**b**) Inline placement of portals on alternate ribs (third, fifth, seventh, and ninth) is usually adequate, as the lower ribs are more flexible.

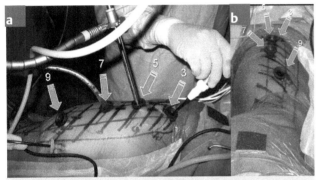

Fig. 37.5 (**a**) From the view of the surgical assistant, the portals in this curve span from the third to the ninth ribs. (**b**) The portals have a sagittal profile corresponding to the apical rotation of the thoracic curve.

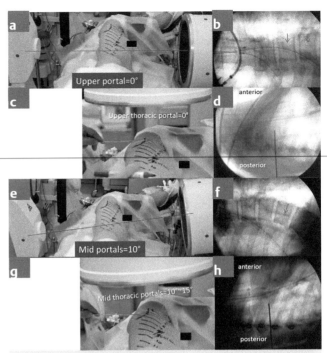

Fig. 37.4 An ideal portal sits directly in line at the midlateral part of the vertebral body. (**a**) At the upper thoracic portal, the rotation is first determined in the lateral position (**b**) under fluoroscopy. Spinous processes (*red arrows*) are verified to be in central positions on the vertebral bodies. (**c**) The fluoroscope is then turned into the lateral position, with the radiological marker pointing at the midlateral position on the vertebral body. (**d**) In mid portals, rotation of 10 to 15° may be required. The fluoroscope is positioned at 10° rotation (**e,f**) to center the spinous process in an anteroposterior view. (**g**) In the lateral position, the 10° rotation is accounted for. (**h**) The radiological marker is then positioned over the midlateral part of the vertebral body. This marks the ideal entry point for the portal.

curve from end vertebra to end vertebra (**Fig. 37.3**). An ideal portal sits directly in line and perpendicular to the midlateral part of the vertebral body. Fluoroscopy is used to assist in locating the point along the rib, taking into consideration vertebral body rotation (**Fig. 37.4**, **Fig. 37.5**). For example, at the upper thoracic portal, fluoroscopy is usually in a neutral position; at the midthoracic portals, 10 to 15° of rotation may be required at the apex of the curve, depending on the axial rotation of the vertebrae. Intermittent direct visualization via the portals allows better depth perception at the surgical field (**Fig. 37.6**).

The patient is cleaned and draped once the points of entry along the ribs are identified and marked.

37.5 Skin Incision and Portal Establishment

The surgeon stands behind the patient. A 3-cm incision is made along the rib on the premarked entry point. The incision is carried down to the rib. The intercostal muscle is detached from the upper border of the rib. Care is taken at the caudal border of the rib to avoid the neurovascular bundle. The rib is detached subperiosteally. An inch of rib is resected and morcellized as autologous bone graft. Parietal pleura is opened sharply. Care

is taken to avoid injuring the potentially undeflated lung or adjacent diaphragm. It is important to avoid making the first entry into the chest through the most caudal portal situated at the ninth or tenth rib, as the risk of injuring the diaphragm and entering the subdiaphragmatic space is high. First entry into the chest should be done through the midthoracic portals situated at the fifth or seventh ribs.

Similar steps are repeated to establish the remaining three portals, and rigid ports 11.5 to 15 mm in diameter are inserted (**Fig. 37.6**). Wound protectors, such as Alexis wound protectors (Applied Medical, Rancho Santa Margarita, CA), are useful at the portals to protect the skin edges and to prevent blood from the portal edges from dripping into the chest cavity.

A fifth and smaller portal that accepts a 5-mm diameter rigid port is then made by a stab incision at the seventh or eighth intercostal space at the anterior axillary line under direct vision. This portal allows the use of a thoracoscopic peanut for diaphragmatic retraction. It is also used for the chest tube insertion at the end of the surgery. The retracted diaphragmatic dome exposes the underlying spinal column for adequate visualization. The spine can thus be exposed laterally from T4 to the T12–L1 disk space. With a further crural detachment at the vertebral body using an ultrasonic dissector (Harmonic scalpel—Ethicon Endo-Surgery Inc.), the L1 vertebral body can be exposed to the level where the segmental vessel crosses the L1 vertebral body.

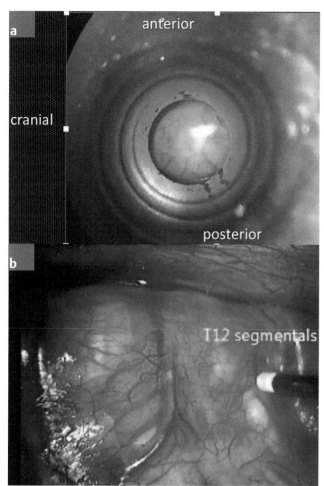

Fig. 37.6 Views through (a) the portal directly and (b) the thoracoscope. T12 segmental vessels are identified. This is further confirmed with fluoroscopy for level identification.

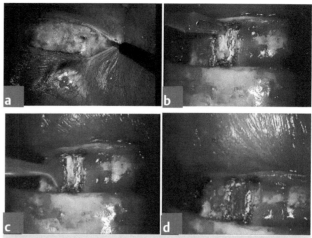

Fig. 37.7 (a) Parietal pleura is dissected with an ultrasonic dissector. Segmental vessels are controlled. (b) Diskectomy is performed. (c) Separation of the disk is done with a Cobb elevator. (d) The appearance of the exposed bony end plate is clearly illustrated.

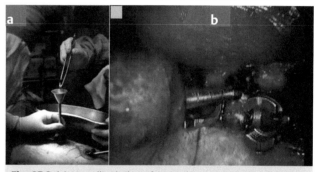

Fig. 37.8 (a) Morcellized rib grafts are placed into the intervertebral space using a funnel through the thoracoscopic portal; (b) the grafts are then compacted into the disk space.

Where needed, access to the L2 or L3 level can be performed through a separate mini-open retroperitoneal approach to the thoracolumbar area.

37.6 Segmental Vessel Ligation, Diskectomy, and Bone Grafting (Video 37.1)

The vertebral level is confirmed with fluoroscopy. The ultrasonic dissector (Harmonic scalpel) is used to dissect the visceral and parietal pleura in a "paintbrush sweeping" manner at the vertebra in the anterior to posterior direction to create an elliptical plane (**Fig. 37.7**). Segmental vessels are cauterized and dissected along its length using the ultrasonic dissector. The dissection is kept anterior to the rib heads and exposes the underlying entry points of the screws to the vertebrae.

In the event of uncontrolled bleeding from the segmental vessels, a thoracoscopic peanut is used to tamponade the bleeding points temporarily before further cautery. Open thoracotomy is rarely required to control the bleeding.

Diskectomy is performed at each segmental level (**Fig. 37.7**). The diskectomy is started with a rectangular incision using diathermy followed by a surgical scalpel with a long handle.

The posterior margin of the incision is kept anterior to the corresponding rib head. Removal of the disk is achieved with a combination of pituitary rongeur, curet, and Cobb elevator. In a skeletally mature patient, an osteotome may be used to separate the fused periphery of the vertebral end plate. Adequate exposure of the bony vertebral end plates is necessary to ensure fusion and to avoid pseudarthrosis. The anterior longitudinal ligament (ALL) and annulus on the left side are preserved as a safety measure. In pediatric patients, segmental mobility is easily achieved after each level of diskectomy.

Morcellized autologous bone graft from the ribs is inserted at each level using a funnel (**Fig. 37.8**). This can also be done after screw placement.

In cases where growth modulation is desired, diskectomy and spinal fusion are not necessary.

37.7 Thoracic Screw Placement (Video 37.1)

Each round-tipped thoracic screw is inserted perpendicular to the vertebral body to achieve bicortical purchase under image intensifier control. The entry point is anterior to the corresponding rib head (**Fig. 37.9**). At the midthoracic vertebrae, the entry point is in line with the anterior border of the rib head. At T11

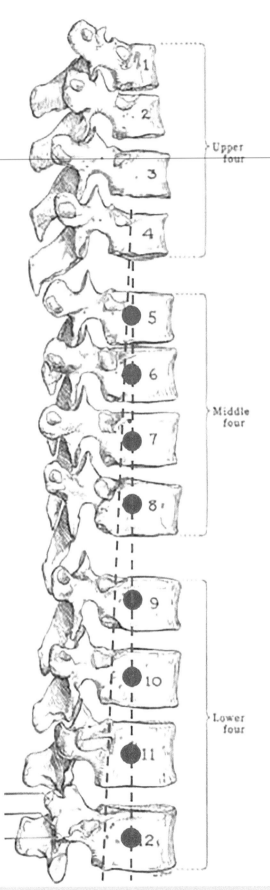

Fig. 37.9 The entry points of the vertebral screws are shown.

and T12, the entry point is midway between the rib head and anterior vertebral border. The array of screws should be placed in line to facilitate rod reduction.

An anterior view of the vertebral body on the image intensifier is used to guide this step. Regional axial rotation is adjusted accordingly for an anatomical anterior view. A pilot hole is first created with an awl and is tapped accordingly (**Fig. 37.10**). The trajectory is perpendicular to the direction of the image intensifier beam. A typical screw has a diameter of 5 or 6 mm, and its length ranges from 25 to 40 mm.

In cases where growth modulation is desired, diskectomy and fusion are not necessary. These immature patients are usually graded Risser 0 on the iliac apophysis and may have open triradiate cartilage of the hip. A vertebral staple is used together with the vertebral screw to improve bony purchase. A braided polyethylene tether is used instead of a solid metal rod.

37.8 Rod Insertion and Cantilever Curve Correction

The rod length is measured with the aid of the image intensifier using a template rod placed outside the body. A titanium 5.5-mm diameter rod is cut to length. A slight bend is placed at the cephalic end to accommodate the cephalic two or three screws on the coronal profile. A rod holder secured at the caudad end of the rod is used to control rod rotation.

The rod is inset into the tulip heads of the cephalic two or three screws (**Fig. 37.11**). The rod is visually checked thoracoscopically for adequate cephalic purchase. The cephalic two or three screws are locked in situ. Reduction is performed using the cantilever method with the aid of reduction towers inserted through the portals under intermittent fluoroscopic guidance. This is done progressively from cephalad to caudad. De-rotation of the vertebral bodies occurs during the reduction maneuver (**Fig. 37.12**).

Final orthogonal X-rays are taken to check the position of the screws after reduction, with particular attention to screw plowing, particularly the cephalad screws. Standing PA and lateral X-rays are obtained two weeks postoperatively (**Fig. 37.13**).

37.9 Skin Closure

The thoracic cavity is washed with warm normal saline to remove debris. Pleura is not routinely repaired.

The 5-mm port is removed. A purse-string stitch using an absorbable 2/0 suture is created. A chest tube (size 28 Fr) is inserted into the thoracic cavity and exited via the wound occupied by the 5-mm port along the costal margin. The chest tube is anchored to the skin using sutures. The right lung is re-inflated.

Muscle layers are approximated. Skin is closed in layers.

37.10 Postoperative Care

The double-lumen endotracheal tube is replaced by a single-lumen endotracheal tube. Bronchoscopy suctioning is performed to minimize mucous plugs. The chest tube is connected to a drain that is water-sealed. The patient is kept intubated and is monitored in the intensive care unit overnight.

The patient is extubated on postoperative day 1. The chest tube is removed on the third postoperative day. A chest X-ray is done before removal of the chest tube. The patient is monitored

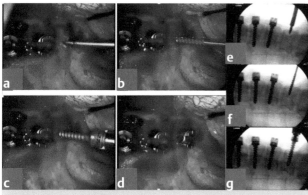

Fig. 37.10 The entry point of the vertebral screw is first identified and should be in line with the cephalad array of screws. (**a**) An awl is used at the point of entry, (**b**) followed by a screw tap. (**c**) The screw is then inserted. (**d**) The appearance of an array of in-line screws. (**e, f, g**) The steps are guided by fluoroscopy.

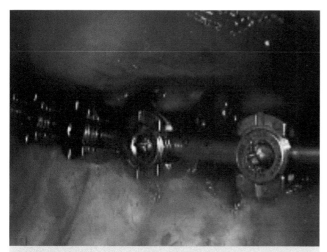

Fig. 37.12 Final appearance of the instrumentation.

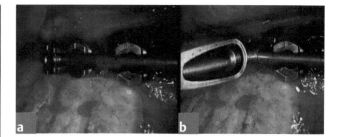

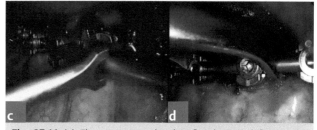

Fig. 37.11 (**a**) The precontoured rod is first bent and fit into the cephalad three screws. (**b**) The set screw is inserted with the aid of an alignment guide. (**c**) The rod is reduced via a cantilever maneuver. (**d**) Further reduction is achieved with compression across the screws under fluoroscopic guidance.

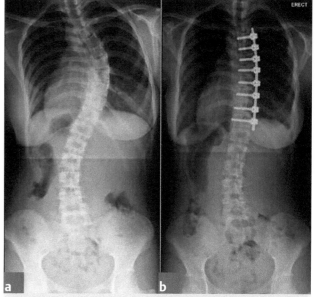

Fig. 37.13 (**a**) Preoperative X-ray and (**b**) postoperative X-ray of a patient with scoliosis. The curve is balanced postoperatively.

clinically and with the aid of pulse oximetry for 24 hours after removal of the chest tube.

Mobility is encouraged once the chest tube is removed. Patients can be discharged on and after the fourth postoperative day. A supportive rigid brace is made and is worn over the next two months.

References

1   Wong HK, Hee HT, Yu Z, Wong D. Results of thoracoscopic instrumented fusion versus conventional posterior instrumented fusion in adolescent idiopathic scoliosis undergoing selective thoracic fusion. *Spine* 2004;*29*(18):2031–2038

2   Newton PO, Upasani VV, Lhamby J, Ugrinow VL, Pawelek JB, Bastrom TP. Surgical treatment of main thoracic scoliosis with thoracoscopic anterior instrumentation. A five-year follow-up study. *J Bone Joint Surg Am* 2008;*90*(10):2077–2089

3   Lonner BS, Auerbach JD, Estreicher MB, et al. Pulmonary function changes after various anterior approaches in the treatment of adolescent idiopathic scoliosis. *J Spinal Disord Tech* 2009;*22*(8):551–558

4   Lonner BS, Auerbach JD, Estreicher M, Milby AH, Kean KE. Video-assisted thoracoscopic spinal fusion compared with posterior spinal fusion with thoracic pedicle screws for thoracic adolescent idiopathic scoliosis. *J Bone Joint Surg Am* 2009;*91*(2):398–408

5   Kishan S, Bastrom T, Betz RR, et al. Thoracoscopic scoliosis surgery affects pulmonary function less than thoracotomy at 2 years postsurgery. *Spine* 2007;*32*(4):453–458

38 Thoracoscopic Approaches to Deformity Correction [2]

Rudolph J. Schrot and George D. Picetti III

38.1 Introduction

This chapter presents the thoracoscopic approach to deformity correction in a progressive manner, each part building on the techniques of the previous part.

38.2 Thoracoscopic-Assisted Arthrodesis for Posterior Deformity Correction

38.2.1 Indications

- Rigid scoliotic curves with Cobb angles greater than 75° and with less than 50° of lateral bending on anteroposterior radiographs[1]
- Lesser curves in immature patients at risk for differential anteroposterior (AP) growth after posterior arthrodesis ("crankshaft phenomenon")

38.2.2 Case Presentation

The patient was a 7-year-old female (20.4 kg) with progressive, severe postlaminectomy kyphosis after resection of a spinal cord anaplastic astrocytoma (**Fig. 38.1a**). The patient underwent T1–L1 Ponte osteotomies, pedicle screw instrumentation, deformity correction, and fusion (**Fig. 38.1b**).

Pseudarthrosis resulted in implant failure, with rod fractures and re-creation of the kyphotic deformity (**Fig. 38.1c**).

The patient underwent redo posterior exploration of the fusion, hardware removal, and redo deformity correction and fusion from T4 to T8 with iliac crest bone graft (**Fig. 38.1d**).

38.2.3 Preoperative Plan

- It was determined that, due to the prior laminectomies, the patient lacked adequate posterior fusion surface and was at high risk for repeat pseudarthrosis. Therefore, anterior diskectomies and fusion with autologous rib graft were planned.

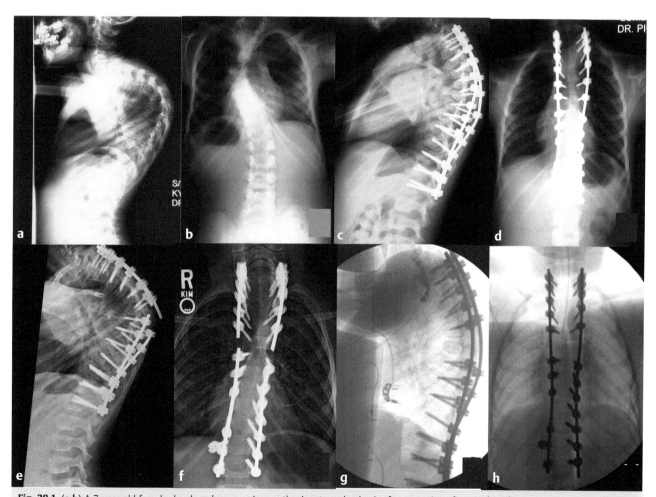

Fig. 38.1 (**a,b**) A 7-year-old female developed progressive postlaminectomy kyphosis after resection of a spinal cord astrocytoma at ages 2 and 3. (**c,d**) A postoperative X-ray shows the deformity correction at age 6. (**e,f**) A follow-up X-ray revealed hardware failure and loss of correction. (**g,h**) Redo posterior surgery was performed.

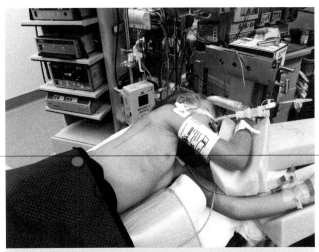

Fig. 38.2 The patient is in the direct left lateral decubitus position. The arms and hips are taped onto the operating table to maintain this position throughout the procedure.

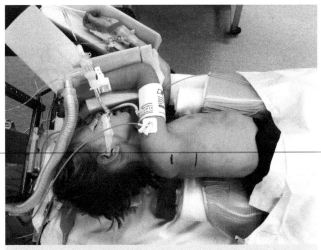

Fig. 38.3 The projection of the intervertebral disks is marked on the skin.

- A minimally invasive thoracoscopic approach was selected to minimize blood loss and recovery time, and to optimize cosmesis, shoulder girdle function, and pulmonary function.

38.2.4 Position and Anesthesia

- Selective intubation of the left bronchus with a single-lumen endotracheal tube was achieved. The patient was placed in a direct lateral decubitus position with the right side up. An arterial line was placed. The pelvis was protected with a lead apron (**Fig. 38.2**).
- AP C-arm fluoroscopy was used to mark the projection of the intervertebral disks on the skin. In this case, the scapula and shoulder girdle could be mobilized superiorly for access to T4–T5. Three portal sites were planned at T4 and T8, with an additional site at T10 for the inflatable lung retractor (**Fig. 38.3**).
- Two video monitors were positioned at the head of the bed 180° apart to afford an endoscopic view to both the surgeon and the assistant holding the endoscope. The surgeon was positioned posterior to the patient, and the assistant stood anterior to the patient.

38.2.5 Thoracoscopic Access (Video 38.1)

- After preparation of the skin and draping, a skin incision is made at T7–T8 and carried through the subcutaneous tissue over the superior surface of T8 to avoid the neurovascular bundle along the inferior surface. A 5-mm portal was inserted.
- The 30° endoscope was inserted into the pleural cavity.
- Under direct endoscopic vision, a second portal for the working channel was placed at T4 and a final portal was placed at T10 to accommodate the lung retractor.
- The lung retractor was placed and inflated and manipulated to afford a view of the anterolateral pleural angle between the thoracic spine and rib heads.

- Instruments and suction were exchanged through the working channel at T4 as needed.

38.2.6 Pleural Dissection

- After the level was confirmed fluoroscopically, the parietal pleura was incised longitudinally with electrocautery, starting at the disk and then along the length of the spine requiring diskectomies and fusion. A hook electrocautery was placed on the pleura overlying the intervertebral disk, and a pleural opening was made. The pleura was elevated off the spine and incised. This maneuver allowed for incision of the pleura along the spine segments to be fused and avoided injury to the segmental vessels.
- The pleura was further dissected anteriorly from the anterior longitudinal ligament and posteriorly from the rib heads.

38.2.7 Rib Head Resection and Diskectomies

- Partial resection of the rib head was performed with osteotomes and rongeurs to gain access to the posterior part of the disk. This maneuver is not required in older patients.
- The intervertebral disk annulus was incised with electrocautery. A complete diskectomy was performed using specialized curets and rongeurs to expose the chondral end plates. The removal of the disk and annulus extended anteriorly to the anterior longitudinal ligament and posteriorly to just behind the remaining rib head.
- In cases performed for anterior release prior to posterior fusion, the anterior longitudinal ligament is thinned so that it can no longer limit spinal mobility but still provides structural support to contain the bone graft.
- The chondral end plates were removed, and the bony end plates were rasped to a homogenous bleeding surface. The disk space was packed with Surgicel for hemostasis.
- The working channel and endoscopic port were interchanged as needed to provide optimal access to the disk spaces.

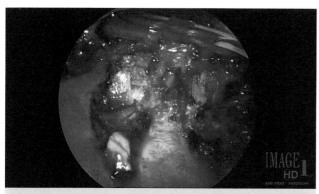

Fig. 38.4 The disk spaces are filled with morcellized autologous bone graft harvested from the rib resection. The chest tube can be seen superiorly.

38.2.8 Bone Graft Harvest

- Attention is directed to rib graft harvest. In this case, because the patient was young, a complete rib block could be resected with expected regrowth.
- A proximal section of the T8 rib was dissected subperiostially and circumferentially to avoid the neurovascular bundle.
- The rib was cut with an endoscopic rib cutter.
- A second rib graft was harvested at T6 after skipping the T7 rib. It is crucial to skip levels when harvesting rib grafts to avoid a flail chest.
- The rib grafts were milled to produce morcellized autologous bone graft.
- For bone graft harvest in older patients, a perpendicular cut using the endoscopic rib cutter is made in the superior aspect of the rib at the anterior and posterior extent of the rib dissection. The cuts are connected with a straight osteotome, thus removing the superior portion of the rib. This technique maintains the integrity of the rib and protects the intercostal nerve.

38.2.9 Arthrodesis

- After the Surgicel was removed from each disk space, the endoscopic bone funnel and plunger were used to pack morcellized local autologous bone graft into each of the disk spaces (**Fig. 38.4**).
- The disk was partially filled, then a small tamp was used to push the graft to the opposite side to ensure complete filling of the space.
- After the disk space was filled, more graft was placed over the space and the adjoining area where the periosteum had been elevated for improved fusion surface.

38.2.10 Closure

- The chest cavity was irrigated, and the lung retractor was removed. The lung was allowed to re-inflate.
- The portals were removed. A 20-French chest tube was placed out of the opening from the inferior portal.
- The portals were closed in layers with absorbable suture. A 2–0 nylon purse-string suture was placed around the chest

tube exit site. Steri-Strips (Nexcare), Xeroform gauze, and sterile dressings were placed. The chest tube was attached to suction.

38.2.11 Results

- Intraoperative blood loss was 30 mL. There were no intraoperative or perioperative complications. The chest tube was removed on postoperative day 1, and the patient was discharged home in stable condition on postoperative day 2.

38.2.12 Notes

- Although fully posterior deformity corrections and fusions are more common with the advent of fourth-generation spinal instrumentation, in this case a lack of posterior fusion surface resulted in failure of the initial treatment with posterior fusion and necessitated an anterior arthrodesis.
- Endoscopic transthoracic diskectomy and fusion provided a minimally invasive option that resulted in minimal blood loss and a short hospital stay.
- The procedure was feasible even in a patient weighing less than 30 kg. A double-lumen endotracheal tube was not required.
- For young patients with low Risser stage, anterior diskectomy and fusion reduce the risk of the crankshaft phenomenon from expansion of the anterior growth plates.
- The key to successful fusion is a total diskectomy and complete removal of the end plate.
- A retrospective comparison review (Level III evidence) showed that Scheuermann's kyphosis was more effectively treated through a completely posterior approach.[2]

38.3 Fully Endoscopic, Completely Transthoracic Deformity Correction

38.3.1 Indications

Progressive primary idiopathic thoracic scoliosis (Lenke type 1 and 2 curves).[3]

38.3.2 Position and Anesthesia

- Positioning and anesthesia are as for the thoracoscopic-assisted arthrodesis for posterior deformity correction described above.
- Double-lumen intubation is used in adults and children weighing more than 45 kg. Children weighing less than 40 to 45 kg require selective intubation of the ventilated lung.
- Intraoperative somatosensory evoked potential (SSEP) and motor evoked potential (MEP) monitoring is established.
- The patient is placed in the lateral decubitus position with the concave side of the scoliotic curve down. The C-arm is used to mark the portal sites, spanning the inferior and superior ends of the Cobb angle. The portal placement must account for spinal rotation as determined with C-arm fluoroscopy.

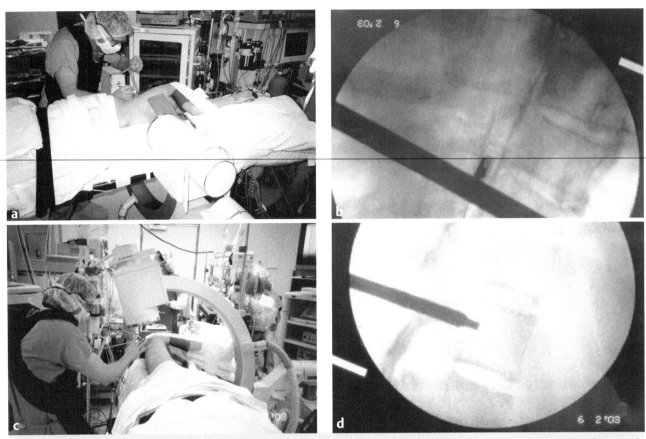

Fig. 38.5 (a) The C-arm is placed in the posteroanterior plane at the distal level to be instrumented with a rod as a marker. A skin marker is used to indicate the levels to be instrumented. (b) Posteroanterior C-arm image of the rod marker parallel to the end plates of the distal level. (c) Photo demonstrating the C-arm in position in the lateral plane using the rod marker to determine the portal location. (d) Lateral C-arm image demonstrating the rod marker at the level of the rib head; the portal will be made just anterior to this mark.

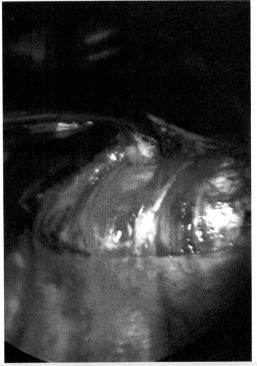

Fig. 38.6 Intraoperative view through the endoscope. The pleura has been incised along the midline of the vertebral bodies and is reflected off the anterior longitudinal ligament.

Three to five incisions are planned, depending on the number of levels to be instrumented (**Fig. 38.5**).

- The position of the operating surgeon at the patient's back allows anatomical orientation of the landmarks visualized through the endoscope and also allows the instruments to be directed away from the spinal cord, enabling the surgeon to safely place vertebral body screws in line with the spinal rotation.

38.3.3 Thoracoscopic Access

- The upside lung is deflated. A 1.5-cm incision is made at the level of the sixth or seventh intercostal space in line with the spine. Placement of the initial portal at this level will avoid injury to the more caudal diaphragm. Digital palpation through the portal ensures lung deflation and the absence of pleural adhesions.
- The endoscope is inserted into the initial portal and is used to place additional portals under endoscopic monitoring. The portals are placed over the superior surface of the rib, avoiding the neurovascular bundle along the inferior surface.
- Portals are separated by two interspaces. Each portal allows access to the interspace above and below the rib.

38.3.4 Pleural Dissection

- Pleural dissection proceeds as already described for thoracoscopic-assisted arthrodesis for posterior deformity correction (**Fig. 38.6**).

38.3.5 Diskectomy

- Diskectomy proceeds as already described for thoracoscopic-assisted arthrodesis for posterior deformity correction (**Fig. 38.7**).

38.3.6 Bone Graft Harvest

- Autologous bone is harvested from ribs as already described for thoracoscopic-assisted arthrodesis for posterior deformity correction.

38.3.7 Screw Placement

- Body position and rotation are rechecked. The sterilely draped C-arm is brought into the operating field with the base parallel to the vertebral body at the superior end of the Cobb angle.
- The segmental vessels are cauterized at the midvertebral level. Larger segmental vessels and the azygous system may be ligated with endoscopic vascular staples and transected.

The undisturbed segmental vessels are grasped at the midvertebral body level and are ligated with the electrocautery. The vessels are located in the valley or middle of the vertebral body and serve as an anatomical guide for screw placement.

- The K-wire triple guide is placed anterior to the rib head, parallel to the end plates, and central on the vertebral body. A slight posterior to anterior inclination of the guide ensures that the K-wire is directed away from the spinal canal (**Fig. 38.8**).
- Once the guide is correctly aligned, a K-wire is advanced into the vertebral body, engaging the opposite cortex. Fluoroscopic monitoring is used to avoid penetration of the opposite cortex and potential penetration of the K-wire into the contralateral segmental vessels and lung (**Fig. 38.9**).
- The screw length is measured on the scale at the upper section of the K-wire or is based on preoperative imaging. The K-wire guide is removed, and the cannulated screw tap is advanced only into the near cortex of the vertebral body (**Fig. 38.10**). If the use of a staple or a washer is desired, it can be inserted at this time. The K-wire is grasped to avoid cortical penetration during screw tap and screw advancement.

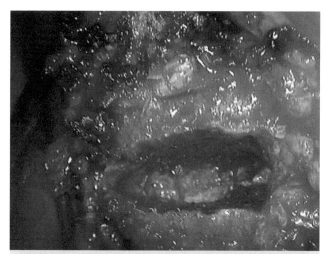

Fig. 38.7 Intraoperative view through the endoscope of a diskectomy. The cartilage has been removed from the end plates, and the anterior longitudinal ligament has been thinned from inside the disk space.

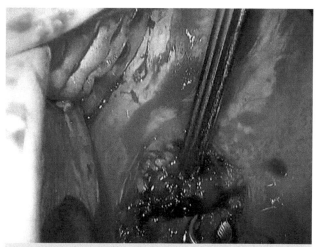

Fig. 38.8 Intraoperative view through the endoscope showing the K-wire guide inserted onto the vertebral body.

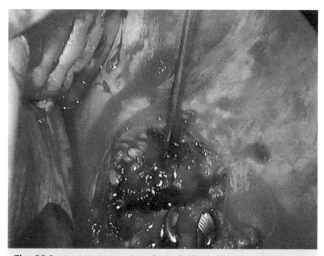

Fig. 38.9 Intraoperative view through the endoscope showing the K-wire inserted into the vertebral body.

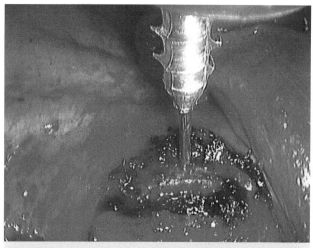

Fig. 38.10 Intraoperative view through the endoscope showing the tap placed over the K-wire ready to be inserted into the vertebral body.

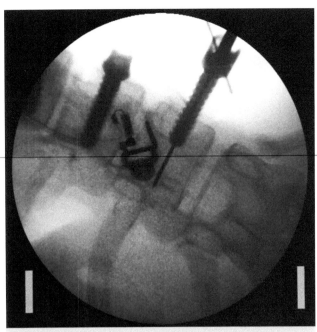

Fig. 38.11 Intraoperative fluoroscopic view showing a screw being inserted into the vertebral body over the K-wire.

- The appropriately sized screw is advanced over the guidewire, engaging the opposite cortex and seating the head against the valley of the vertebral body (**Fig. 38.11**). The guidewire is removed once the screw is advanced three-fourths of the distance across the vertebral body.
- Successive screw placement uses the rib heads as a reference to ensure appropriate screw alignment and effective derotation during rod reduction. Screw heads that end in a V pattern will aid in derotation.
- Screw depth placement must be accurate and at similar levels; otherwise, seating of the rod will be difficult.

38.3.8 Arthrodesis

- Placement of bone graft proceeds as described above for thoracoscopic-assisted arthrodesis for posterior deformity correction (**Fig. 38.12**).

38.3.9 Rod Placement and Deformity Reduction

- The rod length is measured with the ball-and-cable endoscopic rod gauge (**Fig. 38.13**).
- A 4.5-mm titanium rod is cut to the premeasured length and placed freely within the chest cavity through the inferior incision. The rod is placed flush with the inferior screw saddle to avoid protrusion into the diaphragm. The plug introduction tube is placed over the screw saddle, temporarily securing the rod. The plug inserter is advanced through the plug guide and the plug is inserted into the vertebral screw, to secure the rod and the plug is completely tightened (**Fig. 38.14**).
- The rod is next sequentially reduced into the saddles of the remaining screws with the rod pusher, and plugs are placed but not tightened.

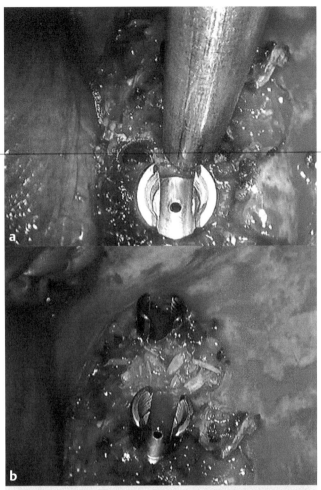

Fig. 38.12 (a) Intraoperative view through the endoscope showing the bone graft funnel inserted into the disk space. **(b)** Intraoperative view demonstrating a disk space filled with bone graft and graft placed over the adjacent vertebral bodies.

- Compression between each screw is performed. The compressor is placed freely into the chest cavity and over the screw heads on the rod at the inferior end of the construct (**Fig. 38.15**). Turning the driver clockwise to bring the two screws closer together performs compression. Segmental compression is sequentially performed from inferior to superior until all levels have been compressed. Plugs are completely tightened after compression.

38.3.10 Closure

- Lateral and AP fluoroscopy is used to confirm adequate reduction and construct integrity.
- The chest cavity is irrigated, and the lung is inflated under endoscopic visualization to confirm that the entire lung is reinflated.
- A chest tube is placed through the inferior portal, and the incisions are closed in layers in standard fashion.

38.3.11 Notes

- Surgeons should not attempt fully endoscopic, completely transthoracic deformity correction until sufficient experience with thoracoscopic diskectomy has been attained.

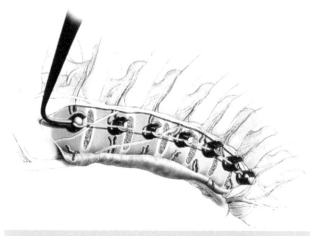

Fig. 38.13 Schematic view of the screws in place, with the endoscopic rod measurer inserted through all of them. The rod length is determined by reading the scale at the top of the measurer.

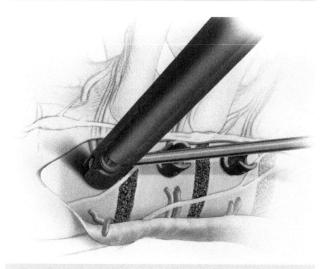

Fig. 38.14 Diagram of the rod as it is inserted into the most inferior screw, with the plug introduction tube over the screw. The window at the tip of the tube on the screw shows the plug inserted into the screw.

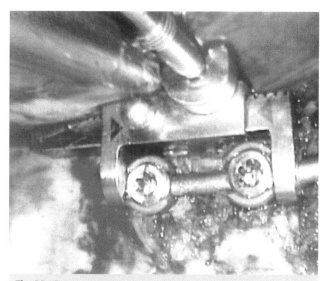

Fig. 38.15 Intraoperative view via the endoscope, with the endoscopic compressor on the rod compressing two screws together.

- Fully endoscopic, completely transthoracic deformity correction has become less popular in recent years with the excellent reductions possible using posterior approaches combining Ponte osteotomies with fourth-generation segmental instrumentation.[4]
- Anterior transthoracic deformity correction and instrumentation may reduce the number of segments included in the construct compared with a fully posterior approach.[5]
- Anterior transthoracic deformity correction may help restore normal thoracic kyphosis after derotation better than posterior approaches can.[6]

38.4 Partially Endoscopic, Completely Anterior Combined Thoracoscopic and Retroperitoneal Thoracolumbar Deformity Correction

38.4.1 Indications

- Progressive thoracic and lumbar/thoracolumbar structural scoliosis (Lenke types 3, 4, and 6)

38.4.2 Procedure

- Proceed as already described for fully endoscopic, completely transthoracic deformity correction.
- A minimum of three portals must be used in the pleural cavity to accommodate the endoscope, the working channel, and the inflatable lung retractor.
- The T12–L1 disk may also be removed from the thoracic cavity if the diaphragm inserts below the T12–L1 disk space. However, if the diaphragm inserts above the T12–L1 disk, the disk must be removed from the retroperitoneal approach.
- Vertebral levels are marked on the skin in lateral fluoroscopic projection for every level to be instrumented (**Fig. 38.16**).

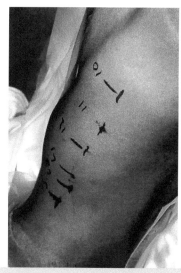

Fig. 38.16 Photograph of a patient with skin markings for a T10–L3 minimally invasive instrumentation correction and fusion.

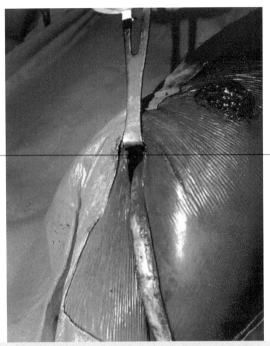

Fig. 38.17 Photograph of the retroperitoneal incision. The eleventh rib has been amputated at its cartilaginous junction. With the endoscopic rib cutter, the rib can now be amputated at the rib head.

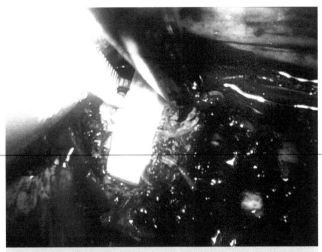

Fig. 38.18 Intraoperative view of the retroperitoneal approach. A femoral ring filled with autograft is inserted into the L1–L2 disk space. To the left of the femoral ring is the diaphragm, and above the femoral ring is the peritoneum.

38.4.3 Skin Incision and Eleventh Rib Harvest

- The lumbar retroperitoneal incision is performed over the previously marked skin site via an eleventh rib approach.
- For constructs extending to L2, the incision should be placed over the L1–L2 disk space, allowing access from T12–L1 to L2.
- For constructs extending to L3, the incision is placed directly over the center of the L2 vertebral body, allowing access from L1 to L3.
- For constructs extending to L1, the incision is placed over the T12–L1 disk space. The approach to L1 is always attempted through the thoracic cavity first, although extensive retraction of the diaphragm may be required.
- A minimal 3- to 4-cm incision is performed over the predetermined location.
- After subperiosteal dissection to expose the eleventh rib, the entire floating eleventh rib is harvested (**Fig. 38.17**). Once the rib has been subperiosteally dissected, it is removed nearly to entirety with the endoscopic rib cutter.

38.4.4 Retroperitoneal Exposure

- Dissection is carried through the muscle into the retroperitoneal space and onto the psoas muscle. The peritoneum is reflected off the psoas, spine, and diaphragm.
- Lighted retractors are inserted. The psoas is retracted posteriorly.

38.4.5 Lower Thoracic and Lumbar Diskectomy

- The disks and end plates are exposed and removed in the standard fashion.

- Once all the disks have been removed, more rib graft can be harvested from the thoracic portal sites, as described in the thoracic technique.

38.4.6 Lower Thoracic and Lumbar Arthrodesis

- The disk spaces from the lower thoracic level through the lumbar level are sized.
- Femoral ring allograft is cut and contoured for lordosis. The amount of taper is decreased for more proximal levels (**Fig. 38.18**).
- The center is packed with the morcellized rib graft and impacted into the disk space. Morcellized graft is inserted into the disk space prior to placement of the femoral ring and then over the ring once it is in place.
- Humeral ring allograft can be used if lower thoracic levels will not accommodate a femoral ring.
- Interbody cages packed with morcellized autologous bone graft can be used instead of allograft bone.

38.4.7 Placement of Vertebral Body Screws

- Using C-arm fluoroscopy, screws are placed thoracoscopically as already described for fully endoscopic, completely transthoracic deformity correction (**Fig. 38.19**).
- In a similar fashion, vertebral body screws are placed in the lower thoracic and lumbar levels through the retroperitoneal exposure.
- The screw should penetrate the opposite cortex for bicortical fixation and should be seated in the valley of the vertebral body.

38.4.8 Thoracic Arthrodesis

- Morcellized autologous bone graft from the rib harvest is packed into the thoracic interspaces using the graft funnel and plunger. The disk spaces should be completely filled to the opposite side.

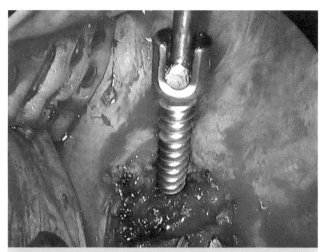

Fig. 38.19 Intraoperative view through the endoscope showing a screw placed over the K-wire, ready to be inserted into the vertebral body.

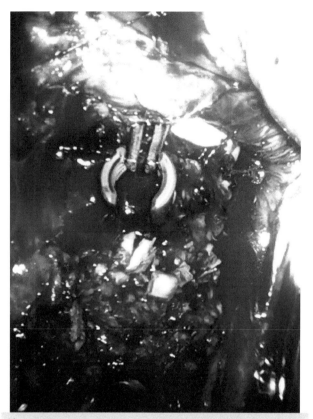

Fig. 38.20 Intraoperative view through the endoscope showing the right-angle clamp under the diaphragm with the tips in the T12 screw.

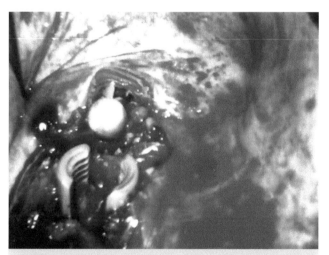

Fig. 38.21 Intraoperative view through the endoscope showing the ball end of the endoscopic rod measurer coming through the small opening under the diaphragm.

38.4.9 Crossing the Diaphragm for Rod Placement and Deformity Reduction

- With a clear endoscopic view of the diaphragmatic attachment to the spine from within the pleural cavity, a right-angle clamp is inserted from the retroperitoneal space to the pleural cavity (**Fig. 38.20**). A small opening under the diaphragm is made at the center of the vertebral body to permit passage of the rod measurer, the rod, and the compressor arm.

- The endoscopic rod measurer is used to determine the rod length, as already described (**Fig. 38.21**).

- The 4.5-mm rod is cut and inserted into the chest cavity through the most inferior port, then is partially pulled into the retroperitoneal space with the right-angle clamp (**Fig. 38.22**, **Fig. 38.23**).

- The rod is placed into the inferior screw flush with the saddle and is locked in place using the plug introduction tube and plug.

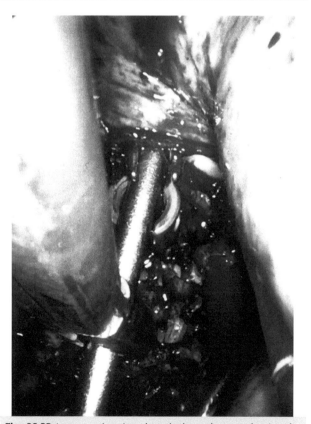

Fig. 38.22 Intraoperative view through the endoscope showing the right-angle clamp under the diaphragm grasping the rod and pulling it into the retroperitoneal space.

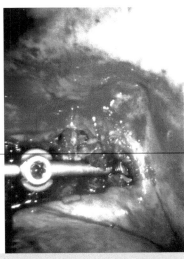

Fig. 38.23 Intraoperative view through the endoscope demonstrating the construct going through the small opening under the diaphragm as the diaphragm is tented over the construct.

- The rod is sequentially reduced into the screw saddles with the rod pushers and then plugs are partially tightened.
- Compression between the screws is performed with the endoscopic compressor. Compression is accomplished from caudal to cranial, and plugs are locked down after each sequential compression.

38.4.10 Closure

- The ports are removed, and a chest tube is placed. The thoracic and retroperitoneal incisions are closed in layers.

38.4.11 Notes

- Sagittal balance and anterior column support are critical in treating thoracolumbar scoliosis. This can be addressed with contoured femoral ring allograft or cages (**Fig. 38.24**).
- Novel dual-head screws allow a two-rod construct with a single set of vertebral body screws and add torsional stability (**Fig. 38.25**).

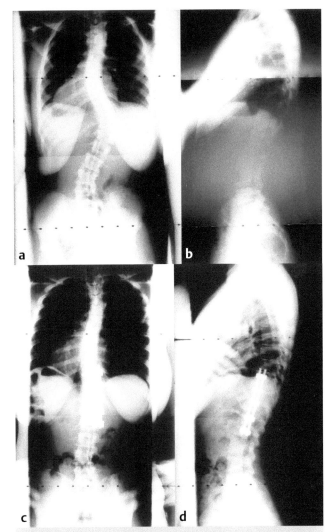

Fig. 38.24 (**a**) Anteroposterior and (**b**) lateral preoperative X-rays of a 14-year-old female with a 26° T5–T10, 54° T10–L2, and 32° L2–L5 curve. Postoperative (**c**) anteroposterior and (**d**) lateral views of the same patient after a minimally invasive instrumentation, correction, and fusion with the new dual-head screws.

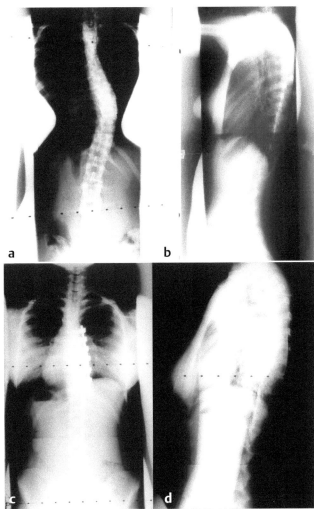

Fig. 38.25 (**a**) Anteroposterior and (**b**) lateral preoperative X-rays of a 14-year-old female with a 48° thoracic and 25° lumbar curve. Postoperative (**c**) anteroposterior and (**d**) lateral views of the same patient after an endoscopic instrumentation, correction, and fusion with the new dual-head screws.

References

1   Arlet V. Anterior thoracoscopic spine release in deformity surgery: a meta-analysis and review. *Eur Spine J* 2000;*9*(Suppl 1):S17–S23

2   Lee SS, Lenke LG, Kuklo TR, et al. Comparison of Scheuermann kyphosis correction by posterior-only thoracic pedicle screw fixation versus combined anterior/posterior fusion. *Spine* 2006;*31*(20):2316–2321

3   Picetti GD III, Ertl JP, Bueff HU. Endoscopic instrumentation, correction, and fusion of idiopathic scoliosis. *Spine J* 2001;*1*(3):190–197

4   Arunakul R, Peterson A, Bartley CE, Cidambi KR, Varley ES, Newton PO. The 15-year evolution of the thoracoscopic anterior release: does it still have a role? *Asian Spine J* 2015;*9*(4):553–558

5   Lonner BS, Kondrachov D, Siddiqi F, Hayes V, Scharf C. Thoracoscopic spinal fusion compared with posterior spinal fusion for the treatment of thoracic adolescent idiopathic scoliosis. *J Bone Joint Surg Am* 2006;*88*(5):1022–1034

6   Lonner BS, Auerbach JD, Levin R, et al. Thoracoscopic anterior instrumented fusion for adolescent idiopathic scoliosis with emphasis on the sagittal plane. *Spine J* 2009;*9*(7):523–529

39 Applied Anatomy for Percutaneous Approaches to the Cervical Spine

Gun Choi, Alfonso García, Akarawit Asawasaksakul, and Ketan Deshpande

39.1 Introduction

To understand the surgical technique of percutaneous endoscopic cervical diskectomy (PECD) and to produce successful outcomes, it is imperative to have a thorough knowledge of the regional anatomy of the neck. The approach to the cervical disk in PECD is always anterior; hence this chapter focuses on the anterior triangle of the neck in describing the surgical anatomy.[1,2,3,4]

39.2 Surface Anatomy

Orientation to surface anatomy helps to locate the surgical level and proper needle trajectory to the disk space (**Fig. 39.1**). The sternocleidomastoid (SCM) muscle separates the anterior and posterior triangles of the neck. The landmarks are described below from the midline and beginning with the top of the neck and moving downward.

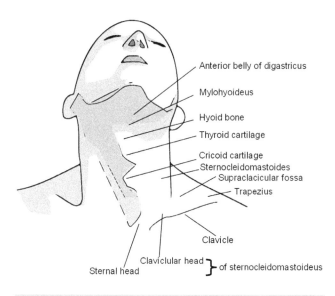

Fig. 39.1 Surface anatomy of the cervical region.

Labels: Anterior belly of digastricus; Mylohyoideus; Hyoid bone; Thyroid cartilage; Cricoid cartilage; Sternocleidomastoides; Supraclacicular fossa; Trapezius; Clavicle; Claviclular head; Sternal head; of sternocleidomastoideus

39.2.1 Hyoid Bone

- About 1.5 cm above the thyroid cartilage
- Corresponds with level of C3 vertebra

39.2.2 Thyroid Cartilage

- Most prominent midline structure, especially in postpubertal males
- Corresponds with C4–C5 level
- Also corresponds with the carotid artery bifurcation into external and internal carotids

39.2.3 Cricoid Cartilage

- Located just below the thyroid cartilage
- Corresponds to the C6 vertebral level
- A horizontal plane approximately at the junction of C6–C7 has the following associations:
- Pharyngoesophageal junction
- Laryngotracheal junction
- Inferior thyroid artery, carotid sheath, and omohyoid muscle
- Entrance of the inferior laryngeal nerve (recurrent nerve) into the larynx
- Entrance of the vertebral artery into the transverse foramen of C6
- The thyroid isthmus and the greatest height of the thoracic duct are located at the C7 level.

39.3 Topographic Anatomy of the Cervical Spine

The neck is divided into anterior and posterior triangles. The following description presents the surgical anatomy of the anterior triangle of the neck (**Fig. 39.2**, **Fig. 39.3**).

39.4 Boundaries of the Anterior Triangle

- Lateral: SCM muscle
- Superior: inferior border of the mandible
- Medial: anterior midline of the neck

The anterior triangle is further subdivided into the following sections:

- Submandibular
- Submental
- Carotid
- Muscular

39.4.1 Submandibular Triangle

Boundaries

- Superior: inferior border of the mandible
- Inferior: anterior and posterior bellies of the digastric muscle

Content

The submandibular gland is the largest structure of the triangle. The roof is formed by skin, superficial fascia composing platysma, and the underlying mandibular and cervical branches of the facial nerves. Below the roof, from superficial to deep, lie the retromandibular vein, part of the facial artery, the submental

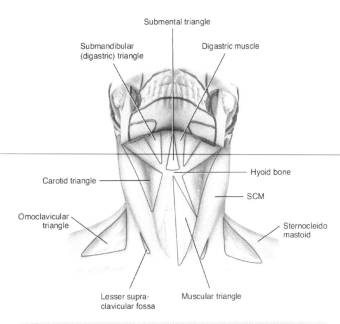

Fig. 39.2 The surgical anatomy of the anterior triangle of the neck.

39.4.2 Submental Triangle

Boundaries

- Lateral: anterior belly of digastric
- Inferior: hyoid bone
- Medial: midline
  - Floor: mylohyoid muscle
  - Roof: skin and superficial fascia, platysma, cutaneous nerves
  - Contents: lymph nodes

39.4.3 Muscular Triangle

The inferior carotid triangle (muscular triangle) is bounded superolaterally by the anterior belly of the omohyoid, inferolaterally by the SCM, and medially by the midline of the neck from the hyoid bone to the sternum. The roof is formed by the superficial fascia, platysma, deep fascia, and branches of the supraclavicular nerves. Beneath these superficial structures are the sternohyoid and sternothyroid muscles, which, along with the medial (anterior) border of the SCM, protect the lower part of the common carotid artery. This vessel is enclosed within the carotid sheath with the internal jugular vein and vagus nerve. The veins lie lateral to the artery on the right side but overlap below on the left side. The nerve lies between the artery and vein in a plane posterior to both. In front of the sheath are a few descending filaments of ansa hypoglossus; behind the sheath are the inferior thyroid artery and recurrent laryngeal nerve and the sympathetic trunk; and on its medial side lie the esophagus, trachea, thyroid/parathyroid glands, and lower part of the larynx. Most of the anterior cervical approach is done in this triangle.

branch of fascia (deep cervical fascia), the lymph nodes, the deep layer of the deep cervical fascia, and the hypoglossal nerve. Below this lie the mylohyoid muscle with its nerve, the hypoglossus muscle, and the middle constrictor muscle of the pharynx. Farther down lie the deep portion of the submandibular gland, the submandibular duct, the lingual nerve, the sublingual vein, the sublingual gland, the hypoglossal nerve, and the submandibular ganglion.

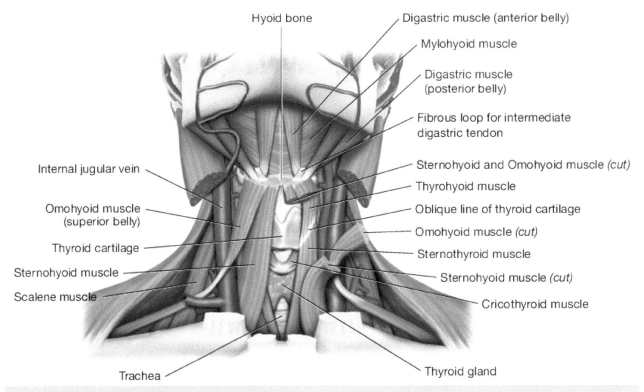

Fig. 39.3 The infrahyoid and suprahyoid muscles of the neck.

39.4.4 Carotid Triangle

Boundaries

- Posterior: bounded by the SCM
- Anterior: anterior belly of the omohyoid
- Superior: posterior belly of digastric muscle
- Roof: Consists of the superficial fascia, platysma, and deep fascia with superficial cutaneous nerve
- Floor: Formed by part of the thyroid, hypoglossus, and medial constrictor of the pharynx
  - The triangle contains the upper part of the carotid artery, which bifurcates opposite to the upper border of the thyroid cartilage into the external and internal carotid arteries. The external and internal carotids lie side by side, the external carotid being the more anterior of the two. The following major branches of the external carotid artery are located in the triangle:
- Superior thyroid artery: running forward and downward
- Lingual artery: running directly forward
- Facial artery: coursing forward and upward
- Occipital artery: running backward
- Ascending pharyngeal artery: coursing upward on the medial side of the internal carotid artery
  - The internal jugular vein lies on the lateral side of the common carotid and internal carotid arteries. It receives the superior thyroid vein, lingual vein, common facial vein, ascending pharyngeal vein, and occasionally the occipital vein. The following nerves are found in the triangle:
- In front of the sheath of the common carotid is the ramus descendens hypoglossi.
- The hypoglossal nerve crosses both the interior and the exterior carotids above.
- The vagus nerve is in the carotid sheath.
- The accessory nerve and superior laryngeal nerve are also found in the triangle.

The upper portion of the larynx and the lower portion of the pharynx are also found in this region (**Fig. 39.4**).

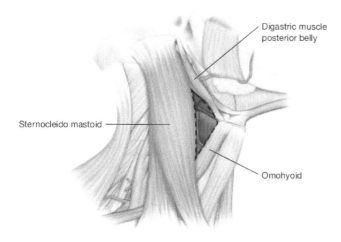

Fig. 39.4 Carotid triangle.

Fasciae of the Neck

The superficial cervical fascia and deep cervical fascia of the neck compartmentalize the neck to form various separate, more or less mobile, compartments. Because of this arrangement, the medial visceral compartment can be safely pushed away and a safe needle trajectory can be created between the visceral and vascular compartments (**Fig. 39.5**).

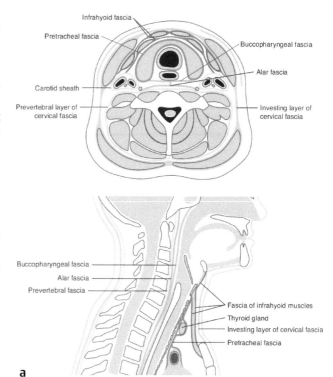

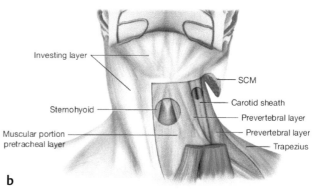

Fig. 39.5 (a) Diagrammatic cross section of the neck, demonstrating fascial layers of the neck. (b) Fascial layers from anterior view.

Superficial Fascia

The superficial fascia lies beneath the skin and is composed of loose connective tissue, fat, platysma, cutaneous branches of the cervical plexus, the cervicofacial division of the facial nerve, and small cutaneous blood vessels. It is important to remember that the cutaneous nerve of the neck and the anterior and external jugular vein are between the platysma and the deep cervical fascia.

Deep Cervical Fascia

The deep cervical fascia is further divided into three layers:

- Investing layer: Originates above from the occipital bone, temporal bone, and mandible. Extends posteriorly to the spinous and supraspinous ligaments, and below to the clavicle, scapula, and manubrium sterni. It splits to envelop the trapezius, SCM, and salivary glands (submandibular and parotid). It forms the roof of the anterior and posterior triangle.
- Pretracheal layer: The pretracheal layer extends medially, in front of the carotid vessels, and assists in formation of the carotid sheath. It continues behind the depressor muscles of the hyoid bone, and after enveloping the thyroid gland (forming a pseudocapsule) is prolonged in front of the trachea to meet the corresponding layer from the opposite side.
- Above, it is attached to the hyoid bone, and below it is carried downward in front of the trachea and large vessels at the roof of the neck, and ultimately blends with the fibrous pericardium.
- The layer is fused on either side with the prevertebral fascia, completing a compartment composed of the larynx, trachea, thyroid/parathyroid glands, and pharynx-esophagus.
- Prevertebral fascia: The prevertebral fascia extends medially behind the carotid vessels, forming a part of the carotid sheath, and passes in front of the prevertebral muscles. It is fixed above to the base of the skull and below extends behind the esophagus into the posterior mediastinal cavity of the thorax.
  - The prevertebral fascia is prolonged downward and laterally behind the carotid vessels and in front of the scalene and forms a sheath for the brachial nerves and subclavian vessels in the posterior triangle of the neck; it continues under the clavicle as the axillary sheath and is attached to the deep surface of the coracoclavicular fascia.

39.5 Anatomical Considerations in the Cervical Percutaneous Approach

When performing the cervical disk puncture, one must give careful attention to the carotid artery medial to the SCM muscle laterally and the trachea and esophagus medially. The pretracheal fascia is fused on either side with the prevertebral fascia, completing a compartment composed of the larynx, trachea, thyroid/parathyroid gland, and pharynx-esophagus. When moved medially, all of these components move together, increasing the safety zone for the initial disk puncture. Laterally, the carotid artery has an almost vertical path, overlying the SCM muscle obliquely. The carotid artery is placed more medially from the medial edge of the SCM at the C3–C4 level and more laterally at the C6-C7 level. A more lateral puncture increases the risk of carotid puncture, whereas a more medial puncture

increases the risk of injury to the hypopharynx and esophagus. The safest needle entry point is between the airway and the pulsating point of the carotid artery.

39.6 Anatomical Structures Related to Levels

39.6.1 C3–C4: Inferior Border of Hyoid Bone

Between the hyoid bone and the thyroid cartilage there is a narrow safety zone. The hypopharynx is broader and the carotid artery is bifurcated medially. The superior thyroidal artery is located in the trajectory of the C3–C4 puncture. Translational movement of the pretracheal fascia enclosing the thyroid gland may change the course of the superior thyroidal artery more horizontally.

39.6.2 C4–C5: Middle of Thyroid Cartilage

The hypopharynx is placed more medially to the lateral margin of the thyroid cartilage, protecting it from injury.

39.6.3 C5–C6: Between Inferior Thyroid Cartilage and Cricoid Ring (Carotid Tubule: C6 Transverse Process), and C6–C7: Inferior to Cricoid Ring

The safety zone is larger at these levels. With correct retraction of the carotid artery and the pharynx–esophagus, there are no endangered vital structures. The right lobe of the thyroid gland is in this area.

39.6.4 C7–T1

A slightly more medial approach is advised, to avoid lung apex injury.

References

1   An HS. Anatomy and the cervical spine. In: An HS, Simpson JM, eds. *Surgery of the Cervical Spine*. Baltimore: Williams & Wilkins; 1994:1–40
2   An HS, Gordin R, Renner K. Anatomical considerations for plate-screw fixation to the cervical spine. *Spine* 1988;*13*:813–816
3   Rauschning W. Anatomy and pathology of the cervical spine. In: Frymoyer JW, ed. *The Adult Spine*. New York: Raven Press; 1991:907–929
4   Zhang J, Tsuzuki N, Hirabayashi S, Saiki K, Fujita K. Surgical anatomy of the nerves and muscles in the posterior cervical spine: a guide for avoiding inadvertent nerve injuries during the posterior approach. *Spine* 2003;*28*(13):1379–1384

40 An Endonasal Approach to the Craniocervical Junction

Juan Barges Coll, Luis Alberto Ortega-Porcayo, and Gabriel Armando Castillo Velázquez

40.1 Background

Several surgical approaches have been used to reach the craniovertebral junction (CVJ), which has a unique anatomy and important vital structures that need to be preserved. The surgical approach utilized depends on the type of lesion, its extent, and its location. The endonasal endoscopic approach (EEA) to reach the CVJ is ideal for ventral and ventrolateral lesions, while posterior and posterolateral lesions are better reached through posterior approaches. The EEA provides adequate medial exposure from the frontal crest to the CVJ. With chordomas, which could have a lateral extension, the corridor can be expanded through maxillary osteotomies or a midline mandibulotomy.[1] The extent of ventral exposure can be anticipated by the naso-palatine, naso-axial, and palatine lines, while the exposure of the CVJ is delineated by the dorsal position of the hard palate (**Fig. 40.1**).[2,3,4] In children, the size of the nares in some cases limits the approach; they may require a sublabial incision to facilitate endoscopic passage into the nose.[5] After the description of expanded endonasal endoscopic odontoidectomy by Kassam et al[6] and the anatomical endoscopic study by Messina et al,[7] a substantial number of publications have described an EEA to reach the CVJ.

Assessment of CVJ stability and motion must be performed prior to surgery. The occipitoatlantal junction contributes 23 to 24.5° of flexion and extension, 3.4 to 5.5° of lateral bending, and 2.4 to 7.2° of axial rotation. The atlantoaxial joint contributes 10.1 to 22.4° of flexion and extension, 6.7° of lateral bending, and 23.3 to 38.9° of axial rotation.[8,9] The atlantoaxial joint is the most mobile of all joints in the body[10] and is potentially the most unstable in response to trauma, tumor, and inflammatory or degenerative processes. Disruption of the craniovertebral complex joints (i.e., occipitoatlantal and atlantoaxial joints) and/ or principal ligaments (i.e., the transverse cruciate ligament, alar ligament, or the tectorial membrane) determines the need for internal fixation before or after EEA of the ventral CVJ. Recently, in the case of degenerative and inflammatory processes, we prefer to perform a C1–C2 fixation because these pathologies are associated with atlantoaxial instability, and it is unnecessary to include the occipital bone if there is no occipitoatlantal joint involvement. Furthermore, with tumor pathology in which one condyle has been invaded more than 75%,[11] a craniocervical fusion is preferred before EEA.

40.2 Craniocervical Junction Endoscopic Anatomical Landmarks

The CVJ is a complex region defined by the axis, atlas, and occiput. It protects the cervicomedullary junction and the vertebral arteries. The majority of the spine's flexion, extension, and rotation occur in the CVJ.[9] Understanding the complex

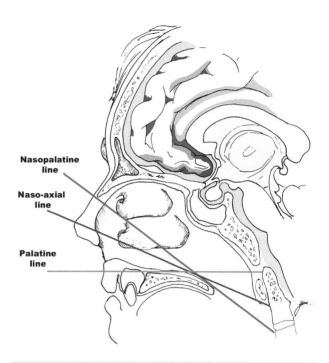

Nasopalatine line

Naso-axial line

Palatine line

Fig. 40.1 A schematic representation of the naso-axial, nasopalatine, and palatine lines in the midsagittal plane. The nasopalatine line is created by connecting the inferior border of the nasal bone to the posterior edge of the hard palate. The extrapolation of the line shows the inferior extension of the endonasal approach. The naso-axial line begins at the midpoint of a line between the rhinion and the anterior nasal spine to the posterior edge of the hard palate. The palatine line is drawn parallel along the superior edge of the palatine process.

anatomy of the ventral CVJ is essential to safe performance of an extended EEA.

The CVJ contains several important neurovascular structures: the cervicomedullary junction, the vertebrobasilar system, and the lower cranial nerves and the cranial nerve VI, which is medially located during EEA and seems to be frequently involved in chordoma pathology.[12] Therefore, total resection of any tumors involving these structures is difficult to accomplish without significant morbidity. A standard preoperative work-up, including computed angiotomography (CT) and gadolinium-enhanced MRI, helps to precisely delimit the tumor and its position in relation to neural and vascular structures.

40.2.1 Anatomical Landmarks

Sphenoid Sinus Ostium and Sphenopalatine Foramen

The sphenoid sinus ostium is located in the anterior sphenoid sinus wall approximately 12 mm from the upper edge of the posterior choanae at the entrance to the sphenoid sinus. The sphenopalatine foramen is ~ 7 mm from the ostium; it is an important landmark for the prevention of bleeding from the sphenopalatine artery.[13]

Vidian Canal

The vidian canal is an important landmark below the floor of the sphenoid sinus between the pterygoid process and the body of the sphenoidal bone. The canal follows the anterolateral edge of the anterior genu of the petrous carotid artery. The anterior genu and the foramen lacerum are medial to the posterior end of the vidian canal.[14]

Torus Tubarium and Fossa of Rosenmüller

The torus tubarium is a prominence derived from the medial cartilaginous end of the eustachian tubes. Behind the torus is the lateral pharyngeal recess or the fossa of Rosenmüller, and at the apex of this fossa, a layer of fibroconnective tissue separates the nasopharyngeal mucosa from the internal carotid artery (ICA).[15] Near the ICA is the anterior pharyngeal artery, which gives rise to three or four branches that supply the parapharyngeal structures.[16] The ICA is an average of 23.7 mm from the midline (minimum 11.5 mm). The eustachian tube is 23.5 mm from the ICA (minimum 10.4 mm), and the distance between the fossa of Rosenmüller and the ICA is minimal, with the closest distance being 0.2 mm.[17] The foramen lacerum is positioned above the fossa of Rosenmüller, and the tensor veli palatini muscle and the levator palatini muscle sit laterally behind the medial pterygoid plate.[16]

The medial working space needed to access the ventral CVJ is limited caudally by the soft palate, rostrally by the floor of the sphenoid sinus, and laterally the eustachian tubes surrounding the nasopharyngeal mucosa.[6]

Longus Capitis

Posterior to the nasopharyngeal mucosa is the basipharyngeal fascia, which covers the longus capitis, a key muscular landmark medial to the internal carotid artery. The longus capitis has its origin at the anterior tubercles of the transverse processes of the third to sixth cervical vertebrae and has its insertion at the ventral surface of the lower clivus. Deep and lateral to the longus capitis is the rectus capitis anterior, which has its origin at the transverse process and lateral mass of C1 and its insertion at the inferior surface of the lower clivus. The hypoglossal nerve and branches of the ascending pharyngeal artery course along the lateral borders of these muscles.[18] The longus colli muscles are encountered deep at the level of the anterior arch of C1. Behind these muscles the craniocervical junction is exposed, including the inferior clivus, the anterior arch of C1, and the dens.

40.3 Indications for an Endonasal Approach to the Craniocervical Junction

- Cervicomedullary ventral compression
  - Irreducible bone compression
  - Rheumatoid pannus compression
  - Lesion above the nasopalatine line

- Extradural tumors (chordoma, chondrosarcoma, nasopharyngeal carcinoma)
- Intradural tumors with limited lateral extension and no vascular encasement (anterior foramen meningiomas)

40.3.1 Endonasal Approach to the Craniocervical Junction

Preoperative Planning

All patients should have a complete medical history, CT, MRI, and otoneurological evaluation. MRI allows for the complete identification and determination of the position of the nerves and vascular structures. Instability must be addressed prior to surgery. Large tumors and extensive drilling of the lower clivus can cause chronic instability. Stability of the occipitoatlantal joint is provided by the configuration of the occipitoatlantal joint and the thick articular capsule, along with the anterior and posterior atlantooccipital membranes. If instability is detected, a second staged surgery must be performed.

The nasal mucosa is prepared with topical 0.05% oxymetazoline. The surgical field is prepared by applying povidone-iodine to the nose and the lateral thigh region, in the event that an autologous fascia lata free graft is required for reconstruction. Broad-spectrum prophylactic perioperative antibiotics (ceftriaxone 1 g and clindamycin 600 mg) are administered and continued for the next 5 days. The operating room setup is demonstrated in **Fig. 40.2**.

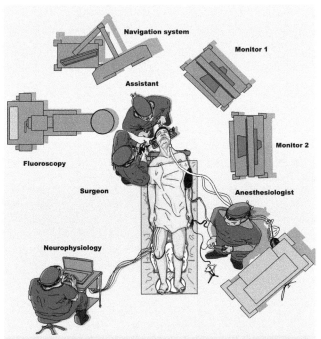

Fig. 40.2 An efficient and organized operating room setup is critical for success. Two monitors are used for the comfort of the surgeon and the assistant. Neurophysiology and anesthesia are usually performed at the feet of the patient to allow sufficient space for the fluoroscope to maneuver freely. We use a two-surgeon binostril technique. No endoscopic holder is used, and the first assistant drives the endoscope and irrigates when needed. This setup allows for an extra hand from the assistant to help with graspers or suction.

Surgical Technique

An EEA is achieved using rod lens endoscopes (Karl Storz, 4 mm, 18 cm, Hopkins II) attached to an HD system (**Video 40.1**). An expanded EEA approach is performed. The right middle turbinate is removed only if needed, and the left middle turbinate is compressed and fractured laterally (**Fig. 40.3a,b**). A posterior septectomy is performed to disarticulate the posterior septum from the rostrum of the sphenoid bone (**Fig. 40.3c,d,e**).

The entire rostrum is removed so that the lateral walls of the sphenoid sinuses are in the same plane as the medial orbital wall and the roof of the sphenoid sinus is in the same plane as the roof of the nasal cavity. The lateral margins of the sphenoidotomies are extended to the level of the medial pterygoid plates to expose the vidian canal, which represents the junction of the most medial aspect of the pterygoid plates with the floor of the sphenoid sinus. The lateral sphenoid recess (the component of the sphenoid recess lateral to the medial pterygoid plates) is also opened to provide a wide bilateral exposure of the structures at the lateral wall of the sphenoid sinus. This exposes the vertical paraclival ICA canal (**Fig. 40.3f**). The canal extends to the antero-lateral edge of the anterior genu of the petrous carotid artery. The anterior genu and the foramen lacerum are medial to the posterior end of the vidian canal (**Fig. 40.4**).

With a combination of high-speed drilling (4-mm diamond bur with a length of at least 18 cm) and Kerrison rongeurs, the sphenoid floor and middle and lower clivus can be removed, depending on the extent of the lesion. In patients for whom an odontoidectomy is required, a focal endoscopic approach to the lower clivus and the anterior arch of C1 is performed without exposing and drilling the mid- and superior clivus.

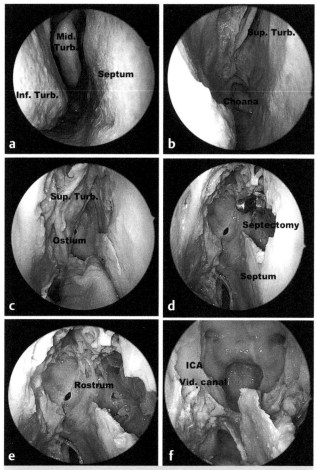

Fig. 40.3 Endonasal endoscopic approach. (**a**) The first stage of the endoscopic approach, localizing the inferior and middle turbinate, reveals the choanae at the end of the endoscopic view, which is the initial landmark for the CVJ. The foramen magnum and the C1 arch typically lie between the choanae, just behind the basipharyngeal fascia. (**b,c**) Posterior to the superior turbinate, the ostium sphenoidale comes into the field. (**d**) Posterior septectomy is performed using a backbiter rongeur. Once the rostrum is totally exposed, it can be removed using a high-speed drill. (**e**) The vomer is also resected to obtain access to the sellar floor and the lower clivus. (**f**) Lateral extension of the approach is performed by first localizing the vidian canal at the pterygoid wedge; the vidian canal leads to the lacerum segment of the ICA. Mid. Turb., middle turbinate; Inf. Turb., inferior turbinate; Sup. Turb., superior turbinate; Vid. canal, vidian canal; ICA, internal carotid artery.

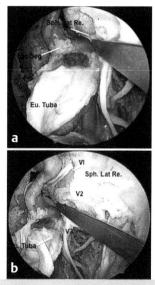

Fig. 40.4 Lateral extension of the EEA. (**a**) Opening the lateral recess of the sphenoid sinus allows exposure of the supracondylar space. (**b**) Some tumors extend into the infratemporal fossa and pterygopalatine fossa, which can be reached using the EEA by drilling out the pterygoid wedge and the posterior wall of the maxillary sinus. Sph. Lat Re., lateral recess of the sphenoid sinus; Eu. Tuba, eustachian tube; Lac Seg, lacerum segment of the internal carotid artery; VI, sixth cranial nerve; V2, maxillary ramus of the trigeminal nerve; V3, mandibular ramus of the trigeminal nerve.

Odontoidectomy

After the aforementioned approach, the C1 anterior tubercle is localized by surgically navigating between the choanae (**Fig. 40.5a**). The anterior portion of the foramen magnum is exposed, along with the transition of the odontoid process and the body of C2 (**Fig. 40.5b**). A longitudinal incision over the midline mucosa and basipharyngeal fascia is made using a long-needle Bovie tip. Dissection of the longus capitis and longus colli exposes the bony structures of the CVJ laterally, and a high-speed drill is used to perform a partial resection of the C1 anterior arch and to completely expose the odontoid process (**Fig. 40.5c**). The odontoid process is drilled out until an eggshell-thick layer of bone is left over the transverse ligament, then a Kerrison rongeur is used to remove the thin layer of bone that remains

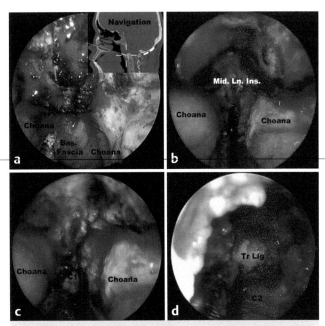

Fig. 40.5 An odontoidectomy performed through an EEA. (**a**) The identification and adequate exposure of the basipharyngeal fascia between the choanae. (**b**) The midline incision over the basipharyngeal fascia. (**c**) Exposure of the anterior arch of C1. (**d**) The complete removal of the upper part of the odontoid process until the transverse ligament is clearly visualized. Mid. Ln. Ins., midline incision; Bas. Fascia, basipharyngeal fascia; Tr Lig, transverse ligament.

(**Fig. 40.5d**). If there is extensive pannus, it is easily removed with a pituitary rongeur. Once the complete removal of the odontoid tip is achieved, the surgical field is covered with Gelfoam and fibrin glue (**Fig. 40.6**). Although a CSF leak has been reported as a complication, it is very unlikely using the eggshell technique (**Fig. 40.7**). The extent of the odontoid resection is confirmed using image guidance and fluoroscopy.[19]

Chordomas

Chordomas extending to the lower clivus are a surgical challenge. They typically extend to the retrocondylar space posterior to the fossa of Rosenmüller. Morera et al[20] described a medially expanded endonasal approach to the lower clivus that provides a unique corridor to the ventrolateral surface of the ponto-medullary and cervicomedullary junctions, and they described the surgical landmarks for the transcondylar and transjugular medial extensions.

The previously described approach is followed at first, but in these cases, a nasoseptal flap is performed at the first stage of the surgery and is left at the maxilla contralateral to the extension of the tumor. After the pterygoid wedge is drilled and the ICA is isolated, the center of the chordoma is removed using an ultrasonic aspirator and sharp dissection. The lateral portion of the chordoma that extends into the posterior fossa requires drilling of the condyle, which is usually required to reach the posterior part of the tumor (**Fig. 40.8a–d**). Cranial nerve XII limits the lateral extension of the condyle resection; a groove over the condyle marks the exit of CN XII and can be used as a landmark, although it is sometimes difficult to spot. In some cases, an intradural component is identified, and widening the opening of the dura is necessary to perform intradural tumor

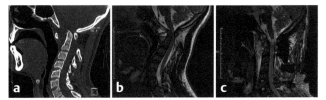

Fig. 40.6 An odontoidectomy case. (**a**) Preoperative T2 MRI, showing the complete disruption of the apical and transverse ligaments, with a 17-mm severe atlantoaxial luxation. (**b**) CT scan showing severe atlantoaxial luxation. (**c**) Postoperative MRI showing adequate decompression after C1–C2 fusion and endoscopic endonasal odontoidectomy.

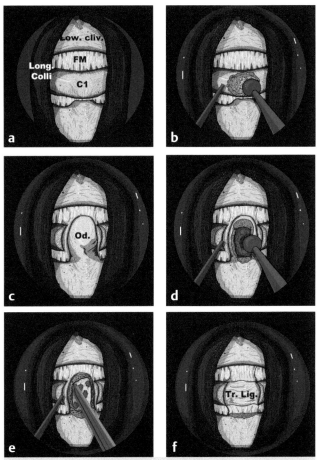

Fig. 40.7 Schematic drawing of an endoscopic endonasal odontoidectomy. (**a**) After longitudinal incision along the midline, lateral dissection of the longus colli is performed to expose the foramen magnum and the anterior arch of C1. (**b,c**) High-speed drilling of the anterior arch of C1 is performed until the odontoid process is exposed. (**d**) Central cavitation with a round diamond bur is performed until only an eggshell remains. (**e**) The eggshell bone is removed using a 1-mm Kerrison rongeur. (**f**) An adequate view of the transverse ligament after odontoidectomy. FM, foramen magnum; Low. cliv., lower clivus; Long. Colli, longus colli muscle; C1, anterior arch of first cervical vertebrae.

resection and dissection from the brainstem and the vertebral arteries (**Fig. 40.8e**). However, localization of the vertebrobasilar system is essential using CT- and MRI-guided navigation (**Fig. 40.8f**). Inferior extension into the cervical spine depends on preoperative planning using the nasopalatine line (**Fig. 40.1**).

In cases in which the hard palate does not allow proper maneuverability of the instruments, a transoral approach is preferred to achieve a total resection. Once the tumor has been removed, hemostasis is achieved with a combination of hemostatic agents and bipolar coagulation. Reconstruction is performed using a collagen matrix (DuraGen) and a fascia lata graft that is harvested and placed over the dural defect. The nasoseptal flap is attached to the bony defect and is covered with fibrin glue.

40.4 Conclusion

Expanded EEA to the CVJ is a feasible, safe, and well-tolerated procedure. Understanding the complex anatomy of the ventral CVJ is essential to safely performing an extended EEA. This approach facilitates a direct route to the ventral CVJ without mobilizing neural and vascular structures. New reconstruction techniques using a nasoseptal flap decrease the risk of CSF leak, providing an advantage over posterior and posterolateral approaches.

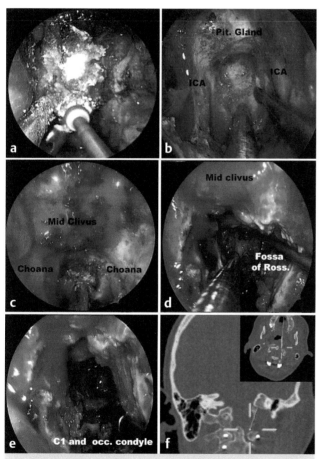

Fig. 40.8 Resection of a chordoma of the lower clivus. **(a)** Removal of the vomer and drilling the sellar floor to expose the mid- and lower clivus. **(b)** Complete exposure of both paraclival ICAs and the clivus. In this particular case, the entire chordoma was retroclival. **(c)** An inverted U incision over the basipharyngeal fascia with a monopolar tip. **(d,e)** Resection of the tumor and the exposure of the condyle and C1 anterior arch. **(f)** Navigation showing the condyle partially eroded by the tumor. The condyle is drilled to gain access to the retrocondylar space, and removal of the tumor located at the fossa is achieved. Pit. Gland, pituitary gland; Fossa of Ross., fossa of Rosenmüller; occ. condyle, occipital condyle.

References

1 Ortega-Porcayo LA, Cabrera-Aldana EE, Arriada-Mendicoa N, Gómez-Amador JL, Granados-García M, Barges-Coll J. Operative technique for en bloc resection of upper cervical chordomas: extended transoral transmandibular approach and multilevel reconstruction. *Asian Spine J* 2014;8(6):820–826

2 de Almeida JR, Zanation AM, Snyderman CH, et al. Defining the naso-palatine line: the limit for endonasal surgery of the spine. *Laryngoscope* 2009;119(2):239–244

3 El-Sayed IH, Wu JC, Dhillon N, Ames CP, Mummaneni P. The importance of platybasia and the palatine line in patient selection for endonasal surgery of the craniocervical junction: a radiographic study of 12 patients. *World Neurosurg* 2011;76(1-2):183–188

4 Aldana PR, Naseri I, La Corte E. The naso-axial line: a new method of accurately predicting the inferior limit of the endoscopic endonasal approach to the craniovertebral junction. *Neurosurgery* 2012;71

5 Kassam A, Thomas AJ, Snyderman C, et al. Fully endoscopic expanded endonasal approach treating skull base lesions in pediatric patients. *J Neurosurg* 2007; 106(2, Suppl)75–86

6 Kassam AB, Snyderman C, Gardner P, Carrau R, Spiro R. The expanded endonasal approach: a fully endoscopic transnasal approach and resection of the odontoid process: technical case report. *Neurosurgery* 2005

7 Messina A, Bruno MC, Decq P, et al. Pure endoscopic endonasal odontoidecto-my: anatomical study. *Neurosurg Rev* 2007;30(3):189–194

8 Panjabi M, Dvorak J, Duranceau J, et al. Three-dimensional movements of the upper cervical spine. *Spine* 1988;13(7):726–730

9 Lopez AJ, Scheer JK, Leibl KE, Smith ZA, Dlouhy BJ, Dahdaleh NS. Anatomy and biomechanics of the craniovertebral junction. *Neurosurg Focus* 2015;38(4):E2

10 Goel A. Craniovertebral junction instability: a review of facts about facets. *Asian Spine J* 2015;9(4):636–644

11 Perez-Orribo L, Little AS, Lefevre RD, et al. Biomechanical evaluation of the craniovertebral junction after anterior unilateral condylectomy: implica-tions for endoscopic endonasal approaches to the cranial base. *Neurosurgery* 2013;72(6):1021–1029

12 Barges-Coll J, Fernandez-Miranda JC, Prevedello DM, et al. Avoiding injury to the abducens nerve during expanded endonasal endoscopic surgery: anatomic and clinical case studies. *Neurosurgery* 2010;67(1):144–154

13 Wang S, Zhang J, Xue L, Wei L, Xi Z, Wang R. Anatomy and CT reconstruction of the anterior area of sphenoid sinus. *Int J Clin Exp Med* 2015;8(4):5217–5226

14 Osawa S, Rhoton AL Jr, Seker A, Shimizu S, Fujii K, Kassam AB. Microsurgical and endoscopic anatomy of the vidian canal. *Neurosurgery* 2009;64(5, Suppl 2):385–411

15 Amene C, Cosetti M, Ambekar S, Guthikonda B, Nanda A. Johann Christian Rosenmüller (1771–1820): a historical perspective on the man behind the fossa. *J Neurol Surg B Skull Base* 2013;74(4):187–193

16 Wen YH, Wen WP, Chen HX, Li J, Zeng YH, Xu G. Endoscopic nasopharyngec-tomy for salvage in nasopharyngeal carcinoma: a novel anatomic orientation. *Laryngoscope* 2010;120(7):1298–1302

17 Bergin M, Bird P, Cowan I, Pearson JF. Exploring the critical distance and posi-tion relationships between the Eustachian tube and the internal carotid artery. *Otol Neurotol* 2010;31(9):1511–1515

18 Funaki T, Matsushima T, Peris-Celda M, Valentine RJ, Joo W, Rhoton AL Jr. Focal transnasal approach to the upper, middle, and lower clivus. *Neurosurgery* 2013; 73

19 Ponce-Gómez JA, Ortega-Porcayo LA, Soriano-Barón HE, et al. Evolution from microscopic transoral to endoscopic endonasal odontoidectomy. *Neurosurg Focus* 2014;37(4):E15

20 Morera VA, Fernandez-Miranda JC, Prevedello DM, et al. "Far-medial" expanded endonasal approach to the inferior third of the clivus: the transcondylar and transjugular tubercle approaches. *Neurosurgery* 2010

41 Endoscopic Transnasal Approaches to the Craniocervical Junction

Sarfaraz Mubarak Banglawala, Jenna Rebelo, Kesava (Kesh) Reddy, and Doron Sommer

41.1 Introduction

The craniovertebral junction is considered a challenging anatomical region for surgical access due to the deep location and close proximity of multiple important neural and vascular structures.

German first demonstrated the feasibility of a transoral approach in dogs in 1930.[1] However, the approach was not used for treatment of spinal pathology until the 1940s and only gained wide acceptance with the advent of the operating microscope in the 1960s.[2] The transoral microscopic approach went on to become the gold standard for odontoidectomy.[3] Despite offering a wide field of view, however, the transoral approach is limited vertically, often requiring a palatal split and/or mandibulotomy to afford access to higher cervical and clival lesions.[4,5,6]

The addition of endoscopic assistance to the transoral route was thus described by Frempong-Boadu et al in 2002 to improve visualization while minimizing the need for palate splitting and mandibulotomy.[2]

The anatomical feasibility of an endoscopic, transnasal approach was demonstrated in cadavers by Alfieri et al,[7] and a fully endoscopic transnasal odontoid resection was first described by Kassam et al in a patient with cervicomedullary compression secondary to rheumatoid arthritis.[8]

This chapter describes the endoscopic transnasal approach and its indications, advantages, and limitations in relation to the transoral (described in Chapter 32) and transcervical approaches.

41.2 Indications for Surgery of the Craniovertebral Junction

- Basilar invagination (**Fig. 41.1**), radiologically defined as:
  - Odontoid tip protrusion[3] 4.5 mm above McGregor's line (line drawn from the posterior hard palate to base of the occiput on sagittal imaging)
  - Tip protrusion[3] 6 mm above Chamberlain's line (line drawn from the posterior hard palate to the anterior lip of the foramen magnum)[9,10]
- Soft tissue pannus due to rheumatoid arthritis (**Fig. 41.2**)[3,8]
- Biopsy or resection of odontoid tumors (**Fig. 41.3**, **Fig. 41.4**)[8,11]
  - Primary or metastatic
  - Intradural or extradural
- Odontoid fracture or nonunion[8]
- Vertebrobasilar aneurysm[8]
- Other craniovertebral junction pathologies, including lesions due to gout, ganglion cyst, and os odontoideum[12]

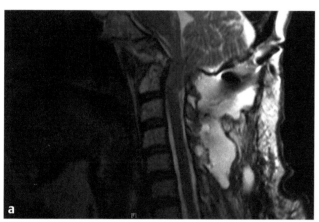
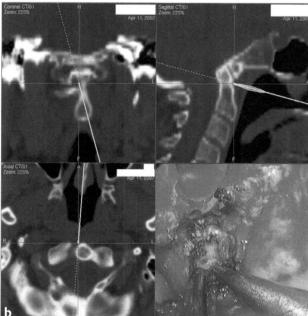

Fig. 41.1 (a,b) Basilar invagination.

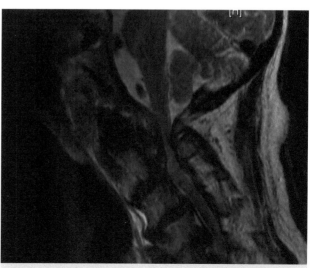

Fig. 41.2 Soft tissue pannus due to rheumatoid arthritis.

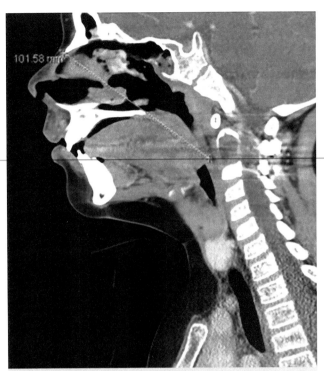

Fig. 41.3 A 7-year-old boy with an osteolytic C2 lesion.

41.3 Approaches

Transnasal Endoscopic Approach

Preoperative Planning

CT angiography is done to study the anatomy of the tumor and to facilitate the use of stereotactic image guidance. The patient is positioned in a slight neck flexion position (as tolerated) to simulate neck position during surgery, as any significant difference will affect the accuracy of the image guidance system. Inferior extent of surgical access may be estimated by the nasopalatine line (**Fig. 41.3**), a line extending from the bottom of the nasal bones to the back of the hard palate.[6]

Preoperative Preparation

The patient is endotracheally intubated.

Using a headlight and nasal speculum, the surgeon prepares the nasal cavity by gentle packing with 1:1000 epinephrine ribbon gauze. This is done very soon after intubation to give the epinephrine ample time to decongest the nasal cavity prior to surgery. There is an option to gently retract the soft palate inferiorly using a small rubber catheter inserted via a nostril and exiting via the oral cavity.

The patient's head is rigidly fixed (via pin fixation) to the operating table in slight neck flexion (as tolerated, trying to emulate the patient's preoperative CT scan position to optimize access and image guidance system accuracy).

The table is placed in reverse Trendelenburg position to decrease venous return and to reduce intraoperative bleeding.

Heights of the table and monitors are adjusted to the surgeon's comfort level. Otolaryngologist and neurosurgeon positioning is similar to that for other expanded endonasal cases (**Fig. 41.5**).

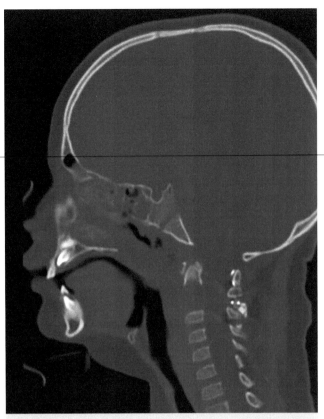

Fig. 41.4 Resection of odontoid tumors.

Image guidance is registered, calibrated and verified prior to draping the patient.

Neurophysiologic monitoring is set up at this time.

The patient is given preoperative antibiotics to cover for nasal contamination into the surgical field.

Operative Steps

● *Exposure*

1. Using a 0° endoscope, the middle turbinate is lateralized or partially resected. Inferior turbinates are lateralized.

2. Sphenoid ostia are identified and wide sphenoidotomies are performed.

3. Use of a long, insulated needle cautery gives the option to develop a large, posteriorly based, nasoseptal flap. This may be performed routinely or only in cases of likely CSF leak. The flap can be raised from the sphenoid face to as far anterior as just behind the columella, extending inferiorly to include partial floor of the nose. Care is taken not to remove the olfactory mucosa superiorly by staying at the level of the sphenoid ostia until the middle turbinate is reached, before then heading superiorly. The flap may be stored in the maxillary sinus to avoid injury during surgery.

4. A posterior, inferior septectomy is performed to allow greater freedom of movement with two-nostril instrumentation.

5. The rostrum is drilled down with a size-4 diamond drill bit or fractured out with Kerrison rongeurs. Bleeding may ensue at the palato-vaginal canal region.

6. A wide exposure is now obtained, with soft palate caudal, and eustachian tubes lateral, to the field.

7. Care should be taken not to injure the vidian nerve or to violate the carotid canals.

8. An inferiorly based U-shaped flap is raised in the nasopharynx and is reflected caudally to the level of the soft palate. The flap is planned well medial to the eustachian tubes—i.e., medial to the internal carotid arteries. See **Fig. 41.6** and **Video 41.1**.

9. The pharyngobasilar fascia is elevated from the inferior sphenoid floor to the ventral clivus.

10. The sphenoid floor is drilled flush with the clivus.

11. Using insulated cautery and periosteal elevators/Freer elevators, the fascia and paraspinal muscles/longus capitis and longus colli are reflected inferiorly (this is partially achieved during step 8, above). Care is taken to avoid heat injury posteriorly to the spinal cord by limiting the cautery setting and avoiding prolonged cautery during this step. Ensure that the trajectory is inferior (not posterior along the clivus) toward C1.

12. The ring of C1 is identified and is verified with image guidance.

● *Resection*

1. Depending on the pathology, various portions of the C1 ring and odontoid process are resected (**Fig. 41.7**, **Fig. 41.8**). This is generally performed with an elongated diamond drill and irrigation. It is advisable to perform the vast majority of drilling prior to freeing up most ligamentous attachments of odontoid, so as to avoid drilling a mobile structure. Other instruments, including Kerrison rongeurs, are also utilized. See **Video 41.2** and **Video 41.3**.

2. The amount of dens that will need to be removed depends on the location and extent of the compression. This predicts how much overlying ring of C1 will need to be resected.

3. The dens is followed from the C2 body to its tip and is removed laterally. The cap is removed using sharp dissection.

4. Drilling and dissection are kept to a median and paramedian location (medial to the occipital condyles). Anatomical landmarks and image guidance are used to ensure the correct trajectory. Surrogate landmarks for the parapharyngeal carotid artery include the eustachian tube orifice. Midline landmarks include the posterior hard palate notch and the rostral portion of the nasal septum/sphenoid (although this is partially excised for access). The tubercle of C1 is also confirmed via image guidance.

5. In rheumatoid disease, as C1 ligaments and odontoid are removed, hypertrophic pannus (**Fig. 41.9**) is identified, which is removed with an ultrasonic aspirator.

6. Decompression is adequately achieved when good CSF pulsations (seen through intact dura) are re-established along the entire length of the affected region.

7. The nasopharyngeal flap is re-approximated with fibrin glue. The nasoseptal flap is used if CSF leak is encountered; otherwise, the flap is replaced onto the septum where it was originally raised.

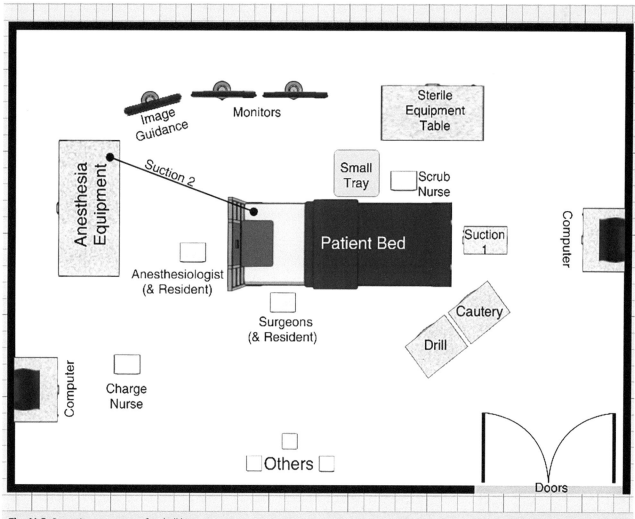

Fig. 41.5 Operating room setup for skull base.

287

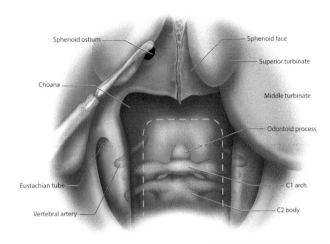

Fig. 41.6 Flap is raised.

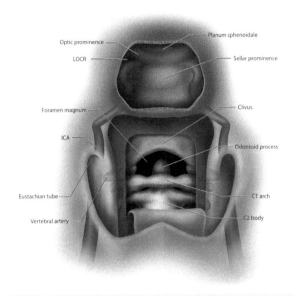

Fig. 41.7 Bony exposure.

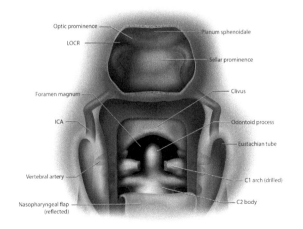

Fig. 41.8 Exposure of odontoid after C1 is drilled out.

8. The posterior nasopharynx is lightly packed with Gelfoam or other absorbable (hemostatic) packing material.
9. The nasal cavity may be packed with various materials (Silastic sheets, Doyle splints, other removable or absorbable nasal packing) to prevent synechiae and to facilitate mucosal healing. The authors' preference is Doyle splints, which are covered with topical antibiotic ointment and sutured to the septum.
10. The patient is awakened from general anesthesia, and efforts are made to prevent the patient's coughing and bucking during this phase.
11. When the patient is alert, he or she is examined for any cranial nerve or peripheral deficits.

Postoperative Notes

1. Posterior instrumented fusion is often indicated for these patients due to instability. Many centers perform this during the same anesthetic session or within 1 week of the initial surgery. However, timing and need vary considerably and depend on patient factors, degree of instability, and individual surgeon preference.
2. Nasal saline irrigations (high volume—e.g., 100–240 mL) are utilized BID to QID for the first few weeks, then once daily for several months until all crusting has stopped.
3. Otolaryngology follow-up is arranged to remove Silastic nasal stents at 1 to 2 weeks, then two or three more visits are scheduled at several-week intervals (more as indicated) to ensure that no crusting, adhesions, or other sinonasal concerns arise.
4. The spinal surgery team follows the patient to monitor for any instability or weakness.

Transoral Approach

1. The tongue is retracted inferiorly and the uvula and soft palate superiorly. Occasionally glossectomy, mandulotomy, and hard palate division are needed to gain access.
2. The oropharyngeal mucosa is incised in the midline.
3. The superior pharyngeal constrictors are divided.
4. The longus capitis and longus colli muscles from C1 to C3 are exposed, displaced, and retracted to give access from the clivus to C3.
5. Resection of lesion/decompression is done in a fashion similar to that described above for the transnasal approach.

Transcervical Approach

1. A high, linear, vertical incision is made along the anterior neck from above the level of the hyoid to the cricoid.
2. The platysma is divided, and the anterior aspect of the sternocleidomastoid muscle is identified and retracted laterally.
3. The strap muscles are retracted medially.
4. The trachea and esophagus are retracted medially, and great vessels are retracted laterally. The digastric is mobilized to provide increased superior exposure.
5. Self-retaining retractors are placed once exposure of the cervical spine is obtained.
6. Care is taken not to injure the recurrent laryngeal nerve or to cause perforation of the esophagus during resection.
7. Exposure is excellent for the C4–C5 level but can be obtained for upper levels as well in certain cases.
8. Resection of the lesion is carried out as indicated.

41.4 Transoral Approach—Advantages and Disadvantages

Advantages

- Well-established procedure
- Wide surgical field
- Access as caudal as the C3 body

Disadvantages

- Oral retraction commonly leads to tongue edema
- Prophylactic tracheotomy common
- Surgical wound contamination due to oral secretions (possibly causing infection, dehiscence, and meningitis)
- Palate splitting or glossectomy for more rostral exposure
- Dysphagia requiring nasogastric feeding tube
- Velopharyngeal incompetency (VPI)
- Dental injury
- Difficulty in micrognathic patients

41.5 Transcervical Approach—Advantages and Disadvantages

Advantages

- Wider exposure
- Avoidance of (contaminated) upper aerodigestive mucosa

Disadvantages and Complications

- Limited exposure of upper cervical spine
- Skin incision
- Risk to nearby structures:
  - Esophagus, trachea
  - Carotid sheath
  - Cranial nerves

41.6 Transnasal Approach—Advantages and Disadvantages

Advantages

- Improved visualization
  - Endoscopy
  - Access to high clival lesions
- Avoids oral retraction
  - No tongue edema
  - No tracheotomy
- Avoids palate splitting
  - No VPI, no dysphonia

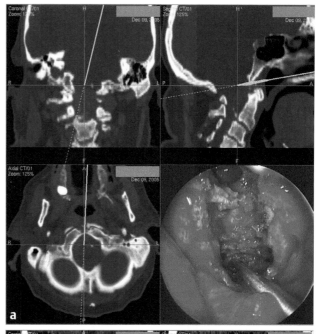

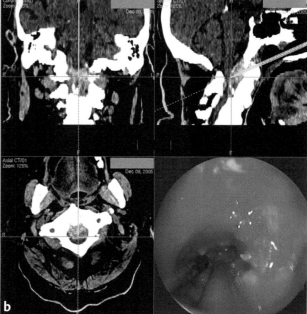

Fig. 41.9 (a,b) Hypertrophic pannus.

  - No dysphagia, and no need for nasogastric feedings
- Decreased exposure to oral microflora in surgical field
- Theoretical decreased risk of infection, dehiscence

Disadvantages and Complications

- Learning curve
  - Loss of 3D view
  - Loss of depth perception
  - Longer operative duration
- Risk to surrounding structures
  - Eustachian tube
  - Parapharyngeal carotid

- o Vidian nerve
- Intranasal complications
  - o Crusting, sinusitis
  - o Epistaxis
  - o Septal perforations

41.7 Limitations of the Endonasal Approach

- Hard palate restricts exposure below C2. (Note: Use nasopalatine line to define inferior limit of resection.[6])
- Can be challenging to new surgeons, especially with perceived loss of 3D and depth perception with endoscope (as compared to microscope).
- There is a surgical learning curve.
- Requires two-person team consisting of neurosurgeon and otolaryngologist. Teams should be experienced with working together and have experience with simpler cases, such as pituitary tumors or CSF leak repair.
- Tumors/lesions posterior to neurovascular structures may not be accessible, and an open approach may be warranted instead.
- Generally contraindicated if a major vessel needs to be resected or reconstructed.

41.8 Limitations of the Transoral Approach

- Can be challenging to get access, depending on oropharyngeal anatomy, such as large tongue/uvula, etc.
- Difficult or sometimes impossible in micrognathic patients
- Limited clival exposure
- Complications, such as VPI, airway concerns (possibly requiring tracheostomy), and swallowing concerns (possibly requiring feeding tube)
- Possible contamination of surgical field with oral microflora

41.9 Limitations of the Transcervical Approach

- Limited exposure of upper cervical spine

- Obesity or short neck may make dissection and exposure difficult.
- Risk of injuring various cranial nerves and great vessels in neck with dissection/retraction
- Injury to esophagus carries high risk of infection and breakdown of any instrumentation placed.

41.10 Conclusion

The transnasal endoscopic approach has been demonstrated to be effective in the management of craniovertebral junction pathologies, while avoiding the airway, speech, and swallowing-related morbidity of transoral surgery.[12] In addition, the approach extends the field of visualization further superiorly than is possible with other routes and should be considered in the management of clival and upper cervical spine lesions.[13]

References

1. Greenberg AD, Scoville WB, Davey LM. Transoral decompression of atlanto-axial dislocation due to odontoid hypoplasia. Report of two cases. *J Neurosurg* 1968;28(3):266–269
2. Frempong-Boadu AK, Faunce WA, Fessler RG. Endoscopically assisted transoral-transpharyngeal approach to the craniovertebral junction. *Neurosurgery* 2002;51(5, Suppl):S60–S66
3. Ponce-Gómez JA, Ortega-Porcayo LA, Soriano-Barón HE, et al. Evolution from microscopic transoral to endoscopic endonasal odontoidectomy. *Neurosurg Focus* 2014;37(4):E15
4. Crockard HA. The transoral approach to the base of the brain and upper cervical cord. *Ann R Coll Surg Engl* 1985;67(5):321–325
5. Menezes AH, VanGilder JC. Transoral-transpharyngeal approach to the anterior craniocervical junction. Ten-year experience with 72 patients. *J Neurosurg* 1988;69(6):895–903
6. Menezes AH. Surgical approaches: postoperative care and complications "transoral-transpalatopharyngeal approach to the craniocervical junction." *Childs Nerv Syst* 2008;24(10):1187–1193
7. Alfieri A, Jho H-D, Tschabitscher M. Endoscopic endonasal approach to the ventral cranio-cervical junction: anatomical study. *Acta Neurochir (Wien)* 2002
8. Kassam AB, Snyderman C, Gardner P, Carrau R, Spiro R. The expanded endonasal approach: a fully endoscopic transnasal approach and resection of the odontoid process: technical case report. *Neurosurgery* 2005
9. de Almeida JR, Zanation AM, Snyderman CH, et al. Defining the nasopalatine line: the limit for endonasal surgery of the spine. *Laryngoscope* 2009;119(2):239–244
10. Wu JC, Mummaneni PV, El-Sayed IH. Diseases of the odontoid and craniovertebral junction with management by endoscopic approaches. *Otolaryngol Clin North Am* 2011;44(5):1029–1042
11. Lee A, Sommer D, Reddy K, Murty N, Gunnarsson T. Endoscopic transnasal approach to the craniocervical junction. *Skull Base* 2010;20(3):199–205
12. Goldschlager T, Härtl R, Greenfield JP, Anand VK, Schwartz TH. The endoscopic endonasal approach to the odontoid and its impact on early extubation and feeding. *J Neurosurg* 2015;122(3):511–518
13. Seker A, Inoue K, Osawa S, Akakin A, Kilic T, Rhoton AL Jr. Comparison of endoscopic transnasal and transoral approaches to the craniovertebral junction. *World Neurosurg* 2010;74(6):583–602

42 Endoscopic Transoral Approaches to the Craniocervical Junction

James H. Stephen and John Y. K. Lee

42.1 Introduction

Surgical access to the craniovertebral junction (CVJ) is challenging because of its deep, anatomically protected location. The pathology that can involve the CVJ is diverse and includes rheumatoid odontoid pannus, basilar invagination, congenital skull base malformations, lower clival chordomas and chondrosarcomas, metastatic disease, infection, and even intradural pathologies, such as meningiomas. The most direct route to the anterior CVJ is by the ventral transoral approach.[1,2] This approach was refined by Menezes, Crockard, and Hadley[3,4,5] and was adopted as the preferred approach for treating pathology of the anterior CVJ. However, the traditional transoral approach has several limitations. Given the deep, narrow working channel, the operating microscope may not provide adequate visualization of the pathology. While the extended transoral variants may achieve improved visualization and greater access, they are achieved at the expense of greater morbidity.

Given the significant morbidity with the traditional transoral approach, endoscopic approaches to the CVJ have been pioneered. Compared with the narrow column of illumination and visualization provided by the operative microscope, the endoscope can provide direct illumination deeper and closer to the target. Modern endoscopes can capture a field of view up to 80° and provide a panoramic view of the anatomy. Another current advantage of endoscopes is their worldwide availability. Unlike microscopes, however, most endoscopes remain two-dimensional, with resolution that is limited by the camera and the display screen, but these limitations are being addressed with three-dimensional endoscopes and improved video technology. The feasibility of transoral robotic surgery (TORS) as a tool to address pathology of the craniocervical junction has been demonstrated.[6] In TORS, the dual-channel endoscope provides stereoscopic (3D) visualization with excellent illumination and there are two articulating robotic arms to work at depth in the deep narrow channel. However, there are limitations to TORS that prevent the entire procedure, especially bony removal, from being performed endoscopically by the robot. As surgeons continue to pioneer the endoscopic transoral approach, improvements in technology and instrumentation over time will allow a greater range of pathology to be tackled through this approach (**Video 42.1**).

42.2 Surgical Anatomy

- The endoscopic transoral approach provides access from the lower third of the clivus down to the C2–C3 disk space.
- Surgical exposure and the size of the working channel are limited by mouth opening. In addition, the hard palate is the physical barrier that limits superior access, while the mandible and tongue limit inferior access. However, given that endoscopy provides panoramic illumination and visualization not limited to the line of sight, these geometric limitations are less of a hindrance than in traditional transoral approaches.[7]
- Identification of the midline is very important for the transoral approach. The anterior arch of the atlas can be palpated and visualized behind the pharynx.
- Aberrant vertebral arteries or retropharyngeal carotid arteries are a possibility, although both usually lie more than 1 cm off the midline. This affords a safe working zone up to 1 cm laterally on either side of the midline.

42.3 Preoperative Planning

- Patients with trismus (inability to fully open the mouth), prior temporomandibular joint (TMJ) injuries, or prior TMJ surgery may not be candidates for transoral surgery. An inability to open the mouth at least 25 mm (average mouth opening is 40 mm) preoperatively is a relative contraindication to transoral surgery.
- A fixed chin-on-chest deformity is also a contraindication to the transoral approach. Other contraindications include dental/periodontal infections or anomalous anatomy that results in vital neurovascular structures' being ventral to the pathology.
- Lesions that are reducible from a posterior approach should undergo a simple posterior decompression and fusion rather than undergoing a transoral approach.
- Preoperative CT may be utilized to assess the limits of surgical access in each individual patient. The length of the hard palate and the position of the CVJ relative to the hard palate help determine access. If the pathology is located above the hard palate, then an endonasal approach may be a better choice.
- Vascular imaging with CT angiography (CTA) may be helpful where a tumor has distorted the anatomy or when lateral dissection is required.
- The transoral approach is limited by providing decompression only. Pathology at the CVJ may lead to instability, and this can be further destabilized by the procedure. Often, posterior surgical stabilization may also be required, and reconstruction/stabilization should be considered preoperatively.
- Preoperative trach or percutaneous endoscopic gastrostomy (PEG) may be required in patients with existing lower cranial nerve dysfunction, and this possibility should be evaluated as part of the preoperative work-up.
- A lumbar drain can also be placed preoperatively if intradural pathology is the surgical target or if a CSF leak is expected.
- The patient should be adequately counseled preoperatively about the potential complications and morbidities of the transoral approach.

42.4 Patient Positioning and Anesthesia

- The patient is positioned supine with slight neck extension. Care should be taken to avoid head rotation to prevent surgical disorientation that may result from rotation of the atlas—and vertebral artery—in relation to the midline.
- The patient's head may be fixed in a Mayfield head holder or a halo vest, depending on the stability of the CVJ.
- The airway is of critical importance, and collaboration with anesthesia should ensure proper choice of, and technique for, the endotracheal tube (ETT). We prefer a midline armored ETT that exits inferiorly toward the patient's feet.
- Intraoperative monitoring, including somatosensory evoked potentials and motor evoked potentials, is utilized to prevent any positioning-related neurological compromise.
- Lateral fluoroscopy is utilized for localization of the bony anatomy. Neuronavigation may also be used for intraoperative localization.
- For endoscopic procedures, surgeons are positioned on either side of the head, with the display monitor at the head of the bed.
- For TORS, the da Vinci surgical robot (Intuitive Surgical, Sunnyvale, CA) is positioned at the head of the bed. A 12-mm, 0° endoscope is used, although a 30° endoscope may be used to enhance the superior or inferior visualization as needed. The binocular endoscopic arm is kept midline, with one articulating arm on either side.

42.5 Surgical Procedure

- There are several options for retraction during the transoral approach, including the Dingman retractor or a Crowe-Davis retractor.
- Care should be taken not to overdistract the jaw, dislocating or injuring the TMJ. We limit the opening to 4 cm.
- The soft palate can also obscure the view, but it may be retracted superiorly using two red rubber catheters placed through the nose and out of the mouth (**Fig. 42.1**). Alternatively, a stitch can be placed in the uvula, which is then retracted out through the nose.
- While it is rarely necessary, the soft palate may be split, incising from the uvula up to the hard palate.
- Teeth guards should be used and care should be taken to avoid tongue compression against the teeth by the retractor or ETT tube.
- The anterior arch of the atlas may be palpated with gentle pressure.
- We prefer a midline incision in the posterior pharyngeal mucosa, where there is a relatively avascular plane. This avoids critical vascular and neural structures that may be damaged with a U-shaped incision (**Fig. 42.2**).
- Using TORS, a midline incision is taken down to the anterior arch of C1 and then is extended inferiorly to the body of C2. At this point, localization is confirmed with lateral fluoroscopy. The anterior longitudinal ligament is taken down to expose the anterior atlantooccipital membrane, the arch of C1, and the base and dens of C2 (**Fig. 42.3**).

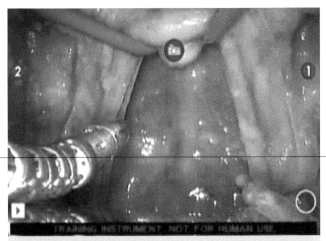

Fig. 42.1 Endoscopic view with uvula and soft palate retracted superiorly by red rubber catheter.

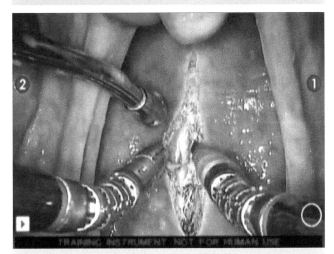

Fig. 42.2 Midline incision made in posterior pharyngeal mucosa.

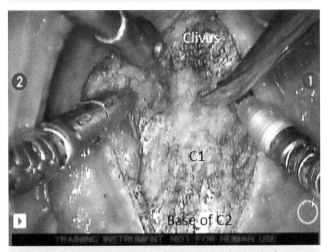

Fig. 42.3 View of craniovertebral junction after removal of anterior longitudinal ligament and subperiosteal dissection of clivus, C1, and base of the dens.

- The eustachian tubes, relatively fixed in the skull, are a useful landmark that represents the lateral extent for carrying out the subperiosteal dissection along C2. However, care should be taken to avoid damage to the eustachian tubes.

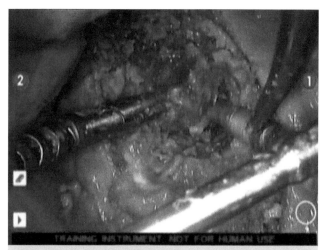

Fig. 42.4 Removal of the tip of the dens.

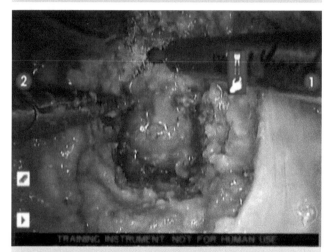

Fig. 42.5 Drilling of inferior clivus is possible if treating intradural pathology.

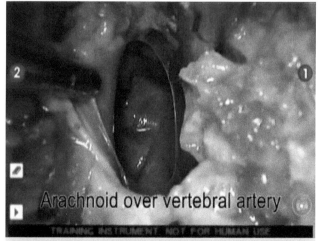

Fig. 42.6 Endoscopic intradural view of vertebral artery overlying the medulla.

- Once soft tissue dissection is completed, we switch to an endoscope-assisted procedure. Due to the lack of a drill attachment for the da Vinci, the endoscope is left in place and traditional bone removal progresses utilizing the endoscopic

monitor for visualization. The primary surgeon may remain at the robot station to assist in bone removal under the 3D optics.

- The C1 arch is removed by drilling two troughs. The maximum width of bone removal should not extend laterally beyond the medial border of the lateral mass (~ 16 mm maximum).
- The dens is removed after the removal of the apical and alar ligaments (**Fig. 42.4**).
- With clival or intradural pathology, the inferior clivus can be removed with further high-speed drilling (**Fig. 42.5**).
- For intradural pathology, the surgeon once again utilizes TORS, using the articulating surgical arms to continue to work in the deep, narrow channel with the benefit of 3D visualization (**Fig. 42.6**).
- With TORS, the dura may be closed with 4–0 suture utilizing the articulating robotic arms. A dural patch or fibrin glue may also be used. For a purely endoscopic approach, a mucosal flap may be used.
- The mucosa is then closed with interrupted sutures.

42.6 Limitations

- Obtaining a watertight dural closure in a deep, narrow working channel is a major limitation in addressing intradural pathology or repairing CSF leaks through the transoral approach.
- TORS offers the ability to perform this closure with dexterity at depth, as the articulated robotic arms can manipulate stitches easily in the deep, narrow working space. A tight, layered closure of the dura and pharyngeal mucosa is key to prevention of CSF leaks and subsequent infections.
- Another limitation of the TORS approach is the lack of bone-cutting instruments, such as drills or rongeurs, and of intradural tools for the current version of the da Vinci robot. This limits the current utility of TORS to improved dexterity during exposure and closure. After bone-removal and intradural instruments are developed, pioneering surgeons will be able to further utilize TORS to address more widespread pathology at the CVJ.

42.7 Complications

- Complications are similar to those in the classic transoral approach and include airway compromise, edema, dysphagia, damage to the TMJ, infection, CSF leak, neurovascular injury, and increased spinal instability.
- CSF leaks, a known complication of the transoral approach, can be challenging to repair and may lead to serious infections if not addressed properly.
- Patients should remain intubated postoperatively to allow edema to subside. Prior to extubation, patients should pass an ETT cuff leak test. Extubation should occur in a monitored setting with access to surgical airway equipment and an otolaryngologist.
- Preoperative stabilization with a halo vest or posterior fusion reduces the risk of postoperative spinal instability at the CVJ.

References

1   Crockard HA, Pozo JL, Ransford AO, Stevens JM, Kendall BE, Essigman WK. Transoral decompression and posterior fusion for rheumatoid atlanto-axial subluxation. *J Bone Joint Surg Br* 1986;*68*(3):350–356

2   Sen CN, Sekhar LN. Surgical management of anteriorly placed lesions at the craniocervical junction—an alternative approach. *Acta Neurochir (Wien)* 1991;*108*(1-2):70–77

3   Menezes AH, VanGilder JC. Transoral-transpharyngeal approach to the anterior craniocervical junction. Ten-year experience with 72 patients. *J Neurosurg* 1988;*69*(6):895–903

4   Crockard HA. The transoral approach to the base of the brain and upper cervical cord. *Ann R Coll Surg Engl* 1985;*67*(5):321–325

5   Hadley MN, Spetzler RF, Sonntag VK. The transoral approach to the superior cervical spine. A review of 53 cases of extradural cervicomedullary compression. *J Neurosurg* 1989;*71*(1):16–23

6   Lee JY, O'Malley BW, Newman JG, et al. Transoral robotic surgery of cranio-cervical junction and atlantoaxial spine: a cadaveric study. *J Neurosurg Spine* 2010;*12*(1):13–18

7   Lega BC, Kramer DR, Newman JG, Lee JY. Morphometric measurements of the anterior skull base for endoscopic transoral and transnasal approaches. *Skull Base* 2011;*21*(1):65–70

43 Foramen Magnum Decompression of Chiari Malformation Using Minimally Invasive Tubular Retractors

Renée Kennedy, Mohammed Aref, Jetan Badhiwala, Brian Vinh, Saleh Almenawer, and Kesava (Kesh) Reddy

43.1 Clinical Case Example

A 50-year-old male presented with a 6-month history of occipital headaches and paresthesias affecting both hands. The headache was worsened by the Valsalva maneuver and had not been relieved by any medical therapy. CT demonstrated a 12-mm cerebellar tonsillar descent below the foramen magnum (**Fig. 43.1**). MRI of the brain and spine suggested impaired flow of CSF across the foramen magnum secondary to tonsillar herniation (**Fig. 43.2**), with no evidence of syringomyelia (**Video 43.1**).

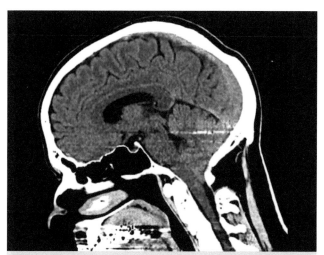

Fig. 43.1 Head CT demonstrating cerebellar tonsillar descent.

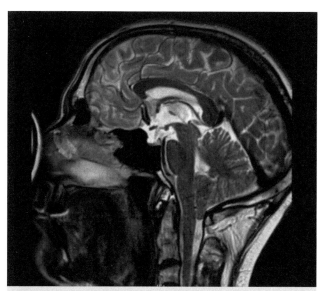

Fig. 43.2 MRI of the brain confirming the diagnosis of Chiari I malformation.

43.2 Preoperative Plan

- The patient was selected to undergo foramen magnum decompression through a minimally invasive technique using the operative microscope and METRx (minimal exposure tubular retractor) tubular retractor system (Medtronic, Memphis, TN).
- Under general anesthesia and endotracheal intubation, the patient was positioned in the prone position with the head in a three-pin Mayfield frame and the cervical spine slightly flexed. Care was taken to ensure that ventilation was not compromised and that the endotracheal tube was accessible to the anesthesiologist.
- The hair was appropriately shaved, and the skin from the occipital protuberance to the spinous process of C2 was prepped and draped in the usual sterile fashion.
- Somatosensory evoked potentials (SSEPs) and motor evoked potentials (MEPs) were monitored throughout the procedure.

43.3 Surgical Procedure

- A small midline incision was made over the suboccipital region through the skin, subcutaneous tissue, and fascia.
- Under fluoroscopic guidance, a K-wire was introduced above the foramen magnum onto the inferior aspect of the occipital bone, with care taken to avoid entry into the occiput–C1 junction (**Fig. 43.3**). Once appropriate K-wire position was confirmed on fluoroscopic views, the skin and fascia incision was extended to accommodate the first tubular dilator. The first dilator was placed in position, and the K-wire was removed.
- Tubular dilators of progressively increasing diameter were sequentially placed to a depth appropriate for the thickness of the

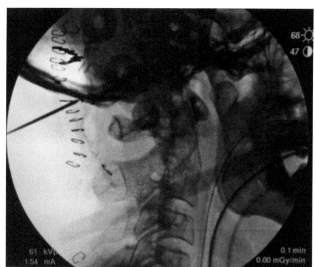

Fig. 43.3 Fluoroscopic image demonstrating insertion of a K-wire onto the inferior aspect of the occipital bone.

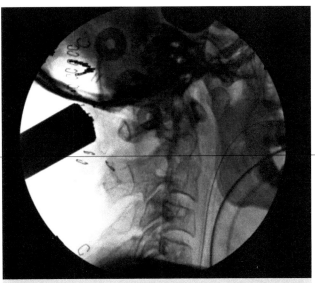

Fig. 43.4 Gradual distraction of soft tissue using sequential dilation technique with progressively larger diameter tubular retractors under fluoroscopic guidance.

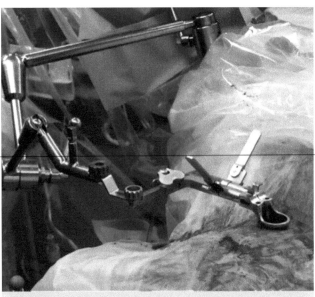

Fig. 43.5 The 22-mm Quadrant tube is attached to the flexible arm to fix it in stable position.

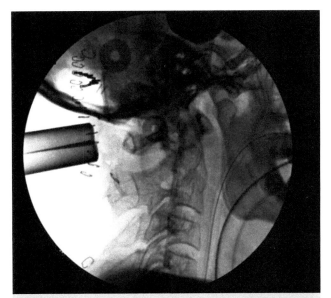

Fig. 43.6 Angulation of the final tubular retractor under fluoroscopic guidance to allow access to a wide working area without increasing soft tissue exposure.

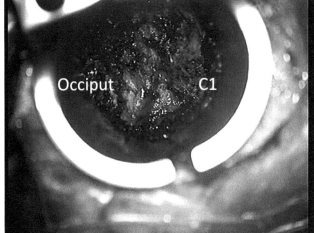

Fig. 43.7 Microscopic view of the occiput (*left*) and C1 (*right*) at the occipitocervical junction.

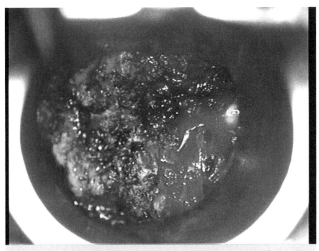

Fig. 43.8 Microscopic view after removal of the posterior arch of C1 (*right*).

underlying tissue and muscle (**Fig. 43.4**). The goal was to gradually distract the soft tissues to provide a final viewing diameter of 22 mm prior to opening the two leaves of the Quadrant system.

- The final tubular retractor (METRx Quadrant) was attached to the flexible arm, which keeps the retractor in a fixed position (**Fig. 43.5**) while also allowing it to be directed in variable angles (**Fig. 43.6**) required for bony removal and dural opening/closure.

43.4 Microscopic Findings

- The microscope was brought into the operating field.
- The occiput–C1 junction was identified (**Fig. 43.7**), and the bony edges of the occiput and C1 were freed from the surrounding soft tissue.

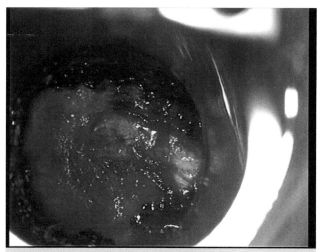

Fig. 43.9 Microscopic view after removal of the posterior arch of C1 (*right*) and the inferior aspect of the occipital bone (*left*).

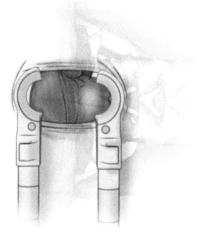

Fig. 43.10 Schematic diagram after removal of the posterior arch of C1 and inferior aspect of the occipital bone.

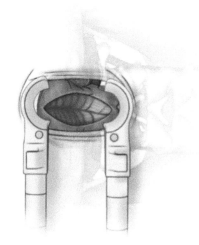

Fig. 43.11 Schematic diagram after elliptical durotomy.

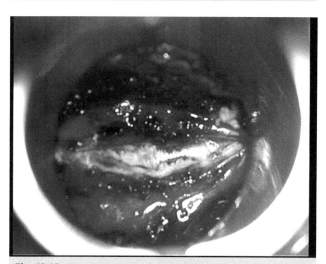

Fig. 43.12 Microscopic image showing the opening through the outer layer of dura.

- Using a cutting bur, the posterior arch of C1 was carefully removed by the "eggshell" technique, with the high-speed drill being directed in a medial-to-lateral direction, back and forth. Any remaining bone was removed with a Kerrison rongeur, and the underlying dura was then fully exposed (**Fig. 43.8**).

- The occipital bone was drilled down using the same technique to provide a bony opening of 3 × 3 cm (**Fig. 43.9**).

- After a satisfactory bony decompression was achieved (**Fig. 43.10**), an elliptical durotomy was fashioned using a No. 11 scalpel (**Fig. 43.11**).

- In the described case, only the outer layer of dura was opened, and this was deemed to be a sufficient decompression (**Fig. 43.12**). However, a duraplasty may be performed

if desired. The goal is to enlarge the space at the foramen magnum to ameliorate obstruction to CSF flow. Using 7–0 Prolene suture with a very small needle, the dural graft is approximated to the margins of the durotomy in a simple, continuous fashion (**Fig. 43.13**). Fibrin sealant is applied liberally over the closure.

- A Valsalva maneuver was induced at this point to confirm watertight dural closure under direct visualization.

- The blades of the tubular retractor were closed, and the instrument was withdrawn.

- The fascia and overlying skin were re-approximated in the usual fashion (**Fig. 43.14**).

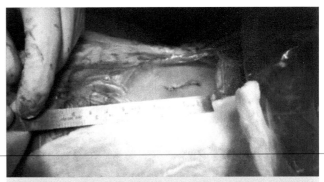

Fig. 43.14 The relatively smaller incision with the minimally invasive technique compared to the incision needed for the conventional open approach.

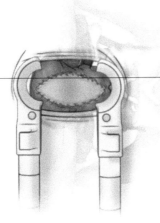

Fig. 43.13 Schematic diagram demonstrating the expansile duraplasty closure.

43.5 Results

Postoperative head CT demonstrated satisfactory bony removal (**Fig. 43.15**). MRI of the area with CSF flow study is performed routinely to assess change in the size of the syrinx, when one is present preoperatively, and to ensure good CSF flow across the foramen magnum.

43.6 Tips

- Carefully start over the lower occipital area under fluoroscopic guidance when inserting the K-wire and subsequent dilators to avoid entering the occiput–C1 junction.
- Use the METRx Quadrant as the final tubular retractor to provide a wide exposure that will facilitate adequate bony decompression and expansile duraplasty.

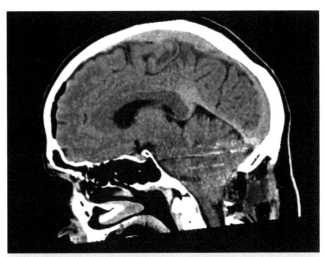

Fig. 43.15 Postoperative CT demonstrating posterior fossa decompression with removal of C1 and the inferior aspect of the occiput.

- The use of a microscope, endoscope, or exoscope through the tubular retractor depends on surgeon preference and recognition of the limitations of each system.
- Perform a Valsalva maneuver to ensure watertight dural closure and to prevent postoperative CSF leak.

44 Percutaneous Endoscopic Cervical Diskectomy

Gun Choi, Alfonso García, Akarawit Asawasaksakul, and Ketan Deshpande

44.1 Introduction

First described by Robinson and Cloward, anterior cervical diskectomy and fusion has become an established, commonly performed operation for subaxial cervical disk prolapse.[1,2] Although anterior cervical diskectomy and fusion (ACDF) still remains the mainstay of the surgical options for cervical disk prolapse, it requires entrance into the spinal canal, with the accompanying risk of complications, such as epidural bleeding, perineural fibrosis, graft-related problems, dysphagia, and hoarseness. Indirect decompression using minimally invasive laminoforaminotomy fails to address the pathology anteriorly. The successful use of percutaneous endoscopic cervical diskectomy (PECD) has been reported by several authors.[3,4,5,6] In the long-term outcome reported by Lee and Lee, the reduction of disk height and progression of disk degeneration did not have any effect on clinical symptoms.[7] Also, Kim et al stated that cervical curvature did not worsen after posterior PECD.[8] These findings proved that PECD can be an excellent alternative for treating various cervical disk problems with meticulous selection of patients.[9] Indications for PECD include soft cervical disk prolapse without cervical instability or evidence of central canal or foraminal stenosis. PECD and thermodiskoplasty can effectively treat diskogenic cervical headaches due to soft disk herniation.[10] PECD is not advisable above the C3 level because of the broader hypopharynx and carotid artery bifurcation. It is also not recommended for patients with previous anterior surgery, axial neck pain, cervical infection, or tumor. Relative contraindications to PECD include bilateral cervical radiculopathy.[11] The advantage of PECD is that it can accomplish both a decompressive surgery and thermal neurotomy/denaturation with the use of radiofrequency (**Video 44.1**).

44.2 Indications

- Low cervical (C3–C7) soft disk herniations without segmental instability
- Cervicogenic headache

44.3 Contraindications

PECD is not recommended for:
- Patients with previous anterior cervical surgery
- Patients with dominant axial neck pain
- Cervical instability
- Cervical infection or tumor
- High cervical level pathology (above C3)

Relative contraindications are:
- Bilateral cervical radiculopathy
- Calcified disk and/or foraminal stenosis
- Cervical stenosis not related to soft disk herniation

44.4 Technique

44.4.1 Anatomical Considerations

When performing anterior cervical disk puncture, one must take into consideration and give careful attention to the carotid artery, which is located medial to the sternocleidomastoid muscle laterally to the entry point and both the trachea and esophagus medially. The pretracheal fascia is fused on either side with the prevertebral fascia, completing a compartment composed of the larynx, trachea, thyroid, and pharynx-esophagus. When moved together, all of these structures displace as one piece, increasing the safety zone for initial disk puncture. The carotid artery runs medially at the C3–C4 level and more laterally at the C6–C7 level. The safest entry point is between the airway and the pulsating carotid artery.

44.4.2 Anatomical Structures Related to Levels of PECD

C3–C4: Inferior Border of Hyoid Bone
- Between the hyoid bone and the thyroid cartilage.
- There is a narrow safety zone. The hypopharynx is broader, and the carotid artery is bifurcated medially.
- The superior thyroid artery is located in the trajectory of C3–C4 puncture.
- Translation movements of the pretracheal fascia enclosing the thyroid gland may change the course of the superior thyroid artery more horizontally.

C4–C5: Middle of Thyroid Cartilage
- The hypopharynx is placed more medially to the lateral margin of the thyroid cartilage, protecting it from injury.

C5–C6 (Between the Thyroid Cartilage and Cricoid Ring) and C6–C7 (Inferior to Cricoid Ring)
- The safety zone is larger at these levels.
- With correct retraction of the carotid artery and pharynx-esophagus, there are no endangered vital structures.

C7–T1
- Slightly more medial approach is advised to avoid lung apex injury.

44.5 Surgical Technique

44.5.1 Settings for PECD

- Laser settings: Energy of 1 to 1.5 J (Joules), 10 to 15 Hz (pulse/sec)
- Radiofrequency cautery: 35 for ablation and 30 for coagulation
- Irrigation pump: Flow at 100% and pressure of 30 mm Hg

44.5.2 Anesthesia

The patient is under conscious sedation with propofol and remifentanil intravenously via a target-controlled infusion pump (**Fig. 44.1**). This anesthesia modality is preferred, because it allows intraoperative feedback directly from the patient, which makes the procedure safer by informing the surgeon if neural structures are being stimulated.

44.5.3 Patient Position

- The patient is placed supine on a radiolucent table.
- The neck is slightly extended by placing a towel roll under the neck.
- The head can be stabilized by applying plaster tape across the forehead.
- A plastic tent is placed over the patient's face to prevent the feeling of suffocation after draping and to facilitate communication during the procedure (**Fig. 44.2a,b**).
- Neck and shoulder padding is done to keep the cervical spine in slight extension (**Fig. 44.3a**).
- The shoulders are pulled down and the arms are fixed to the sides of the table with plaster tape for better visualization under fluoroscopic lateral view (**Fig. 44.3b**).

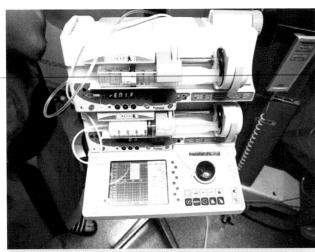

Fig. 44.1 Target-controlled infusion pump.

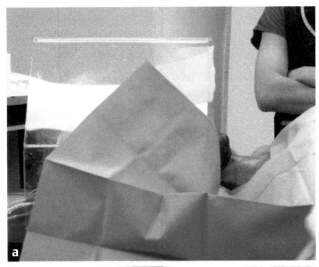

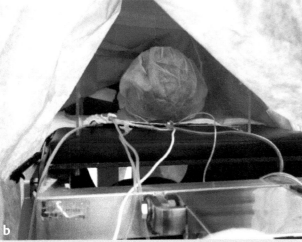

Fig. 44.2 Plastic tent for patient's comfort. (**a**) Lateral view and (**b**) the anesthesiologist's view.

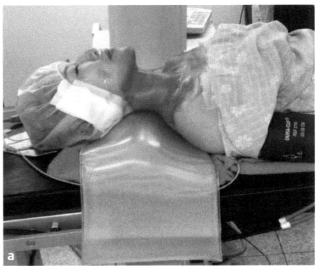

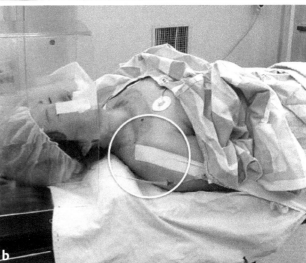

Fig. 44.3 (**a**) Neck and shoulder padding to keep the cervical spine in slight extension. If the patient has a short neck or (**b**) when approaching the C6–C7 level, bilateral arm traction is recommended. The authors use adhesive tape.

44.5.4 Procedure

- The level and midline are marked with the help of the C-arm fluoroscope (**Fig. 44.4a,b**).
- For lower cervical levels, the C-arm may have to be tilted obliquely to avoid the shoulder girdles.
- The anterior cervical skin is prepared and draped.
- Lidocaine (1%) is infiltrated into the skin and subcutaneous tissue at the entry point (**Fig. 44.5**).
- In foraminal disk herniation, approach from the contralateral side is preferable; for a midline herniation, entry from the right side is preferable for a right-handed surgeon.

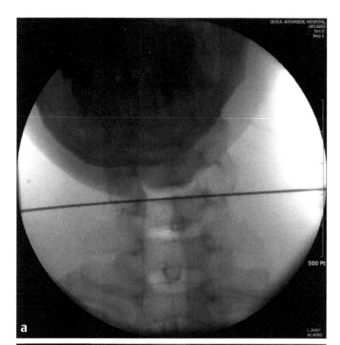

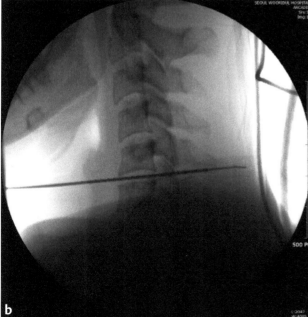

Fig. 44.4 Fluoroscopic view of level marking between C5 and C6 with the use of intraoperative C-arm. (**a**) AP view; (**b**) lateral view.

- Carotid pulse is palpated with the left hand and the tracheo-esophageal complex is gently pushed away while applying soft pressure and alternating movements with the fingertips of either the index and middle fingers or the middle and ring fingers until the anterior portion of the cervical vertebral body is felt. The anatomical relationship of the tracheoesophageal complex makes it possible to retract both the esophagus and trachea as a single structure (**Fig. 44.6**).
- When displacing the tracheoesophageal complex medially and the carotid sheath laterally, it is very important to maintain hand position while holding the guide needle between the third and fourth fingers before insertion. Confirmation of needle position and minor adjustments are made with the aid of the C-arm view, making certain the needle is aimed at the target disk space (**Fig. 44.7a,b**).
- With the fingers kept in place, a 90-mm 18 G needle is inserted into the interval between the carotid sheath and the tracheoesophageal complex up to the anterior margin of the targeted disk space under fluoroscopic guidance in AP and lateral views (**Fig. 44.7c**).
- Access to the disk is done between the longus colli muscles. This helps to prevent bleeding and sympathetic chain injury. As a reminder, note that the sympathetic chain is located more medially in the lower cervical vertebrae than in the upper cervical vertebrae.
- Diskography (indigo carmine solution mixed with normal saline and contrast media in a 1:2:2 ratio) is done to stain the pathological disk fragment and for confirmation of needle position (**Fig. 44.8**).

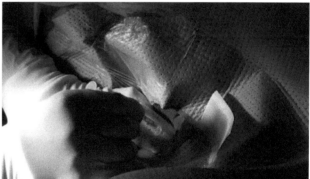

Fig. 44.5 Skin and deep tissue infiltration with 1% lidocaine.

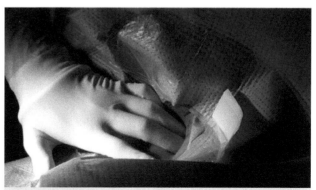

Fig. 44.6 Guarding the carotid artery laterally while displacing the tracheoesophageal complex to the medial side.

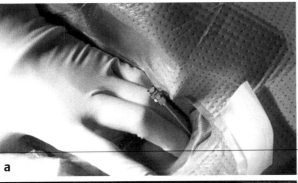

- A guidewire is then passed through the needle and the needle is withdrawn. While the needle is withdrawn, the guidewire should be firmly secured to prevent it from slipping out of the disk space (**Fig. 44.9**).
- A 5-mm transverse skin incision is made following the skin crease of the neck (**Fig. 44.10**).

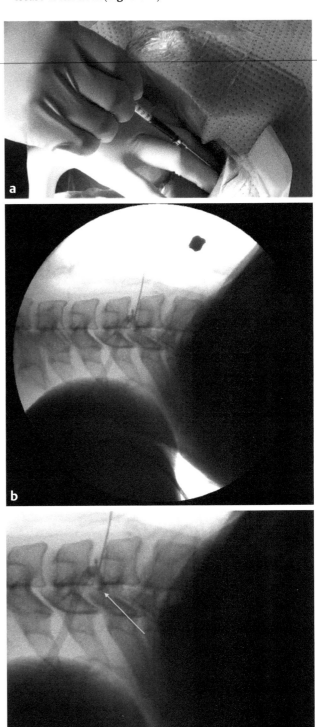

Fig. 44.7 (**a**) In displacing the tracheoesophageal complex medially and the carotid sheath with artery laterally, it is very important to keep that positioning while holding the guide needle between the third and fourth fingers before insertion. (**b**) Note that on the AP view on C-arm that the needle is close to the disk space but not exactly at the intended level yet. (**c**) Lateral view on C-arm, showing the 18 G spinal needle following a line parallel to the upper end plate of C6.

Fig. 44.8 (**a**) Diskography is done with a 2:1:2 mixture of normal saline, indigo carmine, and radiopaque contrast media. (**b**) Intraoperative lateral C-arm view shows the distribution of contrast in the disk and herniated fragment. (**c**) A zoom view of the same image shows the limit of the herniated disk (*arrow*).

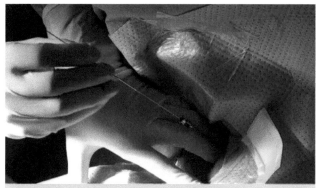

Fig. 44.9 Insertion of guidewire and removal of the 18 G needle. Be careful and gentle while making this simultaneous movement. The guidewire is inserted until subtle resistance is felt, and the needle is removed slowly with rotational movements.

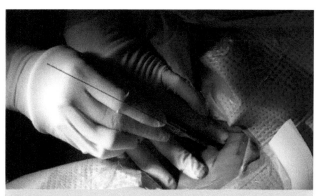

Fig. 44.10 A horizontal incision is made following the skin crease on the neck, while holding the guidewire position.

- Serial dilators (starting at 1 mm) are passed over the guidewire. This maneuver is done while the left hand is firmly guarding the carotid artery laterally and one finger is displacing the tracheoesophageal complex medially. C-arm verification of the correct positioning of the guidewire is mandatory while inserting the dilators. A second dilator is lightly tapped until its tip is close and in line with the posterior vertebral wall on lateral C-arm view (**Fig. 44.11**).

- The working portal can now be established using the 5-mm circular-tip working cannula inserted over the final dilator. The end position of the working cannula should be at the posterior vertebral body line in the lateral view. On the AP view, the midline position can vary slightly according the location of the herniated disk fragment (**Fig. 44.12**).

- For any type of disk herniation, the tip of the working cannula should always start at midline on the AP view. Once entry is gained inside the disk space, the tip can be tilted toward the respective foramen to aim toward a foraminal disk herniation.

- For a right-handed surgeon, we suggest holding the endoscope with the left hand and the working instruments with the dominant hand (**Fig. 44.13**).

- The cervical endoscope (**Fig. 44.14**) is passed through the working cannula. Once inside, usually the first structure that comes into sight is a portion of the annulus, with blue-stained disk material initially (**Fig. 44.15a**).

- Irrigation is done by cold normal saline solution. Initial localization of the fragment may be difficult. Soft tissue clearance with forceps is done first, and side-firing Ho:YAG laser is used to widen the annular opening. This helps in ablating the annulus, thus creating an opening for the advancement of the endoscope, making it easier to locate the fragment. Once the annular and posterior longitudinal ligament (PLL) opening is enlarged, we can visualize the disk fragment clearly and use gentle movements to grab and pull the herniated tissue (**Fig. 44.15b,c,d**).

- The temptation to remove the fragment at this stage should be avoided until a sufficient portion of the annulus is widened. The ruptured fragment itself acts as a shield to protect the neural tissue.

- While holding the disk fragment, always confirm the position of the forceps under C-arm lateral view to avoid undesirable neural tissue damage (**Fig. 44.15e**). While removing the disk fragment, make sure to retract the tissue slowly, since negative pressure is created (**Fig. 44.15f**).

- If the fragment is too large, laser can be used to downsize the fragment before removal. Sometimes the tail of the herniated fragment is seen very clearly (**Fig. 44.15g**). If there are any remaining fragments behind the PLL, the PLL can be partially cut using the Ho:YAG laser with side-firing probe to expose them.

- Some bleeding may ensue after fragment removal; it can be controlled by continuous irrigation and by waiting 10 to 20 seconds until it stops by itself.

- The adequacy of decompression can be confirmed by seeing the free course of the nerve root/dural pulsations (**Fig. 44.15h**). Also, remember that patient's symptoms can be assessed easily due to conscious sedation.

- Skin closure is done with single nylon suture and dressing is applied as a final step.

44.6 Possible Complications

- Neural tissue damage and dural tear: With meticulous handling of disk tissue, the possibility of inadvertent dural tear is very minimal. If a larger dural tear is observed, the PECD may need to be converted to an open procedure.

- Carotid artery puncture: In a very few cases, this might occur because of weak pulsations.

- Infection: The infection rate for PECD is less than 0.1%.

- Airway edema and hematoma: Overall incidence of edema is less than 0.2%.

- Revision surgery for remnant disk herniation: Because of the use of an endoscope, optics and illumination are of very high quality, making the disk fragments easily recognized. Additionally, the disk material is blue-stained, adding another visual indicator. The use of the side-firing laser has eased access through the PLL and annulus. The reported incidence of revision surgery is less than 5%.

44.7 Postoperative Management Protocol

- The patient is shifted to the postoperative recovery room for observation.

- Ambulation is allowed 1 hour after the surgical procedure. Sitting with back support is allowed immediately.

- Patients can eat regular food 1 hour after the procedure.

- There is no need for postoperative bracing.
- First dressing is done at the time of discharge and final dressing is advised at the time of suture removal (usually on the seventh postoperative day).

- Patients are observed in the hospital for the first 24 hours postoperatively and are discharged on the next day with oral antibiotics and analgesics.
- First postoperative office visit is recommended at 1 month, and follow-up is done with plain-film X-rays and MRI.

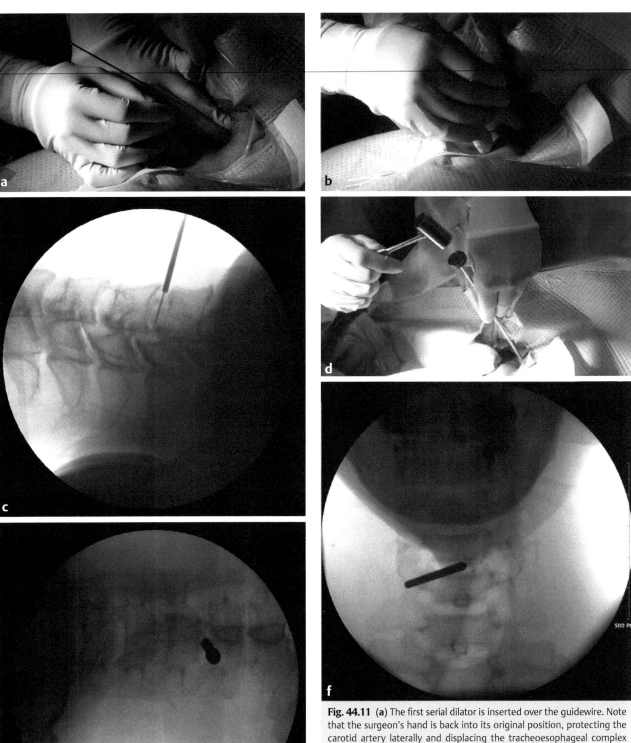

Fig. 44.11 (**a**) The first serial dilator is inserted over the guidewire. Note that the surgeon's hand is back into its original position, protecting the carotid artery laterally and displacing the tracheoesophageal complex medially. (**b**) A second dilator is inserted over the first one and is advanced to the disk space. (**c**) C-arm verification of the correct positioning of the guidewire while inserting the serial dilator. (**d**) The second dilator is hammered until it reaches the posterior vertebral body line on a lateral view, while maintaining the midline position on AP view on C-arm. (**e**) C-arm lateral view of dilator in place. Note that the tip is at the posterior vertebral body line. (**f**) AP view of dilator still in midline position.

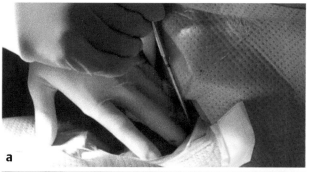

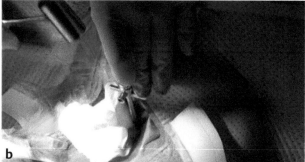

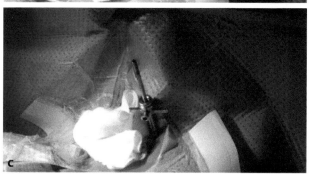

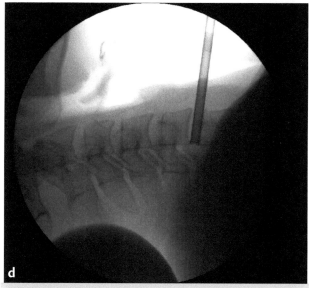

Fig. 44.12 (**a**) The cannula is inserted over the dilator with slow, firm, and gentle rotational movements. (**b**) It will be necessary to hammer the cannula into final position. This is better accomplished by applying short and steady taps while checking closely on lateral C-arm view. Make sure that the tip of the cannula ends at the posterior vertebral body line. (**c**) Position of the cannula on lateral view. Note that the tip is exactly at the posterior vertebral body line. (**d**) AP view on C-arm verifying the midline final position of the working cannula.

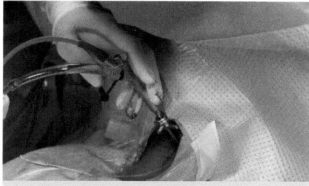

Fig. 44.13 Surgeon holding cervical endoscope. Note the hand position used during PECD.

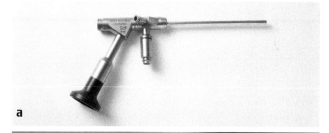

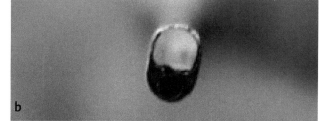

Fig. 44.14 (**a**) Cervical endoscope (Spine Doctors, Seoul, South Korea). (**b**) Tip of the cervical endoscope.

44.8 Case Example

44.8.1 History

A 24-year-old male patient presented with neck discomfort and left radiating arm pain for 2 months. He reported no history of trauma or other underlying diseases. He had undergone conservative treatment with no significant improvement. On physical examination he showed limited neck movements due to left arm pain, with no neurologic deficits or signs of myelopathy.

Imaging included C-spine plain radiographs, CT, and MRI. Plain radiograph lateral view showed loss of cervical lordosis, with focal kyphosis at the C4–C5 level but no other signs of degeneration or instability (**Fig. 44.16a–c**). CT and MRI showed left paramedian soft disk herniation at C5–C6 without cord signal alteration (**Fig. 44.17a,b**).

44.8.2 Results

After PECD, radiating arm pain was relieved and neck pain was clinically improved. MRI of the cervical spine showed complete removal of the disk fragment. (**Fig. 44.18a,b**). Follow-up at 3, 6, and 12 months showed no complications or development of new symptoms.

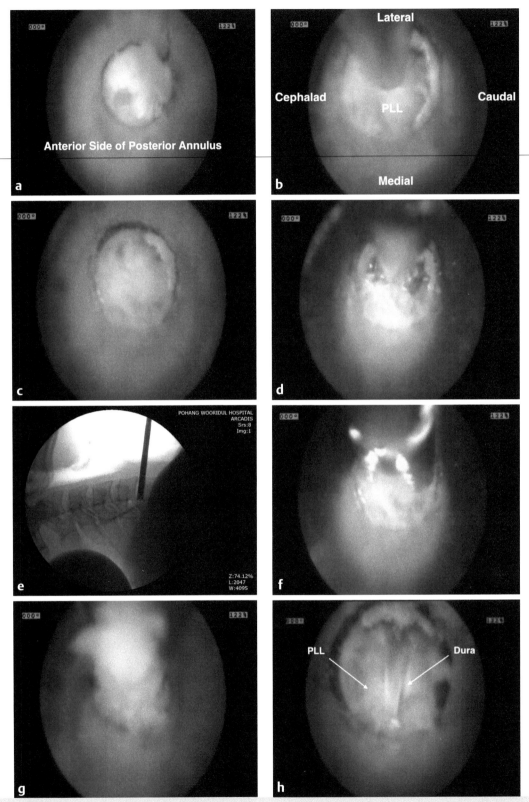

Fig. 44.15 Sequence of still images taken during PECD. (**a**) Initial view when putting the scope through the working cannula. In the depth of the viewing field, the most anterior part of the annulus can be seen with herniated disk material stained blue with indigo carmine. (**b**) Use of the 90° side-firing holmium:yttrium-aluminum-garnet (Ho:YAG) laser is mandatory for PECD. Here the laser probe is used to dissect through the annulus and posterior longitudinal ligament (PLL) to access the herniated disk fragment. (**c**) View after PLL is removed with Ho:YAG laser. Note the blue-stained disk in the bottom of the view field; it is ready for grasping with specialized forceps. (**d**) Forceps grasping the disk fragment. (**e**) Lateral C-arm view of forceps grasping the herniated disk fragment. It is advisable to confirm with fluoroscopic view when the forceps are first introduced to avoid any undesirable injury to neural tissue. (**f**) When removing the disk fragment, ensure that you retract the tissue slowly, since negative pressure is created. (**g**) The tail of the herniated fragment has come into view through the cannula. (**h**) After complete decompression, the dura is visible and free from any disk fragments.

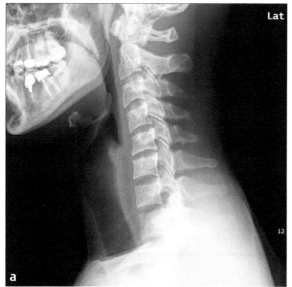

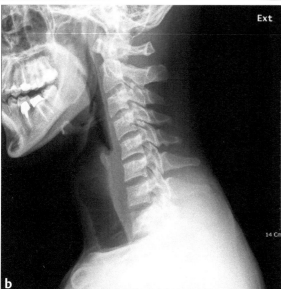

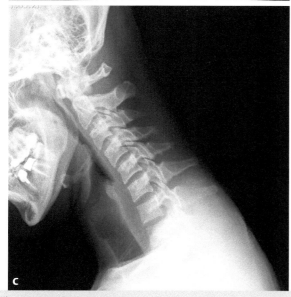

Fig. 44.16 (a,b,c) Lateral plain films demonstrating loss of cervical lordosis without instability.

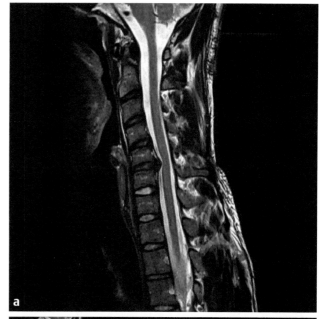

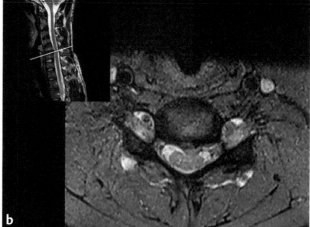

Fig. 44.17 (a) Sagittal T2 MRI shows soft disk herniation at the C5–C6 level. (b) Confirmation of left paramedian soft disk herniation at the C5–C6 level on axial T2 MRI.

44.9 Tips and Pearls

- Make it a routine to confirm the mobility of the tracheo-esophageal complex every time before needle insertion. Try to simulate the hand positioning and make an effort to feel the anterior aspect of the cervical spine before draping the patient.
- Remember to keep the guarding position of the hand until passing the second dilator.
- When pathology is located at the paramedian or foraminal region, approaching from the contralateral side makes it easier to reach the desired endpoint.

44.10 Authors' Opinion

To understand the surgical technique and to produce successful outcomes, knowledge of proper surgical anatomy is a must. With careful patient selection and training, PECD yields better results than ACDF. Further research is necessary to prove its neuromonitoring are the most outstanding advantages of PECD.[11]

44.11 Conclusion

PECD is an excellent alternative to conventional open anterior cervical diskectomy and fusion. This minimally invasive approach is designed to make a targeted decompression while preserving motion of the treated segment. Current developments in optics and endoscopic instruments make it possible to aim only at the herniated fragment. Conscious sedation makes it possible to elicit the patient's response when inadvertent neural tissue handling occurs, eliminating the need for neuromonitoring.

Contraindications to PECD are the presence of bony ridges and spurs, as well as a disk fragment that compresses the exiting nerve root, making it difficult to fully decompress. A steep learning curve and the need for highly specialized equipment and instruments make this technique very demanding. PECD is a good alternative to ACDF in patients unfit for general anesthesia or with other comorbidities.

References

1   Cloward RB. The anterior approach for removal of ruptured cervical disks. *J Neurosurg* 1958;*15*(6):602–617
2   Smith GW, Robinson RA. The treatment of certain cervical-spine disorders by anterior removal of the intervertebral disc and interbody fusion. *J Bone Joint Surg Am* 1958;*40-A*(3):607–624
3   Choi G, Lee SH. *Textbook of Spine*. Korean Spinal Neurosurgery Society; 2008:1173–1185
4   Lee SH, Lee JH, Choi WC, Jung B, Mehta R. Anterior minimally invasive approaches for the cervical spine. *Orthop Clin North Am* 2007;*38*(3):327–337, abstract v
5   Ruetten S, Komp M, Merk H, Godolias G. Full-endoscopic cervical posterior foraminotomy for the operation of lateral disc herniations using 5.9-mm endoscopes: a prospective, randomized, controlled study. *Spine* 2008;*33*(9):940–948
6   Ahn Y, Lee SH, Shin SW. Percutaneous endoscopic cervical discectomy: clinical outcome and radiographic changes. *Photomed Laser Surg* 2005;*23*(4):362–368
7   Lee JH, Lee SH. Clinical and radiographic changes after percutaneous endoscopic cervical discectomy: a long-term follow-up. *Photomed Laser Surg* 2014;*32*(12):663–668
8   Kim CH, Shin KH, Chung CK, Park SB, Kim JH. Changes in cervical sagittal alignment after single-level posterior percutaneous endoscopic cervical diskectomy. *Global Spine J* 2015;*5*(1):31–38
9   Ahn Y, Lee SH, Lee SC, Shin SW, Chung SE. Factors predicting excellent outcome of percutaneous cervical discectomy: analysis of 111 consecutive cases. *Neuroradiology* 2004;*46*(5):378–384
10 Ahn Y, Lee SH, Chung SE, Park HS, Shin SW. Percutaneous endoscopic cervical discectomy for discogenic cervical headache due to soft disc herniation. *Neuroradiology* 2005;*47*(12):924–930
11 Choi G, Garcia A. Motion preserving techniques for treating cervical radiculopathy. *J Spine* 2015;*4*(4):1–3

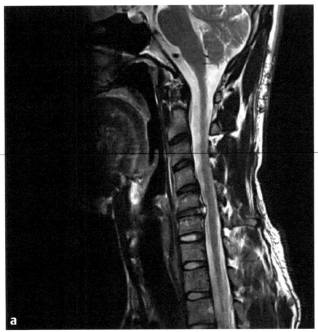

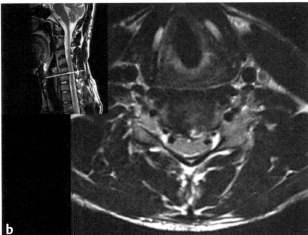

Fig. 44.18 **(a)** Postoperative T2 MRI, sagittal view, clearly shows complete C5–C6 decompression. **(b)** Complete removal of herniated disk fragment confirmed by axial T2 MRI.

long-term clinical outcomes are superior to those of the open anterior diskectomy. Short surgical time, less blood loss, use of local anesthesia, and no need for continuous intraoperative

45 Endoscopic Anterior Cervical Diskectomy and Cord Decompression

Shrinivas M. Rohidas

45.1 Introduction

Degenerative changes at vertebrae and the intervertebral disks occur due to wear and tear after constant use of the spine, among other reasons accelerating the degeneration. Degenerative changes in the spine have two main effects. One is compression of the neural structures, and the other is increased motion at the joints involved. Neural compression can be either with or without instability at the motion segment. When there is a compressed nerve or cord, the surgical treatment is to create more space for the nerve or cord. At the same time, the surgical procedures for decompression should not compromise the stability of the motion segment. In the cervical spine, Endospine makes it possible to treat endoscopically the compressed nerve and the cervical cord. In 1996, Jho described a microscopic anterior cervical foraminotomy procedure where the transverse process and uncovertebral joint were exposed and the decompression was performed with gradual removal of the uncinate process so as to reach the nerve root.[1,2]

45.2 Surgical Indications

Degenerative cervical pathology includes nerve compression, causing radiculopathy; cord compression, causing myelopathy; or nerve and cord compression, causing myeloradiculopathy. In young patients, most of the time the compression is due to soft disk herniation, and in elderly patients, compression is due to osteophytes, hard disks, and hard posterior longitudinal ligament.

Endospine can be used for anterior endoscopic cervical foraminotomy with Jho's approach and anterior endoscopic cervical foraminotomy and partial vertebrectomy with Jho's approach. This is indicated for soft or hard foraminal disk herniations. In elderly patients, the disk can be very small, or hard, or nonexistent, but the nerve and cord are compressed, leading to myelopathy and/or myeloradiculopathy. In these pathologies, anterior endoscopic foraminotomy can be easily extended to the opposite side, up to the midline or where the foramen begins (**Fig. 45.1**, **Fig. 45.2**).[3,4,5]

45.3 Technique

We use Endospine, a straight, rigid, 0°,18-cm endoscope, a high-definition (HD) camera, an endoscopic drill, 2-mm and 3-mm tip burs, ultrasonic bone dissector, and endoscopic bipolar cautery. The rest of the instruments are similar to those used in conventional cervical spine surgery—for example, a 2-mm Kerrison punch, 45° and 90° nerve hook, Penfield dissector No. 4, scissors, etc. Bone removal is performed with 3-mm and 2-mm cutting high-speed drills, which can be used through the working channel of Endospine. The ultrasonic bone dissector is used to remove bone near the vertebral artery, nerve root, and cervical cord, so as to protect these important structures.

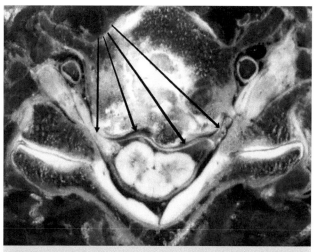

Fig. 45.1 Cervical nerve root and cord compression due to degenerative changes. Courtesy of Dr. W. Rauschning.

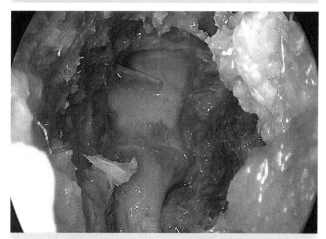

Fig. 45.2 Cervical nerve root and cord decompression through transuncal approach with Endospine in cadaver dissection.

The ultrasonic bone dissector will emulsify bone and will not damage the soft tissue nearby.

45.4 Patient Positioning

All operations are performed with the patient under general endotracheal anesthesia. Patient positioning is similar to that for conventional anterior cervical discectomy, with the head straight without turning and the neck neutral without turning to opposite side. For patients with a short neck, we use shoulder traction bilaterally to pull both shoulders caudally. In some patients who have a short neck, slight neck extension is used. Precaution during neck positioning is important to prevent position-induced injury to the cervical cord, especially if the patient experiences aggravation of symptoms upon neck extension preoperatively.

45.5 Use of Cervical Localization Pin

For the endoscopic anterior cervical approach, exact localization of the disk level is very important to minimize approach-related tissue trauma. The special localizing pin can be moved in three spatial planes. After exactly localizing the pathological disk level, the entry point is determined, as well as the direction of the disk space, so that the anteroposterior foraminotomy can be aimed to reach the nerve root and cord. In spite of the exact localization of the disk space, the level is confirmed with the help of the C-arm after exposure of disk space, before starting bone removal (**Fig. 45.3**, **Fig. 45.4**).

45.6 Skin Incision

Skin incision is horizontal, as in an open cervical approach. After exact localization of the disk level, the incision is approximately one-third lateral and two-thirds medial to the

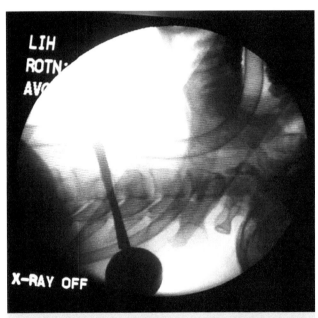

Fig. 45.3 Cervical localizing pin to localize disk space and disk direction.

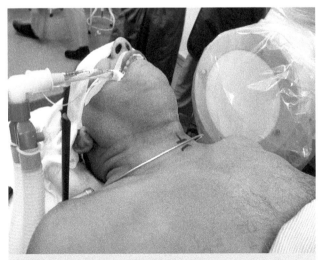

Fig. 45.4 Patient with cervical localizing pin.

sternocleidomastoid muscle. Then the platysma is cut, and the soft tissues are dissected between the carotid laterally and the trachea-esophagus medially, with the help of fingers. The anterior aspect of the cervical spine is exposed. At this point, the transverse processes can be palpated with the finger under longus colli muscle. The C6 transverse process can be easily identified with the help of the bony prominence of the carotid tubercle. Two thin blades of the cervical retractor system are used to retract the carotid artery laterally and the trachea and esophagus medially. Then the outer tube of the Endospine with an obturator is placed between the retractor blade switch are retracting the vascular and visceral axis. The blades of cervical retractor system are used without the holding arms of the retractor. Through the outer tube, with the help of scissors, the medial part of longus colli is cut over the disk space concerned. One to two millimeters must be removed from the medial part of the longus colli muscle. This will avoid trauma to the sympathetic chain, which is located more laterally, and will expose the disk space and the uncovertebral joint laterally. At this point, once again the C-arm is used to confirm the disk space level to be targeted.

45.7 Endoscopic Foraminotomy

Now the working insert with the 4-mm rigid telescope is introduced through the working channel of the Endospine. With the help of HD vision, the disk space, uncovertebral joint, and transverse processes of the cranial and caudal vertebrae are defined (**Fig. 45.5**).

The working area for the surgeon is between the two transverse processes and medial to the vertebral artery. The nerve root leaving the dural sleeve and reaching the vertebral artery measures approximately 6 mm. Then bone removal is performed using the 2- or 3-mm cutting/diamond pencil-grip high-speed drill (**Fig. 45.6**).

The bony window measures approximately 8 to 10 mm in the craniocaudal direction and 5 to 8 mm in the transverse direction. During creation of the bony window, part of the disk medial to the uncovertebral joint is removed. The Endospine with endoscope is at an angle of 15 to 30°, in order to reach the lateral part of the disk and vertebral bodies. The disk has to be followed laterally and cranially toward the uncovertebral joint. The uncovertebral joint is cranial to the disk space concerned.

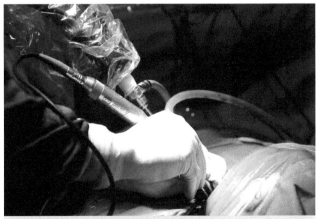

Fig. 45.5 Endospine with endoscopic drill.

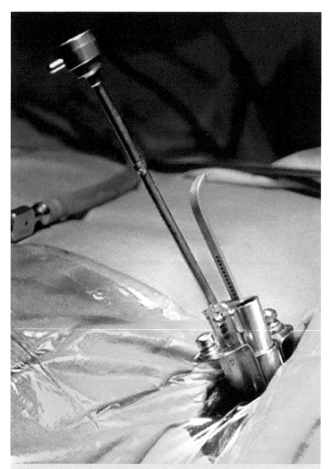

Fig. 45.6 Endospine working insert with outer tube without any fixation system.

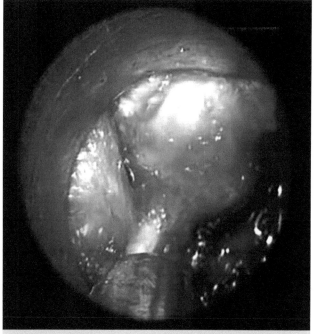

Fig. 45.7 Endoscopic exposure of uncovertebral joint on left side.

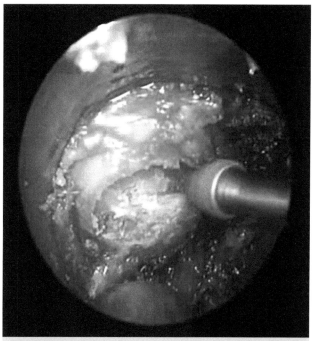

Fig. 45.8 Drilling of bone at uncovertebral joint with endoscopic drill.

While widening the bony window, we drill out the osteophytes from the cranial and caudal vertebral bodies, which opens the neural foramen. The spinal canal is reached just at the medial part of the neural foramen, where the herniated soft disk is most often found. The nerve root is exposed and is decompressed from the spinal canal or lateral edge of the dural sac until the nerve crossing the vertebral artery is reached. This tunnel is ~ 6 mm in diameter and follows the oblique direction of the nerve root. Therefore, it enlarges the intervertebral foramen in front of the nerve root (**Fig. 45.7**). Left-sided C4–C5 foraminotomy and nerve root decompressed from the dural sac are shown in **Fig. 45.8** and **Fig. 45.9**. The preoperative left-side C4–C5 disk herniation sagittal and axial views are shown in **Fig. 45.10** and **Fig. 45.11**, and postoperative sagittal and axial views are shown in **Fig. 45.12** and **Fig. 45.13**.

45.8 Endoscopic Foraminotomy and Vertebrectomy for Cord Decompression

In elderly patients presenting with compressive myelopathy and/or myeloradiculopathy, there is compression of the cervical cord due to hard structures, such as hard disks situated centrally and/or laterally, thick osteophytes, calcified and/or thick posterior longitudinal ligament, etc. Hence, along with nerve root compression, there is cord compression and a hyperintense signal in the cord due to myelomalacia. In these cases, once the exiting root is decompressed, Endospine with the endoscope is still angulated medially to reach the anterior surface of the cord. We use a 2-mm drill tip so that the drill tip is under constant vision while drilling the vertebral bodies craniocaudally. This will expose the posterior longitudinal ligament. Unless adequate craniocaudal decompression in the transverse direction is achieved, the posterior longitudinal ligament is not opened. When there is a central disk herniation, one can see the tear in the posterior longitudinal ligament. Then the OPLL is removed

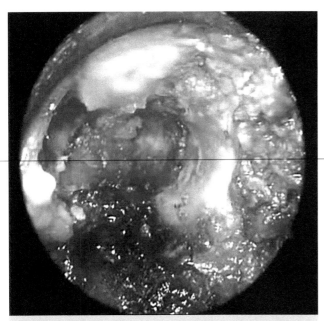

Fig. 45.9 Endoscopic foraminotomy to decompress the nerve root medial to the vertebral artery.

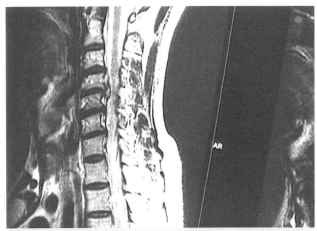

Fig. 45.11 Left C4–C5 decompressed nerve root with cord and vertebral artery.

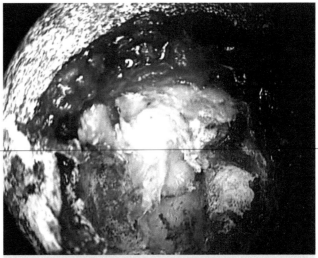

Fig. 45.10 Left C4–C5 transuncal drilling to follow the disk.

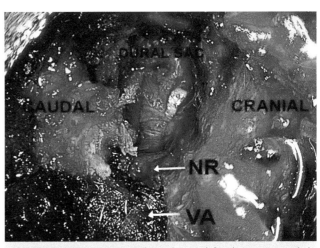

Fig. 45.12 Preoperative sagittal MRI showing left-side C4–C5 extruded disk compressing nerve root.

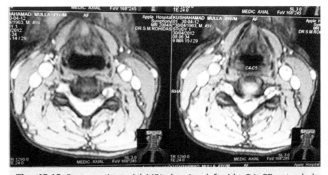

Fig. 45.13 Preoperative axial MRI showing left-side C4–C5 extruded disk compressing nerve root and cord.

with the help of the 2-mm Kerrison punch. Here the ultrasonic bone dissector/rasp is used to widen the bony window safely. Accidental slippage or kick-back of the drill tip can be life-threatening in the cervical region when working close to the cord. For the safety of the important neural and vascular structures, the ultrasonic bone dissector/rasp is used to remove bone. The bone window is widened until the lateral edge of the opposite dural sac is seen (**Fig. 45.14**, **Fig. 45.15**).

45.9 Closure

A small piece of Gelfoam is kept in the foraminotomy. The outer tube is taken out. Platysma is sutured with 3–0 Vicryl and the skin is closed with subcuticular sutures of 3–0 Vicryl (**Fig. 45.16**, **Fig. 45.17**, **Fig. 45.18**).

45.10 Results

Between 2006 and 2013, we used Jho's technique with the Endospine for endoscopic anterior cervical microforaminotomy, diskectomy, and cord decompression in 35 cases. The patients' demographics, clinical presentations, and surgical outcome data were recorded. Twenty-one patients were male, and 14 were female. Patients' ages ranged from 24 to 65 years. There were

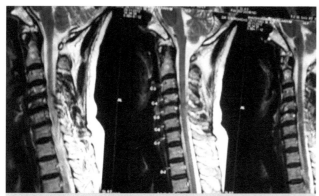

Fig. 45.14 Postoperative sagittal MRI showing excision of disk compressing root and cord.

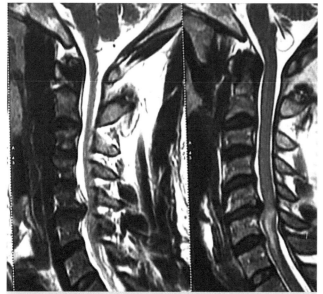

Fig. 45.16 MRI showing C5–C6 disk compressing cervical cord with cord edema causing compressive myeloradiculopathy.

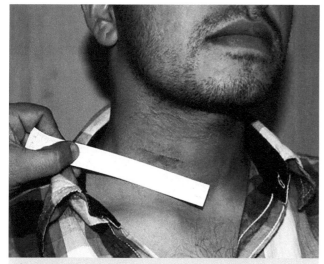

Fig. 45.18 Photograph showing skin incision with Endospine, a disk-preserving technique.

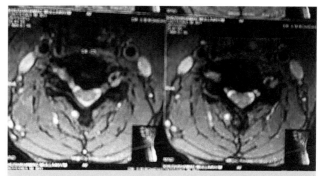

Fig. 45.15 Postoperative axial MRI showing decompressed nerve root and cervical cord.

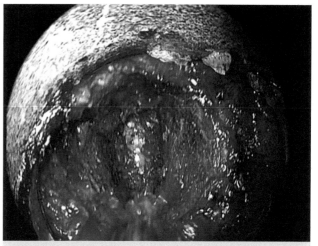

Fig. 45.17 Endoscopic transuncal view of adequately decompressed cervical cord with anterior two-thirds of the disk still intact.

16 disk herniations at C5–C6, 10 disk herniations at C4–C5, four nerve root compressions at C6–C7, and one patient with C3–C4 disk herniation leading to root compression. Of these, three had myeloradiculopathy at C4–C5 and one each had myeloradiculopathy at C5–C6 and C6–C7. Three patients had two-level nerve root compression at C3–C4 and C4–C5, C4–C5 and C5–C6, and C5–C6 and C6–C7. One patient had a mass at the C6 body, and we took biopsy using this approach with Endospine. Seventeen patients had neck pain, 13 had motor weakness, 25 had radicular pain, and 20 had paresthesias. Five had myeloradiculopathy with spasticity in the lower limbs, ataxia, KJ exaggerated, ankle clonus, with BJ and BR jerk inverted, and Hoffman's sign positive, along with finger flexion positive. All the patients had sufficient conservative treatment (~ 6 months to 1 year). All underwent MRI of the cervical spine with screening of the whole spine. Plain-film X-rays of the cervical spine in AP and lateral views, in flexion and extension, and right and left oblique views, were used to evaluate instability and bony foraminal compression due to foraminal osteophytes.

Thirty-two patients had excellent results, with good results in two patients, and one had fair results. Dural puncture was seen in one patient. A muscle piece with fibrin glue was used to seal the puncture. Two had Horner's syndrome. Two patients had transient recurrent laryngeal nerve paresis, which recovered completely within 2 to 8 weeks. Pseudoaneurysm of the vertebral artery was reported in one case. This case was not included in the study reported here but is mentioned for the purpose of covering technique-related complications.[6]

45.11 Discussion

Conventional anterior cervical disk surgery has evolved over last five decades into complete disk removal without bone graft, with bone graft for fusion, and with use of a metal implant to support the idea of fusion. More recent advancements using arthroplasty with an artificial disk have attempted to restore the mobile motion segment but still require diskectomy. Anterior endoscopic cervical diskectomy and foraminotomy is a new surgical technique using an uncovertebral trajectory, with the novel concept of "functional spine surgery."[3] The aim of functional spine surgery is to preserve the motion segment of the spine while achieving direct removal of the compressing pathology, with preservation of the rest of the normal disk.[7]

Generally, the cervical intervertebral disks in the sagittal plane incline cranially from an anterior to posterior direction. Therefore, we have to follow the disk space from an anterolateral region until the lateral edge of the dural sac. Also, according to the cranial or caudal migration of the herniated disk, we might have to widen the bony window to expose the disk herniation.

Although the surgical risks of anterior cervical foraminotomy and cord decompression have been minimal in our experience, permanent and serious complications are a possibility, as in any type of anterior cervical spine surgery. The major concerns include Horner's syndrome, laryngeal nerve injury, vertebral artery injury, spinal instability, and recurrent disk herniation. The cervical sympathetic nerve and chain pass along the lateral margin of the longus colli muscle, and Horner's syndrome can occur if the sympathetic nerve is damaged while retracting the structures or is completely sectioned during dissection of the longus colli. Hence we remove a small part of the longus colli muscle medially to expose the disk space. There is no treatment for Horner's syndrome and it can be temporary or permanent. We had two patients with Horner's syndrome, and both recovered completely over 6 weeks. Vertebral artery injury is a risk in any anterior cervical approach. To avoid this injury, one has to know the variations in the entry point of the vertebral artery, which usually enters at the C6 level. The level of vertebral artery entry into the transverse foramen should be identified on preoperative MRI to avoid this injury.

Medial to lateral dissection is used for foraminotomy. First, the drilling is started from the medial edge, and then once the disk space is entered, one can proceed laterally, rather than going from lateral to medial while drilling. This will keep a thin film of bone over the medial aspect of the vertebral artery. For removal of this bone, we use a 2-mm Kerrison punch with the cutting edge of the punch directed medially away from the vertebral artery. The author uses the ultrasonic bone dissector to remove bone covering the vertebral artery. The ultrasonic bone dissector safely removes bone without any thermal trauma to the vertebral artery. During removal of bone medial to the vertebral artery with the Kerrison punch there can be significant bleeding from the venous plexus around the vertebral artery. It is not helpful to use endoscopic bipolar cautery to stop oozing from the venous plexus. The best approach is to put a small piece of Surgicel medial to the vertebral artery between the two adjacent transverse processes.

Another possible relevant complication is cerebrospinal fluid leakage. The author has had one dural puncture. To prevent CSF leak, fibrin glue is used over a small piece of muscle pushed into the puncture carefully and lightly. Furthermore, hoarseness can be due to trauma to the laryngeal nerve caused by the retractor or during finger dissection. Because this is blind dissection, it can happen. We have had two patients with postoperative hoarseness. One developed hoarseness immediately after surgery. Intravenous methylprednisolone for 3 days effected complete recovery. The other patient had hoarseness at 2 weeks when she came for follow-up. Oral steroids for 3 weeks in tapering doses aided complete recovery of the voice over the next 6 weeks.

45.12 Postoperative Management

Eighty percent of patients are discharged after 24 hours. No cervical brace or collar is advised. Four hours after surgery, patients are mobilized with oral lozenges to reduce throat pain around the trachea and esophagus. All patients are followed every 15 days for 2 months, every 2 months for 6 months, and then every 4 to 6 months for the next year. Postoperative cervical spine X-ray for instability evaluation and MRI are performed.

45.13 Advantages of the Surgical Approach

- Direct access to the compressing lesion, allowing targeted surgery
- Preservation of most of the noncompressive disk
- Does not require any sort of fusion
- Direct decompression of the nerve root and cord
- Can treat either soft or hard disk and root and/or cord compression

45.14 Advantages to the Patient

- No need for cervical brace/collar after surgical procedure
- Hospital stay is shorter
- Less postoperative neck or arm pain
- Quick return to normal life

45.15 Advantages of Endospine System

- Mobility of the operating system, because the endoscope, suction, and instrument move as a single piece in constant relation to each other
- HD vision with zoom provides good-quality panoramic vision.
- Surgeon obtains a wide view of the operative field, and with zoom, anatomical structures can be enlarged.

45.16 Conclusion

Endoscopic anterior cervical nerve root decompression with foraminotomy and diskectomy is a minimally invasive technique allowing one to remove the compressing pathology with minimal bone and disk removal. The method avoids osteoarthrodesis and arthroplasty with an artificial disk.[8,9,10,11] The technique is efficient, with good results and low morbidity. The technique requires a long learning curve, but it is rewarding given its advantage of preservation of the disk and motion segment, so as to decelerate the ongoing age-related spinal degeneration.

References

1 Jho HD. Microsurgical anterior cervical foraminotomy for radiculopathy: a new approach to cervical disc herniation. *J Neurosurg* 1996;*84*(2):155–160

2 Jho HD, Kim WK, Kim MH. Anterior microforaminotomy for treatment of cervical radiculopathy: part 1—disc-preserving "functional cervical disc surgery." *Neurosurgery* 2002;*51*(5, Suppl):S46–S53

3 Jho HD. Decompression via microsurgical anterior foraminotomy for spondylotic cervical myelopathy. *J Neurosurg* 1997;*86*:121–126

4 Jho HD. Spinal cord decompression via microsurgical anterior foraminotomy for spondylotic cervical myelopathy. *Minim Invasive Neurosurg* 1997;*40*(4):124–129

5 Jho HD, Ha HG. Anterior cervical microforaminotomy. *Oper Tech Orthop* 1998;*8*:46–52

6 Kuttner H. Die Verletzungen und traumatischen Aneurysmen der Vertebral-gef-isse am Halse und ihre operative Behandlung. *Beitr Klin Chir* 1917;*108*:1–60

7 Bruneau M, Cornelius JF, George B. Microsurgical cervical nerve root decompression by anterolateral approach. *Neurosurgery* 2006;*58*

8 Edwards CC II, Heller JG, Murakami H. Corpectomy versus laminoplasty for multilevel cervical myelopathy: an independent matched-cohort analysis. *Spine* 2002;*27*(11):1168–1175

9 Emery SE, Fisher JR, Bohlman HH. Three-level anterior cervical discectomy and fusion: radiographic and clinical results. *Spine* 1997;*22*(22):2622–2624

10 Lunsford LD, Bissonette DJ, Zorub DS. Anterior surgery for cervical disc disease. Part 2: Treatment of cervical spondylotic myelopathy in 32 cases. *J Neurosurg* 1980;*53*(1):12–19

11 Wada E, Suzuki S, Kanazawa A, Matsuoka T, Miyamoto S, Yonenobu K. Subtotal corpectomy versus laminoplasty for multilevel cervical spondylotic myelopathy: a long-term follow-up study over 10 years. *Spine* 2001;*26*(13):1443–1447

46 Video-Assisted Anterior Cervical Diskectomy and Instrumentation

Keith A. Kerr, Victor Lo, Ashley E. Brown, Alissa Redko, and Daniel H. Kim

46.1 Introduction

Anterior cervical diskectomy and fusion was first developed in the 1950s as a treatment for cervical disk disease.[1] The advent of the operating microscope (OM) and microsurgical techniques improved the visualization, lighting, and ease of dissection of this approach and provided satisfactory results.[2] The endoscope has been used more and more frequently in neurosurgery for operations traditionally done with the OM, including spine surgery.[3,4,5] The senior author has applied this technology in anterior approaches to the cervical spine for a variety of pathologies.

The video telescope operating monitor (VITOM) has comparable capabilities to the OM with respect to focal length (25–75 cm compared to 20–40 cm) and magnification (both at 12x), while having the advantage of a larger depth of field (3.5–7.0 cm versus 1.2 cm). In addition, there are cost, ergonomic, and educational advantages provided by the system. The cost of the typical neurosurgical microscope is over $200,000, while the VITOM system costs less than $75,000.[6] This makes it a more widely affordable technology. Ergonomically, the VITOM system is much smaller and attaches to the operating table, making it usable even in smaller operating rooms. Other ergonomic advantages include less frequent adjustments to the scope due to the larger depth of field and no need to adjust one's posture to look into eyepieces. Since the OM is utilized only during the deepest portion of dissections, the field is viewable by others in the room for only a brief period of the operation. The VITOM can be used even in the more superficial portion of the dissection, making it a superior educational tool.

This chapter describes the use of the VITOM for anterior cervical diskectomy and instrumentation (**Video 46.1**).

46.2 Equipment Specific to This Approach

- Autoclavable rigid lens 0° telescope (VITOM SPINE HOPKINS; Karl Storz Endoscopy, Tutlingen, Germany)
- C-mount coupler (Stryker, San Jose, CA)
- 1280 × 1024 high-definition camera (1288 HD Video Camera; Stryker)
- Light-emitting diode (LED) system (L9000; Stryker)
- Two 26-inch, 1920 × 1080 resolution, 1 billion colors monitors (Vision Pro 26" LED; Stryker)
- Pneumatic endoscope holder (Point Setter, Mitaka Kohki, Tokyo, Japan)
- Optional archiving system (SDC3; Stryker) for documentation

46.3 Procedure

46.3.1 Operating Room Setup

- In addition to the typical operating room setup, a tower including a high-definition (HD) screen and a power source for the scope, camera, and Mitaka arm are placed opposite the surgeon. An additional HD screen is placed opposite the assistant (**Fig. 46.1**).
- The patient is placed in a supine position on a regular operating table with the head held in slight extension. The use of bolsters or a shoulder roll underneath the shoulder blades facilitates the position
- The incision is then marked from near the midline to the edge of the sternocleidomastoid at the appropriate level identified using either external landmarks or X-ray guidance. Using a skin crease or fold can provide a superior cosmetic result.
- The Mitaka Point Setter is attached to the side rail by the OR table adapter prior to sterile preparation and draping of the patient. The nitrogen source is then connected with the provided cables, and an operational and range-of-motion check is performed prior to draping (**Fig. 46.2**).
- In addition to the normal draping, prior to attachment of the VITOM, the Mitaka arm is draped with a sterile bag provided by the manufacturer, and is secured with adhesive tape.
- The endoscope and its attached camera are then attached to the arm by the endoscope holder and the illumination source's fiberoptic cables are connected to its power source. The endoscope and arm can then be positioned out of the way of the surgeon during the superficial dissection (**Fig. 46.3**).

46.3.2 Superficial Dissection

- After an appropriate time out, an incision is made using a No. 10 blade down to the level of the fat overlying the platysma.
- Careful hemostasis is obtained, and a Weitlaner retractor is positioned over the platysma. The platysma is dissected in the orientation of the incision sharply or by monopolar cautery, and is undermined extensively both superiorly and inferiorly.
- The sternocleidomastoid and omohyoid muscles are then identified. The dissection proceeds between the muscles, with careful attention paid not to injure the trachea and esophagus medially, and the carotid sheath and its contents laterally. The omohyoid can be mobilized superiorly for access to the most caudal levels of the cervical spine.

46.3.3 Deep Dissection and Retractor Placement

- The prevertebral fascia and longus colli are encountered next, and a handheld retractor can be placed on top of the vertebral bodies and intervertebral disks to gently retract the esophagus and trachea to the contralateral side.
- The prevertebral fascia can then be bluntly dissected off the anterior portion of the vertebral bodies by a Kittner.
- After confirmation of the correct level by use of X-ray and a spinal needle, the longus colli can be dissected off the anterior vertebral body by monopolar cautery at the needed levels. This is performed to the medial uncovertebral joint,

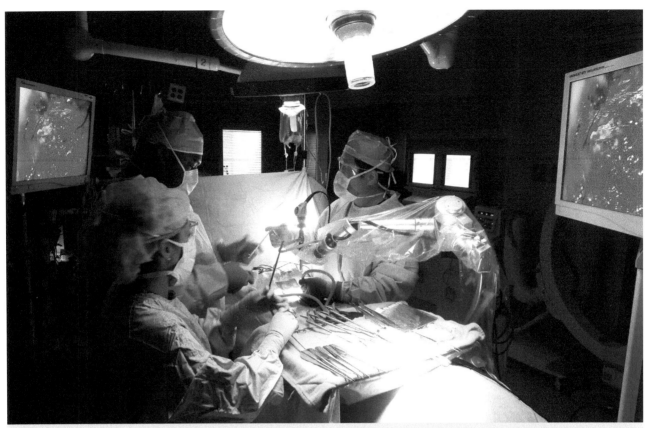

Fig. 46.1 Operating room setup with monitors across from both the operator and the assistant. A tower containing the power source for the camera, Mitaka arm, and HD screens is positioned at the end of the bed on either side.

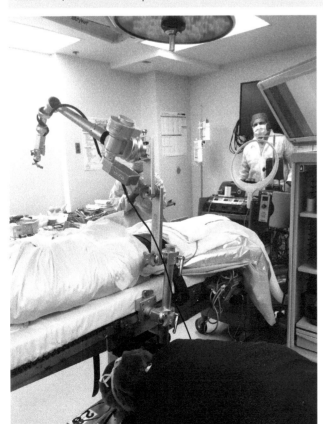

Fig. 46.2 The Mitaka arm is attached directly to the bed prior to draping of the patient.

facilitating the formation of a lip of muscle that will hold the retractor system in place

- Caspar pins can be placed into the midportion of the vertebral bodies of the involved levels to aid in distraction. Once this is complete, the Mitaka arm and VITOM can be moved into place.

46.3.4 Optimal Positioning of the Mitaka Arm and VITOM

- The working distance of the scope is anywhere between 25 and 75 cm above the surgical field. It should be placed above the field with enough room for the longest instruments (such as a high-speed drill, Leksell rongeurs, and Kerrison punches) to be used underneath it (**Fig. 46.4**).
- The depth of field is anywhere from 3.5 to 7 cm, depending on a shorter or longer working distance. This allows for a great depth of the operative field to remain in focus with the initial positioning, requiring minimal adjustment and zoom.

46.3.5 Diskectomy

- A transverse incision is made into the disk space with a No. 15 blade. The disk can be curetted with a combination of straight and angled curets and can be removed with an appropriately sized pituitary rongeur. The overlying lip of the end plate can be removed by Kerrison rongeurs. Disk removal by this method is performed until the posterior longitudinal ligament (PLL) is encountered (**Fig. 46.5**).

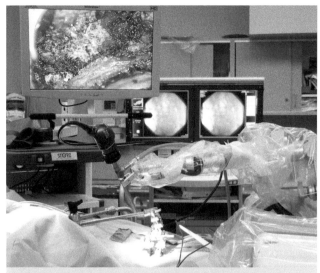

Fig. 46.3 The arm is sterilely draped and the camera is attached.

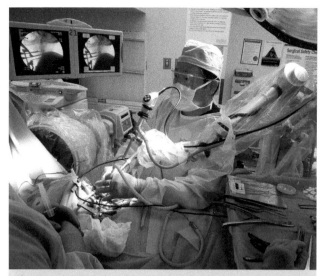

Fig. 46.4 The VITOM has a long focal length, allowing it to be positioned far enough from the surgical field to allow for instruments to be passed and used underneath the scope.

- When the PLL is a source of spinal cord compression or pathology is present posterior to the PLL and its removal is required, it can be entered and elevated by a nerve hook. No. 1 and 2 Kerrison punches can be subsequently used to remove it and any osteophyte material that overlies the dura.
- The above steps are repeated at all planned levels. Due to the wide object field of the VITOM, minimal adjustment of the scope is required when changing levels.

46.3.6 Hardware Placement

- Appropriately sized PEEK implants, autografts, or artificial disks can be placed within the disk spaces. Once this is completed, the VITOM is moved out of position for the rest of the procedure, and the remaining steps are completely under direct visualization (**Fig. 46.6**).
- At this time, the Caspar pins are removed, and the hole left behind is sealed with bone wax.
- An appropriately sized plate to traverse the needed levels is then selected. Large anterior osteophytes often require removal by a Leksell rongeur so that the plate can sit flush along the anterior spine. A gentle curve to match the cervical lordosis should be employed for longer constructs.
- Screws are then placed to secure the plate in position. A 5 to 10° medial trajectory and 15° superior or inferior trajectory is favored for the superior- and inferior-most screws, respectively (**Fig. 46.7**).

46.3.7 Closure

- The wound is then copiously irrigated with antibiotic irrigation. The retractors are removed and the entire surgical field is searched for any evidence of bleeding. Hemostasis is obtained.
- The platysma is the first layer closed, which is done with interrupted absorbable suture. A one- or two-layer subcutaneous closure is then used to approximate the skin. Steri-Strips are applied to the wound, and a coverlet completes the dressing.

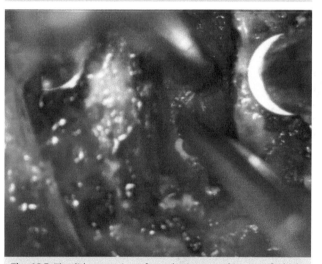

Fig. 46.5 The diskectomy is performed using a combination of a high-speed drill and pituitary and Kerrison rongeurs.

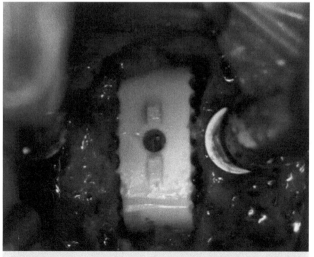

Fig. 46.6 Placement of an appropriate spacer prior to removal of the Caspar pins and placement of the plate and screws.

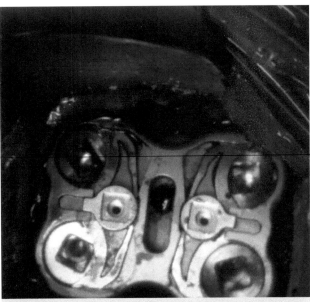
Fig. 46.7 Final positioning of the instrumentation prior to closure.

46.4 Conclusion

Use of the endoscope is an alternative to use of surgical loupes or the operating microscope. Its strengths include a more ergonomic operating position for the surgeon, the ability for other members of the operative team to see the surgical field, its compact design, and a large depth of field. These characteristics have increased its popularity in neurosurgery, and this chapter presents another approach for which it can be used.

References

1. Cloward RB. The anterior approach for removal of ruptured cervical disks. *J Neurosurg* 1958;*15*(6):602–617
2. Hankinson HL, Wilson CB. Use of the operating microscope in anterior cervical discectomy without fusion. *J Neurosurg* 1975;*43*(4):452–456
3. Dickman CA, Karahalios DG. Thoracoscopic spinal surgery. *Clin Neurosurg* 1996;*43*:392–422
4. Khoo LT, Fessler RG. Microendoscopic decompressive laminotomy for the treatment of lumbar stenosis. *Neurosurgery* 2002;*51*(5, Suppl):S146–S154
5. Sandhu FA, Santiago P, Fessler RG, Palmer S. Minimally invasive surgical treatment of lumbar synovial cysts. *Neurosurgery* 2004;*54*(1):107–111
6. Shirzadi A, Mukherjee D, Drazin DG, et al. Use of the video telescope operating monitor (VITOM) as an alternative to the operating microscope in spine surgery. *Spine* 2012;*37*(24):E1517–E1523

47 Cervical Laminoforaminotomy with Working Channel Endoscope

Gun Choi and Akarawit Asawasaksakul

47.1 Introduction

Posterior cervical foraminotomy has been applied extensively in the management of unilateral cervical radiculopathies, either due to a foraminal disk or due to bony spurs projecting into the foramen.[1] Keyhole laminoforaminotomy with the use of an operating microscope has limited morbidity of the paraspinal soft tissue and enhanced safety of the neural structures.[1,2,3] Sequential dilator systems like the METRx have also reduced intraoperative bleeding and surgical times. The results are equivalent between open and minimally invasive approaches.[3,4,5,6,7] To further benefit the patient in terms of the most minimally invasive approach possible, we have combined keyhole surgery with a working channel endoscope (**Video 47.1**).

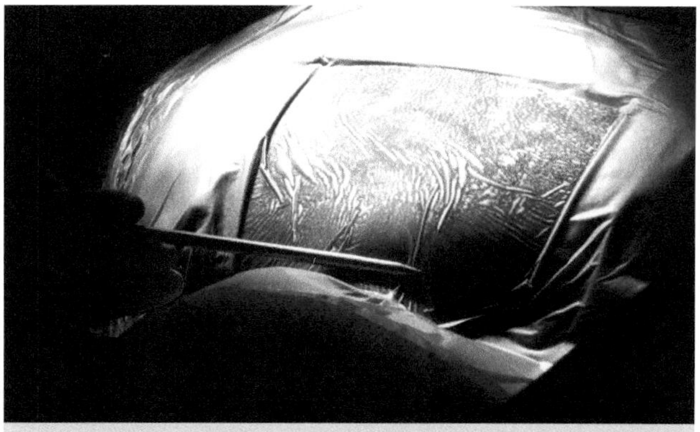

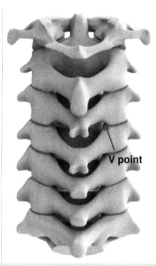

Fig. 47.1 Patient in prone position with slight neck flexion. Also shown is initial level marking.

47.2 Surgical Technique

47.2.1 Position and Anesthesia

- The patient is placed in the prone position and general anesthesia is preferred (**Fig. 47.1**).
- The patient is positioned on a radiolucent table with the neck in either neutral or slight flexion to facilitate interlaminar approach and drilling.
- Shoulders need to be strapped and pulled caudally to allow visualization of lower cervical levels on lateral view fluoroscopy.
- Level marking is done before scrubbing/draping to facilitate changes in position if needed.

47.2.2 Needle Insertion

- The target point for the needle tip is the V point of the cranial lamina on the symptomatic side—i.e., the lateral-most part of the lamina approximately correlating with the location of the pedicles (**Fig. 47.2**).
- It is always safe to target the needle toward the inferior margin of the cranial lamina, because in the cervical spine the laminae are significantly overlapped and targeting the caudal lamina may result in inadvertent entry of the needle into the interlaminar space toward the spinal cord.
- An 18 G 90-mm spinal needle is directed toward the target point under lateral view fluoroscopy (**Fig. 47.3**).
- Inclination of the needle trajectory is highly variable depending on the level, but the needle should be perpendicular to the lamina, in the mediolateral plane, and slightly cranial to caudal.
- The needle advancement is stopped when the bone is encountered and the needle is replaced with a 0.9-mm guidewire.

V point

Fig. 47.2 The V point of the cervical lamina is formed where the inferior border of the upper lamina and the superior border of the lower lamina converge.

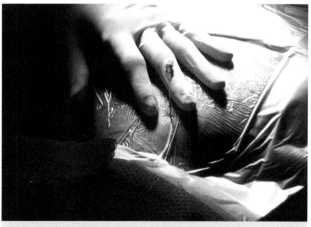

Fig. 47.3 Skin entry point for needle insertion.

47.2.3 Instrument Placement

- A 1-cm skin incision allows passage of sequential dilators over the guidewire (**Fig. 47.4**).
- It is essential to ensure that the serial dilators are held securely against the lamina to make sure that no soft tissue obliterates the endoscopic view.
- Serial dilators avoid the need for soft tissue dissection by pushing the tissue away, resulting in reduced postoperative pain and bleeding.
- The dilators are followed by the passage of a 7.5-mm round working cannula, which accommodates the working channel endoscope, and continuous-pressure cold irrigation with antibiotic-instilled normal saline (**Fig. 47.5**).

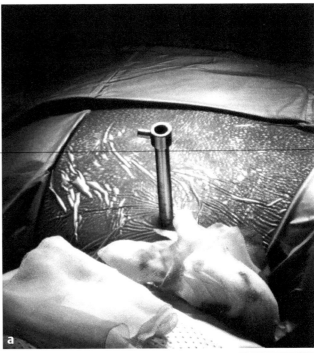

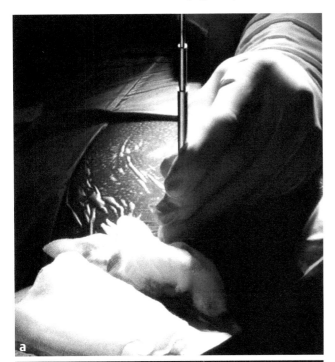

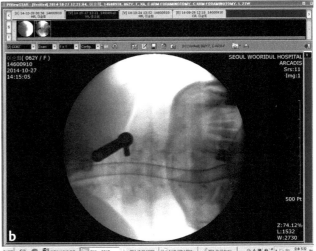

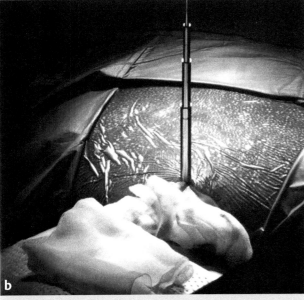

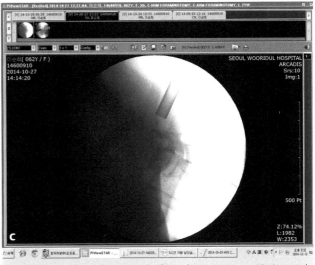

Fig. 47.4 (a,b) Sequential serial dilators are used for splitting the paraspinal muscles before establishing the working portal.

Fig. 47.5 (a) The working cannula, **(b)** anchoring point on AP view, and **(c)** anchoring point on lateral view.

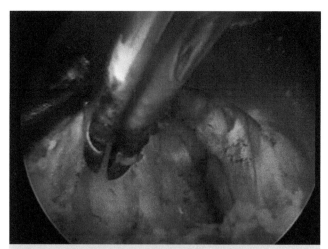

Fig. 47.6 Endoscopic view of bleeding control using the bipolar RF probe.

47.2.4 Laminoforaminotomy

- The rest of the procedure is similar to open or key-hole foraminotomy. Initial hemostasis and soft tissue clearance are done with a radiofrequency (RF) probe (**Fig. 47.6**).

- An endoscopic drill (bur) is used to begin the decompression from the V point of the cranial lamina extending laterally toward the apex of the interlaminar space and caudally on to the inferior lamina (**Fig. 47.7**).

- The skin elasticity is used to move the working cannula, along with the endoscope and the drill, for better visualization and safety in achieving sufficient bony decompression.

- We recommend approaching the root from the axilla, and bony decompression should be limited to exposing the concerned region only.

- One more tip to prevent excessive facetectomy is to tilt the working channel to undermine the facet instead of complete removal. For the same reason, the author prefers to stand on the contralateral side, which facilitates ease of access to the apex.

- This exposes the ligamentum flavum, which needs to be removed piecemeal with the help of an endoscopic punch (**Fig. 47.8**).

- The lateral margin of the dura and the root can be identified. A blunt-tipped probe is used to palpate the axilla of the root for any loose disk fragments, and a pituitary forceps is used to remove the same (**Fig. 47.9**).

- In addition, a side-firing holmium:yttrium-aluminum-garnet (Ho:YAG) laser is used to further extend the soft tissue dissection in the axilla and along the nerve root laterally (**Fig. 47.10**).

- The endpoint of the procedure is determined when direct visual endoscopic confirmation of a freely mobile nerve root is accomplished. The skin is closed with a single nonabsorbable suture with or without a drain (**Fig. 47.11**).

47.3 Complication Avoidance

- We stress the importance of needle insertion and a trajectory to the target point. Targeting the needle to the V point together with the lower lamina prevents injury to the dural sac and cervical cord.

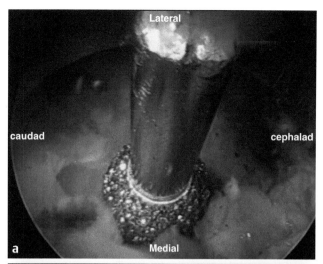

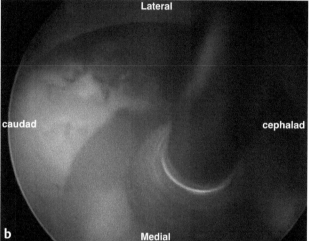

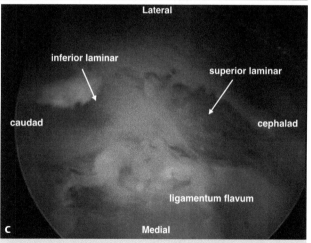

Fig. 47.7 (**a**) Endoscopic view of diamond bur touching laminae at V point; (**b**) initial starting point and drilling; (**c**) view after partial removal of lamina.

- Standing on the side contralateral to the lesion is more comfortable and ergonomic in foraminal decompression.

- The Ho:YAG laser is a great help for dissection of the soft tissue beneath the ligamentum flavum.

- Clearing an axilla of the nerve root with the blunt-tipped probe can also remove some of the entrapped disk fragments without injury to the exiting root.

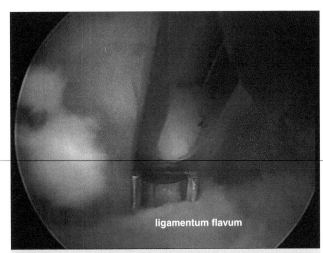

Fig. 47.8 Removal of ligamentum flavum with the use of a specialized endoscopic punch.

47.4 Case Demonstration

47.4.1 History

A 62-year-old female presented a 2-month history of right arm pain and neck discomfort without any numbness or neurologic deficit. Conservative treatment showed no improvement.

There were no signs of myelopathy during physical examination. Cervical spine MRI showed right foraminal disk herniation at C6–C7 (**Fig. 47.12**). CT showed no calcification.

Treatment options were discussed with the patient, advantages and disadvantages were carefully explained, and finally the patient decided to undergo posterior endoscopic foraminotomy.

47.4.2 Surgical Procedure

- The patient was positioned prone with slight neck flexion on a radiolucent operating table. She was given general anesthesia.
- Strapping the shoulder was really important in this case because the pathology was in lower cervical vertebrae. Also, the head was stabilized before draping.
- Level marking was done by C-arm fluoroscopy.
- Under C-arm guidance on AP view, we identified the V point according. Needle insertion was directed toward this point. From the lateral view, the needle was aimed at the superior edge of the lower lamina.
- After the lamina was reached, the guidewire was inserted through the needle and then was followed by dilation with serial dilators.
- Final docking point of the working channel was posterior to the lamina on the lateral view and at the V point on AP view.

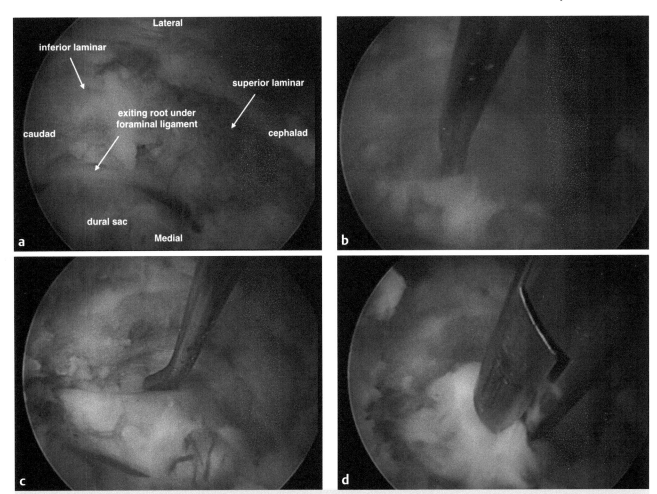

Fig. 47.9 (a) Endoscopic anatomy; (b,c) blunt-tipped probe palpating at the axilla of exiting root; (d) removal of disk fragment by endoscopic forceps.

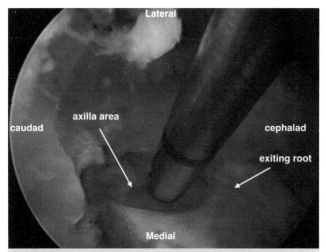

Fig. 47.10 Endoscopic view of side-firing Ho:YAG laser used to dissect soft tissue laterally.

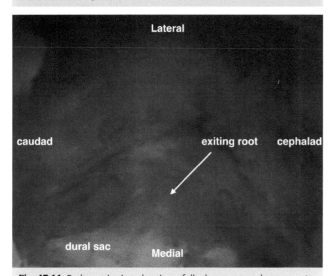

Fig. 47.11 Endoscopic view showing a fully decompressed nerve root.

47.5 Endoscopic Findings

- Soft tissue clearance and bleeding control were done before reaching the lamina.
- Bony decompression began with the use of the diamond-tipped bur, starting at the cranial lamina where the V point is located, continuing with the lateral portion, and finishing at the caudal lamina.
- After partially removal of the lamina, we could see the ligamentum flavum, and it was now to safe remove it using a specialized Kerrison rongeur to expose the nerve root.
- At this point we could see the C7 exiting root and clearly identified the other related structures (**Fig. 47.13**).
- For most of our cases, an axillary approach is chosen, and a blunt-tipped probe is then used to bring the fragments into view so they can be safely removed with endoscopic forceps (**Fig. 47.14**).
- After removal of the disk, we also partially remove the foraminal ligament that is compressing the exiting root with the help of Ho:YAG laser (**Fig. 47.15**).

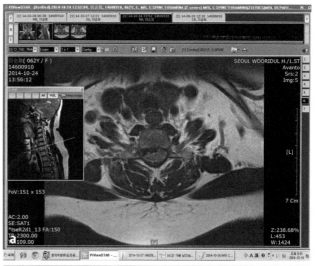

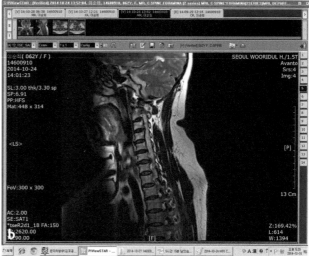

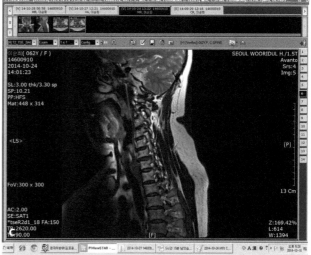

Fig. 47.12 MRI of the cervical spine demonstrates a right foraminal disk at C6–C7. (**a**) AP view, (**b,c**) right sagittal oblique view.

- After decompression, the nerve root was clearly free of compression.

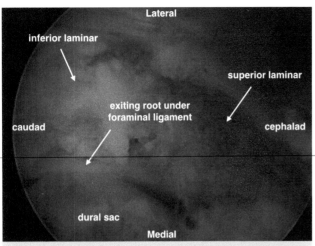

Fig. 47.13 Root is clearly visualized after removal of ligamentum flavum.

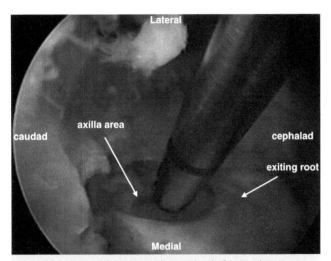

Fig. 47.15 The use of the Ho:YAG laser with side-firing probe to remove the foraminal ligament.

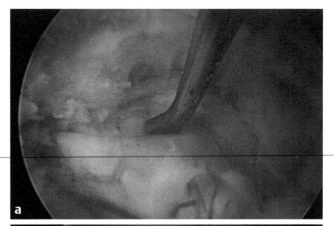

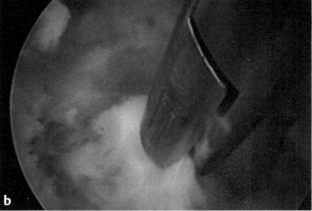

Fig. 47.14 **(a,b)** Removing the disk fragment with endoscopic forceps and the aid of a blunt-tipped probe.

47.6 Results

- The postoperative MRI showed a fully decompressed right C6–C7 foramen (**Fig. 47.16**).
- The patient's right arm pain was alleviated, and no complications were observed.

47.7 Tips

- Needle position at the cranial lamina is crucial to avoid accidentally penetrating the interlaminar space.
- Start from the V point, and moving laterally, avoid excessive removal of the medial part of the lamina.
- Be aware that a partial facetectomy may be needed.
- The authors recommend the axilla approach, because there is a broader space.

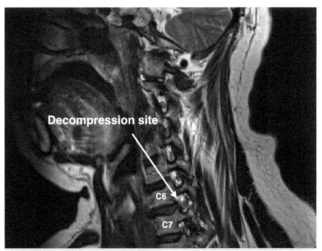

Fig. 47.16 Postoperative MRI confirms a fully decompressed right C6–C7 foramen.

References

1. Celestre PC, Pazmiño PR, Mikhael MM, et al. Minimally invasive approaches to the cervical spine. *Orthop Clin North Am* 2012;*43*(1):137–147, x
2. O'Toole JE, Sheikh H, Eichholz KM, Fessler RG, Perez-Cruet MJ. Endoscopic posterior cervical foraminotomy and discectomy. *Neurosurg Clin N Am* 2006;*17*(4):411–422
3. Winder MJ, Thomas KC. Minimally invasive versus open approach for cervical laminoforaminotomy. *Can J Neurol Sci* 2011;*38*(2):262–267
4. Burke TG, Caputy A. Microendoscopic posterior cervical foraminotomy: a cadaveric model and clinical application for cervical radiculopathy. *J Neurosurg* 2000; *93*(1, Suppl):126–129
5. McAnany SJ, Kim JS, Overley SC, Baird EO, Anderson PA, Qureshi SA. A meta-analysis of cervical foraminotomy: open versus minimally-invasive techniques. *Spine J* 2015;*15*(5):849–56
6. Ruetten S, Komp M, Merk H, Godolias G. A new full-endoscopic technique for cervical posterior foraminotomy in the treatment of lateral disc herniations using 6.9-mm endoscopes: prospective 2-year results of 87 patients. *Minim Invasive Neurosurg* 2007;*50*(4):219–226
7. Ruetten S, Komp M, Merk H, Godolias G. Full-endoscopic cervical posterior foraminotomy for the operation of lateral disc herniations using 5.9-mm endoscopes: a prospective, randomized, controlled study. *Spine (Phila Pa 1976)* 2008;*33*(9):940–948

48 Posterior Percutaneous Endoscopic Cervical Foraminotomy and Diskectomy: Case Presentation and Surgical Technique

Chi Heon Kim and Chun Kee Chung

48.1 Case Presentation

The patient, a 41-year-old female, presented with the chief complaints of right arm pain and triceps weakness (onset was 6 months earlier). Several epidural injections had been performed, but her pain was not relieved. The intensity of pain was 10/10 on neck/arm, and the neck disability index was 35/50.

Neurological examination revealed right triceps weakness (manual motor test IV/V) and Spurling's test was positive. The MRI showed disk protrusion and slight superior migration at the C6–C7 right neural foramen (**Fig. 48.1**).

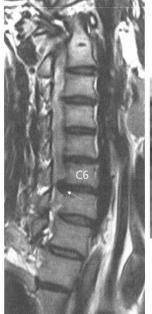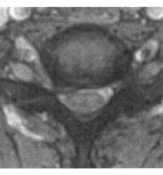

Fig. 48.1 Preoperative MRI. Left, foraminal view; right, axial view.

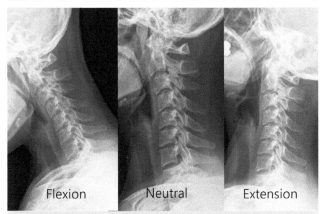

Fig. 48.2 Preoperative plain radiographs. Left to right: flexion, neutral, and extension positioning.

Plain-film standing lateral cervical radiographs showed kyphosis at neutral and limited extension (**Fig. 48.2**).

48.2 Literature Review

- Anterior cervical diskectomy and fusion (ACDF) is currently the standard treatment for cervical disk disease.[1,2] However, there are problems associated with fusion, such as limitation of motion and possible adjacent-segment pathology.[1,2]

- Artificial disk replacement was introduced to address issues of ACDF. However, various problems associated with artificial cervical disks, such as heterotopic ossification, mechanical failure, and spontaneous fusion, have been reported.[3,4,5,6]

- Motion preservation surgeries may be an alternative depending on patient age and activity level. Traditional posterior foraminotomy and diskectomy could be performed with full endoscopic techniques.[7,8,9,10,11,12,13]

- If cervical kyphosis is caused by pain, the curvature may be improved with alleviation of neck/arm pain.[7] Therefore, in this case, posterior percutaneous endoscopic cervical foraminotomy and diskectomy (P-PECD) may be considered.

48.3 Surgical Technique[7,8,9] (Video 48.1)

48.3.1 Position and Anesthesia

- P-PECD is performed under general anesthesia in a prone position with three-point pin fixation devices and a table-mounted holder (Mayfield system, Integra, Plainsboro, NJ) or craniocervical traction with a Gardner-Wells tongs skeletal fixation system (**Fig. 48.3**).[7]

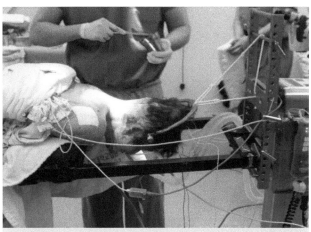

Fig. 48.3 Skeletal traction. Skeletal traction is performed to enlarge the interlaminar space.

48.3.2 Skin Incision and Introduction of Endoscope

- The V point is bounded by the inferior margin of the cephalic lamina, the medial junction of the facet joints, and the superior margin of the caudal lamina (**Fig. 48.4**).[7,8]
- After identification of the V point with the fluoroscope, the skin incision is made with a scalpel, and then the obturator, working channel, and endoscope are introduced sequentially (**Fig. 48.5**).
- The endoscope and working channel are held in one hand, and endoscopic instruments are deployed with the other hand (**Fig. 48.6**).

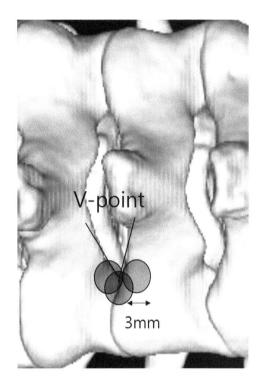

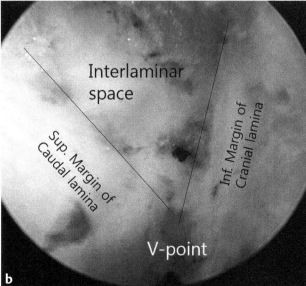

Fig. 48.4 (**a**) The V point in a 3D reconstructed CT scan. (**b**) Operative view.

48.3.3 Preparation of V Point

- Muscles attached around the V point are cleared out with the forceps and coagulator. The ligamentum flavum (LF), inferior margin of the cranial lamina, superior margin of the caudal lamina, and starting point of the facet joint are visualized (**Fig. 48.4b**).

48.3.4 Drilling of Lamina and Facet Joint

- The entire operation is performed under visual control and continuous irrigation with normal saline.[7,8,10,11] The opened bevel of the working channel is directed toward the medial side to avoid accidentally compressing the spinal cord.[7,8]
- Bone drilling is started from the V point with the endoscopic drill. A side-cutting drill (shaver) covered by a protector can be utilized.
- The extent of bone drilling is dependent on the size and location of the herniated disk material, and it is usually within a 3- to 4-mm radius around the V point.[7,8] The size of bone removal can be assessed with the diameter of the endoscopic instrument.[7,8]
- The sequence of drilling is cranial lamina, caudal lamina, and facet joint.
- Thinned inner cortex of lamina is removed with a Kerrison punch.
- Usually, the removal of facet joint is less than 10% of the entire joint for diskectomy (**Fig. 48.7**).

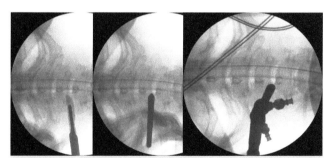

Fig. 48.5 Introduction of endoscopy. Left to right: skin incision with scalpel, insertion of obturator, and insertion of endoscope after insertion of working channel.

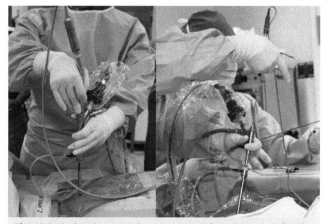

Fig. 48.6 The hand position during surgery. Left, endoscopic drill; right, endoscopic coagulator.

48.3.5 Preparation of Epidural Space

- After removal of the lamina, the thin LF is removed with a Kerrison punch.
- The disk space is exposed and cleared with coagulator and forceps.
- Usually, ruptured disk is located at the axilla of the nerve root (**Fig. 48.8**).

48.3.6 Diskectomy

- The lateral margin of the dura is first identified and dissected from the disk and posterior margin of the vertebral body with the dissector. Then the dissector is moved along the lateral margin and the inferior margin of the nerve root to delineate neural tissue.

- The ruptured disk is removed with endoscopic forceps.
- For contained disk, annulotomy is made with an annulotome and disk material is removed.
- Decompression is confirmed at both the superior (shoulder) and inferior margin (axilla) of the nerve root (**Fig. 48.9**).
- Usually, ruptured disk material is removed and internal decompression of disk is not performed (**Fig. 48.10**).

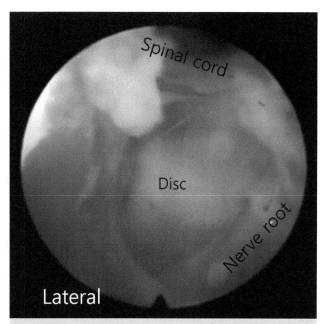

Fig. 48.8 Disk and nerve root after foraminotomy. The bulging annulus compresses the nerve root. Ruptured disk material is located under the dura (*red arrow*).

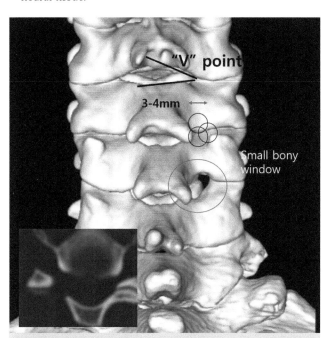

Fig. 48.7 The size of the foraminotomy. The amount of the facet joint removed is around 1 mm (10% of the facet joint).

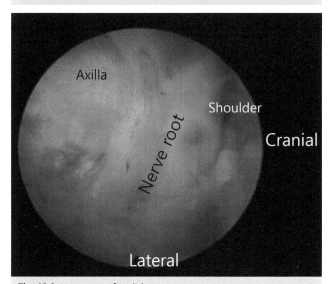

Fig. 48.9 Nerve root after diskectomy.

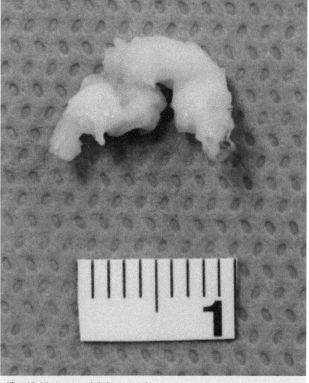

Fig. 48.10 Removed disk material.

48.3.7 Closure

- After the operation, a closed suction drain can be inserted along the working channel, if necessary.
- The wound is closed with nylon (**Fig. 48.11**).

48.4 Hospital Course

- In the case example, the patient's neck and arm pain were improved directly after surgery, with minimal incisional pain.
- Postoperative MRI showed well-decompressed nerve tissue (**Fig. 48.12**).
- The patient was discharged the next day without a neck brace. Cervical motion was not restricted.
- Triceps weakness was normalized 1 week later.
- Standing cervical radiographs taken 1 month after surgery showed that cervical extension was not limited (**Fig. 48.13**).
- One year after surgery, the patient's pain score was 0/0 at neck/arm and the neck disability index was 0/50.

48.5 Tips

48.5.1 Bleeding Control

- Surgical positioning is most important. Reducing abdominal pressure can reduce venous bleeding from the epidural vein.

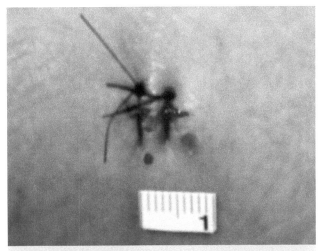

Fig. 48.11 Surgical wound. The skin incision is less than 1 cm.

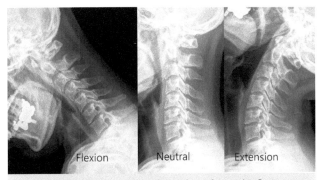

Fig. 48.13 Postoperative plain radiographs. Left to right: flexion, neutral, and extension positioning.

- Usually, continuous irrigation washes out bleeding and bleeding from the perineural venous plexuses can be controlled with a coagulator.
  - If the bleeding is not controllable, applying membrane at the endoscope is effective. However, increased water pressure may cause spinal cord injury or increased intracranial pressure. The application of membrane should be less than several minutes. Increasing water pressure with the water pump is not routinely recommended.

48.5.2 Dual Root

- Dual root is reported in 20% of patients (**Fig. 48.14**).[11]
- To prevent injury at the ventral motor root, the lateral margin of the dura is first identified and dissected from the disk and posterior margin of the vertebral body with a dissector. Then the dissector is moved along the lateral margin and inferior margin of the nerve root to delineate neural tissue.

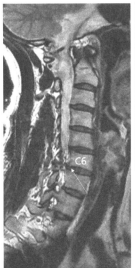
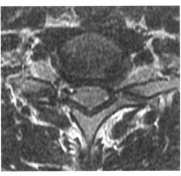

Fig. 48.12 Postoperative MRI. Left, foraminal view; right, axial.

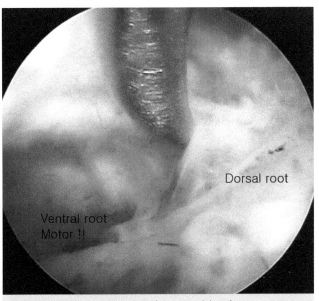

Fig. 48.14 Dual nerve root. Ventral motor and dorsal sensory roots.

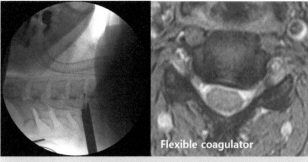

Fig. 48.15 Vertebral artery injury. Left: The flexible coagulator can be inserted to the vertebral foramen. Right: Pathway of flexible coagulator.

48.5.3 Vertebral Artery Injury

- Because the tip of the coagulator is flexible, forceful insertion to the vertebral foramen can irritate or injure the vertebral artery (**Fig. 48.15**).

48.5.4 Kyphosis

- Because the facet joint is violated, progression of cervical kyphosis may be a concern.[14]
- If the extent of removal of the facet joint is around 1 mm (less than 10% of facet joint), it may not cause kyphosis.[8]
- Kyphosis caused by pain may be improved by pain relief.[7]

References

1. Hilibrand AS, Carlson GD, Palumbo MA, Jones PK, Bohlman HH. Radiculopathy and myelopathy at segments adjacent to the site of a previous anterior cervical arthrodesis. *J Bone Joint Surg Am* 1999;*81*(4):519–528
2. Kraemer P, Fehlings MG, Hashimoto R, et al. A systematic review of definitions and classification systems of adjacent segment pathology. *Spine* 2012;*37*(22, Suppl):S31–S39
3. Richards O, Choi D, Timothy J. Cervical arthroplasty: the beginning, the middle, the end? *Br J Neurosurg* 2012;*26*(1):2–6
4. Park SB, Kim KJ, Jin YJ, et al. X-ray based kinematic analysis of cervical spine according to prosthesis designs: analysis of the Mobi C, Bryan, PCM, and Prestige LP. *J Spinal Disord Tech* 2013; E-pub
5. Lee SE, Chung CK, Jahng TA. Early development and progression of heterotopic ossification in cervical total disc replacement. *J Neurosurg Spine* 2012;*16*(1):31–36
6. Cho SK, Riew KD. Adjacent segment disease following cervical spine surgery. *J Am Acad Orthop Surg* 2013;*21*(1):3–11
7. Kim CH, Shin KH, Chung CK, Park SB, Kim JH. Changes in cervical sagittal alignment after single-level posterior percutaneous endoscopic cervical diskectomy. *Global Spine J* 2015;*5*(1):31–38
8. Kim CH, Kim KT, Chung CK, et al. Minimally invasive cervical foraminotomy and diskectomy for laterally located soft disk herniation. *Eur Spine J* 2015;*24*(12):3005–3012
9. Kim CH, Chung CK, Kim HJ, Jahng TA, Kim DG. Early outcome of posterior cervical endoscopic discectomy: an alternative treatment choice for physically/socially active patients. *J Korean Med Sci* 2009;*24*(2):302–306
10. Ruetten S, Komp M, Merk H, Godolias G. Full-endoscopic cervical posterior foraminotomy for the operation of lateral disc herniations using 5.9-mm endoscopes: a prospective, randomized, controlled study. *Spine* 2008;*33*(9):940–948
11. Ruetten S, Komp M, Merk H, Godolias G. A new full-endoscopic technique for cervical posterior foraminotomy in the treatment of lateral disc herniations using 6.9-mm endoscopes: prospective 2-year results of 87 patients. *Minim Invasive Neurosurg* 2007;*50*(4):219–226
12. Yang JS, Chu L, Chen L, Chen F, Ke ZY, Deng ZL. Anterior or posterior approach of full-endoscopic cervical discectomy for cervical intervertebral disc herniation? A comparative cohort study. *Spine* 2014;*39*(21):1743–1750
13. Lubelski D, Healy AT, Silverstein MP, et al. Reoperation rates after anterior cervical discectomy and fusion versus posterior cervical foraminotomy: a propensity-matched analysis. *Spine J* 2015;*15*(6):1277–1283
14. Jagannathan J, Sherman JH, Szabo T, Shaffrey CI, Jane JA. The posterior cervical foraminotomy in the treatment of cervical disc/osteophyte disease: a single-surgeon experience with a minimum of 5 years' clinical and radiographic follow-up. *J Neurosurg Spine* 2009;*10*(4):347–356

49 Posterior Tubular Endoscopic Cervical Diskectomy

Alejandro J. Lopez, Zachary A. Smith, Richard G. Fessler, and Nader S. Dahdaleh

49.1 Introduction

While less commonly performed than anterior cervical diskectomy, posterior approaches to the cervical spine reduce the approach-related risks of esophageal injury, vascular injury, recurrent laryngeal nerve injury, or dysphagia.[1] Before the introduction of the endoscopic technique, a posterior approach involved extensive disruption of the paraspinal musculature that contributed to increased complications, pain, and disability.[2,3] Modern application of blunt tubular retractors has proven as effective as open procedures while preserving the musculature, achieving symptom relief in 87 to 97% of patients while decreasing blood loss, length of stay, and use of postoperative pain medication.[1,4] The application of endoscopic technology enhances visualization and has been increasingly applied during minimally invasive spinal surgery. This chapter focuses on endoscopic posterior cervical decompression and diskectomy (**Video 49.1**).

49.2 Patient Selection

49.2.1 Indications

- Cervical lateral disk herniation (**Fig. 49.1**) or foraminal stenosis causing radiculopathy[5]
- Persistent nerve root symptoms after anterior cervical diskectomy and fusion
- Cervical disk disease in patients for whom anterior approaches are contraindicated (e.g., those with anterior neck infection, tracheostomy, prior irradiation, previous radical neck surgery for neoplasm)

49.2.2 Contraindications

- Pain without neurologic symptoms
- Gross cervical instability
- Central disk herniation
- Excessive burden of ventral compression (diffuse ossification of the posterior longitudinal ligament)
- Kyphotic deformity that would render posterior decompression ineffective or destabilize the cervical spine

49.3 Preparation

49.3.1 Essential Surgical Instruments

- Head fixation device
- Tubular retractor system
- Endoscopic camera system
- Endoscopic spinal instruments, including microcurets and 1- to 2-mm rongeurs
- High-speed drill
- Intraoperative fluoroscopy

49.3.2 Positioning

After induction of anesthesia with the patient in the supine position, the patient is placed in a three-point head fixation device and elevated to a sitting position (**Fig. 49.2**). The head is then flexed until the cervical spine is perpendicular to the floor, ensuring sufficient jugular venous return while preventing

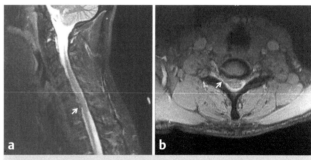

Fig. 49.1 A 30-year-old man presented with neck pain and right upper extremity radiation. On exam his right triceps motor strength was 4/5. MRI of the cervical spine showed a right-sided soft lateral disk herniation at C6–C7 causing impingement of the foraminal nerve at C7 noted on his right parasagittal T2 view (**a**, *arrow*) and axial T2 view (**b**, *arrow*).

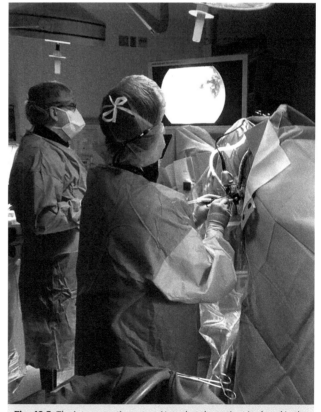

Fig. 49.2 The intraoperative setup. Note that the patient is placed in the sitting position. The monitor is placed facing the surgeon.

airway compromise. This position also accommodates fluoroscopic imagery by allowing the shoulders to fall inferiorly with gravity and decreases the accumulation of blood within the surgical field. Physician fatigue may also be decreased. Air emboli have not been reported as a complication of this position.[1,4]

Alternatively, the patient may be placed in the prone position with the head secured in three-point pin fixation. The neck is then flexed to better expose the interlaminar window. Continuous irrigation of the surgical corridor with normal saline may be employed to improve visualization of the surgical field.[6,7,8]

49.4 Surgical Technique

49.4.1 Preparation

Approach and visualization of the correct operative level should be confirmed with fluoroscopy before beginning sterilization of the site. The neck is then shaved, cleansed, and draped in sterile fashion.

49.4.2 Incision

After again confirming the operative level by fluoroscopy, the incision is planned. For single-level procedures, an 8- to 18-mm vertical incision offset 1.5 cm from the midline (toward the side to be operated) is sufficient, depending on the final width of the dilator system chosen. The length of the incision should be approximately equal to or slightly greater than the diameter of the final tubular retractor. When operating at two levels, the incision should straddle the affected levels. If bilateral access is planned, the incision can be made directly on the midline. The planned incision site is injected with local anesthesia, and an initial blade-length incision is made at the midpoint of the marked area.

49.4.3 Dilation

Under fluoroscopy, a Kirschner wire (K-wire), guidewire over needle, or obturator is introduced and guided toward the inferomedial edge of the superior lateral mass of the affected level and is docked. Bone must be identified by palpation to ensure that the interlaminar space has not been violated. The cervical fascia is then opened to allow for less forceful introduction of the muscle dilators.

Under fluoroscopy, the initial dilator is placed (**Fig. 49.3**). The instrument may be placed over a K-wire, or guidewire if preferred; however, extra care is needed to ensure that the K-wire does not violate the interlaminar space. To avoid this potential complication, we introduce the smallest dilator and dock it perpendicular to the facet/lateral mass, after which serial dilation then proceeds according to the dilator system chosen until the final tubular retractor overlies the laminofacet junction (**Fig. 49.4**, **Fig. 49.5**). Operative windows from 7.9 to 18 mm have been described.[5,9] The retractor arm is then fixed and the inner dilators are removed, allowing for introduction and attachment of the endoscope to the final retractor (**Fig. 49.6**).

49.4.4 Exposure

Endoscopic dissection begins in the lateral aspect of the field over palpable bone. Monopolar cautery and pituitary rongeurs are employed to complete visualization of the lamina and lateral

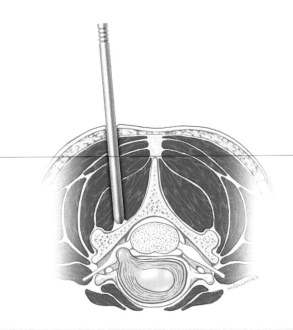

Fig. 49.3 Initial dilation is performed following exposure of the laminofacet junction. Care should be taken to avoid violation of the interlaminar space by the K-wire or the smallest dilator.

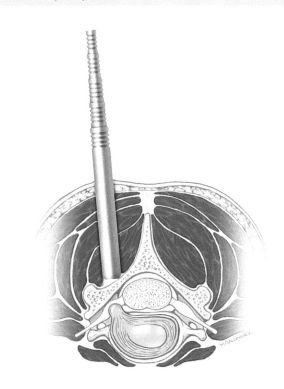

Fig. 49.4 Sequential dilators are introduced under fluoroscopic guidance to dilate the paraspinal muscles

mass (**Fig. 49.7**).[1] The ligamentum flavum is then removed from the inferior edge of the lamina using an up-angled curet.

A Kerrison punch and high-speed drill with fine bit and adjustable guard sleeve are employed to develop the laminotomy. The lateral edge of the dura and proximal portion of the nerve root are visualized by detaching the ligamentum flavum medially. The medial aspect of the facet is then removed along

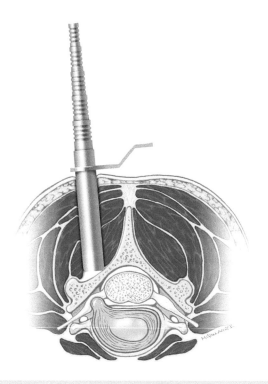

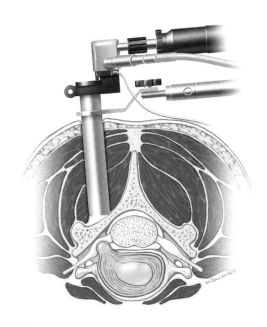

Fig. 49.6 The tubular retractor is mounted to the operative table, and the endoscopic apparatus is then attached to it.

Fig. 49.5 The tubular retractor is docked at the laminofacet junction, and the dilators are then removed.

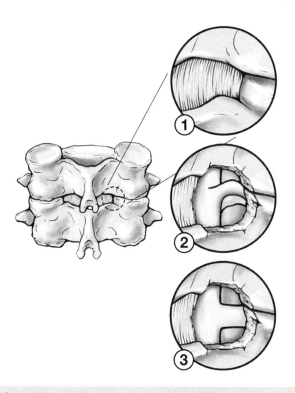

Fig. 49.7 The endoscopic view after subperiosteal removal of the paraspinal musculature. (**a**) Note the interlaminar space and the lamina facet junction. (**b**) Following the laminotomy and resection of the medial aspect of the lateral mass and the ligamentum flavum, the nerve root and the soft lateral disk herniation at the level of the axilla of the nerve are exposed. (**c**) The disk herniation is then resected.

the course of the nerve root. Facet resection should be limited to less than 50% to preserve function (**Fig. 49.7**).[2,10]

49.4.5 Decompression

The nerve root is denuded of any obscuring venous plexus using bipolar cautery. Disk fragments and any osteophytes should now be palpable with an angled dissector. Supplemental resection of the pedicle may be required to adequately expose the pathology and to reduce retraction of the nerve root. Osteoid osteomas have been excised in a similar fashion.[11] Removal of the disk herniation is accomplished by separating the nerve root and disk with a nerve hook before extracting the fragment with pituitary rongeurs (**Fig. 49.7**).[3]

49.4.6 Closure

After inspecting for sufficient decompression, the operative corridor is irrigated with antibiotic solution and hemostasis is achieved. Applying a methylprednisolone-soaked pledget to the root has been suggested to reduce ensuing inflammation. A closed suction drain may be employed if epidural bleeding is expected.

The retractor tube is removed and visible musculature and fascia is infiltrated with local anesthetic. The fascia is closed simply with absorbable suture, while the subcutaneous tissue receives inverted stitching. A running subcuticular stitch is performed on the skin and overlaid with skin adhesive. The wound is dressed and the table is leveled such that the patient resumes the preoperative position. Head fixation is then removed.

49.4.7 Recovery

The patient is allowed to recover from anesthesia and may be discharged in as little as 2 to 3 hours with an opioid analgesic, nonsteroidal anti-inflammatory drug, and muscle relaxant.

49.5 Complications

The overall complication rate of this procedure is 2 to 9%.[1] The most commonly encountered complication is incidental durotomy with cerebrospinal fluid leak. When the small operative corridor precludes primary closure of a durotomy, small defects may be amenable to closure using muscle, fat, or dural substitute secured with fibrin glue or synthetic sealant. Larger defects may require lumbar drainage of the CSF for 2 to 3 days.

Nerve root and spinal cord injury are possible during the dilation and decompression stages. The vertebral artery may also be subject to injury if dilation proceeds lateral to the facet or if dissection is carried too far laterally.

Long-term loss of sagittal alignment has not been demonstrated in the posterior endoscopic approach,[9] as it has in the anterior endoscopic procedures.[7,12,13] This may be due to the preservation of muscle and facet anatomy afforded by the posterior approach.

49.6 Discussion

While anterior cervical diskectomy and fusion is the current standard of treatment for cervical disk disease, the procedure is associated with multiple approach-related complications.[14,15] Fusion alone comes at the expense of motion loss and potential risk for adjacent segment disease.[16,17] Posterior endoscopic cervical diskectomy offers a less invasive, motion-segment-sparing approach for the treatment of lateral disk herniation or foraminal stenosis.

Studies have shown that 87 to 97% of patients who undergo posterior endoscopic cervical diskectomy have demonstrated favorable improvement for greater than 2 years as measured by clinical outcome and disability indices.[6,7,9] Moreover, comparative studies have shown outcome measures similar to those for anterior endoscopic cervical diskectomies.[6,13,18,19] While no single approach can address the entirety of cervical disk disease, in the correct patient, the posterior endoscopic approach to diskectomy may prove a valuable alternative to more invasive procedures.

References

1 Fessler RG, Khoo LT. Minimally invasive cervical microendoscopic foraminotomy: an initial clinical experience. *Neurosurgery* 2002;51(5, Suppl):S37–S45
2 Ratliff JK, Cooper PR. Cervical laminoplasty: a critical review. *J Neurosurg* 2003;98(3, Suppl):230–238
3 Hosono N, Yonenobu K, Ono K. Neck and shoulder pain after laminoplasty. A noticeable complication. *Spine* 1996;21(17):1969–1973
4 Siddiqui AY. Posterior cervical microendoscopic diskectomy and laminoforaminotomy. In: Kim DH, Fessler RG, Regan JJ, eds. *Endoscopic Spine Surgery and Instrumentation: Percutaneous Procedures.* New York: Thieme; 2005
5 Gala VC, O'Toole JE, Voyadzis JM, Fessler RG. Posterior minimally invasive approaches for the cervical spine. *Orthop Clin North Am* 2007;38(3):339–349, abstract v
6 Ruetten S, Komp M, Merk H, Godolias G. A new full-endoscopic technique for cervical posterior foraminotomy in the treatment of lateral disc herniations using 6.9-mm endoscopes: prospective 2-year results of 87 patients. *Minim Invasive Neurosurg* 2007;50(4):219–226
7 Ruetten S, Komp M, Merk H, Godolias G. Full-endoscopic cervical posterior foraminotomy for the operation of lateral disc herniations using 5.9-mm endoscopes: a prospective, randomized, controlled study. *Spine* 2008;33(9):940–948
8 Kim CH, Chung CK, Kim HJ, Jahng TA, Kim DG. Early outcome of posterior cervical endoscopic discectomy: an alternative treatment choice for physically/socially active patients. *J Korean Med Sci* 2009;24(2):302–306
9 Kim CH, Shin KH, Chung CK, Park SB, Kim JH. Changes in cervical sagittal alignment after single-level posterior percutaneous endoscopic cervical diskectomy. *Global Spine J* 2015;5(1):31–38
10 Raynor RB, Pugh J, Shapiro I. Cervical facetectomy and its effect on spine strength. *J Neurosurg* 1985;63(2):278–282
11 Nakamura Y, Yabuki S, Kikuchi S, Konno S. Minimally invasive surgery for osteoid osteoma of the cervical spine using microendoscopic discectomy system. *Asian Spine J* 2013;7(2):143–147
12 Yi S, Lim JH, Choi KS, et al. Comparison of anterior cervical foraminotomy vs arthroplasty for unilateral cervical radiculopathy. *Surg Neurol* 2009;71(6):677–680
13 Ahn Y, Lee SH, Shin SW. Percutaneous endoscopic cervical discectomy: clinical outcome and radiographic changes. *Photomed Laser Surg* 2005;23(4):362–368
14 Frempong-Boadu A, Houten JK, Osborn B, et al. Swallowing and speech dysfunction in patients undergoing anterior cervical discectomy and fusion: a prospective, objective preoperative and postoperative assessment. *J Spinal Disord Tech* 2002;15(5):362–368
15 Jung A, Schramm J, Lehnerdt K, Herberhold C. Recurrent laryngeal nerve palsy during anterior cervical spine surgery: a prospective study. *J Neurosurg Spine* 2005;2(2):123–127
16 Hilibrand AS, Carlson GD, Palumbo MA, Jones PK, Bohlman HH. Radiculopathy and myelopathy at segments adjacent to the site of a previous anterior cervical arthrodesis. *J Bone Joint Surg Am* 1999;81(4):519–528
17 Kraemer P, Fehlings MG, Hashimoto R, et al. A systematic review of definitions and classification systems of adjacent segment pathology. *Spine* 2012;37(22, Suppl):S31–S39
18 Yang JS, Chu L, Chen L, Chen F, Ke ZY, Deng ZL. Anterior or posterior approach of full-endoscopic cervical discectomy for cervical intervertebral disc herniation? A comparative cohort study. *Spine* 2014;39(21):1743–1750
19 Riew KD, Cheng I, Pimenta L, Taylor B. Posterior cervical spine surgery for radiculopathy. *Neurosurgery* 2007;60(1 Suppl 1):S57–S63

50 Posterior Tubular Endoscopic Cervical Laminectomy and Foraminotomy

Albert P. Wong, Youssef J. Hamade, Zachary A. Smith, Nader S. Dahdaleh, and Richard G. Fessler

50.1 Introduction

Cervical spondylosis is a degenerative spinal condition that can result in progressive foraminal or central stenosis of the spine, leading to radiculopathy or cervical spondylotic myelopathy.[1,2,3] A minimally invasive posterior cervical approach through a tubular retractor may maximize the benefits of surgical decompression while minimizing soft-tissue trauma, resulting in improved neurologic outcomes with a decrease in surgical morbidity or spinal instability.[4,5,6,7,8,9,10,11] This chapter describes the surgical technique for a posterior cervical minimally invasive microendoscopic foraminotomy (cMEF) and laminectomy (cMEL) (**Video 50.1**).

50.2 Patient Selection

Prior to surgical intervention, a thorough history and physical examination, with review of pertinent imaging (X-rays or MRI of the cervical spine), is always completed. Any ambiguity in the surgical level may be clarified with adjunctive tests: nerve conduction studies (NCS), electromyography (EMG), and selective nerve root blocks may be helpful in confirming the level of the pathologic nerve root.[12,13,14,15,16]

50.2.1 Indications

- Upper-extremity weakness, pain, numbness, or tingling (cMEF)[17,18]
- Radiographic evidence of cervical foraminal stenosis correlating with clinical presentation without spinal cord compression (cMEF)
- Clinical signs or symptoms of spinal cord compression (cMEL)
- Radiographic evidence of cervical spinal cord compression primarily from dorsal pathology, such as hypertrophic ligamentum flavum or hypertrophic facets (cMEL)

50.2.2 Contraindications

- Axial neck pain as the primary complaint with minimal upper-extremity symptoms (cMEF or cMEL)[18]
- Trauma patient with cervical spine fractures (cMEF or cMEL)
- Cervical instability based on dynamic flexion–extension X-rays (cMEL)
- Radiographic evidence of cervical spinal cord compression primarily from ventral pathology, such as a central disk herniation, osteomyelitis, tumor, ossified posterior longitudinal ligament (OPLL), or cervical kyphosis (cMEL)

50.3 Surgical Technique

Note that setup is the same for cMEF and cMEL.

50.3.1 Positioning

- The patient may be placed in either the prone or the sitting position with the head secured by a three-point pin fixation system. The sitting position allows the operative blood to drain away from the surgical field.
- Neuromonitoring may be used to decrease the risk of potential neurologic injury.
- The surgical level is marked with lateral fluoroscopy.
- The entry point is 1.5 cm lateral to the midline. The incision is ~ 18 mm long.
- Skin infiltration is done with local anesthetic (1% lidocaine).

50.3.2 Surgical Approach

See **Fig. 50.1 through Fig. 50.13** and **Video 50.1**.

- The skin is incised with a scalpel and electrocautery is used to dissect through the posterior cervical fascia until the muscle fibers are exposed.
- Blunt scissors are used to gently separate the muscle fibers, while the index finger may be used to bluntly dissect the surgical planes until the laminofacet junction is palpated.
- The smallest tubular dilator is guided onto the laminofacet junction with the index finger and the surgical level confirmed with fluoroscopy.
- Sequential tubular dilators are used to bluntly separate the muscle fibers in a nontraumatic fashion until the final tubular retractor is secured with a robotic arm.

50.3.3 Microendoscopic Foraminotomy

- Residual soft tissue overlying the ipsilateral laminofacet junction is removed with a combination of electrocautery and pituitary rongeurs.
- A high-speed drill and Kerrison rongeurs are used to perform a limited ipsilateral laminotomy and medical facetectomy.
- One-third to one-half of the medial inferior and superior articular processes of the surgical level may be removed until the "shoulder" of the nerve root is clearly exposed.
- Residual ligamentum flavum is removed with rongeurs until the nerve root is completely mobile.

50.3.4 Microendoscopic Laminotomy

- Once the ipsilateral laminectomy and facetectomy are completed, the cMEL procedure continues with decompression of the contralateral lamina and ligament.
- The endoscope is repositioned medially to visualize the ventral surface of the spinous process and contralateral lamina.
- A high-speed drill with a guarded drill tip is used to undercut the ventral surface of the spinous process and contralateral lamina.
- The bony resection is continued until the contralateral foramen is visualized or palpated with a bayoneted Penfield-4.
- Kerrison rongeurs may be used to complete the bony decompression.
- Fluoroscopy may be used to confirm entrance into the contralateral foramen.
- Once the bony decompression is complete, the contralateral ligamentum flavum is removed with rongeurs.
- After the contralateral ligamentum flavum is removed, the endoscope is repositioned to remove the residual ipsilateral ligamentum flavum.
- Hemostasis is achieved with electrocautery and thrombin-soaked agents.
- The tubular retractor is removed and soft-tissue bleeding is coagulated under direct visualization.
- The fascia is approximated with absorbable sutures, and the dermis is closed with a skin adhesive.

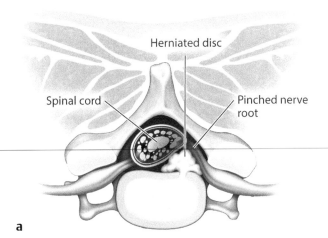

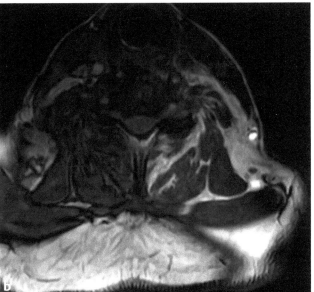

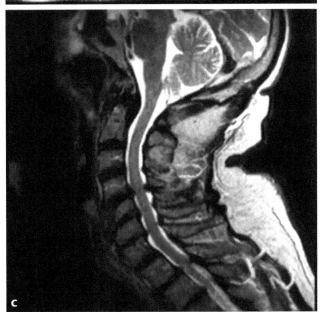

Fig. 50.1 (a,b,c) Drawing of a paracentral cervical disk herniation with compression of the traversing nerve root. T2-MRI axial and sagittal views demonstrate moderate central and lateral recess stenosis treatable with a minimally invasive posterior laminotomy/foraminotomy.

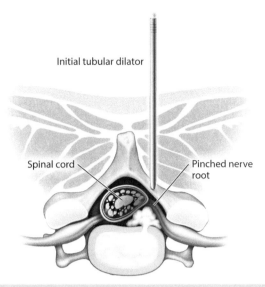

Fig. 50.2 The initial tubular dilator is placed on the ipsilateral laminofacet junction. The K-wire is not used due to the potential risk of plunging through the interlaminar space.

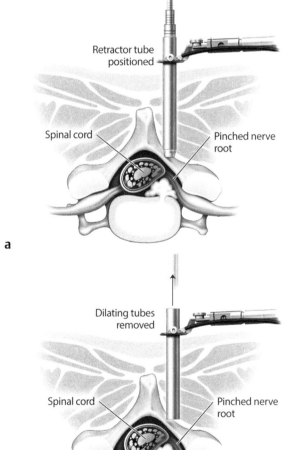

Fig. 50.4 (a,b) The dilating tubes are removed after the final tubular retractor is placed over the surgical site and secured to the operating table with a flexible robotic arm.

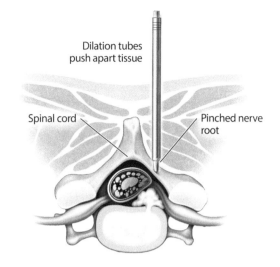

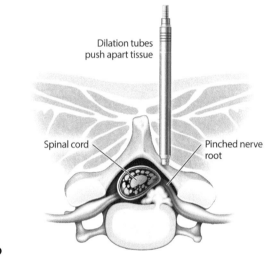

Fig. 50.3 (a,b) Sequential muscle-splitting tubes are inserted to separate the paraspinal muscle fibers in an atraumatic fashion.

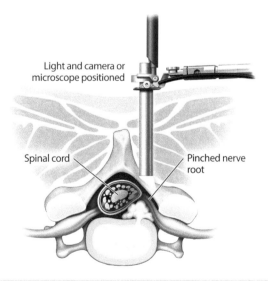

Fig. 50.5 An endoscope with a lighted tip is positioned within the tubular retractor to visualize the ipsilateral laminofacet junction.

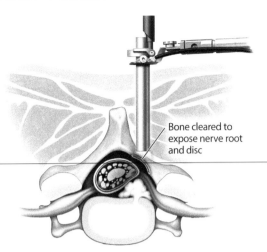

Fig. 50.6 The ipsilateral hemilaminotomy is performed to expose the underlying ligamentum flavum. Kerrison rongeurs may be used to complete the laminotomy and ligament resection.

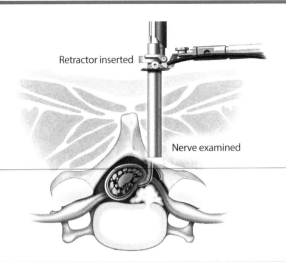

Fig. 50.7 Gentle retraction with a nerve root retractor may be used to expose the compressed traversing nerve root and the disk herniation. Caution should be exercised when retracting against the cervical spinal cord, due to the potential risk of injury to the spinal cord.

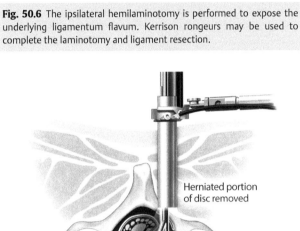

Fig. 50.8 The annulus is incised with a bayoneted scalpel and the disk herniation is removed with a combination of pituitary rongeurs and curets.

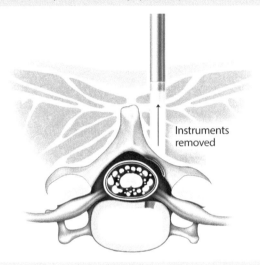

Fig. 50.9 The compressed nerve will return to its normal position after the disk herniation is resected. The tubular retractor is removed, and the paraspinal muscles return to their normal anatomic position.

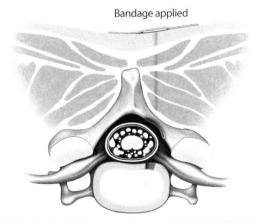

Fig. 50.10 Once the fascia and skin are closed with absorbable sutures, the dermis is re-approximated with a skin adhesive. The final incision is ~ 18 mm in length.

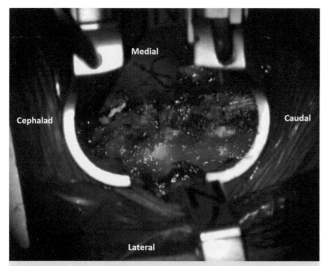

Fig. 50.11 Intraoperative view after the three-level ipsilateral hemila-minotomy has been completed. The thecal sac is visible lateral to the residual laminae.

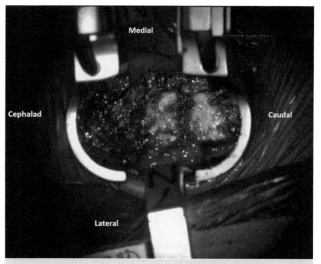

Fig. 50.12 The tubular retractor and endoscope are rotated medially to expose the ventral undersurface of the spinous processes and contralateral laminae.

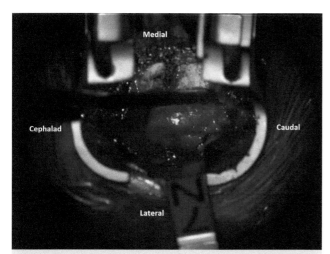

Fig. 50.13 The ventral undersurface of the spinous processes and contralateral laminae are removed with a high-speed drill and Kerrison rongeurs to reveal the complete dorsal aspect of the cervical thecal sac.

References

1 Karadimas SK, Erwin WM, Ely CG, Dettori JR, Fehlings MG. Pathophysiology and natural history of cervical spondylotic myelopathy. *Spine* 2013;*38*(22 Suppl 1):S21–S36

2 Shedid D, Benzel EC. Cervical spondylosis anatomy: pathophysiology and biomechanics. *Neurosurgery* 2007;*60*(1, Suppl 1):S7–S13

3 Tracy JA, Bartleson JD. Cervical spondylotic myelopathy. *Neurologist* 2010;*16*(3):176–187

4 Caralopoulos IN, Bui CJ. Minimally invasive laminectomy in spondylolisthetic lumbar stenosis. *Ochsner J* 2014;*14*(1):38–43

5 Clark JG, Abdullah KG, Steinmetz MP, Benzel EC, Mroz TE. Minimally invasive versus open cervical foraminotomy: a systematic review. *Global Spine J* 2011;*1*(1):9–14

6 McAnany SJ, Kim JS, Overley SC, Baird EO, Anderson PA, Qureshi SA. A meta-analysis of cervical foraminotomy: open versus minimally-invasive techniques. *Spine J* 2015;*15*(5):849–56

7 Mobbs RJ, Li J, Sivabalan P, Raley D, Rao PJ. Outcomes after decompressive laminectomy for lumbar spinal stenosis: comparison between minimally invasive unilateral laminectomy for bilateral decompression and open laminectomy: clinical article. *J Neurosurg Spine* 2014;*21*(2):179–186

8 Nerland US, Jakola AS, Solheim O, et al. Minimally invasive decompression versus open laminectomy for central stenosis of the lumbar spine: pragmatic comparative effectiveness study. *BMJ* 2015;*350*:h1603

9 Popov V, Anderson DG. Minimal invasive decompression for lumbar spinal stenosis. *Adv Orthop* 2012;*2012*:645321

10 Skovrlj B, Gologorsky Y, Haque R, Fessler RG, Qureshi SA. Complications, outcomes, and need for fusion after minimally invasive posterior cervical foraminotomy and microdiscectomy. *Spine J* 2014;*14*(10):2405–2411

11 Steinberg JA, German JW. The effect of minimally invasive posterior cervical approaches versus open anterior approaches on neck pain and disability. *Int J Spine Surg* 2012;*6*:55–61

12 Blankenbaker DG, De Smet AA, Stanczak JD, Fine JP. Lumbar radiculopathy: treatment with selective lumbar nerve blocks—comparison of effectiveness of triamcinolone and betamethasone injectable suspensions. *Radiology* 2005;*237*(2):738–741

13 Chung JY, Yim JH, Seo HY, Kim SK, Cho KJ. The efficacy and persistence of selective nerve root block under fluoroscopic guidance for cervical radiculopathy. *Asian Spine J* 2012;*6*(4):227–232

14 Hong CZ, Lee S, Lum P. Cervical radiculopathy. Clinical, radiographic and EMG findings. *Orthop Rev* 1986;*15*(7):433–439

15 Nardin RA, Patel MR, Gudas TF, Rutkove SB, Raynor EM. Electromyography and magnetic resonance imaging in the evaluation of radiculopathy. *Muscle Nerve* 1999;*22*(2):151–155

16 Pawar S, Kashikar A, Shende V, Waghmare S. The study of diagnostic efficacy of nerve conduction study parameters in cervical radiculopathy. *J Clin Diagn Res* 2013;*7*(12):2680–2682

17 Lawrence BD, Brodke DS. Posterior surgery for cervical myelopathy: indications, techniques, and outcomes. *Orthop Clin North Am* 2012;*43*(1):29–40, vii–viii

18 Rhee JM, Basra S. Posterior surgery for cervical myelopathy: laminectomy, laminectomy with fusion, and laminoplasty. *Asian Spine J* 2008;*2*(2):114–126

51 Endoscopic Approaches to Cervical Tumors, Trauma, and Infection

Christopher C. Gillis and John O'Toole

51.1 Introduction

As the decreased morbidity of minimal access (minimally invasive surgery, or MIS) approaches is increasingly presented in the literature, the techniques continue to evolve and to be expanded to include approaches to the cervical spine.[1] Traditional approaches to the dorsal cervical spine continue to require extensive periosteal stripping of the paraspinal musculature that leads to increased postoperative pain, spasm, and dysfunction that can lead to muscular ischemia and can be persistently disabling in 18 to 60% of patients.[2,3,4,5] Furthermore, preoperative loss of lordosis and long-segment decompressions increase the risk for postoperative sagittal plane deformity,[3,6,7] a complication that frequently prompts instrumented arthrodesis at the time of laminectomy. Employing these extensive posterior fusion techniques increases operative risks, time, and blood loss, exacerbates early postoperative pain, and potentially contributes to adjacent-level degeneration.

To reduce the complication of deformity and avoid fusion after cervical decompression, minimally invasive cervical decompression was described as an adaption of MIS lumbar laminectomy techniques and can be adapted to approach both intradural and extradural lesions in the cervical spine, be they tumor or infection.[8,9,10] Additionally, minimally invasive dorsal cervical foraminotomy is a well-described and practiced technique that can be adapted to decompression of nerve roots in the face of impinging pathology.[2,3,11,12] With respect to trauma, MIS lateral mass screw placement has been described, as well as MIS screw placement for traumatic spondylolisthesis of the axis.[3,5,13] Combining these techniques, a wide variety of traumatic, infectious, or neoplastic pathology in the cervical spine can be approached in an MIS fashion, tailored to the specific case. This chapter discusses the basics of these techniques and how to use them.

51.2 Choice of Patient

51.2.1 Indications

Intradural lesions, extradural lesions, dorsal spinal pathology involving the facet, lamina, lateral mass or any of the posterior elements, pathology along the nerve root, and even more laterally located ventral lesions are all appropriate for a minimally invasive approach. Generally, the MIS approach works best with lesions spanning less than two spinal levels. In cases where fusion is required, such as in trauma, it can be done with MIS lateral mass screws or percutaneous screws.

51.2.2 Contraindications

Generally, lesions spanning more than two spinal segments or tumors with a significant ventral portion are too difficult to

approach with MIS techniques, due to the size limitation of the expandable retractor, even with angling of the retractor.[8,9,14,15] Open approaches are often considered in these cases. Tumor and trauma cases that are in the vertebral body in the cervical spine are best approached through anterior approaches, due to the presence of the vertebral artery. The traditional anterior cervical approach takes advantage of natural tissue planes and thus is best for these cases.

51.3 Procedure

The basic tools of MIS in the lumbar spine are adapted to use in the cervical spine. The approaches are performed using muscle dilators and tubular retractors (which can include either fixed or expandable tubular retractors), and visualization can be achieved through use of an endoscope, loupes, and a headlight, or even the operating room microscope. The patient is usually positioned prone; however, the sitting position is an option when performing endoscopic foraminotomy.

51.3.1 Foraminotomy

With prone patient positioning, the head is held with a Mayfield pin holder or Gardner-Wells tongs, with the neck in slight flexion, which allows for rigid holding of the cervical spine during muscle dilation. Also with the prone position, the operating table is tilted in a reverse Trendelenburg position to ensure that the cervical spine is parallel to the floor. For the sitting position, the patient's head is fixed in a Mayfield head holder. The table is manipulated to place the patient in a semisitting position with the chin flexed and the neck straight and perpendicular to the floor, and the table is turned either 90° or 180° relative to the anesthesiologist.

For foraminotomy, the general approach is paramedian. The operative level(s) and entry point are confirmed on lateral fluoroscopy with a Kirschner (K)-wire or the inner muscle dilator. A 2-cm longitudinal incision is marked out ~ 1.5 cm off the midline on the operative side and is injected with local anesthetic. For two-level procedures, the incision should be placed midway between the targeted levels. Once an optimal trajectory is established, using fluoroscopy as the guide, due to the thicker fascial and muscle attachments in the cervical spine, dissection is taken down to the fascia, which is then incised with a scalpel or electrocautery to accommodate dilators. Metzenbaum scissors are used to bluntly dissect to the level of the facets to enable "force-free" insertion of the tissue dilators. The fascia is retracted, and the smallest dilator is placed through the posterior cervical musculature under fluoroscopic guidance and is docked on the facet at the level of interest. A slightly lateral trajectory is advised to avoid the spinal canal and to ensure contact with the lateral mass. Successive tubular muscle dilators are carefully and gently inserted, remembering that the axial forces that are

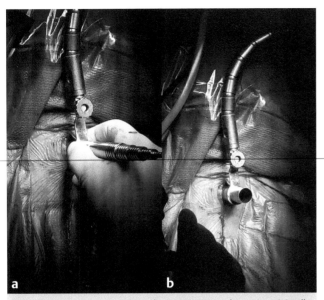

Fig. 51.1 Intraoperative view during sitting endoscopic minimally invasive cervical foraminotomy. (**a**) Paramedian incision in the cervical spine with insertion of the fixed retractor over the dilators. (**b**) The fixed tubular dilator in the final position after removal of the dilators, affixed to the rigid retractor arm.

routinely applied during muscle dilation in the lumbar spine are hazardous in the cervical spine (**Fig. 51.1**).

After dilation, the final tubular retractor is placed and is secured over the laminofacet junction with a table-mounted flexible retractor arm. The following steps are performed under microscopic magnification or using loupes and headlight or an endoscope attached to the tubular retractor. Tissue is cleared off the bone to expose the underlying lamina and lateral mass using monopolar cautery and a pituitary rongeur, taking care to start and maintain the dissection laterally and over solid bone.

The medial facet/interlaminar space junction is identified. Using a high-speed drill, a partial laminotomy-facetectomy is performed, beginning at the medial facet/interlaminar space and going laterally, removing less than 50% of the facet, to maintain biomechanical integrity. The dorsolateral portion of the superior lamina and the medial part of the inferior articular facet are removed first. This will permit the removal of the lateral corner of the inferior lamina and the medial part of the superior articular facet, exposing the medial border of the caudal pedicle. The nerve root is located directly above the caudal pedicle and anterior to the superior articular facet. The ligamentum flavum can be removed medially after the foraminotomy to expose the lateral edge of the dura and proximal portion of the nerve root. Progressive lateral dissection can then proceed along the root as it enters the foramen. The venous plexus overlying the nerve root should be carefully coagulated with bipolar cautery and incised. With the root well visualized, a fine-angled dissector can be used to palpate ventrally to the nerve root for compressive lesion or tissue. Gentle dissection along the root can allow removal of material ventral and inferior to the root. If there is a large portion of lesion or bony fragment ventral to the root, additional drilling of the superomedial quadrant of the caudal pedicle allows greater access while avoiding the need for excessive nerve root retraction.

51.3.2 Laminectomy/Decompression/ Tumor Resection

Laminectomy or decompression is more often done through a laterally to medially oriented approach. A skin incision to accompany the size of retractor desired is made one finger breadth off the dorsal midline, with the incision centered on the level of the disk space. Larger incisions extending over two segments may be necessary for larger lesions and allowing for angulation of the tubular retractor. The operative level(s) and entry point are confirmed with lateral fluoroscopy. The fascia is again incised under direct vision and Metzenbaum scissors used to carry out subfascial dissection down to the level of bone for easy docking of the tubular dilators. Sequential muscle dilation and insertion of the tubular retractor follow, and, again depending on the lesion, an expandable tubular retractor can be placed. The remaining steps are performed under microscopic magnification or using loupes and a headlight or with an attached endoscope. Starting close to the midline is useful in cases of anatomical distortion to maintain orientation given the limited visualization.

Ipsilateral laminotomy of the level of interest is performed using a high-speed drill and the ligamentum flavum is left in place to protect the dura until bony removal is finished. The tube is then angled ~ 45° off the midline so that the tube is oriented to allow visualization and decompression of the contralateral side. The contralateral drilling can be tailored to the lesion; for example, if the lesion is located only ipsilateral, then complete contralateral decompression is not required, and exposure of at least the midline to allow space for enough durotomy and closure is recommended. To safely drill along the underside of the spinous process, a tissue plane can be developed between the ligamentum flavum and undersurface of the spinous process through dissection with a fine curet. Either using the suction to retract the ligamentum away from the drill or using an adjustable guard sleeve extended to cover the tip of the drill allows for safe drilling along the undersurface of the spinous process and contralateral lamina all the way to the contralateral facet. This initial decompression allows greater working space within which to remove hypertrophied ligament while avoiding downward pressure on the dura and spinal cord. Dissection and removal of the ligamentum flavum with curets and Kerrison rongeurs may now proceed safely. Any compressive elements of the contralateral facet or the superior edge of the caudal lamina may also be drilled off or removed with Kerrison rongeurs at this time, because their compression on the dura is most apparent once the ligament is removed. After confirming decompression of the contralateral foramen with a fine probe, the tube is returned to its original position to complete the ipsilateral removal of ligament and bone. This should then reveal completely decompressed and pulsatile dura. If indicated, ipsilateral foraminotomy, as described earlier, also may be performed at this time. Decompression and irrigation may be all that is required in cases of infection.

For intradural work, it is important to ensure enough bony decompression and dural exposure to allow for the durotomy and its closure. The operating room microscope is used for cases of tumor resection. An ultrasound with a long, small tip can be used to help guide the extent of decompression needed. The durotomy is carefully started with a long-handled scalpel, and

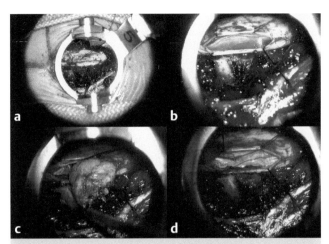

Fig. 51.2 Intraoperative views of sequential resection of intradural extramedullary tumor. For all views, rostral is to the reader's left, caudal to the right, medial superior, and lateral inferior: **(a)** Tubular retractor in place with laminectomy performed and thecal sac visible through the retractor. **(b)** Microscope view through the tubular retractor with dural tack-up sutures in place exiting outside of the tubular retractor and durotomy performed, exposing the arachnoid. **(c)** Extramedullary lesion being delivered away from the spinal cord. **(d)** Intradural exposure after removal of the lesion.

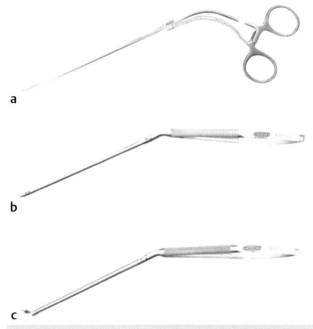

Fig. 51.3 Minimally invasive dural closure instruments. **(a)** Curved locking needle holder. **(b)** Jacobson needle holder. **(c)** Knot pusher.

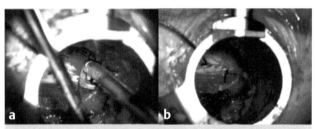

Fig. 51.4 Intraoperative view of **(a)** knot pusher in use, pushing the knot in durotomy closure, and **(b)** final closure of durotomy.

a favored technique is to use straight hooks to open the dura longitudinally while preserving the arachnoid plane. Preserving the arachnoid is ideal to minimize early flooding of the exposure with CSF and epidural blood. The dural edges can be held open with tack-up sutures pulled up out of the tube retractor and held with hemostats (**Fig. 51.2**).

After carrying out intradural work in standard microsurgical fashion, specialized instruments can be used for primary dural closure. These instruments consist of a long, locking, curved needle driver, a Jacobson needle driver, and a knot pusher that allows tight knot placement on the dura (**Fig. 51.3**). The curved needle driver, either Jacobson or locking driver, can be used to maneuver the suture into the tube, and both can be combined to help in instrument tying of the suture. The sutures are tied with the knots thrown outside of the tube and the knot is pushed down into the tube slowly with the specialized knot pusher (**Fig. 51.4**).

The closure is checked after suturing with a Valsalva maneuver, and if the repair is not watertight, a small piece of locally harvested muscle can be sutured in place to buttress the defect. Following dural closure, the exposure is covered in fibrin glue. A Hemovac drain is not used.

51.3.3 Lateral Mass Fixation

Following decompression and foraminotomy, or in cases requiring only fusion, lateral mass screws can be placed through an expandable tubular retractor. To place screws, it is important to visualize both the medial and lateral extent of the lateral mass to ensure a proper entry point and trajectory through the tube. After exposure of the facet joint, a hand drill is used to create a pilot hole with a 2.5-mm drill and a 14-mm stopping length. Care is taken to avoid disruption of facet capsules that are not to be fused. The tubular retractor should be angled 15° cephalad for optimal screw placement. The starting point is 1 mm medial to the midpoint of the lateral mass in the medial–lateral plane

and in the middle of the lateral mass in the cephalad-caudad plane, and the trajectory will be 15° cephalad and 30° lateral and parallel to the facet joint. Polyaxial screws of 3.5-mm diameter are inserted after tapping, and a rod is fixed with set screws. The retractor can be angled and adjusted to reach each level to be fused. The screws are inserted on the side of the decompression and foraminotomy through the same incision used to approach the pathology. Given that MIS is usually limited to cases of one to two spinal segments, the rod can often be placed into the screw heads through the expandable retractor.

51.4 Closure and Postoperative Care

Local anesthetic is injected into the fascia and muscles surrounding the incision. The wound is closed using one or two absorbable stitches for the fascia, two or three inverted stitches for the subcutaneous layer, and a running subcuticular stitch and Dermabond on the skin with or without additional dressing. The patient is usually mobilized on the morning of postoperative day 1—even with durotomy we do not recommend maintaining the patient on prolonged bedrest. No collar is necessary.

51.5 Complication Avoidance

The most common complication of MIS approaches remains durotomy. This can be minimized through meticulous dural closure, the technique of which is described and demonstrated in **Video 51.1**.[8] When the leak is not repairable, dural adjuncts, such as fibrin glue or onlay grafts, can be of use, and the benefit of the remaining muscle and tissue re-expanding over the defect often leaves the leak as an asymptomatic pseudomeningocele that improves with time.[9,16]

51.6 Case Examples

51.6.1 Case 1

A 47-year-old male presented with left arm tingling, numbness, and pain in the left neck and shoulder. MRI of the cervical spine showed a gadolinium-enhancing intradural extramedullary lesion on the left side at the C3 level (**Fig. 51.5**). The size of the lesion in a rostral–caudal direction was limited to one spinal level and it was located along the left side of the spinal cord.

Due to the length of the lesion, an MIS cervical approach was deemed appropriate. With use of a 26-mm fixed dilator, a C2–C4 left-side hemilaminectomy was performed, with removal of only the caudal portion of C2, all of C3, and the top C4. Visualization was obtained with the operating room microscope. A midline durotomy was performed, dural sutures were used to tack it open, and the tumor was removed in a piecemeal fashion. Once the tumor was removed, the dura was closed using specialized dural closure instruments, which include a MIS knot pusher,[8]

and 6-0 Gore-Tex suture. Intraoperative monitoring was used throughout the case without changes. Pathology returned as Schwannoma grade 1. Six weeks postoperative MRI was performed and showed minimal tissue disruption, limited to only the left side at the C3 level (**Fig. 51.6**).

51.6.2 Case 2

A 58-year-old female presented with increasing difficulty maintaining her balance as well as left leg numbness and right leg weakness. She had also noticed numbness in her left trunk. Examination revealed hemisensory loss on the left from her trunk through her leg and mild (MRC 4/5) weakness in her right leg. MRI (**Fig. 51.7**) illustrated a homogeneously enhancing right-sided intradural extramedullary lesion at C6 with a suggestion of a dural tail. The lesion encompassed the right side of the spinal canal, causing severe spinal cord compression.

Given the lesion's size, it was deemed amenable to an MIS approach. The patient underwent a right-sided C5–C7 MIS laminectomy and resection of an intradural extramedullary meningioma. The incision was ~ 3 cm in length, made 2 cm off midline, and an expandable tubular retractor was used. Intraoperative view of the tumor underneath the midline durotomy is shown in **Fig. 51.8**.

51.6.3 Case 3

A 41-year-old female presented with symptoms of gradually progressive cervical myelopathy along with neck pain. Physical

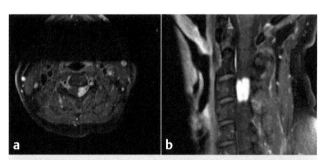

Fig. 51.5 T1-weighted MRI post gadolinium contrast showing (**a**) axial and (**b**) sagittal view of contrast-enhancing intradural extramedullary lesion at the C3 level.

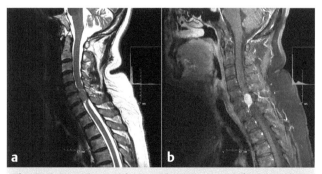

Fig. 51.7 Sagittal MRI: (**a**) T2-weighted image and (**b**) T1-weighted image with gadolinium showing right-sided C6 homogeneously enhancing lesion with ventral and caudal dural tail. The lesion can be seen to extend to encompass the entire right side of the spinal canal.

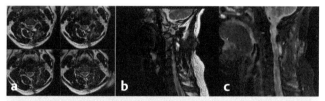

Fig. 51.6 MRI taken 6 weeks postoperatively: (**a**) sequential T2-weighted axial images from the C3 to C4 level with only minimal left-sided focal tissue disruption and edema; (**b**) sagittal T2-weighted image; and (**c**) sagittal STIR gated image further illustrating the focal nature of the postoperative tissue disruption with increased signal intensity behind the C3 spinal level on the left.

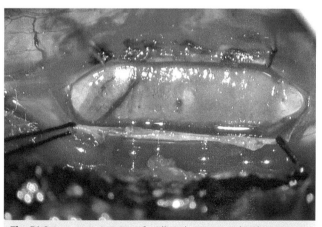

Fig. 51.8 Intraoperative view of midline durotomy and tack-up sutures in place. The tumor is visible as a reddish gray mass immediately upon dural opening.

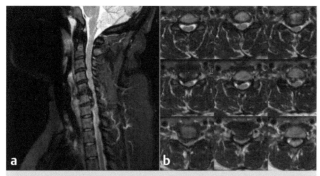

Fig. 51.9 MRI (**a**) sagittal and (**b**) sequential axial images illustrating C5–C6 large caudally migrated disk herniation along with disk osteophyte and posterior longitudinal ligament hypertrophy causing severe spinal cord stenosis and cord compression.

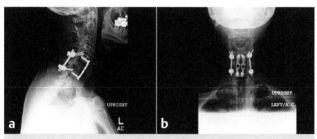

Fig. 51.10 (**a**) Lateral and (**b**) anteroposterior radiographs showing instrumentation after C6 anterior cervical corpectomy and fusion with plate and posterior MIS lateral mass screw insertion at C5–C7.

exam revealed Hoffman's sign present on the right and mild weakness (MRC 4+/5) in the bilateral hand intrinsic muscles and lower extremities. MRI (**Fig. 51.9**) demonstrated C5–C6 disk herniation and disk osteophyte complex as well as extensive hypertrophy of the posterior longitudinal ligament behind C6.

The patient underwent a staged procedure with a standard C6 anterior cervical corpectomy and fusion to decompress the spinal cord, followed by posterior MIS lateral mass instrumentation

~ 1 week later. MIS lateral mass instrumentation was inserted through a midline incision made just caudal to the C7 level, followed by bilateral midline incision through the cervicodorsal fascia and subsequent bilateral (one side at a time) muscle dilation, insertion of expandable retractor, and then placement of instrumentation. Postoperative images are seen in **Fig. 51.10**.

References

1   Ross DA. Complications of minimally invasive, tubular access surgery for cervical, thoracic, and lumbar surgery. *Minim Invasive Surg* 2014;*2014*:451637
2   Fessler RG, Khoo LT. Minimally invasive cervical microendoscopic foraminotomy: an initial clinical experience. *Neurosurgery* 2002;*51*(5 Suppl):S37–S45
3   Mikhael MM, Celestre PC, Wolf CF, Mroz TE, Wang JC. Minimally invasive cervical spine foraminotomy and lateral mass screw placement. *Spine* 2012;*37*(5):E318–E322
4   Fong S, Duplessis S. Minimally invasive lateral mass plating in the treatment of posterior cervical trauma: surgical technique. *J Spinal Disord Tech* 2005;*18*(3):224–228
5   Wang MY, Levi AD. Minimally invasive lateral mass screw fixation in the cervical spine: initial clinical experience with long-term follow-up. *Neurosurgery* 2006;*58*(5):907–912
6   Albert TJ, Vacarro A. Postlaminectomy kyphosis. *Spine* 1998;*23*(24):2738–2745
7   Deutsch H, Haid RW, Rodts GE, Mummaneni PV. Postlaminectomy cervical deformity. *Neurosurg Focus* 2003;*15*(3):E5
8   Tan LA, Takagi I, Straus D, O'Toole JE. Management of intended durotomy in minimally invasive intradural spine surgery: clinical article. *J Neurosurg Spine* 2014;*21*(2):279–285
9   Gandhi RH, German JW. Minimally invasive approach for the treatment of intradural spinal pathology. *Neurosurg Focus* 2013;*35*(2):E5
10 Hur JW, Kim JS, Shin MH, Ryu KS. Minimally invasive posterior cervical decompression using tubular retractor: The technical note and early clinical outcome. *Surg Neurol Int* 2014;*5*:34
11 Mansfield HE, Canar WJ, Gerard CS, O'Toole JE. Single-level anterior cervical discectomy and fusion versus minimally invasive posterior cervical foraminotomy for patients with cervical radiculopathy: a cost analysis. *Neurosurg Focus* 2014;*37*(5):E9
12 Eicker SO, Mende KC, Dührsen L, Schmidt NO. Minimally invasive approach for small ventrally located intradural lesions of the craniovertebral junction. *Neurosurg Focus* 2015;*38*(4):E10
13 Buchholz AL, Morgan SL, Robinson LC, Frankel BM. Minimally invasive percutaneous screw fixation of traumatic spondylolisthesis of the axis. *J Neurosurg Spine* 2015;*22*(5):459–465
14 Tredway TL, Santiago P, Hrubes MR, Song JK, Christie SD, Fessler RG. Minimally invasive resection of intradural-extramedullary spinal neoplasms. *Neurosurgery* 2006;*58*
15 Tredway TL. Minimally invasive approaches for the treatment of intramedullary spinal tumors. *Neurosurg Clin N Am* 2014;*25*(2):327–336
16 Stadler JA III, Wong AP, Graham RB, Liu JC. Complications associated with posterior approaches in minimally invasive spine decompression. *Neurosurg Clin N Am* 2014;*25*(2):233–245

52 Three-Dimensional Spine Surgery: Clinical Application of 3D Stereo-Tubular Endoscopic Systems

Dong Hwa Heo and Jin Sung Luke Kim

52.1 Introduction

Although there have been great advances in biotechnology and the development of specialized instruments, such as improved micro-endoscopes, digital video equipment, and percutaneous systems, minimally invasive spinal surgery (MISS) based on the endoscope still has drawbacks because of its two-dimensional (2D) images. Three-dimensional (3D) images or techniques have been popularly used in ordinary life, such as television, movie, video games, and education programs. Also, 3D vision has already been applied in video-assisted laparoscopic surgeries in urology, gynecology, and general surgery.[1,2,3]

The vision or images with existing video-assisted surgical devices for spinal operations are two-dimensional. Video-assisted thoracoscopic spinal approaches, percutaneous endoscopic spine surgery, and micro-endoscopic spine surgery have used 2D vision in the operative field. Although endoscopic systems have the advantage of magnified images, distortion and lack of depth perception are disadvantages of 2D endoscopic systems.[1,2,3,4]

Endoscopic surgery using 3D vision recently has been attempted in the field of minimally invasive brain and spine surgery.[4,5] In particular, 3D stereo-vision endoscopic spinal surgery has been tried in MISS using tubular retractor systems. Three-dimensional real-time images permit depth perception and improve hand–eye coordination during operations.[1,2,3]

52.2 Equipment

- The 3D endoscope systems: The system (VISIONSENSE, Philadelphia, PA) consists of a 3D high-definition endoscope, a processing console, and 3D glasses. The console processes pictures input via the endoscopic camera to 3D real-time visual information, and 3D images are presented on a large monitor. The operator wears specialized 3D glasses during the operation for 3D vision sensation. The 3D endoscope for the spine has a light source and a 4-mm camera (**Fig. 52.1**). There are two types of endoscope: one is rigid and the other is flexible.

- Tubular retractor system: There are many tubular retractor systems in spinal surgery. Any tubular retractor system can be used in 3D stereo-tubular endoscopic surgery.

- Robotic arm: For the prevention of swaying of the 3D endoscope, the authors recommend the application of a robotic arm for fixation of the 3D endoscope.

52.3 Surgical Procedures

The operative procedures are similar to those for micro-endoscopic spine surgery or microscopic spine surgery using a tubular retractor system. The surgical anatomy and view are same as with microscopic surgery and are familiar to the spine surgeon. In posterior lumbar approaches, a 2.5-cm skin incision is made after skin marking using fluoroscopic guidance. After fascia incision, serial dilators are inserted under C-arm guidance. The tubular retractor is finally inserted and fixed with the flexible arm system, and then the 3D endoscope is applied in the tubular retractor and is fixed with the robotic arm (**Fig.**

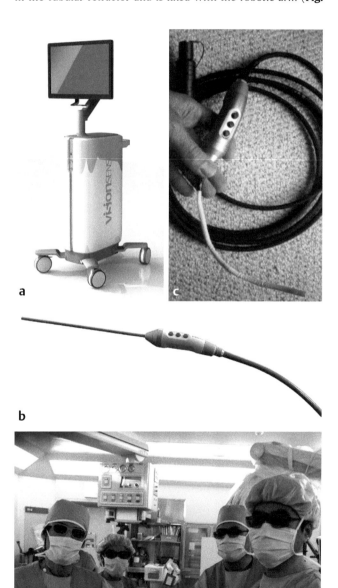

Fig. 52.1 The VISIONSENSE 3D vision endoscopic system. (**a**) Processing console with monitor. The 3D endoscope has a camera and a light source, and there are (**b**) rigid and (**c**) flexible types. (**d**) 3D glasses. Operation participants must wear 3D glasses for stereo vision during surgery.

52.2a). Routine laminotomy and diskectomy are performed while watching the 3D video monitor (**Fig. 52.2b**). Specialized bayonet-type surgical instruments for the tubular retractor are easier to work. General spine instruments are also available for these procedures (**Fig. 52.3**). All pictures present real-time 3D images. All participants, including the operator, the assistant, and nurses, should wear 3D glasses during the operation.

52.4 Clinical Applications

If a tubular retractor is available, 3D vision endoscopic spine surgery can be applied from the cervical to the lumbosacral spine. The posterior approach may be better than the anterior or lateral approaches in these procedures. Favorable indications for 3D stereo-tubular endoscopic spine surgery are posterior cervical

laminectomy (**Fig. 52.4**, **Fig. 52.5**), posterior cervical laminoforaminotomy, anterior cervical diskectomy, video-assisted thoracoscopic spine surgery, posterior thoracic diskectomy (transfacetal-transpedicular approach), lumbar decompressive laminectomy or foraminotomy, lumbar diskectomy, transforaminal lumbar interbody fusion (TLIF) (**Fig. 52.6**), and the lumbar paramedian approach (Wiltse approach) (**Fig. 52.7**).

52.5 Indications

- Cervical spine: posterior laminectomy, posterior foraminotomy, anterior diskectomy
- Thoracic spine: posterior diskectomy
- Lumbar spine: posterior diskectomy with laminotomy, paramedian Wiltse approach, posterior decompressive

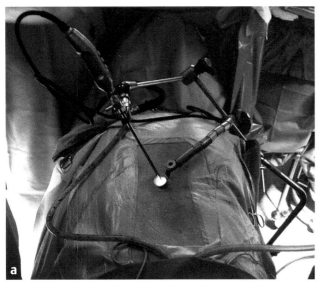

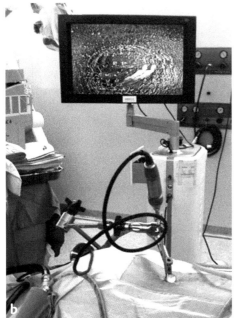

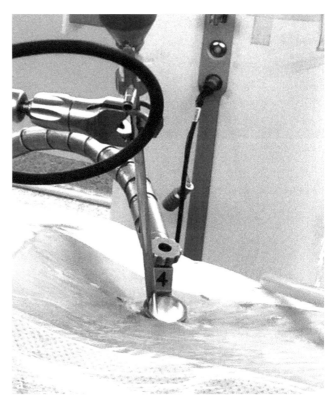

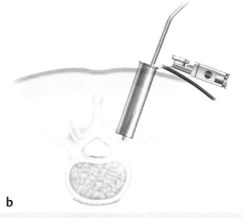

Fig. 52.2 Intraoperative full setting feature of 3D stereo-tubular endoscopic system. **(a)** The 3D endoscope was fixed with a robotic arm and **(b)** the operation was performed while participants watched the 3D video monitor system.

Fig. 52.3 (a) The 3D endoscope is inserted into the tubular retractor. **(b)** The small diameter of the 3D endoscope allows enough working space for surgical procedures and instruments.

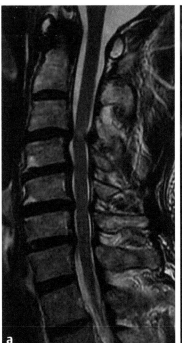
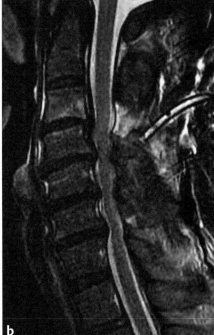
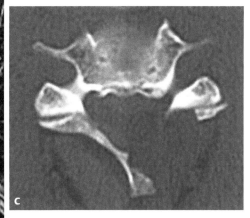

Fig. 52.4 **(a)** Preoperative MRI showed spinal canal stenosis with cord signal change due to hypertrophied ligamentum flavum at C3–C4. **(b,c)** Postoperative images revealed well-decompressed status.

laminectomy and foraminotomy, bilateral decompression via unilateral approach for lumbar stenosis, minimally invasive fusion surgeries (e.g., minimally invasive TLIF)

52.6 Case Presentations

52.6.1 Case 1

A 62-year-old male presented with bilateral arm weakness and tingling sensation. MRI showed cord signal change with stenosis at the C3–C4 level (**Fig. 52.4a**). We performed posterior decompression using the 3D stereo-tubular endoscopic system (**Video 52.1**). Postoperative imaging showed the stenosis at C3–C4 was completely decompressed (**Fig. 52.4b,c**).

52.6.2 Case 2

The patient underwent minimally invasive TLIF (**Fig. 52.5**).

52.6.3 Case 3

The patient required lateral foraminotomy via a right-sided paramedian approach for L5–S1 stenosis with extraforaminal disk herniation (**Fig. 52.6**).

52.7 Advantages of 3D Vision Surgery

The most important advantages are depth perception and 3D spatial perception during the operation.[1,3,5] Depth perception is difficult in 2D endoscopic surgery.[1,4] Fluoroscopic guidance and a long learning curve may be necessary for depth perception and anatomical orientation in 2D endoscopic spine surgeries. Too

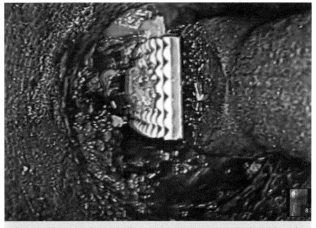

Fig. 52.5 A case of minimally invasive TLIF at L4–L5 on the right side. A cage was inserted after diskectomy and unilateral facetectomy via tubular retractor.

shallow manipulation under 2D vision can result in incomplete decompression or diskectomy, and too deep manipulation has the risk of neural or vascular damage. The intraoperative view in a 3D stereo-tubular operation is similar to that in microscopic spine surgery. The 3D spatial perception improves hand–eye coordination and makes it easier to perform the surgery.[1,3] Easy and early adoption of 3D vision may result in shortening of the learning curve for MISS using tubular systems. Real-time 3D pictures can be shared on the monitor with all participants, such as scrub, assistants, and medical students. Therefore, the 3D vision system is also good for teaching purposes. In summary, the advantages of 3D endoscopic surgery are:

- Depth perception and 3D spatial perception
- Better visual cues
- Volumetric orientation
- Easy adaptation

- Familiar anatomical orientation
- Shortened learning curve
- 3D views aid in education

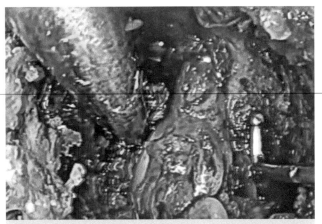

Fig. 52.6 Good decompression status of the right-side L5 nerve root after paramedian approach to L5–S1.

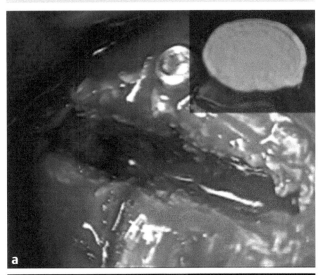

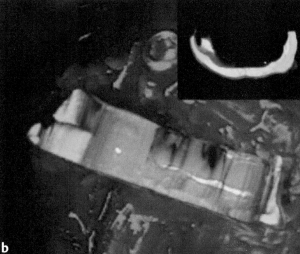

Fig. 52.7 (**a**) Volumetric measurement of disk removal area in anterior cervical diskectomy using integration technique of 3D vision and navigation. (**b**) The software can measure the remnant volume of disk after anterior cervical diskectomy.

52.8 Advanced Applications

In the near future, 3D vision and navigation systems may be integrated and fused completely. Advanced software development and fusion technique for navigation and 3D images can permit intraoperative 2D and 3D volumetric measurement. For example, the software can measure the remnant volume of disk and the size of laminectomy (**Fig. 52.7**). Furthermore, the technical development of navigation integration will help with insertion of spinal instruments, such as the cervical artificial disk, cage, and various kinds of screws.

52.9 Conclusion

The technique of 3D stereo-tubular endoscopic spine surgery can overcome the limitations of 2D endoscopic surgeries using tubular retractors. The authors anticipate the development of a 3D camera for percutaneous endoscopic lumbar operations.

References

1. Feng X, Morandi A, Boehne M, et al. 3-Dimensional (3D) laparoscopy improves operating time in small spaces without impact on hemodynamics and psychomental stress parameters of the surgeon. *Surg Endosc* 2015;29(5):1231–1239
2. Sinha RY, Raje SR, Rao GA. Three-dimensional laparoscopy: principles and practice. *J Minim Access Surg* 2016
3. Usta TA, Gundogdu EC. The role of three-dimensional high-definition laparoscopic surgery for gynaecology. *Curr Opin Obstet Gynecol* 2015;27(4):297–301
4. Zaidi HA, Zehri A, Smith TR, Nakaji P, Laws ER Jr. Efficacy of three-dimensional endoscopy for ventral skull base pathology: a systematic review of the literature. *World Neurosurg* 2016;86:419–431
5. Anichini G, Evins AI, Boeris D, Stieg PE, Bernardo A. Three-dimensional endoscope-assisted surgical approach to the foramen magnum and craniovertebral junction: minimizing bone resection with the aid of the endoscope. *World Neurosurg* 2014;82(6):e797–e805

53 Minimally Invasive Microsurgical Resection of Spinal Intradural Extramedullary Lesions

Dragos Catana, Mohammed Aref, Jetan Badhiwala, Brian Vinh, Saleh Almenawer, and Kesava (Kesh) Reddy

53.1 Minimally Invasive Resection of T9–T10 Intradural Extramedullary Spinal Tumor

53.1.1 Clinical Findings

- A 24-year-old male presented with left-sided abdominal pain and paresthesias.
- The pain began insidiously but progressively worsened over several months. It followed a bandlike distribution at the level of the umbilicus.
- There were no signs or symptoms of myelopathy, and there was no history of urinary or fecal incontinence.
- MRI of the spine showed a left-sided intradural, extramedullary lesion at the T9–T10 level causing mass effect on the spinal cord and near-complete obliteration of the CSF spaces (**Fig. 53.1**). The lesion avidly enhanced with gadolinium administration (**Fig. 53.2**). There was no obvious dural tail.
- The differential diagnosis included schwannoma, neurofibroma, and meningioma (**Video 53.1**).

53.1.2 Preoperative Plan

- The patient was selected to undergo minimally invasive microsurgical resection of the T9–T10 intradural spinal lesion using the METRx (Minimal Exposure Tubular Retractor) tubular retractor system (Medtronic, Memphis, TN), with possible sacrifice of the left T9 nerve root.
- Lower limb and sphincteric somatosensory evoked potentials (SSEP) and motor evoked potentials (MEP) were monitored throughout the operation.

- The patient was positioned prone on a Jackson table. The upper limbs were flexed at the elbow, with the forearms oriented cranially. Pressure points were carefully padded.

53.1.3 Surgical Procedure

- The T9 lamina was localized using lateral fluoroscopy and counting from the sacrum up to the lower thoracic region.
- Under fluoroscopic guidance, a 2-mm K-wire was advanced through a small skin incision over the left T9 lamina, starting 2 cm off midline and aiming medially. The smallest size tubular retractor was guided over the K-wire, and the paraspinal muscles were dissected off the lamina in the subperiosteal plane in a mediolateral fashion. The K-wire was removed, and tubular retractors were sequentially placed over each other to dilate and distract the soft tissues. The mediolateral blunt dissection was repeated at each step, along with fluoroscopic confirmation of placement (**Fig. 53.3**).
- The depth of the surgical corridor was measured using the markings on the dilators, and an appropriate length of final tubular METRx Quadrant retractor was chosen.
- The flexible arm attached to the table rail was used to secure the final tubular retractor in place and to allow for appropriate angulation.

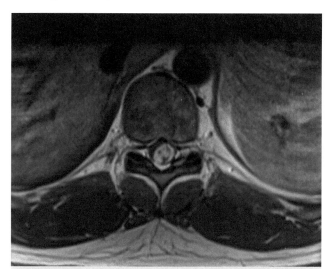

Fig. 53.1 Axial T1-weighted MRI with gadolinium contrast demonstrating an intradural left-eccentric enhancing lesion with associated mass effect on the spinal cord.

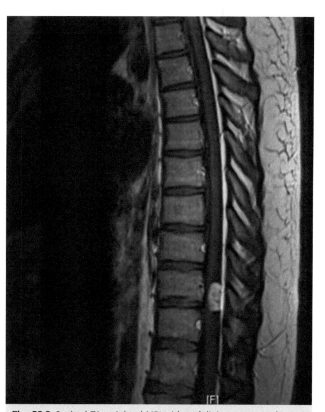

Fig. 53.2 Sagittal T1-weighted MRI with gadolinium contrast demonstrating an enhancing intradural lesion at the T9–T10 level.

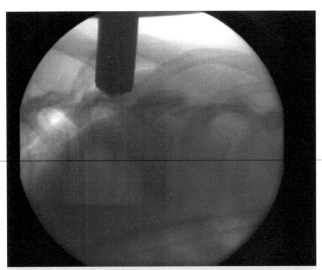

Fig. 53.3 Fluoroscopic image demonstrating the insertion of the final tubular retractor over the T9 lamina.

53.1.4 Microscopic Findings

- The microscope was brought into the surgical field and appropriately positioned over the surgical corridor. Paraspinal muscles not displaced with the sequential dilation technique were dissected with monopolar electrocautery to expose the bony lamina. The lamina was thinned out with a high-speed pneumatic drill; the thinned bone was then resected with Kerrison rongeurs along the epidural plane. The exposure was extended by undercutting the upper and lower laminae. Bone wax was applied for hemostasis.

- A sharp hook and a bayoneted blade were used to perform the initial durotomy. (Sutures may be used at the dural edges for epidural hemostasis to prevent blood from entering the intradural space. Alternatively, the dural edge may be lifted up using a micro hook.)

- A nerve stimulator was used to identify neuronal tissue. The tumor margins were identified in a systematic fashion. The left T9 nerve root could not be dissected off the tumor mass. Therefore, a decision was made to sacrifice the root.

- The tumor capsule was cauterized with low-setting bipolar electrocautery and was sharply dissected. The mass was debulked in a piecemeal fashion using standard bimanual technique. The resulting mobile capsule was dissected from surrounding structures using standard microsurgical techniques and hemostasis was achieved.

- The dural edges were re-approximated with 7–0 Prolene suture, starting just above the apex. An angled bayoneted microdriver was used in conjunction with microforceps. The assistant provided gentle countertraction using a bayoneted suture pusher during the repair. A Valsalva maneuver confirmed watertight closure, and a fibrin sealant (e.g., Tisseel) was used to augment the repair.

- The tubular retractor was gently removed and soft tissue hemostasis was achieved with bipolar electrocautery. The fascia was re-approximated with 2–0 Vicryl interrupted sutures. Finally, the skin was re-approximated with a 3–0 Monocryl running subcuticular suture.

- The final incision was ~ 25 mm long.

53.1.5 Results

- The patient was discharged home on the following day (postoperative day 1). On follow-up, the patient's pain, numbness, and paresthesias had improved significantly. Postoperative MRI showed complete tumor resection.

53.1.6 Tips

- Careful study of preoperative MRI and fluoroscopic images for exact level identification is essential.

- The shortest possible final tubular retractor length provides more degrees of freedom for microinstruments when working in the tubular corridor.

- Lateral bone removal is limited by the facet to avoid destabilizing the spine.

- Use of the flexible arm is essential to angle the tube superomedially, superolaterally, inferomedially, and inferolaterally to improve visualization throughout the procedure.

- It is important to use fluoroscopic guidance when inserting the K-wire and subsequent tubes to avoid entering the interlaminar space and causing secondary neuronal injury.

53.2 Minimally Invasive Resection of L3 Intradural Spinal Tumor

53.2.1 Clinical Findings

- A 59-year-old male with a history of resection of an L3 intradural dermoid tumor 5 years earlier presented with a history of worsening back pain, along with difficulty ambulating and paresthesias in both legs (but more intense on the right side), and recent urinary incontinence.

- MRI of the lumbar spine showed recurrence of the intradural lesion at L3 (**Fig. 53.4**, **Fig. 53.5**).

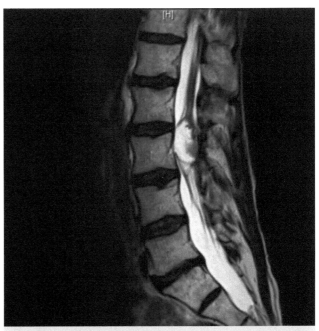

Fig. 53.4 Sagittal T2-weighted MRI demonstrating the recurrence of intradural tumor at the L3 spinal level.

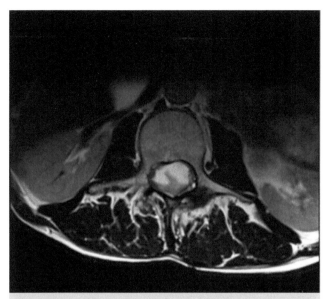

Fig. 53.5 Axial T2-weighted MRI showing the recurrence of intradural tumor that occupies most of thecal sac and compresses the nerve roots of the cauda equina.

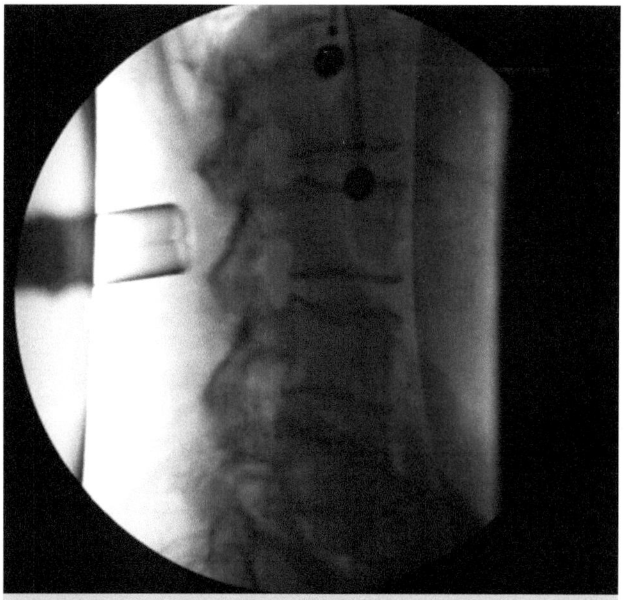

Fig. 53.6 Fluoroscopic image demonstrating insertion of the final tubular retractor over the right lamina.

53.2.2 Preoperative Plan

- The patient was scheduled for minimally invasive microsurgical tumor resection using the METRx tubular retractor system. It was decided to approach the tumor through the right side, contralateral to the previous surgical site, to avoid fibrotic adhesions.
- Neurophysiological monitoring was employed throughout the operation, including monitoring of electromyography (EMG), motor evoked potentials (MEPs), and somatosensory evoked potentials (SSEPs).

53.2.3 Surgical Procedure

- The patient was positioned prone on a Jackson table.
- A superficial cut was made along the old left-sided incision and the skin was retracted toward the right side. This avoided making a new incision.
- Under fluoroscopic guidance, a K-wire was inserted over the right lamina and the sequential tubular dilators were introduced, gradually dilating and distracting the soft tissues (**Fig. 53.6**).
- The METRx Quadrant tube was used as the final tubular retractor to provide an expanded operative view of the previously resected tumor.

53.2.4 Microscopic Findings

- Using the microscope, a right-sided hemilaminectomy was performed using a high-speed bur to thin the bone, followed by Kerrison rongeurs to resect the thinned bone (**Fig. 53.7**).
- The dura was then opened using a sharp hook and bayoneted blade (**Fig. 53.8**).
- A nerve stimulator was used to identify neuronal tissue and to delineate the tumor margins (**Fig. 53.9**).

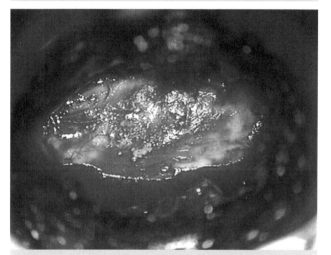

Fig. 53.7 Microscopic view through the tubular retractor demonstrating the removed right hemilamina and exposed dura.

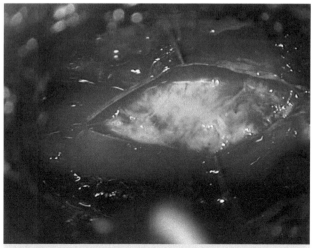

Fig. 53.8 Microscopic view through the tubular retractor demonstrating the opened dura and exposed tumor.

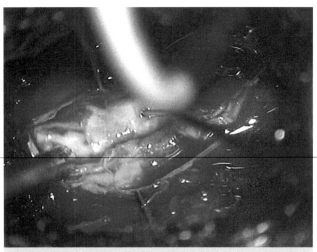

Fig. 53.9 Microscopic view through the tubular retractor demonstrating the nerve stimulator over the exposed tumor.

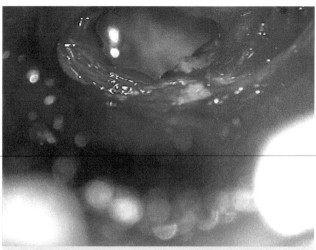

Fig. 53.10 Microscopic view through the tubular retractor after tumor resection.

- Tumor resection was performed using standard microsurgical techniques (**Fig. 53.10**).
- The dura was closed through the tubular retractor using a continuous 7–0 Prolene suture (**Fig. 53.11**).
- Fibrin sealant (Tisseel) was used as an adjunct for watertight closure. A Valsalva maneuver was done at the end to ensure absence of CSF leak.

53.2.5 Results

- Postoperative MRI showed the tumor was completely resected.
- The patient was discharged home the following day (postoperative day 1) with significant improvement in his motor and sensory deficits, along with minimal back pain. His incontinence continued to be present 2 months postoperatively.

53.2.6 Tips

- Preoperative planning is essential, including neuromonitoring and proper level identification.
- Fluoroscopy is essential when introducing the K-wire and sequential dilators to avoid interlaminar insertion and resultant neuronal injury.

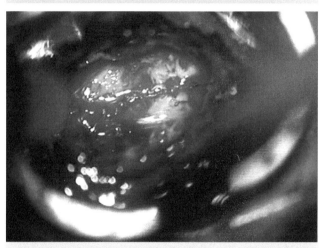

Fig. 53.11 Microscopic view through the tubular retractor demonstrating dural closure.

- The Quadrant tube facilitates a wider operative view, which helps in achieving a watertight dural closure.

Index

Note: Page numbers followed by *f* and *t* indicate figures and tables, respectively.